Antioxidants in Male Infertility

Sijo J. Parekattil • Ashok Agarwal
Editors

Antioxidants in Male Infertility

A Guide for Clinicians and Researchers

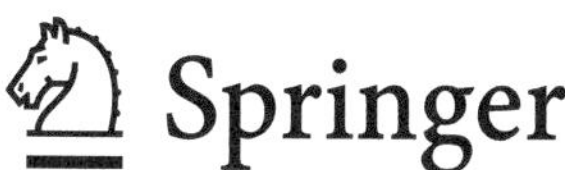 Springer

Editors
Sijo J. Parekattil, M.D.
Director of Urology
Winter Haven Hospital
University of Florida
Winter Haven, FL, USA

Ashok Agarwal, Ph.D., H.C.L.D. (ABB)
Director, Center for Reproductive Medicine
Glickman Urological and Kidney Institute
Cleveland Clinic
Cleveland, OH, USA

ISBN 978-1-4614-9157-6
Springer New York Heidelberg Dordrecht London

Library of Congress Control Number: 2013953261

Printed on acid-free paper

Springer is part of Springer Science+Business Media (www.springer.com)

Preface and Acknowledgments

The field of male infertility truly illustrates the need of a multispecialty approach to the effective diagnosis and management of such conditions. From the initial referral possibly from a reproductive endocrinology gynecologist and embryologist to the male infertility urologist, andrologist, researcher and alternative medicine specialist—this multidisciplinary team really needs to work as a cohesive unit to provide our patients with the most effective and highest quality care.

This book was an attempt to gather experts from each of these fields and present an integrated clinical management approach with detailed descriptions of topics ranging from the initial clinical diagnosis, management, new treatment options, and scientific rational for the various approaches. This book initially focuses on the clinical diagnosis of male infertility and then dives into spermatozoa metabolism, common infertility conditions, and then the role of antioxidants in male infertility. The authors come from leading institutions from around the globe in an attempt to capture a wide range of techniques and approaches. We are hoping that this text may serve as a reference guide for specialists across this team to further enhance dialogue, discussion, and refinement in our multidisciplinary approach.

We would like to thank the authors for their contributions and our families for their patience in allowing us to put together this project. We would like to acknowledge the Glickman Urological Institute at the Cleveland Clinic Foundation and the Department of Urology at University of Florida for institutional support for this endeavor as well. We would also like to thank Richard Lansing, executive editor, for his support and advice, Margaret Burns, publishing manager, for her tireless efforts in reviewing and editing each of the manuscripts, and Kristopher Spring, Associate Editor for his work in putting together this book.

We hope that this book will provide a concise, consolidated reference for clinical male infertility.

Winter Haven, FL, USA

Cleveland, OH, USA

Sijo J. Parekattil

Ashok Agarwal

Contents

Contributors

Ashok Agarwal, Ph.D. Center for Reproductive Medicine, Glickman Urological and Kidney Institute, Cleveland Clinic Foundation, Cleveland, OH, USA

Ignacio S. Alvarez, Ph.D. Department of Cell Biology, School of Life Sciences, University of Extremadura, Badajoz, Spain

Juan G. Alvarez, M.D., Ph.D. Centro de Infertilidad Masculina Androgen, La Coruña, Harvard Medical School, Boston, Spain

Monica Antinori, M.D. Department of Infertility, RAPRUI Day Surgery, Rome, Italy

Giancarlo Balercia, M.D. Andrology Unit, Endocrinology, Department of Internal Medicine and Applied Biotechnologies, Umberto I Hospital, School of Medicine, Rome, Italy

Department of Clinical and Molecular Sciences, Marche Polytechnic University, Ancona, Italy

Edson Borges Jr., M.D. Department of Fertility, Center for Assisted Fertilization, Sao Paulo, Brazil

Nancy L. Brackett, Ph.D. H.C.L.D. The Miami Project to Cure Paralysis, University of Miami Miller School of Medicine, Lois Pope Life Center, Miami, FL, USA

Stephanie Cabler, B.Sc. Center for Reproductive Medicine, Glickman Urological and Kidney Institute, Cleveland Clinic Foundation, Cleveland, OH, USA

Aldo E. Calogero, M.D. Department of Medical and Pediatrics Sciences, University of Catania, Catania, Italy

Shereen Cynthia D'Cruz, M.Phil. Department of Biochemistry and Molecular Biology, Pondicherry University, Kalapet, Pondicherry, India

Stefan S. du Plessis, Ph.D., M.B.A. Department of Medical Physiology, Faculty of Health Sciences, Stellenbosch University, Tygerberg, Western Cape, South Africa

Sandro C. Esteves, M.D., Ph.D. ANDROFERT, Andrology and Human Reproduction Clinic, Center for Male Reproduction, Campinas, SP, Brazil

Mark A. Faasse, M.D. Department of Urology, University of Illinois at Chicago, Chicago, IL, USA

Sandra García-Herrero, Ph.D. IVIOMICS, Valencia, Spain

Nicolas Garrido, Ph.D. Andrology Laboratory and Sperm Bank, Instituto Universitario IVI Valencia, Valencia, Spain

Túlio M. Graziottin, M.D., Ph.D. Andrology Section of Fertilitat – Human Reproduction Center, Department of Urology, Santa Casa Hospital and Federal University of Health Sciences, Porto Alegre, RS, Brazil

Sonja Grunewald, M.D. Department of Dermatology, Venerology and Allergology, European Training Center of Andrology, University of Leipzig, Leipzig, Germany

Ralf Henkel, B.Ed., Ph.D. Department of Medical Biosciences, University of the Western Cape, Bellville, South Africa

Tung-Chin Hsieh, M.D. Department of Urology, Baylor College of Medicine, Houston, TX, USA

Kathleen Hwang, M.D. Department of surgery (Urology), Brown University, Providence, RI, USA

Viacheslav Iremashvili, M.D., Ph.D. Department of Urology, University of Miami Miller School of Medicine, Miami, FL, USA

Samuel Juncal, M.S., M.D. Andrology Section of Fertilitat – Human Reproduction Center, Federal University of Health Sciences, Porto Alegre, RS, Brazil

John C. Kefer, M.D., Ph.D. Alpine Urology, Boulder, CO, USA

Edward D. Kim, M.D. Division of Urology, Department of Surgery, Center for Reproductive Medicine, University of Tennessee Medical Center, Knoxville, TN, USA

Edmund Y. Ko, M.D. Section of Male Infertility, Department of Urology, Glickman Urological and Kidney Institute, Cleveland Clinic, Cleveland, OH, USA

Tobias S. Köhler, M.D., M.Ph. Division of Urology, Southern Illinois University, Springfield, IL, USA

Sandro La Vignera, M.D. Department of Medical and Pediatrics Sciences, University of Catania, Catania, Italy

Dolores J. Lamb, Ph.D. Scott Department of Urology, Baylor College of Medicine, Houston, TX, USA

Fanuel Lampiao, Ph.D. Department of Medical Physiology, Faculty of Health Sciences, Stellenbosch University, Tygerberg, Western Cape, South Africa

Francesco Lanzafame, M.D. Centro Territoriale de Andrologia, Siracusa, Italy

Gian Paolo Littarru, M.D. Dipartimento di Scienze Cliniche Specialistiche ed Odontostomatologiche, Universita Politecnica delle Marche, Ancona, Italy

Charles M. Lynne, M.D. Department of Urology, University of Miami Miller School of Medicine, Miami, FL, USA

Antonio Mancini, M.D. Department of Internal Medicine, Division of Endocrinology, The Catholic University of the Sacred Heart, Rome, Italy

Francisco Javier Martin-Romero, Ph.D. Department of Biochemistry and Molecular Biology, School of Life Sciences, University of Extremadura, Badajoz, Spain

P.P. Mathur, Ph.D. Department of Biochemistry & Molecular Biology, and Center for Bioinformatics, School of Life Sciences, Pondicherry University, Kalapet, Pondicherry, India

Marcos Meseguer, Ph.D. Clinical Embryology Laboratory, Instituto Universitario IVI Valencia, Valencia, Spain

Ryan Mori, M.D., M.S. Cleveland Clinic Lerner College of Medicine and Glickman Urological and Kidney Institute, Cleveland clinic Foundation, Cleveland, OH, USA

Craig S. Niederberger, M.D. F.A.C.S. Department of Urology, University of Illinois at Chicago College of Medicine and Department of Bioengineering University of Illinois at Chicago College of Engineering, Chicago, IL, USA

C.J. Opperman, B.Sc. Department of Medical Physiology, Faculty of Health Sciences, Stellenbosch University, Tygerberg, South Africa

Uwe Paasch, M.D., Ph.D. Division of Dermatopathology, Division of Aesthetics and Laserdermatology, Department of Dermatology, Venerology and Allergology, European Training Center of Andrology, Univeristy of Leipzig, Leipzig, Germany

Eleonora Pasqualotto, M.D., Ph.D. Conception—Center for Human Reproduction, Caxias do Sul, RS, Brazil

Department of Clinical Medicine, Center of Health Science, University of Caxias do Sul, Caxias do Sul, RS, Brazil

Fabio Pasqualotto, M.D., Ph.D. Department of Anatomy and Urology, Institute of Biotechnology, University of Caxias do Sul, Caxias do Sul, RS, Brazil

Conception—Center for Human Reproduction, Caxias do Sul, RS, Brazil

Antonio Pellicer, M.D. Department of Gynecology and Obstetrics, School of Medicine, Universidad de Valencia, Assisted Reproduction Unit, Instituto Universitario IVI Valencia, Valencia, Spain

Eulalia Pozo-Guisado, Ph.D. Department of Biochemistry and Molecular Biology, School of Life Sciences, University of Extremadura, Badajoz, Spain

José Remohí, M.D. Department of Gynecology and Obstetrics, School of Medicine, Universidad de Valencia, Assisted Reproduction Unit, Instituto Universitario IVI Valencia, Valencia, Spain

Laura Romany, M.D. Clinical Embryology Laboratory, Instituto Universitario IVI Valencia, Valencia, Spain

Edmund Sabanegh, M.D. Department of Urology, Glickman Urological and Kidney Institute, Center for Reproductive Medicine, Cleveland Clinic, Cleveland, OH, USA

Tamer Said, M.D., Ph.D. Andrology Laboratory and Reproductive Tissue Bank, The Toronoto Institute for Reproductive Medicine, Toronto, ON, Canada

Jay Sandlow, M.D. Department of Urology, Medical College of Wisconsin, Milwaukee, WI, USA

Maria San Gabriel, Ph.D. Division of Urology, Department of Surgery, Royal Victoria Hospital, McGill University, Montreal, QC, Canada

Paul Shin, M.D. Urologic Surgeons of Washington, Washington, DC, USA

Aspinder Singh, B.S. Center for Reproductive Medicine, Glickman Urological and Kidney Institute, Cleveland Clinic Foundation, Cleveland, OH, USA

Adam F. Stewart, M.D. Division of Urology, Department of Surgery, University of Tennessee Medical Center, Knoxville, TN, USA

Claudio Telöken, M.D., Ph.D. Andrology Section of Fertilitat – Human Reproduction Center, Department of Urology, Santa Casa Hospital and Federal University of Health Sciences, Porto Alegre, RS, Brazil

Aaron Thompson Center for Reproductive Medicine, Glickman Urological and Kidney Institute, Cleveland Clinic Foundation, Cleveland, OH, USA

Kelton Tremellen, M.B.B.S.(Hons.), Ph.D., F.R.A.N.Z.C.O.G., C.R.E.I. School of Pharmacy and Medical Sciences, University of South Australia, Dulwich, SA, Australia

S. Vaithinathan, Ph.D. Department of Biochemistry and Molecular Biology, Pondicherry University, Kalapet, Pondicherry, India

Alex C. Varghese, Ph.D. Montreal Reproductive Centre, Montreal, QC, Canada

Herbert J. Wiser, M.D. Division of Urology, Southern Illinois University, Springfield, IL, USA

Armand Zini, M.D. Department of Surgery, St. Mary's Hospital, Montreal, QC, Canada

Part I
Male Infertility Diagnosis

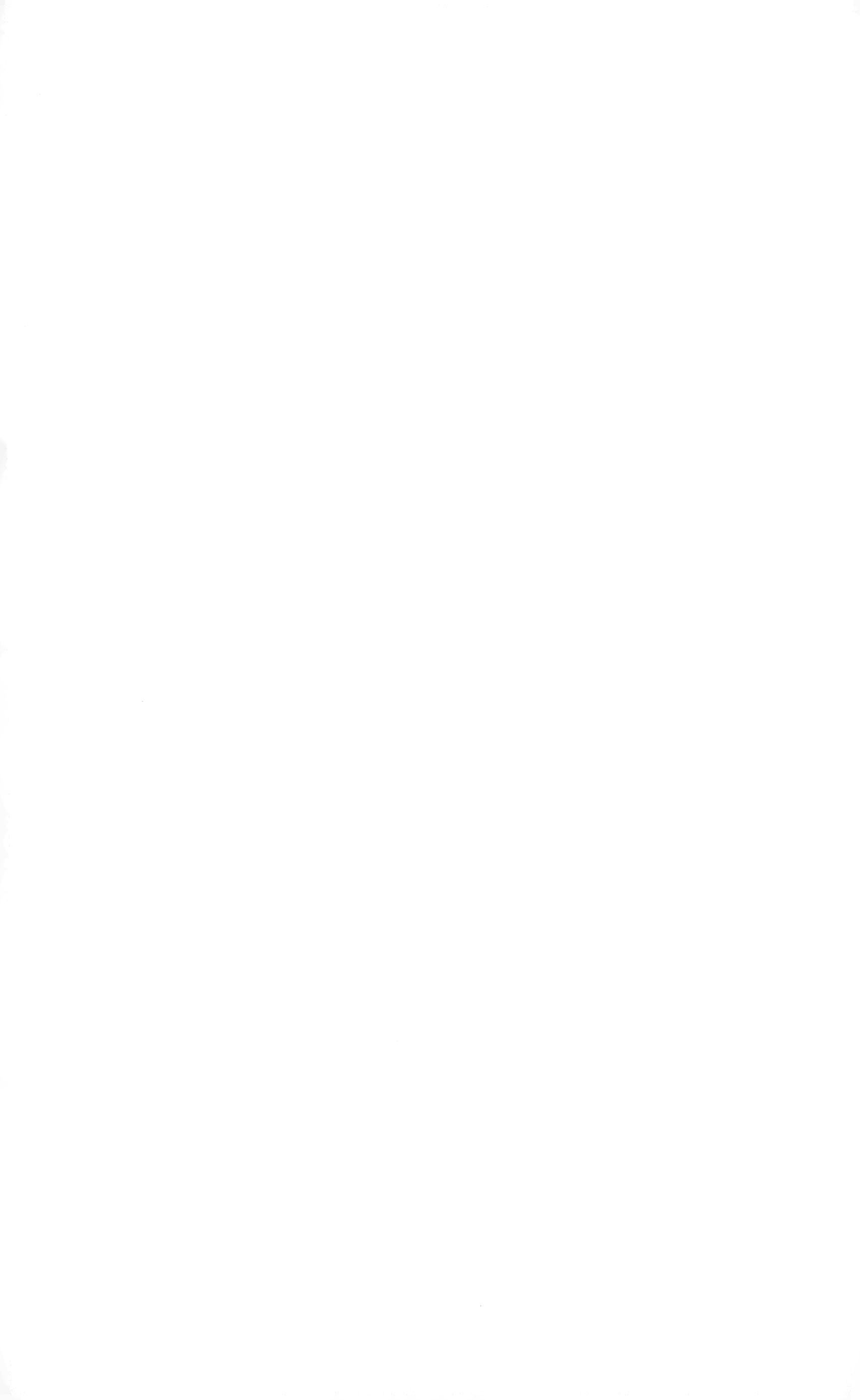

Chapter 1
Causes of Male Infertility

Herbert J. Wiser, Jay Sandlow, and Tobias S. Köhler

Of all sexually active couples, 12–15% are infertile [1]. When broken down by gender, a male component can be identified 50% of the time either in isolation or in combination with a female factor [2]. The majority of the causes of male infertility are treatable or preventable, so a keen understanding of these conditions is paramount. Despite advancements in assisted reproductive technologies, the goal of a male infertility specialist is not simply to retrieve sperm. Instead, the male infertility specialist attempts to optimize a male's reproductive potential and thereby allow a couple to conceive successfully through utilization of less invasive reproductive techniques. Often, this involves the use of sperm or testicular tissue cryopreservation prior to fertility insult. At the same time, the male fertility specialist is wary of underlying or causal, potentially serious medical or genetic conditions that prompted reproductive evaluation. Previous research in a US male fertility clinic analyzing 1,430 patients identified causes of infertility from most to least common: varicocele, idiopathic, obstruction, female factor, cryptorchidism, immunologic, ejaculatory dysfunction, testicular failure, drug effects/radiation, endocrinology, and all others [3]. The focus of this book on the role of reactive oxygen species (ROS) is easily applied to the majority of the listed conditions (described in detail in later chapters) which comprise this chapter's overview of pre-testicular, testicular, and post-testicular causes of male infertility.

H.J. Wiser, MD (✉) • T.S. Köhler, MD, MPh
Division of Urology, Southern Illinois University,
301 N 8th Street, Floor 4, Springfield, IL, USA
e-mail: hwiser@siumed.edu

J. Sandlow, MD
Department of Urology, Medical College of Wisconsin,
9200 West Wisconsin Avenue, Milwaukee, WI, USA

S.J. Parekattil and A. Agarwal (eds.), *Antioxidants in Male Infertility: A Guide for Clinicians and Researchers*, © Springer Science+Business Media New York 2013

Causes of Male Infertility

Pre-testicular

Hypogonadotropic Hypogonadism

Hypogonadotropic hypogonadism affects fertility at multiple levels. Sperm production is deleteriously affected by a lack of testosterone and a lack of a stimulatory effect on the Sertoli/germ cell complex. Sexual function is also negatively impacted with effects seen at the level of erectile function, ejaculatory function, and sexual desire. There are many etiologies of hypogonadotropic hypogonadism. The most common are elevated prolactin, medications, illicit drugs, and pituitary damage. Kallmann syndrome is another, albeit rare, cause of hypogonadotropic hypogonadism.

Elevated Prolactin

Elevated prolactin may cause hypogonadism by suppressing the release of GnRH. Symptoms of hypogonadism, especially erectile dysfunction and loss of libido, are the most common presenting symptoms in males with hyperprolactinemia, though galactorrhea and gynecomastia may also be evident [4].

Elevated prolactin may be secondary to various etiologies. The most common of these is a prolactinoma, which typically arises from the pituitary. Because prolactinomas in men are more likely to manifest through mass effect, visual disturbances and headaches are more likely to be present when compared to women with prolactinomas [5].

There are other significant causes for hyperprolactinemia as well. Prolactin is elevated in renal failure, as well as in patients with hypothyroidism and cirrhosis. Prolactin levels may also be elevated in certain systemic diseases such as systemic lupus erythematosus, rheumatoid arthritis, celiac disease, and systemic sclerosis. Many drugs elevate prolactin levels, especially those which block the effects of dopamine, such as antipsychotics [6].

Pharmacologic

Various medications may cause hypogonadotropic hypogonadism. Estrogens and progestins may cause a decrease in testosterone levels via negative feedback to the hypothalamic-pituitary-gonadal axis. Marijuana is known to decrease testosterone levels by working on the endocannabinoid receptors present at multiple levels of the hypothalamic-pituitary axis [7]. Both ethanol and cannabinoids suppress GnRH secretion at the level of the hypothalamus. Endocannabinoid receptors have also been found in the pituitary and so may also affect the hypothalamic-pituitary axis at that level as well [8]. LHRH agonists and antagonists are used for the treatment of prostate cancer, precocious puberty, and gender reassignment surgeries. In the male, both induce profound hypogonadism. LHRH antagonists directly and intuitively decrease LH and FSH levels. LHRH agonists produce a tonically stimulated state which, unlike the physiologic circadian rhythmicity of normal LHRH stimulation, acts to decrease LH and FSH secretion. Narcotics may also produce profound hypogonadism. Nearly 40% of men using methadone were found to have total testosterone levels less than 230 ng/dL [9].

Kallmann Syndrome

Kallmann syndrome affects between one in 8,000–10,000 males [10, 11]. It is a spectrum of disease in which the primary manifestations are anosmia and hypogonadotropic hypogonadism which leads to an absence of puberty. Multiple genetic defects can lead to Kallmann syndrome [12]. These most commonly manifest through the same mechanism whereby GnRH secreting neurons fail to migrate to the hypothalamus. Lack of these neurons in the hypothalamus results in a lack of GnRH secretion and thus hypogonadism.

Hypergonadotropic Hypogonadism

One of the most common causes of hypergonadotropic hypogonadism is Klinefelter syndrome (Klinefelter's). Klinefelter's affects male fertility by altering spermatogenesis both directly and indirectly by altering the hormonal milieu [13–15]. Interestingly, sex hormone levels are normal until puberty. During puberty, they do rise to low-normal levels, but plateau. By adulthood, serum testosterone levels are typically below normal. Histologic studies demonstrate gradual degeneration of the testes with development, with hyperplasia of poorly functioning Leydig cells [16]. Klinefelter's also directly affects spermatogenesis, as discussed later in this chapter.

Testicular

Varicocele

A varicocele is a dilation of the pampiniform plexus likely caused by the absence or incompetence of the venous valves of the internal spermatic vein. Varicoceles have long been associated with infertility. The first written description is attributed to Celsius who noticed the association between the varicocele and testicular atrophy [17]. In the 1800s, surgical correction was seen to improve semen quality. It is currently seen to be the most common surgically correctable cause of male infertility. Roughly 12% of all men have a varicocele, but this number jumps to 25% in men with abnormal semen parameters [18].

Varicoceles affect multiple semen parameters; total sperm count, sperm motility, and sperm morphology are all negatively affected [19, 20]. There are many theories about the underlying pathophysiology of a varicocele, with heat, renal metabolites, and hormonal abnormalities all playing a role. However, most agree that disruption of the countercurrent heat exchange mechanism in the testis, causing hyperthermia, is the most likely mechanism.

Scrotal temperature in humans is variable during the day, but remains 1–2°C lower than core body temperature at 33–36°C [21]. Thermoregulation of the gonads at a temperature lower than that of body temperature is a trait that is well preserved in homeotherms and especially in mammals [22]. Nearly all mammals have a scrotum. Other mechanisms, such as the efficient heat exchange system in whales, have developed in animals in environments where the scrotum would not be efficient at keeping gonadal heat at a few degrees below body temperature. Besides this teleologic evidence that lower body temperature is necessary for testicular function, numerous studies point to impaired sperm production and a decrease in semen quality when scrotal temperatures are elevated [23–28]. One study showed that men with scrotal skin temperatures above 35°C for >75% of the day had sperm concentrations of 33 million/mL as compared with men with scrotal skin temperatures greater than 35°C for <50% of the day who had sperm concentrations of 92 million/mL [27]. The mechanism by which heat causes decreased sperm counts is poorly understood, but one hypothesis is that increased temperature could increase the metabolic rate of testicular and epididymal sperm, secondarily increasing the amount of oxidative damage to both the structure and the DNA of the spermatocytes and spermatids [22].

Varicoceles are noted to be associated with higher scrotal temperatures [29], and cooling of the scrotum has been shown to improve semen parameters [30]. Interestingly, the temperature of the contralateral testis is also elevated in men with unilateral varicoceles. So the cause of elevated testicular temperatures, which intuitively would seem to be an impaired countercurrent flow mechanism, is less clear [31]. Hormonal abnormalities are a similarly controversial area, with no consistent hormonal changes associated with the presence of a varicocele. Testosterone, SHBG, FSH, and LH have all been examined, and different studies have produced opposing results [17].

Cryptorchidism

Cryptorchidism is well known to affect fertility. The severity of its effect on fertility is directly proportional to the severity of the cryptorchidism, with bilateral cryptorchidism having more severe effects than unilateral, and with higher testes having worse function than lower testes [32–35].

Similarly, orchidopexy has been shown to improve fertility, with the best results obtained with fixation at a young age, especially prior to 1 year of age [36]. Fixation after age 10 may not improve fertility, or may improve it only modestly, suggesting that permanent and progressive damage is done to the testis while in an abnormal position, and this is supported by histologic studies [37, 38]. Actual paternity rates in men who underwent orchidopexy for unilateral cryptorchidism are 89%, slightly less than the non-cryptorchid group, which had a 94% paternity rate. Bilaterally cryptorchid men post-orchidopexy had markedly lower paternity rates, at 62% [34, 35].

The pathophysiology of the effects of cryptorchidism is complex, with heat likely playing a partial but significant role [39, 40]. A number of other factors are also likely to come in to play, including the underlying genetics, hormonal milieu, and environmental exposures which originally led to the cryptorchidism [41–43].

Testicular Cancer

Testicular cancer is strongly associated with infertility. There are multiple ways in which testicular cancer is related to and can contribute to reduced fertility. Both testicular cancer and impaired spermatogenesis may be related in their etiology of embryologic testicular dysgenesis. The testicular dysgenesis syndrome is a spectrum of disease that may involve cryptorchidism, hypospadias, decreased spermatogenesis, and testis cancer. In this syndrome, it is thought that all of these share an origin of abnormal fetal testis development. As a result of this developmental anomaly, any number of these manifestations may be present in a boy [44]. Testicular tumors may also directly contribute to infertility by secreting hormones, which can downregulate sperm production in the contralateral testis [45–48]. This is uncommon but has been seen with Leydig and Sertoli cell tumors as well as seminomas. Tumors may also directly disrupt spermatogenesis by mass effect or by the effects of the inflammatory reaction to the tumor [49]. Cancer treatments may also decrease fertility.

At presentation, roughly 10% of men will be azoospermic, and roughly 50% will be oligospermic. While orchiectomy will result in a rebound in semen parameters in roughly 90% of these men [50], further treatment with surgery, chemotherapy, or radiation can further decrease fertility.

Ionizing Radiation

Excellent data on the effects of ionizing radiation is available from two similar studies, which are unlikely to be repeated. Researchers in these studies prospectively irradiated the testes of prisoners with single or multiple doses of radiation up to 600 cGy [51, 52]. Sperm counts were followed, and serial testicular biopsies were done. These studies showed that sperm counts declined when testes were irradiated and that decline was dose dependant. At low doses of ~7.5 cGy, a mild decline of sperm counts was seen, and this decline increased to severe oligospermia by 30–40 cGy and azoospermia by 78 cGy. The time to recovery was also seen to be dose dependant, with those receiving 20 cGy beginning to have a recovery of sperm counts by 6 months, those with 100 cGy at 7 months, 200 cGy at 11 months, and 600 cGy at 24 months. The percent of men achieving a complete recovery and time to achieve a complete recovery also declined with increasing radiation doses.

Decline to the nadir of sperm counts was seen at roughly 64 days, corresponding roughly to the time required for sperm cell production from spermatogonia.

More rapid declines were seen with higher radiation doses, indicating increased damage to the more highly differentiated cells undergoing spermatogenesis. Biopsy results from these studies showed that spermatogonia numbers nadired at much lower levels with higher doses of radiation and that these nadirs took longer to achieve than those which had received lower doses of radiation.

These studies provide excellent information into the biology of the effects of radiation on spermatogenesis on the healthy young testis. Clinically, however, the effects we see are often more pronounced given the setting of the radiation, namely, cancer patients undergoing radiotherapy. Fractionated radiation has been shown to be more damaging than single dose radiation [53]. One report showed that fractionated radiation with a total dose of 200 cGy may cause permanent azoospermia [54].

As would be expected, Leydig cells are more resistant to radiation than the germinal epithelium [51]. Doses of 20 Gy are known to cause declines in testosterone [55]. Doses on the order of 2 Gy do not cause appreciable drops in testosterone [56].

Chemotherapy

Chemotherapy typically targets rapidly dividing cells and thus has profound effects on the germinal epithelium. As such, the expected outcome of acute chemotherapy is a decline in spermatogenesis, and this has been well documented since the late 1940s [57]. The mechanism by which chemotherapeutics decrease fertility and the rates of recovery is both drug and dose dependent [58–61].

Bleomycin, etoposide, and cisplatin or carboplatin (BEP) is the most commonly used chemotherapy regimen for testicular germ cell tumors. The decrease in fertility seen post-BEP chemotherapy is likely the result of a direct reduction of spermatogenesis and not as a result of any change in the hormonal milieu. Indeed, testosterone levels are not seen to be significantly reduced at 12 months post-chemotherapy, and FSH levels are appropriately elevated. FSH levels decline as spermatogenesis returns over the following 2–4 years [62]. It should be noted, however, that return of spermatogenesis is not guaranteed. In patients who were normospermic prior to chemotherapy, fewer than 4 cycles of BEP have not typically been associated with high rates of permanent infertility [63]. However, high-dose BEP is associated with approximately a 50% of permanent infertility in one study [64]. Notably, even in azoospermic men post-high dose BEP chemotherapy, nests of spermatogenesis have been found on TESE [65].

Genetic Azoospermia/Oligospermia

It is estimated that 2–8% of infertile men have an underlying genetic abnormality, with this number rising to 15% in azoospermic men [66]. Although the majority of male infertility does not have an identifiable genetic cause, two potential etiologies are Y chromosome microdeletions and karyotypic abnormalities. The two most common karyotypic abnormalities are Klinefelter's (47,XXY) and chromosomal translocations.

Y chromosome microdeletions are a common cause of these, occurring in 11–18% of azoospermic men and 4–14% of oligospermic men [67]. Currently, research is focused on the azoospermia factor (AZF) region on the long arm of the Y chromosome at Yq11. This area itself contains three separate regions, AZFa, AZFb, and AZFc, and microdeletions of these areas lead to slightly different phenotypes [68]. Deletions in the AZFa and AZFb regions both cause azoospermia, but histologically, they are different with AZFa deletions resulting in Sertoli cell-only syndrome and AZFb deletions causing an arrest of spermatogenesis at the primary spermatocyte stage [66]. AZFc deletions are the most common of the Y chromosome microdeletions and are found in 5–7% of oligospermic men [68]. Unlike the AZFa/AZFb deletions, they do not uniformly result in azoospermia; rather, a spectrum of phenotypes are seen with partial deletions being found in normospermic men, from oligospermia to azoospermia in some full deletions [66]. In men undergoing micro-TESE sperm extraction with azfC deletions, about 35% have sperm found successfully [69].

Classic and mosaic Klinefelter's are common karyotypic abnormalities found in infertile men. Klinefelter's has a prevalence of one in 660 males; thus, it is the most common genetic cause of male infertility as 75–90% of men with Klinefelter's will be azoospermic, with some with mosaic Klinefelter's being mainly oligospermic [13, 70, 71]. Studies which show higher prevalences of azoospermic men with AZF deletions than Klinefelter's are likely flawed by a selection bias as men with the obvious stigmata of Klinefelter's are not tested and included in these studies [72, 73].

As would be expected, Klinefelter's has much broader effects than Y chromosome microdeletions and affects fertility through two routes, direct effects on spermatogenesis and indirect hormonal effects on spermatogenesis [13–15]. As far as altered spermatogenesis is concerned, the majority of Klinefelter's patients actually do produce sperm, as is witnessed by the 69% TESE sperm retrieval rates [74]; however, the quantity of sperm produced is typically very low. Biopsy studies of Klinefelter's testes have demonstrated that spermatogenesis is halted pre-pachytene in the vast majority of aneuploid cells and that meiosis was seen mainly in cells with normal karyotypes [15].

Robertsonian translocations are a third significant genetic cause of infertility. They occur in 0.8% of infertile men, and this number rises to 1.6% in oligospermic men [75]. Phenotypes are highly variable given the possibilities of recombination [66].

Environmental Factors

Hyperthermia is considered to be a major contributor in the pathogenesis of infertility in men with varicocele and cryptorchidism. Many lifestyle factors also have the potential to increase scrotal temperatures, including underwear type, heated car seats, and occupational heat exposure. The role of underwear style in male infertility has been investigated. One small study of 14 normospermic men, a tight polyester scrotal support, when worn day and night, was shown to make all azoospermic at a mean time of 140 days. After removal of the scrotal support, all men regained function at a mean time of 157 days [76]. However, normal underwear, i.e., boxer or brief style, has not been shown to exert a significant influence on semen parameters [77]. Other types of heat exposure, such as occupational heat exposure in a group of welders, have been shown to decrease semen quality [78]. Sedentary posture, heated car seats, and sauna and hot tub use are all lifestyle factors that increase scrotal temperature as well and may contribute to a decline in fertility [79].

Recently, cell phones have been implicated as possibly playing a role in decreasing male fertility, and several studies show that there may be some basis for this. One observational study assessed semen parameters and cell phone usage in 361 men who presented to an infertility clinic. Sixty percent of the men in this study had greater than 2 h of cell phone use per day, with 30% using their cell phones for more than 4 h per day. They found that sperm counts, motility, viability, and morphology all worsened with increasing cell phone use [80]. The mechanism by which cell phones affect semen parameters has not yet been elucidated, but one hypothesis is that cell phone-generated electromagnetic radiation (CPEMR) alters mitochondrial function and acts to increase reactive oxygen species. This is somewhat corroborated by one study which looked at the effects of CPEMR on semen parameters and found increased levels of reactive oxygen species with decreased viability and motility in the sperm exposed to CPEMR [81].

Tobacco use has been implicated in the pathogenesis of numerous cancers and medical diseases. While the use of tobacco significantly impacts female fertility, its impact on male fertility is less clear. Semen parameters, including sperm density, motility, and morphology, have all been shown to be worsened with tobacco use [82–85]. However, a significant reduction in fertility has not yet been proven.

Testicular Injury

Injury to the testicle can be sustained either directly or indirectly. Direct trauma to the testis is typically managed by debridement of devitalized seminiferous tubules and closure of the tunica albuginea [86]. The resultant loss of volume of seminiferous tubules and possible obstruction from scarring is one possible cause of decreased fertility. Reports on testicular salvage after bilateral trauma indicated that preserved volume of testis is the key to preserving fertility [86–91].

Indirect damage to the testis may be sustained by exposure to infection or inflammation of the testis. The classic infectious agent causing infertility is mumps. Orchitis occurs in roughly 20% of postpubertal males with mumps [92] and is bilateral in 30% of these. Of those postpubertal males with bilateral mumps orchitis, 25% will have resultant infertility. In other words, 1.5% of postpubertal males with mumps may become infertile as a result of the disease. In nations where immunization against mumps is common, this is a rare phenomenon. The mechanism by which mumps causes orchitis is via pressure atrophy. Infection of the testis with the mumps virus causes inflammation and swelling, which is limited by the tunica albuginea; this in turn leads to atrophy [93].

Other bacterial and viral pathogens may also cause infertility at the testicular level, most commonly; this is the result of spread of infection from the epididymis [94, 95]. The mechanism for infertility in these cases may be persistent inflammation which suppresses testicular function or obstruction secondary to resultant sclerosis.

Primary Ciliary Dyskinesia

Ultrastructural defects that affect sperm motility are described under the grouping of primary ciliary dyskinesia (PCD). PCD is a rare and heterogeneous genetic disease which affects one in 20,000–60,000 [96]. Many components of cilia and flagella are affected, though the defect is found in the dynein in over 80% of cases [97]. The key clinical finding is chronic respiratory infections leading to bronchiectasis. When situs inversus is present in addition to the other components, it is termed Kartagener's syndrome. Male infertility secondary to sperm dysmotility is related to the dysfunction of the flagellate tail of the sperm. It is a common finding, though not universal, and this is likely related to the heterogeneity of the genetics.

Sertoli Cell-Only Syndrome

Sertoli cell-only syndrome may be either primary or secondary, and attempts have been made to distinguish these histologically [98]. The primary form is hypothesized to result from a lack of migration of the germ cells to the seminiferous tubules during embryologic development. The secondary form is due to a gonadotoxic insult to the testis after birth. While the different etiologies of these would intuitively suggest a higher likelihood of finding sperm in biopsies of testes with secondary Sertoli cell-only syndrome, this is not borne out in the literature [99].

Antisperm Antibodies

In the normal male, sperm reside in an immunoprivileged site. The blood-testis barrier prevents proteins from the sperm from interacting with the immune system and setting up an immune reaction against them. Trauma, infection, and inflammation all may disrupt this barrier and result in immunity against the germinal epithelium and spermatozoa.

Antisperm antibodies (ASA) are very common, with 8–17% of men and 1–22% women in infertile couples testing positive for serum ASA [100, 101]. As expected, ASA are heterogeneous in their binding sites and, as such, have wide ranging effects on sperm function. Some ASA will not significantly affect fertility, and 0.9–2.5% of fertile men will test positive for serum ASA [102, 103]. ASA targeted against proteins on the head region are more likely to affect zona binding and sperm penetration, whereas ASA targeted against the tails of spermatozoa are more likely to decrease motility and cervical mucus penetration and cause sperm agglutination [104]. Antibody type also plays a significant role in the degree of reduction of fertility. In a study of ASA in men who had undergone vasectomy reversal, IgA ASA were associated with a much more significant reduction in fertility than IgG ASA [105]. While ASA clearly may affect fertility in some cases, serum ASA positivity is not a strong predictor of infertility.

DNA Damage

There are many etiologies of sperm DNA damage. Radiation, toxins, genital tract inflammation, varicocele, advanced paternal age, and testicular hyperthermia all induce significant DNA damage [106, 107] and will be discussed at length elsewhere in this book.

Post-testicular

Absence of the Vas Deferens

Congenital bilateral absence of the vas deferens (CBAVD) is a condition strongly related to cystic fibrosis (CF) and has even been considered as a diagnostic criterion for CF. However, while current dogma states that nearly all patients with CF have bilaterally absent vasa, there is little data to support this. Indeed, two recent articles suggest that CBAVD is present in half or less of CF patients. One series looking at children with CF who were undergoing inguinal hernia repair reported only a 24% (6/25) rate of CBAVD [108]. A series of 20 adults with CF and a mean age around 30 years old had a CBAVD rate of 55% [109]. In this latter series, only one man had a semen analysis consistent with possible fertility, and the more constant finding was atrophy of the seminal vesicles, which was seen in 18/20.

Nevertheless, CBAVD is strongly associated to CF, and the same genetics, mutation of the CFTR, are typically responsible for both phenomenons [110]. So, while men with CF do not necessarily have CBAVD, most men with CBAVD do have a CFTR mutation [111–113]. The pathophysiology of CBAVD thus clearly involves altered chloride transport in the majority of cases, and, like the respiratory and pancreatic sequelae seen with CF, there is evidence that the genital abnormalities and pathology seen are a progressive disease. Namely, intentionally aborted CF fetuses demonstrate normal vas deferens, albeit with secretions filling their lumens. This suggests that the mechanism for CBAVD is atresia, and not aplasia, when a CFTR mutation is present [114]. One interesting sequela of this is that renal agenesis is not associated with CBAVD [115].

Congenital unilateral absence of the vas deferens (CUAVD) is a different entity altogether [116]. While there is still a significant rate of CFTR mutations in men with CUAVD, especially when the obstructive azoospermia is present [110], the majority of CUAVD is the result of an embryologic Wolffian duct aberrancy [117]. As such, renal agenesis is often seen with CUAVD, though CUAVD is not always seen in men with unilateral renal agenesis, as there are many other embryologic missteps that may occur to result in renal agenesis. While there is only a 20% rate of CUAVD seen in those with a unilateral renal agenesis, there is a 79% rate of unilateral renal agenesis seen in men with CUAVD. Since CUAVD not associated with a CFTR mutation is usually a unilateral and isolated phenomenon, fertility is often preserved.

Young's Syndrome

Young's syndrome is a rare disorder which presents clinically as obstructive azoospermia and chronic sinopulmonary infections [118]. Thus, it can be difficult to differentiate clinically from cystic fibrosis variants and primary ciliary dyskinesia. Indeed, definitive diagnosis of Young's syndrome requires negative CFTR genetic testing as well as investigation of ciliary ultrastructure to rule out primary ciliary dyskinesia [119]. Normal spermatogenesis is seen, and the obstructive azoospermia is due to inspissated secretions in the vas deferens.

The etiology of Young's syndrome is unclear with childhood mercury exposure having been postulated to play a role in the past [120]. Interestingly, the incidence of Young's syndrome has plummeted from estimates of one in 500 in the 1980s down to case reports and articles which question the existence of Young's syndrome today [121]. The observation that the reduced incidence over the last 50 years coincides with a decrease in mercury use and poisoning is tempered by the fact that our knowledge of genetics has rapidly advanced. Thus, the decreased incidence of Young's syndrome is more likely due to the increased correct genetic diagnosis of CF spectrum disease.

EjDO/Seminal Vesicle Dysfunction

Ejaculatory duct obstruction is a common etiology of male infertility, occurring in 1–5% of men presenting with infertility [122]. There are many causes of ejaculatory duct obstruction, including cystic fibrosis spectrum disease, Wolffian or Muellerian origin cysts, calcifications, tuberculosis and other GU infections, calculi, and urinary tract instrumentation [123, 124]. Additionally, chronic ejaculatory duct obstruction may affect the seminal vesicle in a manner analogous to the effect of bladder outlet obstruction on the bladder. Namely, with longstanding obstruction, the seminal vesicles may lose contractility, and resolution of the anatomical obstruction may not improve seminal vesicle emptying during ejaculation. Seminal vesicle dysfunction may also be seen in the absence of previous obstruction. This can be secondary to multiple sclerosis, diabetes, spinal cord injury or other neurologic insult, and medications. One interesting physical finding seen in 25–50% of men with spinal cord injuries likely related to seminal vesicle dysfunction is brown semen [125]. This brown coloration is not derived from heme and is not related to semen stasis per se.

Vasectomy and Vasectomy Reversal

Vasectomy is a procedure that is intended to produce infertility, and it is successful in over 90% of cases [126]. Some of the key determinants of success are related to aspects of surgical technique. The main reason for a correctly performed vasectomy to fail is recanalization of the vas deferens, a finding that has been histologically verified [127, 128]. Some debate remains as to which techniques provide the lowest recanalization rates. The manner of ligating the ends, non-ligation versus clipping versus suture ligation, length of vas removed, as well as whether to fold vas ends are all controversial [129, 130]. Two maneuvers which do seem to provide significant benefits are luminal cauterization and fascial interposition [131, 132].

Vasectomy reversal may be performed in an attempt to return fertility to the sterilized man. The outcomes of vasectomy reversal are dependent on a number of factors. Surgical technique is one factor, with use of a microscope significantly improving pregnancy rates over loupe-assisted vasovasostomy [133]. Time elapsed since fertility also plays a significant role with a 97% patency rate and 76% pregnancy rate being achieved if surgery is performed at less than 3 years since vasectomy. Patency and pregnancy rates decline as time elapses, with patency and pregnancy rates of 79% and 44%, respectively, if the vasectomy was between 9 and 14 years prior and 71% and 30% if greater than 15 years elapsed [134]. Type of vasectomy reversal also plays a role with vasoepididymostomy (VE) having lower patency and pregnancy rates than vasovasostomy (VV) [135]. Presence and type of antisperm antibodies also may reduce fertility rates in men after vasectomy reversal [105]. Sperm granulomas were previously thought to decrease testicular pressure and so portend better vasectomy reversal outcomes. Though better sperm quality has been found in the vasa of men with sperm granulomas at the time of surgery, patency and pregnancy rates are not significantly different [134, 136]. Similarly, a testicular vasal remnant of 2.7 cm or longer predicts finding whole sperm in the vasal fluid [137], though research is not available as to its effect on patency and pregnancy rates. Though repeat attempts at vasectomy reversal would intuitively seem less likely to succeed, high success rates have been reported with combined VV/VE patency rates of 89% and pregnancy rates of 58% if the interval of obstruction was less than 10 years [138].

Nerve Injury

Nervous injury affecting ejaculation may occur at many levels and have a diverse etiology ranging from spinal cord injury to neural damage during retroperitoneal or pelvic surgery to neuropathy from systemic diseases. Ejaculatory dysfunction is present in 90% of spinal cord injury patients [139]. The type and severity of ejaculatory dysfunction are dependent on the level and extent of the injury.

Higher cord lesions often result in an intact reflex arc which allows for penile vibratory stimulation to induce ejaculation. Men with sacral lesions or lesions of the efferent parasympathetic nerves are often not responsive to penile vibratory stimulation and may require endorectal electrical stimulation to induce ejaculation [140].

Retroperitoneal lymph node dissection (RPLND) for testicular cancer resulted in a high rate of ejaculatory dysfunction until the development of methods to spare the sympathetic nerve fibers. Both emission and bladder neck contraction are mediated by the sympathetic nervous system, and damage to the sympathetic chain and the hypogastric plexus overlying the great vessels results in a high degree of ejaculatory dysfunction. In the past, RPLND was associated with a 55–60% chance of ejaculatory dysfunction [141, 142]. Modified templates have helped to reduce the rates of retrograde ejaculation, with one study demonstrating an 82% rate of antegrade ejaculation with a modified unilateral template [143]. Another study using a modified bilateral template demonstrated an 88% rate of preservation of antegrade ejaculation [144].

Nerve sparing RPLND, developed in the late 1980s, has reduced the incidence of retrograde ejaculation even further to 0–7% [145, 146]. Nerve sparing RPLND may also be done after chemotherapy, though only 136 of 341 men qualified for this as compared to standard RPLND in one series [147]. Rates of ejaculatory dysfunction were also higher at 21%.

Medications

Medications affecting ejaculation do so by altering adrenergic signaling. This is most clearly seen with alpha-1 antagonists. Tamsulosin and silodosin, especially, are known to cause ejaculatory dysfunction [148, 149]. Previously, this was thought to be retrograde ejaculation. Recent studies have shown that the ejaculatory dysfunction induced by alpha-1 antagonists is actually a failure of emission [150, 151].

Antipsychotics have long been associated with sexual dysfunction, including ejaculatory dysfunction. Antipsychotics have effects on many different neurotransmitters including dopamine, norepinephrine, acetylcholine, and serotonin. Predictably, altered ejaculatory function with antipsychotics use correlates with anti-adrenergic actions of the antipsychotics [152]. Even atypical antipsychotics like risperidone may affect ejaculation [153, 154].

Resection of the Prostate

Surgery of the prostate is well known to cause retrograde ejaculation. Transurethral resection of the prostate as well as the laser photovaporization and enucleation all have a high likelihood of inducing retrograde ejaculation since removal of the proximal prostatic urethra severely diminishes the resistance to backflow of semen.

Coital

Abnormal coital practices may play a role in infertility when they interfere with semen deposition in the vagina or affect their timing with the female reproductive cycle. Similarly, erectile dysfunction and penile abnormalities such as hypospadias and chordee may interfere with semen deposition and thus may play a role in infertility.

Lubricants are commonly used by infertile couples, and many vaginal lubricants have been shown to negatively affect fertility. Many synthetic lubricants not only affect sperm motility but have also been shown to increase the DNA fragmentation index. In one study, FemGlide, Replens, and Astroglide all affected sperm motility, and FemGlide and K-Y jelly increased DNA fragmentation. One lubricant that has not been shown to have a significant impact on sperm motility or DNA fragmentation is Pre-Seed [155]. Another study showed similar findings with decreased motility in sperm exposed to K-Y jelly and Touch. Non-viability was seen in sperm exposed to Replens and Astroglide which was comparable to the non-viability seen when sperm were exposed to the spermicide nonoxylnol-9 [156]. In this study, canola oil was not found to affect sperm motility or viability. Yet another study showed that K-Y jelly, saliva, and olive oil all reduced sperm motility, while baby oil did not significantly affect motility [157].

Expert Commentary

This chapter has described the pre-testicular, testicular, and post-testicular spectrum of conditions known to affect male fertility. Many of the listed causes stem from or are subject to further degradation from reactive oxygen species. Pre-testicular causes often alter the normal hormonal milieu for sperm development, providing a suboptimal environment for sperm and perhaps a greater exposure or sensitivity to free radical damage. Testicular causes of infertility such as radiation, toxins, genital tract inflammation, varicocele, and testicular hyperthermia all induce significant DNA damage and thus increase reactive oxygen species. Finally, post-testicular causes of male infertility often affect sperm transit time, increasing likelihood of free radical damage of sperm. Despite our understanding of many of the conditions leading to male infertility, idiopathic infertility still comprises a large portion of the men evaluated for problems with reproduction. The proportion of idiopathic infertility will likely decrease with further understanding of the role of reactive oxygen species and clarification of the role of DNA integrity assays.

The male partners of all couples presenting with infertility must be examined and evaluated. Infertility itself is an independent risk factor for testicular cancer and genetic disease. Indeed, men of reproductive years often forego visiting physicians, and the infertility visit offers a viable platform for general health screening and recommendations. It must be remembered that the majority of the causes of male infertility are either preventable or treatable. Treatment success goes beyond simply harvesting sperm for assisted reproductive techniques. Facilitating pregnancy through intrauterine insemination with varicocele repair should be viewed with the same regard as facilitating natural pregnancy with vasectomy reversal. Finally, the importance of sperm banking cannot be understated, as cryopreservation of reproductive tissue prior to reproductive insult from chemotherapy or surgery is simple and often is the only chance of preserving future fertility.

Five-Year View

Although details and further understanding of some of the causes of male fertility conditions of male described have been elucidated in recent years, previous and future chapters in reproductive textbooks are and will be very similar to this one. However, the development and refinement of DNA integrity tests and determination of the relative importance of reactive oxygen species will likely obviate the need for male infertility evaluation. For example, if varicocele repair is definitively proven to reduce DNA damage to sperm, and decreased DNA damage to sperm is definitively proven to improve success rates with assisted reproductive techniques, referral from female fertility specialists will likely increase. Additional public and provider education on the rationale for male infertility referral and messages on the need for sperm banking will also increase the need for specialists knowledgeable in the causes and treatment of male infertility. This in itself may bring challenges because in relation to female assisted reproductive technology centers, large areas are greatly underserved by male fertility specialists [158].

Key Issues

- The majority of the causes of male infertility are either preventable or treatable.
- Male infertility is an independent risk factor for testicular cancer and genetic diseases.
- Sperm banking should be utilized liberally prior to potential gonadotoxic exposure.
- Pre-testicular causes of male infertility exert their negative effect via imbalances in the hormonal milieu of sperm production. Sexual function is also negatively impacted with effects seen at the level of erectile function, ejaculatory function, and sexual desire.
- Medications can negatively impact pre-testicular, testicular, and post-testicular function.
- Varicocele is the most common cause of male infertility.
- For fertility potential, cryptorchidism is best treated early, especially if bilateral.
- After testicular trauma, fertility is most dependent on operative testicular volume preservation.

- Severe oligospermia or azoospermia requires genetic screening, given their high associated prevalence of Klinefelter's syndrome, karyotypic abnormalities, and microdeletion of the Y chromosome.
- CBAVD is not always seen with cystic fibrosis; evaluation for renal agenesis in CUAVD is essential.
- Many testicular causes of male infertility (radiation, toxins, environmental factors, genital tract inflammation, varicocele, testicular hyperthermia) lead directly to sperm DNA damage.
- Several post-testicular causes of male infertility stem from surgery.

References

1. Mosher WE. Reproductive impairments in the United States, 1965–1982. Demography. 1985;22:415–30.
2. Tielemans E, Burdorf A, te Velde E, Weber R, van Kooij R, Heederik D. Sources of bias in studies among infertility clients. Am J Epidemiol. 2002;156:86–92.
3. Sigman M. Male Infertility. Med Health R I. 1997;80(12):406–9.
4. Buvat J. Hyperprolactinemia and sexual function in men: a short review. Int J Impot Res. 2003;15(5):373–7.
5. Carter JN, Tyson JE, Tolis G, et al. Prolactin-screening tumors and hypogonadism in 22 men. N Engl J Med. 1978;299(16):847–52.
6. Patel SS, Bamigboye V. Hyperprolactinaemia. J Obstet Gynaecol. 2007;27(5):455–9.
7. Fasano S, Meccariello R, Cobellis G, et al. The endocannabinoid system: an ancient signaling involved in the control of male fertility. Ann N Y Acad Sci. 2009;1163:112–24.
8. Rettori V, De Laurentiis A, Fernandez-Solari J. Alcohol and endocannabinoids: neuroendocrine interactions in the reproductive axis. Exp Neurol. 2010;224(1):15–22.
9. Hallinan R, Byrne A, Agho K, et al. Hypogonadism in men receiving methadone and buprenorphine maintenance treatment. Int J Androl. 2009;32(2):131–9.
10. Dodé C, Hardelin JP. Kallmann syndrome. Eur J Hum Genet. 2009;17:139–46.
11. Fechner A, Fong S, McGovern P. A review of Kallmann syndrome: genetics, pathophysiology, and clinical management. Obstet Gynecol Surv. 2008;63(3):189–94.
12. Hardelin JP, Dode C. The complex genetics of Kallmann syndrome: KAL1, FGFR1, FGF8, PROKR2, PROK2, et al. Sex Dev. 2008;2:181–93.
13. Kamischke A, Baumgardt A, Horst J, et al. Clinical and diagnostic features of patients with suspected Klinefelter Syndrome. J Androl. 2003;24:41–8.
14. Blanco J, Egozcue J, Vidal F. Meiotic behavior of the sex chromosomes in three patients with sex chromosome abnormalities (47, XXY, mosaic 46, XY/47, XXY, and 47, XYY) assessed by flourescence in-situ hybridization. Hum Reprod. 2001;16(5):887–92.
15. Bergere M, Wainer R, Nataf V, et al. Biopsied testis cells of four 47, XXY patients: fluorescence in-situ hybridization and ICSI results. Hum Reprod. 2002;17:32–7.
16. Wikström AM, Dunkel L. Testicular function in Klinefelter syndrome. Horm Res. 2008;69(6):317–26.
17. Nagler HM, Grotas AB. Varicocele. In: Lipshultz LI, Howards SS, Niederberger CS, editors. Infertility in the male. 4th ed. New York City, NY: Cambridge University; 2009.
18. World Health Organization. The influence of varicocele on parameters of fertility in a large group of men presenting to infertility clinics. Fertil Steril. 1992;57:1289–93.
19. MacLeod J. Seminal cytology in the presence of varicocele. Fertil Steril. 1965;16(6):735–57.

20. Paduch DA, Niedzielski J. Semen analysis in young men with varicocele: preliminary study. J Urol. 1996;156:778–90.
21. Hjollund NH, Storgaard L, Ernst E, et al. The relation between daily activities and scrotal temperature. Reprod Toxicol. 2002;16(3):209–14.
22. Ivell R. Lifestyle impact and the biology of the human scrotum. Reprod Biol Endocrinol. 2007;5:15.
23. Paul C, Murray AA, Spears N, et al. A single, mild, transient scrotal heat stress causes DNA damage, subfertility and impairs formation of blastocysts in mice. Reproduction. 2008; 136(1):73–84.
24. Dada R, Gupta NP, Kucheria K. Spermatogenic arrest in men with testicular hyperthermia. Teratog Carcinog Mutagen. 2003;S1:235–43.
25. Esfandiari N, Saleh RA, Blaut AP, et al. Effects of temperature on sperm motion characteristics and reactive oxygen species. Int J Fertil Womens Med. 2002;47(5):227–33.
26. Bedford JM. Effects of elevated temperature on the epididymis and testis: experimental studies. Adv Exp Med Biol. 1991;286:19–32.
27. Hjollund NH, Bonde JP, Jensen TK, et al. Diurnal scrotal skin temperature and semen quality. The Danish first pregnancy planner study team. Int J Androl. 2000;23(5):309–18.
28. Wang C, McDonald V, Leung A, et al. Effect of increased scrotal temperature on sperm production in normal men. Fertil Steril. 1997;68(2):334–9.
29. Zorgniotti AW, MacLeod J. Studies in temperature, human semen quality, and varicocele. Fertil Steril. 1973;24(11):854–63.
30. Jung A, Eberl M, Schill WB. Improvement of semen quality by nocturnal scrotal cooling and moderate behavioral change to reduce genital heat stress in men with oligoasthenoteratozoospermia. Reproduction. 2001;121(4):595–603.
31. Goldstein M, Eid JF. Elevation of intratesticular and scrotal skin surface temperature in men with varicocele. J Urol. 1989;142(3):743–5.
32. Trsinar B, Muravec UR. Fertility potential after unilateral and bilateral orchidopexy for cryptorchidism. World J Urol. 2009;27(4):513–9.
33. Gracia J, Sánchez Zalabardo J, Sánchez García J, et al. Clinical, physical, sperm and hormonal data in 251 adults operated on for cryptorchidism in childhood. BJU Int. 2000;85(9):1100–3.
34. Lee PA, O'Leary LA, Songer NJ, et al. Paternity after unilateral cryptorchidism: a controlled study. Pediatrics. 1996;98:676–9.
35. Lee PA, O'Leary LA, Songer NJ, et al. Paternity after bilateral cryptorchidism. A controlled study. Arch Pediatr Adolesc Med. 1997;151(3):260–3.
36. Canavese F, Mussa A, Manenti M, et al. Sperm count of young men surgically treated for cryptorchidism in the first and second year of life: fertility is better in children treated at a younger age. Eur J Pediatr Surg. 2009;19(6):388–91.
37. Wiser A, Raviv G, Weissenberg R, et al. Does age at orchidopexy impact on the results of testicular sperm extraction? Reprod Biomed Online. 2009;19(6):778–83.
38. Cooper ER. The histology of the retained testis in the human subject at different ages and its comparison to the testis. J Anat. 1929;64:5–10.
39. Murphy F, Paran TS, Puri P. Orchidopexy and its impact on fertility. Pediatr Surg Int. 2007;23(7):625032. Epub 13 Mar 2007.
40. Setchell BP. The Parkes Lecture: heat and the testis. J Reprod Fertil. 1998;114(2):179–94.
41. Leissner J, Filipas D, Wolf HK, et al. The undescended testis: considerations and impact on fertility. BJU Int. 1999;83(8):885–91.
42. Hadziselimovic F, Zivkovic D, Bica DTG, et al. The importance of mini-puberty for fertility in cryptorchidism. J Urol. 2005;174:1536–9.
43. Kurpisz M, Havryluk A, Nakonechnyj A, et al. Cryptorchidism and long-term consequences. Reprod Biol. 2010;10(1):19–35.
44. Jørgensen N, Meyts ER, Main KM, Skakkebaek NE. Testicular dysgenesis syndrome comprises some but not all cases of hypospadias and impaired spermatogenesis. Int J Androl. 2010;33(2):298–303. Epub 4 Feb 2010.

45. Abe T, Takaha N, Tsujimura A, et al. Leydig cell tumor of the testis presenting male infertility: a case report. Hinyokika Kiyo. 2003;49(1):39–42.
46. Shiraishi Y, Nishiyama H, Okubo K, et al. Testicular Leydig cell tumor presenting as male infertility: a case report. Hinyokika Kiyo. 2009;55(12):777–81.
47. Chovelidze S, Kochiashvili D, Gogeschvili G, et al. Cases of Leydig cell tumor in male infertility. Georgian Med News. 2007;143:76–9.
48. Hayashi T, Arai G, Hyochi N, et al. Suppression of spermatogenesis in ipsilateral and contralateral testicular tissues in patients with seminoma by human chorionic gonadotropin beta subunit. Urology. 2001;58(2):251–7.
49. Ho GT, Gardner H, DeWolf WC, et al. Influence of testicular carcinoma on ipsilateral spermatogenesis. J Urol. 1992;148(3):821–5.
50. Carmignani L, Gadda F, Paffoni A, et al. Azoospermia and severe oligospermia in testicular cancer. Arch Ital Urol Androl. 2009;81(1):21–3.
51. Rowley MJ, Leach DR, Warner GA, et al. Effect of graded doses of ionizing radiation on the human testis. Radiat Res. 1974;59(3):665–78.
52. Paulsen CA. The study of radiation effects on the human testis: including histologic, chromosomal and hormonal aspects. Final progress report of AEC contract AT(45-1)-2225, Task Agreement 6. RLO-2225-2. 1973.
53. Speiser B, Rubin P, Casarett G. Aspermia following lower truncal irradiation in Hodgkin's disease. Cancer. 1973;32(3):692–8.
54. Ash P. The influence of radiation on fertility in man. Br J Radiol. 1980;53:271–8.
55. Giwercman A, von der Maase H, Berthelsen JG, et al. Localized irradiation of testes with carcinoma in situ: effects of Leydig cell function and eradication of malignant germ cells in 20 patients. J Clin Endocrinol Metab. 1991;73(3):596–603.
56. Shapiro E, Kinsella TJ, Makuch RW, et al. Effects of fractionated irradiation on endocrine aspects of testicular function. J Clin Oncol. 1985;3(9):1232–9.
57. Spitz S. The histological effects of nitrogen mustard on human tumours and tissues. Cancer. 1948;1(3):383–98.
58. Watson AR, Rance CP, Bain J. Long term effects of cyclophosphamide on testicular function. BMJ. 1985;291:1457–60.
59. Pryzant RM, Meistrich ML, Wilson G, et al. Long-term reduction in sperm count after chemotherapy with and without radiation therapy for non-Hodgkin's lymphomas. J Clin Oncol. 1993;11(2):239–47.
60. da Cunha MF, Meistrich ML, Fuller LM, et al. Recovery of spermatogenesis after treatment for Hodgkin's disease: limiting dose of MOPP chemotherapy. J Clin Oncol. 1984; 2(6):571–7.
61. Meistrich ML, Chawla SP, Da Cunha MF, et al. Recovery of sperm production after chemotherapy for osteosarcoma. Cancer. 1989;63(11):2115–23.
62. Pectasides D, Pectasides M, Farmakis D. Testicular function in patients with testicular cancer treated with Bleomycin-Etoposide-Carboplatin (BEC90) combination chemotherapy. Eur Urol. 2004;45(2):187–93.
63. Pont J, Albrect W. Fertility after chemotherapy for testicular germ cell cancer. Fertil Steril. 1997;68:1–5.
64. Ishikawa T, Kamidono S, Fujisawa M. Fertility after high-dose chemotherapy for testicular cancer. Urology. 2004;63:137–40.
65. Sakamoto H, Oohta M, Inoue K, et al. Testicular sperm extraction in patients with persistent azoospermia after chemotherapy for testicular germ cell tumor. Int J Urol. 2007;14(2):167–70.
66. Ferlin A, Raicu F, Gatta V, Zuccarello D, Palka G, Foresta C. Male infertility: role of genetic background. Reprod Biomed Online. 2007;14(6):734–45.
67. Foresta C, Moro E, Ferlin A. Y chromosome microdeletions and alterations of spermatogenesis. Endocr Rev. 2001;22(2):226–39.
68. Vogt PH. Azoospermia factor (AZF) in Yq11: towards a molecular understanding of its function for human male fertility and spermatogenesis. Reprod Biomed Online. 2005;10(1):81–93.

69. Stahl PJ, Masson P, Mielnik A, et al. A decade of experience emphasizes that testing for Y microdeletions is essential in American men with azoospermia and severe oligozoospermia. Fertil Steril. 2010;94(5):1753–6.
70. Bojesen A, Gravholt CH. Klinefelter syndrome in clinical practice. Nat Clin Pract Urol. 2007;4(4):192–204.
71. Ferlin A, Garolla A, Foresta C. Chromosome abnormalities in sperm of individuals with constitutional sex chromosomal abnormalities. Cytogenet Genome Res. 2005;111:310–6.
72. Zhou-Cun A, Yang Y, Zhang SZ, et al. Chromosomal abnormality and Y chromosome microdeletion in Chinese patients with azoospermia or severe oligozoospermia. Yi Chuan Xue Bao. 2006;33(2):111–6.
73. Foresta C, Garolla A, Bartoloni L, Bettella A, Ferlin A. Genetic abnormalities among severely oligospermic men who are candidates for intracytoplasmic sperm injection. J Clin Endocrinol Metab. 2005;90(1):152–6.
74. Schiff JD, Palermo GD, Veeck LL, et al. Intracytoplasmic sperm injection in men with Klinefelter syndrome. J Clin Endocrinol Metab. 2005;90(11):6263–7.
75. O'FlynnO'Brien KL, Varghese AC, Agarwal A. The genetic causes of male factor infertility: a review. Fertil Steril. 2010;93(1):1–12.
76. Shafik A. Contraceptive efficacy of polyester-induced azoospermia in normal men. Contraception. 1992;45(5):439–51.
77. Munkelwitz R, Gilbert BR. Are boxer shorts really better? A critical analysis of the role of underwear type in male subfertility. J Urol. 1998;160(4):1329–33.
78. Bonde JP. Semen quality in welders exposed to radiant heat. Br J Ind Med. 1992;49(1):5–10.
79. Jung A, Schuppe HC. Influence of genital heat stress on semen quality in humans. Andrologia. 2007;39:203–15.
80. Agarwal A, Deepinder F, Sharma RK, et al. Effect of cell phone usage on semen analysis in men attending infertility clinic: an observational study. Fertil Steril. 2008;89:124–8.
81. Agarwal A, Desai NR, Makker K, et al. Effects of radiofrequency electromagnetic waves (RF-EMW) from cellular phones on human ejaculated semen: an in vitro pilot study. Fertil Steril. 2009;92:1318–25.
82. Collodel G, Capitani S, Pammolli A, et al. Semen quality of male idiopathic infertile smokers and nonsmokers: an ultrastructural study. J Androl. 2010;31:108–13.
83. Calogero A, Polosa R, Perdichizzi A, et al. Cigarette smoke extract immobilizes human spermatozoa and induces sperm apoptosis. Reprod Biomed Online. 2009;19:564–71.
84. Gaur DS, Talekar MS, Pathak VP. Alcohol intake and cigarette smoking: impact of two major lifestyle factors on male fertility. Indian J Pathol Microbiol. 2010;53:35–40.
85. Künzle R, Mueller MD, Hänggi W, et al. Semen quality of male smokers and nonsmokers in infertile couples. Fertil Steril. 2003;79:287–91.
86. Brandes SB, Buckman RF, Chelsky MJ, et al. External genitalia gunshot wounds: a ten-year experience with fifty-six cases. J Trauma. 1995;39:266–71.
87. Cass AS, Ferrara L, Wolpert J, et al. Bilateral testicular injury from external trauma. J Urol. 1988;140:1435–6.
88. Kuhlmann J, Bohme H, Tauber R. Bilateral testicular gunshot injuries. Urologe A. 2005;44:918–20.
89. Tomomasa H, Oshio S, Amemiya H, et al. Testicular injury: late results of semen analyses after uniorchiectomy. Arch Androl. 1992;29:59–63.
90. Lin WW, Kim ED, Quesada ET, et al. Unilateral testicular injury from external trauma: evaluation of semen quality and endocrine parameters. J Urol. 1998;159:841–3.
91. Kukadia AN, Ercole CJ, Gleich P, et al. Testicular trauma: potential impact on reproductive function. J Urol. 1996;156:1643–6.
92. Philip J, Selvan D, Desmond A. Mumps orchitis in the non-immune postpubertal male: a resurgent threat to male fertility? BJU Int. 2006;97:138–41.
93. Masarani M, Wazait H, Dinneen M. Mumps orchitis. J R Soc Med. 2006;99:573–5.

94. Osegbe DN. Testicular function after unilateral bacterial epididymo-orchitis. Eur Urol. 1991;19:204–8.
95. Schuppe HC, Meinhardt A, Allam JP, et al. Chronic orchitis: a neglected cause of male infertility? Andrologia. 2008;40:84–91.
96. Zariwala MA, Knowles MR, Omran H. Genetic defects in ciliary structure and function. Annu Rev Physiol. 2007;69:423–50.
97. Leigh MW, Pittman JE, Carson JL, et al. Clinical and genetic aspects of primary ciliary dyskinesia/Kartagener syndrome. Genet Med. 2009;11:473–87.
98. Terada T, Hatakeyama S. Morphological evidence for two types of idiopathic "Sertoli-cell-only" syndrome. Int J Androl. 1991;14(2):117–26.
99. Weller O, Yogev L, Yavetz H, et al. Differentiating between primary and secondary Sertoli-cell-only syndrome by histologic and hormonal parameters. Fertil Steril. 2005;83(6):1856–8.
100. Collins JA, Burrows EA, Yeo J, et al. Frequency and predictive value of antisperm antibodies among infertile couples. Hum Reprod. 1993;8(4):592–8.
101. Menge AC, Medley NE, Mangione CM, et al. The incidence and influence of antisperm antibodies in infertile human couples on sperm-cervical mucus interactions and subsequent fertility. Fertil Steril. 1982;38:439–46.
102. Sinisi AA, Di Finizio B, Pasquali D, et al. Prevalence of antisperm antibodies by SpermMARtest in subjects undergoing a routine sperm analysis for infertility. Int J Androl. 1993;16:311–4.
103. Heidenreich A, Bonfig R, Wilbert DM, et al. Risk factors for antisperm antibodies in infertile men. Am J Reprod Immunol. 1994;31:69–76.
104. Walsh T, Turek P. Immunologic infertility. In: Lipshultz LI, Howards SS, Niederberger CS, editors. Infertility in the male. 4th ed. New York City, NY: Cambridge University; 2009.
105. Meinertz H, Linnet L, Fogh-Andersen P, et al. Antisperm antibodies and fertility after vaso-vasostomy: a follow-up study of 216 men. Fertil Steril. 1990;54:315–21.
106. Hammiche F, Laven J, Boxmeer J, et al. Semen quality decline among men below 60 years of age undergoing IVF or ICSI treatment. J Androl. 2010;32:70–6. Epub ahead of print.
107. Belloc S, Benkhalifa M, Junca AM, et al. Paternal age and sperm DNA decay: discrepancy between chromomycin and aniline blue staining. Reprod Biomed Online. 2009;19:264–9.
108. Escobar MA, Grosfeld JL, Burdick JJ, et al. Surgical considerations in cystic fibrosis: a 32-year evaluation of outcomes. Surgery. 2005;138:560–71.
109. Wilschanski M, Corey M, Durie P, et al. Diversity of reproductive tract abnormalities in men with cystic fibrosis. JAMA. 1996;276:607–8.
110. Lissens W, Mercier B, Tournaye H, et al. Cystic fibrosis and infertility caused by congenital bilateral absence of the vas deferens and related clinical entities. Hum Reprod. 1996;S4:55–78.
111. Donat R, McNeill AS, Fitzpatrick DR, et al. The incidence of cystic fibrosis gene mutations in patients with congenital bilateral absence of the vas deferens in Scotland. Br J Urol. 1997;79:74–7.
112. Sokol RZ. Infertility in men with cystic fibrosis. Curr Opin Pulm Med. 2001;7:421–6.
113. Dörk T, Dworniczak B, Aulehla-Scholz C, et al. Distinct spectrum of CFTR gene mutations in congenital absence of vas deferens. Hum Genet. 1997;100:365–77.
114. Gaillard DA, Carré-Pigeon F, Lallemand A. Normal vas deferens in fetuses with cystic fibrosis. J Urol. 1997;158:1549–52.
115. Radpour R, Gourabi H, Gilani M, et al. Correlation between CFTR gene mutations in Iranian men with congenital absence of the vas deferens and anatomical genital phenotype. J Androl. 2008;29:35–40.
116. Donohue RE, Fauver HE. Unilateral absence of the vas deferens. A useful clinical sign. JAMA. 1989;261:1180–2.
117. Shapiro E, Goldfarb DA, Ritchey ML. The congenital and acquired solitary kidney. Rev Urol. 2003;5:2–8.

118. Handelsman DJ, Conway AJ, Boylan LM, et al. Young's syndrome. Obstructive azoospermia and chronic sinopulmonary infections. N Engl J Med. 1984;310:3–9.
119. Domingo C, Mirapeix RM, Encabo B, et al. Clinical features and ultrastructure of primary ciliary dyskinesia and Young syndrome. Rev Clin Esp. 1997;197:100–3.
120. Goeminne PC, Dupont LJ. The sinusitis-infertility syndrome: Young's saint, old devil. Eur Respir J. 2010;35:698.
121. Arya AK, Beer HL, Benton J, et al. Does Young's syndrome exist? J Laryngol Otol. 2009;123:477–81.
122. Smith JF, Walsh TJ, Turek PJ. Ejaculatory duct obstruction. Urol Clin North Am. 2008;35:221–7.
123. Paick JS, Kim SH, Kim SW. Ejaculatory duct obstruction in infertile men. BJU Int. 2000;85:720–4.
124. Carson CC. Transurethral resection for ejaculatory duct stenosis and oligospermia. Fertil Steril. 1984;41:482–4.
125. Wieder JA, Lynne CM, Ferrell SM, et al. Brown-colored semen in men with spinal cord injury. J Androl. 1999;20:594–600.
126. Labrecque M, Nazerali H, Mondor M, et al. Effectiveness and complications associated with 2 vasectomy occlusion techniques. J Urol. 2002;168:2495–8.
127. Freund MJ, Weidmann JE, Goldstein M, et al. Microrecanalization after vasectomy in man. J Androl. 1989;10:120–32.
128. Cruickshank B, Eidus L, Barkin M. Regeneration of vas deferens after vasectomy. Urology. 1987;30:137–42.
129. Hallan RI, May AR. Vasectomy: how much is enough? Br J Urol. 1988;62:377–9.
130. Adams CE, Wald M. Risks and complications of vasectomy. Urol Clin North Am. 2009;36:331–6.
131. Sokal DC, Labrecque M. Effectiveness of vasectomy techniques. Urol Clin North Am. 2009;36:317–29.
132. Cook LA, Van Vliet H, Lopez LM, et al. Vasectomy occlusion techniques for male sterilization. Cochrane Database Syst Rev. 2007;2:CD003991.
133. Jee SH, Hong YK. One-layer vasovasostomy: microsurgical versus loupe-assisted. Fertil Steril. 2010;94(6):2308–11. Epub 13 Jan 2010.
134. Belker AM, Thomas Jr AJ, Fuchs EF, et al. Results of 1,469 microsurgical vasectomy reversals by the Vasovasostomy Study Group. J Urol. 1991;145:505–11.
135. Nagler HM, Jung H. Factors predicting successful microsurgical vasectomy reversal. Urol Clin North Am. 2009;36:383–90.
136. Magheli A, Rais-Bahrami S, Kempkensteffen C, et al. Impact of obstructive interval and sperm granuloma on patency and pregnancy after vasectomy reversal. Int J Androl. 2010;41(1):52–7.
137. Witt MA, Heron S, Lipshultz LI. The post-vasectomy length of the testicular vasal remnant: a predictor of surgical outcome in microscopic vasectomy reversal. J Urol. 1994;151:892–4.
138. Hollingsworth MR, Sandlow JI, Schrepferman CG, et al. Repeat vasectomy reversal yields high success rates. Fertil Steril. 2007;88:217–9.
139. Talbot HS. The sexual function in paraplegia. J Urol. 1955;73:91–100.
140. Utida C, Truzzi JC, Bruschini H, et al. Male infertility in spinal cord trauma. Int Braz J Urol. 2005;31:375–83.
141. Narayan P, Lange PH, Fraley EE. Ejaculation and fertility after extended retroperitoneal lymph node dissection for testicular cancer. J Urol. 1982;127:685–8.
142. Lange PH, Narayan P, Vogelzang NJ, et al. Return of fertility after treatment for nonseminomatous testicular cancer: changing concepts. J Urol. 1983;129:1131–5.
143. Pizzocaro G, Salvioni R, Zanoni F. Unilateral lymphadenectomy in intraoperative stage I nonseminomatous germinal testis cancer. J Urol. 1985;134:485–9.
144. Richie JP. Clinical stage 1 testicular cancer: the role of modified retroperitoneal lymphadenectomy. J Urol. 1990;144:1160–3.

145. Donohue JP, Foster RS, Rowland RG, et al. Nerve-sparing retroperitoneal lymphadenectomy with preservation of ejaculation. J Urol. 1990;144:287–91.
146. Heidenreich A, Albers P, Hartmann M, et al. Complications of primary nerve sparing retroperitoneal lymph node dissection for clinical stage I nonseminomatous germ cell tumors of the testis: experience of the German Testicular Cancer Study Group. J Urol. 2003; 169:1710–4.
147. Pettus JA, Carver BS, Masterson T, et al. Preservation of ejaculation in patients undergoing nerve-sparing postchemotherapy retroperitoneal lymph node dissection for metastatic testicular cancer. Urology. 2009;73:328–31.
148. Hellstrom WJ, Sikka SC. Effects of acute treatment with tamsulosin versus alfuzosin on ejaculatory function in normal volunteers. J Urol. 2006;176:1529–33.
149. Marks LS, Gittelman MC, Hill LA, et al. Rapid efficacy of the highly selective alpha1A-adrenoceptor antagonist silodosin in men with signs and symptoms of benign prostatic hyperplasia: pooled results of 2 phase 3 studies. J Urol. 2009;181:2634–40.
150. Hisasue S, Furuya R, Itoh N, et al. Ejaculatory disorder caused by α-1 adrenoceptor antagonists is not retrograde ejaculation but a loss of seminal emission. Int J Urol. 2006; 13:1311–6.
151. Kobayashi K, Masumori N, Hisasue S, et al. Inhibition of seminal emission is the main cause of an ejaculation induced by a new highly selective α1A-blocker in normal volunteers. J Sex Med. 2008;5:2185–90.
152. Smith SM, O'Keane V, Murray R. Sexual dysfunction in patients taking conventional antipsychotic medication. Br J Psychiatry. 2002;181:49–55.
153. Loh C, Leckband SG, Meyer JM, et al. Risperidone-induced retrograde ejaculation: case report and review of the literature. Int Clin Psychopharmacol. 2004;19:111–2.
154. Haefliger T, Bonsack C. Atypical antipsychotics and sexual dysfunction: five case-reports associated with risperidone. Encéphale. 2006;32:97–105.
155. Agarwal A, Deepinder F, Cocuzza M, et al. Effect of vaginal lubricants on sperm motility and chromatin integrity: a prospective comparative study. Fertil Steril. 2008;89:375–9.
156. Kutteh WH, Chao CH, Ritter JO, et al. Vaginal lubricants for the infertile couple: effect on sperm activity. Int J Fertil Menopausal Stud. 1996;41:400–4.
157. Anderson L, Lewis SE, McClure N. The effects of coital lubricants on sperm motility in vitro. Hum Reprod. 1998;13:3351–6.
158. Nangia AK, Likosky DS, Wang D. Distribution of male infertility specialists in relation to the male population and assisted reproductive technology centers in the United States. Fertil Steril. 2010;94(2):599–609.

Further Reading

Blau H, Freud E, Mussaffi H, et al. Urogenital abnormalities in male children with cystic fibrosis. Arch Dis Child. 2002;87:135–8.
Chen-Mok M, Bangdiwala SI, Dominik R, et al. Termination of a randomized controlled trial of two vasectomy techniques. Control Clin Trials. 2003;24:78–84.
Fejes I, Závaczki Z, Koloszár S, et al. Hypothesis: safety of using mobile phones on male fertility. Arch Androl. 2007;53:105–6.

Chapter 2
Laboratory Evaluation for Male Infertility

Ryan Mori and Edmund Sabanegh Jr.

The diagnosis and treatment options for male infertility have recently undergone a sea of change as advancements in technology and understanding in the fields of molecular biology, genetics, and laboratory medicine have grown. Further, advancements in assisted reproductive technologies (ART) have rendered previously subfertile and infertile couples with various options for pregnancy. Such changes in the understanding and treatment of fertility and infertility have necessitated a much more detailed assessment of the couple presenting with infertility. At the basis of this assessment is a sophisticated and methodological evaluation of male factor infertility including laboratory assessment of urine, serum, and semen, as well as radiological and genetic studies.

Conception requires a balanced coordination between the endocrinologic and reproductive systems of both the male and the female partners. Studies in normal individuals demonstrate that within 1 year of unprotected intercourse, 60–75% of couples will achieve conception, whereas 90% will achieve conception after 1 year [1]. Based on such studies, the currently accepted definition of infertility by the American Society for Reproductive Medicine (ASRM) is the absence of conception after 12 months of regular, unprotected intercourse [2].

The workup and diagnosis of infertility is unique in medicine in that it involves multiple organ systems of two individuals. Pathology is often difficult to isolate given this complexity. Isolated male factor has been shown to be causative in 20% of infertility cases and is a contributing factor in conjunction with female factor

R. Mori, MD, MS (✉)
Cleveland Clinic Lerner College of Medicine and Glickman Urological and Kidney Institute, Cleveland Clinic Foundation, Cleveland, OH USA

E. Sabanegh Jr., MD
Department of Urology, Glickman Urological and Kidney Institute, Center for Reproductive Medicine, Cleveland Clinic, 9500 Euclid Avenue/Q10-1, Cleveland, OH 44195, USA
e-mail: sabanee@ccf.org

S.J. Parekattil and A. Agarwal (eds.), *Antioxidants in Male Infertility: A Guide for Clinicians and Researchers*, © Springer Science+Business Media New York 2013

pathology in an additional 30% of cases [3]. These estimates have changed little over time despite great diagnostic advancements [4, 5].

A workup of couples presenting for evaluation of failure to conceive after 12 months of unprotected intercourse should consist of concurrent male and female partner evaluation. Further, as recommended by the practice committees of both the American Urological Association (AUA) and the ASRM, workup for infertility should be started earlier than 12 months in the setting of (1) male risk factors for infertility, (2) advanced maternal age (>35y), or (3) there is concern about male factor infertility [2]. The initial workup of the male partner should be basic, methodological, and cost-effective. Isolated pathology should be isolated and treated when possible given the high cost of ART. The initial evaluation of the male may suggest the need to proceed with more costly advanced testing. Many treatments of male factor infertility and subfertility allow pregnancy using the patient's own sperm with or without ART. Options for uncorrectable causes of male factor infertility include donor sperm insemination in a healthy female partner as well as adoption.

Clinical and Laboratory Evaluation of Male Factor Infertility

Initial Evaluation of Male Factor Infertility

The initial evaluation of a male presenting with infertility mandates a thorough general history, physical exam, and review of systems as well as a focused and targeted reproductive history and physical exam. A plethora of general medical conditions may contribute to infertility or altered sexual function and may be undiagnosed prior to urological evaluation (Table 2.1). Up to 1.3% of men undergoing evaluation for infertility are diagnosed with a significant and potentially life-threatening general medical condition [6]. Basic laboratory testing is a critical component of the initial evaluation of male factor and includes urinalysis, basic semen analysis, and a routine serum hormone analysis. Data from the initial evaluation will guide more advanced testing in infertility and should proceed in a methodological and cost-effective fashion.

History and Review of Systems

A complete medical history is important to obtain as a variety of medical conditions can contribute to abnormal fertility and sexual function in the male, as detailed in Table 2.1. Recent acute systemic illness such as viremia or fever should be noted. The human spermatogenesis cycle has a length of 64 days with an additional 5–10 days needed for epididymal sperm transit [7–9]. Thus, any insult to spermatogenesis such as a febrile illness may not be manifested for 2–3 months in semen analysis. In addition, medical conditions such as diabetes mellitus, hypertension, diseases of the thyroid, certain neoplasms, and diseases of the central and peripheral nervous systems may have substantial impact on fertility, erectile or ejaculatory function.

Table 2.1 Pertinent components of the history for male infertility evaluation

Past medical history
- Infertility
  Previous conceptions
  Duration
  Previous evaluations/treatments
  Female partner fertility status: previous conceptions/outcomes, evaluation, previous treatments
- Sexual
  Erectile/ejaculatory function
  Lubrications
  Intercourse timing/knowledge
- Childhood
  Infectious: mumps orchitis, sexually transmitted infections/urethritis
  Trauma: groin/testicular trauma, torsion, prior inguinal surgery
  Onset of puberty
- Adult
  General/systemic: obesity, hypertension
  Metabolic/endocrinologic: DM, metabolic syndrome, thyroid function
  Infectious: sexually transmitted infections/urethritis, urinary tract infections, epididymo-
    orchitis/prostatitis
  Neoplasms: treatments (radiation, chemotherapy)
  Neurological: spinal cord, MS
  Trauma: testicular, CNS/PNS

Past surgical history
- Inguinal: orchidopexy, herniorrhaphy
- Pelvic/retroperitoneal: prostate, bladder/bladder neck, RPLND
- Scrotal: vasectomy, hydrocele

Social history
- Environmental/occupational exposures
- Tobacco use
- Alcohol use
- Recreational drugs: marijuana, cocaine, anabolic steroids

Family history
- Chromosomal abnormalities: Klinefelter's syndrome
- Infertility
- Cystic fibrosis

Medications
- Ejaculatory dysfunction: antihypertensives, alpha-blockers
- Erectile dysfunction: antidepressants, psychotropics
- Hypogonadism: anabolic steroids
- Spermatogenesis: antibiotics

A reproductive history should focus on identification of primary versus secondary infertility, details of prior conceptions of both partners, previous fertility treatments, and evaluation of libido, erectile function, and ejaculatory function. Primary infertility is by definition the absence of previous conception, whereas secondary infertility represents conception in the past with the current or previous partner.

A sexual history should be addressed and include timing and frequency of coitus. As sperm survive within cervical mucus for 2–5 days [10], optimal timing of intercourse is at least every 48 h during the periovulatory period [11]. Commercially available ovulation prediction kits aid the couple in determining accurate time of ovulation. Attention should also be paid to types of lubricants used as many commercially available sexual lubricants have been shown to adversely affect sperm quality [12, 13].

Attention should be paid to the past medical history of the patient as well as a number of childhood diseases and conditions which may adversely affect future fertility including but not limited to mumps orchitis, cryptorchidism, testicular torsion or trauma, and previous inguinal surgery. Studies suggest that paternity rates for unilateral cryptorchidism are only slightly decreased, but significantly reduced in cases of bilateral cryptorchidism [14]. Controversy exists regarding future sperm quality and paternity after orchidopexy. The timing of the onset of puberty should be assessed as either delayed or precocious puberty may be indicative of underlying endocrinologic abnormalities.

A thorough review of systems and family medical history can identify genetic diseases which may affect fertility including Klinefelter's syndrome, Kallmann syndrome, and cystic fibrosis. The existence of male siblings with infertility may suggest Y chromosome microdeletions or other chromosomal abnormalities, although most genetic diseases present as de novo rather than inherited mutations. Cystic fibrosis (CF) is associated with congenital absence of the vas deferens bilaterally (CBAVD). Genetic causes of infertility can be transmissible, especially with the advent of ART. With the growing use of ART, we can expect the incidence of genetically derived infertility to increase in the future.

Past surgical history should focus on surgery involving the male genitourinary tract, the retroperitoneum, or the inguinal region as such surgeries can be associated with ejaculatory dysfunction or obstruction or erectile dysfunction. Previous exposure to ionizing radiation should be noted as this has been shown to affect sperm quality. Social history should identify any hazardous occupational exposures as well as ingestion of potentially gonadotoxic substances including ETOH, tobacco, marijuana, and other recreational drugs. Use of anabolic steroids or other performance-enhancing drugs should be assessed in appropriate patient populations. A review of medications is valuable and should include both prescribed substances as well as over-the-counter and herbal substances. Specific attention should be given to medications that can lead to impaired ejaculation (alpha-blockers, antihypertensives) or sexual dysfunction (antidepressants, antipsychotic agents).

Physical Examination

The physical examination consists of a general examination as well as a detailed genital examination. The general overall appearance and degree of virilization can offer clues about possibly androgen deficiency. Assessment of body habitus, hair growth patterns, and gynecomastia should be noted and may suggest underlying endocrinological or hormonal abnormalities. A man with a history of primary infertility presenting with disproportionately long extremities and low volume testes is highly suggestive of Klinefelter's syndrome.

The genital exam includes a thorough evaluation of the phallus and testes as well as the paratesticular structures. The phallus should be evaluated for potential causes of altered deposition of ejaculate including penile curvature, hypospadias, or meatal stenosis. The testes should be examined in both the supine and standing positions. The exam is often facilitated by warming of the scrotum via either room temperature or a scrotal warming pack to prevent retraction of the testes from the cremasteric reflex. The testes should be palpated for masses, and attention should be paid to the volume of the testis and any discrepancies in symmetry. Normal adult testis volume should be at least 20 cm^3, or 4 × 3 cm [15], and an orchidometer or calipers can assist in measurement. Enlargement or tenderness of the epididymides may suggest obstruction or inflammation. The spermatic cord should be evaluated with the patient in the upright position to aid in identification of abnormally dilated spermatic veins, which by definition is a varicocele. Classically, a prominent varicocele is described as having a "bag of worms" feel on physical exam. Examination during a Valsalva maneuver is required to correctly grade the varicocele if present. A grade I varicocele is only detectable during the Valsalva maneuver. Grade II varicoceles are palpable without Valsalva maneuver, and grade III varicoceles are visible through the scrotal skin. Varicoceles are common findings, present in up to 15% of normal males. In men presenting for evaluation of infertility, 19–41% have been shown to have varicoceles. Ninety percent of unilateral varicoceles are left sided, thought to be secondary to the more acute insertion of the left gonadal vein into the renal vein. An isolated moderate to severe unilateral right varicocele raises suspicion of a retroperitoneal process obstructing the insertion of the gonadal vein more proximally such as a retroperitoneal mass or large renal mass with a vein thrombus.

During examination of the spermatic cord, the vas deferens should be palpated. Absence of the vas deferens raises suspicion of genetic causes of infertility, such as mutation in cystic fibrosis transmembrane regulator gene (CFTR). The prostate should be palpated for midline cysts, or Mullerian duct cysts, which can be associated with ejaculatory duct obstruction. The seminal vesicles are not normally palpable, but may be in the setting of obstruction.

Laboratory Evaluation of Male Factor Infertility

Basic Testing

The initial assessment of a man presenting for an evaluation of male factor infertility should include a basic laboratory assessment of the semen. Further testing such as serum endocrine assays or genetic tests is suggested and guided by the results of the physical and laboratory evaluations.

Table 2.2 Comparison of 1999 and 2010 WHO normal reference values for semen parameters

Semen parameter	Normal values: 1999 WHO	2010 WHO lower reference limit (5th centile + 95% CI)
Semen volume (mL)	2–6	1.5 (1.4–1.7)
Total motility PR + NP (%)	50+	40 (38–42)
Progressive motility PR (%)	25+	32 (31–34)
Vitality (% live spermatozoa)	50+	58 (55–63)
Sperm number (10^6 sperm/ejaculate)	>40	39 (33–46)
Sperm concentration (10^6 sperm/mL)	20	15 (12–16)
Morphology (% normal)	>30	4 (3.0–4.0)

Data from World Health Organization. WHO Laboratory Manual for the Examination of Human Semen and Sperm-Cervical Mucus Interaction, 1999; World Health Organization, Department of Reproductive Health and Research. WHO Laboratory Manual for the Examination and Processing of Human Semen, 5th edn. 2010; Cooper TG, Noonan E, von Eckardstein S, et al. World Health Organization reference values for human semen characteristics. Hum Reprod Update. 2010; 16(3):231–45

Semen Analysis. A semen analysis is a critical component of the initial workup of male infertility. It can offer great insight into the etiology of infertility or subfertility; however, it serves as a surrogate rather than a true measure of fertility. An abnormal semen analysis can yield a viable pregnancy, and normal semen parameters can be associated with failure to conceive. As few as 15% of men presenting with infertility have currently recognizable abnormalities on semen analysis [16]. Table 2.2 reports a distribution of abnormalities in semen analyses in men presenting for infertility evaluation, and Table 2.3 lists the currently accepted nomenclature of diagnoses set forth by the World Health Organization (WHO). Beyond just the appearance of semen and spermatozoa microscopically, it is often necessary to obtain functional studies of sperm to assess the true fertilizing potential. In addition, guided by the basic semen analysis, more advanced testing may be needed and will be explored in greater depth below.

Evaluation of Basic Semen Analyses

Collection. Prior to analysis, semen must be properly collected into a sterile container. Sperm count and semen volume are variable from day to day; thus, it is essential to evaluate at least 2 samples to characterize baseline data for a patient [17]. Semen parameters and ejaculate volume can also vary widely based on the frequency of ejaculation, and it is currently recommended that a period of 2–5 days of ejaculatory abstinence precede sample collection. This period of abstinence should remain a constant with further semen samples to maintain comparability.

Optimally, the sample should be collected via self-stimulation in a private room near the laboratory to reduce the time between collection and analysis and to ensure constant temperature of the specimen. Lubricants should be avoided if possible as they may lead to altered sperm motility. The semen sample should be complete, and the man should be cautioned to collect all fractions of the ejaculate, as the first

Table 2.3 WHO nomenclature related to semen quality

Aspermia	No semen
Asthenospermia	<32% Progressively motile spermatozoa
Asthenoteratospermia	Percentages of both progressively motile and morphologically normal spermatozoa below the reference limits
Azoospermia	No spermatozoa present in the ejaculate
Cryptozoospermia	Spermatozoa not found in fresh preparations but found in centrifuged pellet
Hematospermia	Erythrocytes in ejaculate
Leukospermia	Presence of leukocytes in ejaculate > threshold (1 mil/cm^3)
Necrospermia	Low percentage of live and high percentage of immotile spermatozoa in ejaculate
Normozoospermia	Within normal limits for spermatozoa number and motility
Oligoasthenospermia	Total number of spermatozoa and percentage of progressively motile spermatozoa below lower reference limits
Oligoasthenoteratospermia	Total number of, percentage of progressively motile, and percentage of morphologically normal spermatozoa below the lower reference limits
Oligoteratospermia	Total number of and percentage of progressively motile spermatozoa below the lower reference limits
Oligospermia	Total number of spermatozoa below the lower reference limit
Teratospermia	Percentage of morphologically normal spermatozoa below the reference limit

Adapted from Appendix 1 Reference values and semen nomenclature. WHO Laboratory manual for the Examination and Processing of Human Semen, 5th edn. 2010, with permission

fraction contains sperm-rich prostatic fluids [18]. Coitus interruptus should be avoided as this first fraction is often loss. Semen collection devices that are free of spermicidal lubricants are less than ideal, but may be necessary if the patient has barriers to conventional collection methods. Semen should be analyzed within 1 h of collection to prevent alteration in semen parameters secondary to delayed analysis. Patients unable to provide a sample on location should be instructed to bring the sample to the lab at a constant temperature near body temperature for analysis within 1 h.

Some patients will be unable to provide a semen sample due to erectile or ejaculatory dysfunction and may require oral or intracavernosal injection therapy to produce a specimen. Discussion of such techniques is beyond the scope of this chapter.

Macroscopic Assessment. Semen analysis begins with a macroscopic assessment after liquefaction occurs. The time to liquefaction should be noted and considered abnormal if greater than 60 min. The five macroscopic variables are semen volume, viscosity, color, coagulation, and pH (Table 2.4).

The semen volume is best measured by weight, but can also be measured directly. The volume of the ejaculate is supplied mainly by the seminal vesicles and prostate gland, with some contribution from the bulbourethral glands and the epididymides. The viscosity can be measured by drawing the sample into a wide-bore 1.5-mm pipette and letting the semen drop. A thread length of greater than 2 cm is abnormally viscous. While viscosity is a consistently measured parameter, the

Table 2.4 Components of the macroscopic semen assessment

Macroscopic variable	Normal quality
Liquefaction	Homogenous, <60 min
Appearance	Homogenous, gray opalescent
Viscosity	Thread < 2 cm
Volume	>1.5 mL
pH	>7.2

Table 2.5 Distribution of semen analysis parameters in men presenting for initial evaluation of infertility

Semen parameter	Incidence (%)
Any abnormality	37
Motility	26
Asthenospermia	24
Oligospermia	8
Agglutination	2
Volume	2
Morphology	1
Azoospermia	8
Normal semen analysis	55

From Lipshultz L. Subfertility. In: Kaufman JJ, editor. Current urologic therapy. Philadelphia: WB Saunders. 1980, with permission of Elsevier

significance of an abnormal assessment is controversial with many experts discounting the importance of this finding. A normal liquefied semen sample is described as homogenous and gray opalescent in color. Seminal pH results from the balance of acidic prostatic secretion and alkaline seminal vesicular secretions. This principle can be clinically valuable in the setting of low semen volume and abnormal pH, as the location of obstruction can be logically deduced to be at the level of the ejaculatory duct.

Microscopic Assessment. A wet prep of the semen next examined under light microscopic magnification. A basic microscopic semen analysis assesses agglutination/aggregation, sperm count, motility, morphology, and presence of non-sperm cells. The World Health Organization has set forth "normal" reference ranges for each of the above semen parameters. There has been some lack of consensus as to the utility and applicability of previously accepted lower limits of normal. The lower reference values have been recently updated based on analysis of semen samples of men with proven fertility and time to pregnancy less than 12 months [19]. Distributions of semen parameters across these men were obtained using standardized WHO laboratory criteria, and the lower reference limit, taken as the 5th centile, is presented in comparison with previous lower limits from the 1999 WHO criteria [20] in Table 2.5.

- Sperm aggregation and agglutination: Semen is first analyzed as a wet prep specimen. Agglutination or clumping of spermatozoa with either sperm or non-sperm semen elements is noted as well as site of binding (head to head, tail to tail, or mixed fashion). Though some degree of sperm agglutination is considered normal, more considerable amounts could represent the presence of antisperm antibodies (ASA) [21]. Aggregation refers to the clumping together of nonmotile spermatozoa. The presence of agglutination may also be suggestive of ASA. Sperm agglutination with non-sperm semen elements may occur in the presence of infection. Thus, the presence of agglutination on microscopic assessment should trigger further testing with seminal white blood cell assessment and antisperm antibody measurement.

- Motility: The degree of progressive sperm motility is related to pregnancy rates [22]. Sperm are classified as either being motile or immotile. Further, motile sperm are assessed for their degree of progressive motility. Movement is considered progressively motile (PR) if the spermatozoa is moving actively either linearly or in a large circle. Nonprogressive motility (NP) refers to motion with absence of progression such as movement in small circles. Total motility (PR + NP) and progressive motility (PR) are reported in the basic semen analysis as percentages of total sperm. Complete absence of motility may be suggestive of ultrastructural cilia abnormalities such as Kallmann syndrome as well as necrospermia. Necrospermia is assessed via sperm vitality testing as detailed below.

- Sperm vitality: Sperm vitality is measured as a function of the membrane integrity of sperm cells and is expressed as a percentage of total sperm. This measurement is especially important when a large number of immotile sperm are present in order to rule out necrospermia [16]. The 2 methods commonly employed to assess the integrity of the cell membrane are the dye exclusion test and hypotonic swelling. The dye exclusion test is based on the principle that an intact membrane will not take in dye. In the latter test, a hypotonic solution is utilized, and spermatozoa with intact membrane swell within 5 min. This test is particularly useful if viable sperm are being identified for use in ICSI. Recently published lower reference limit for sperm vitality is 58% which is in agreement with previous assessments [19].

- Sperm count and concentration: Of paramount importance in the evaluation of male factor infertility is the presence of sperm in the ejaculate. Azoospermia, or the absence of sperm in the ejaculate, may occur from ejaculatory dysfunction, obstruction of the reproductive tract, or as a result of abnormal sperm production. Both the number of sperm per ejaculate and the sperm concentration have been correlated with both time to pregnancy and pregnancy rates [23]. Sperm concentration is directly measured and expressed in terms of millions per milliliter, whereas total sperm number is a calculated value based on semen volume and concentration. The total number of spermatozoa in the ejaculate has been correlated with testis volume; however, the concentration is heavily influenced by the volume of the glandular secretions. The normal sperm concentration is commonly accepted as > 20 million sperm per mL semen based on the 1999 WHO cutoff [20]. However, according to this threshold, 20% of 18-year-old males would be classified as oligospermic [24]. As demonstrated in Table 2.5, more recent data by the WHO sets the lower reference limit of sperm concentration to 15 million/mL in a population of fertile men [19]. Oligospermia is still commonly accepted by definition as a sperm concentration of less than 20 million sperm per mL. For an exhaustive list of current WHO infertility nomenclature and definition, refer to Table 2.3.

- Non-sperm cells: The number of non-sperm cells present in a semen sample should be estimated and may have implications regarding underlying pathology. The most commonly encountered non-sperm cells in semen are epithelial cells, immature germ cells, and leukocytes [25]. The latter two cell types are referred to collectively as round cells due to their appearance microscopically and are not easily differentiated by microscopy alone. If the estimated round cell concentration exceeds 1×10^6/mL, then further testing should be done to assess the nature of the cell types. This is most reliably done by using immunohistochemistry to stain for specific leukocyte markers. However, the Endtz test allows a cost-effective method of identifying leukocytes by measuring peroxidase enzyme activity visualized with orthotoluidine dye [26]. The presence of leukocytes in semen may have detrimental effects on semen quality including reductions in sperm motility and DNA integrity [27, 28] as well as elevations in seminal reactive oxygen species [29].

- Sperm morphology: Sperm cells by nature have varying morphologies during maturation. Assessment is operator dependent and thus more subjective than other components of the basic semen analysis. Studies of sperm taken from post-coital cervical mucus or zona pellucida offer insight about the morphology of sperm with fertilizing potential [30–32]. Multiple classification schemata exist, but the currently most widely used are the WHO criteria and Kruger's strict criteria. Kruger and colleagues demonstrated that in men with sperm concentrations greater than 20 million sperm per mL and greater than 30% motility, fertilization rates were significantly higher for those men with greater than 14% normal sperm by the rigid criteria [13]. By WHO criteria, teratospermia represents less than 15% of sperm with normal morphology [20]. There remains substantial controversy regarding the predictive implications of abnormal morphology on assisted reproductive outcomes with both intrauterine insemination and intracytoplasmic sperm injection.

Normal spermatozoa consist of a head, midpiece, and a tailpiece (Fig. 2.1). A spermatozoa must have both a normal head and tail to be considered morphologically normal. The head should be a smooth ovoid shape with a well-defined acrosomal region (more lightly stained region) comprising about 40–70% of the head volume and containing no large vacuoles. The head should taper into a midpiece aligned along the same axis of the head. The tail should be of uniform caliber and approximately 10 times the length of the head. Looping of the tail is acceptable, but any sharp abnormalities are abnormal. Excess residual cytoplasm is also a morphologic abnormality. Common abnormalities of spermatozoa head, midpiece, and tail are demonstrated in Fig. 2.1.

Abnormal sperm morphology is commonly seen with defective spermatogenesis or with certain epididymal pathologies. They generally have less fertilizing potential and have been linked with increased DNA fragmentation [33] and chromosomal abnormalities [34].

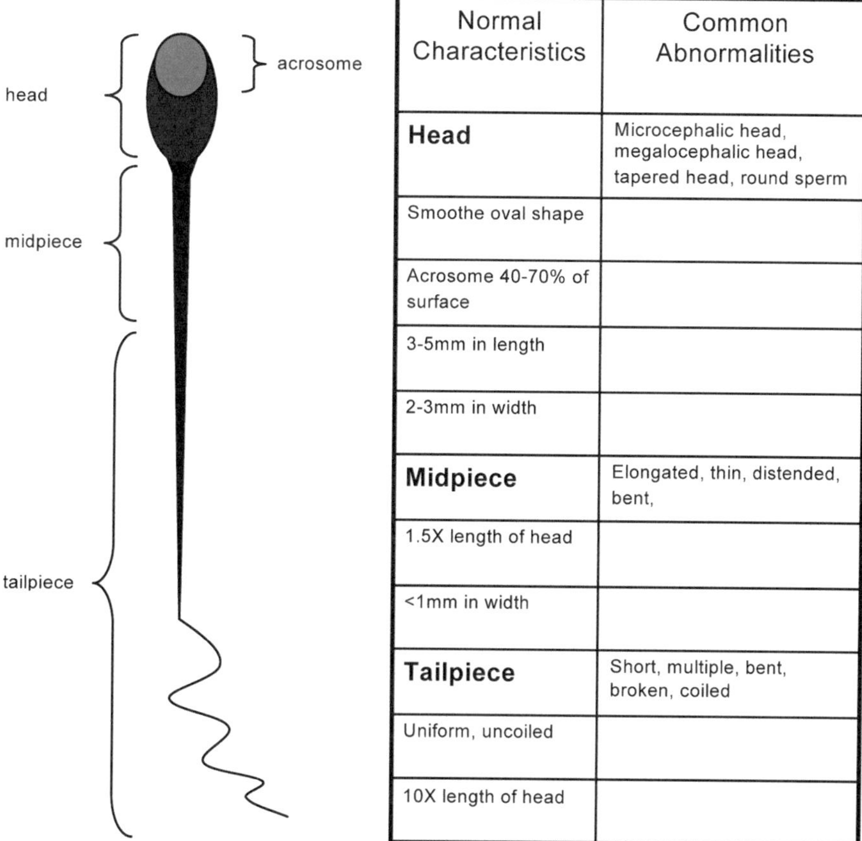

	Normal Characteristics	Common Abnormalities
Head		Microcephalic head, megalocephalic head, tapered head, round sperm
	Smoothe oval shape	
	Acrosome 40-70% of surface	
	3-5mm in length	
	2-3mm in width	
Midpiece		Elongated, thin, distended, bent,
	1.5X length of head	
	<1mm in width	
Tailpiece		Short, multiple, bent, broken, coiled
	Uniform, uncoiled	
	10X length of head	

Fig. 2.1 Sperm morphology (Kruger Strict Criteria)

All intact spermatozoa per area surveyed should be assessed, and the percentage of normal sperm should be recorded. Recently updated lower reference limits for normal forms in fertile men is 4% by strict criteria [19, 21], which is considerably lower than the previously accepted reference range. Some spermatozoa may have multiple defects; thus, percentages of specific defects should be based on total sperm count.

Computer-Assisted Semen Analysis (CASA). With advances in technology, it is now feasible to measure sperm motility, kinematics, and concentration using computer-aided sperm analysis (CASA). The potential advantages over more traditional methods are its precision and ability to quantify the kinematic properties of the spermatozoa. At present, this technology requires costly equipment and training and is more commonly a tool used in research settings rather than basic pathology laboratories.

Functional Sperm Testing

The fertilizing potential of a sperm cell cannot always be inferred from a basic semen analysis. Functional sperm tests assess various processes in the normal fertilization cycle to include sperm transit, penetration of the zona pellucida of the oocyte, and, ultimately, fertilization. Sperm-mucous interaction can be assessed by a cervical mucus migration assay where the rate of sperm transit through mucous is measured. The sperm penetration assay (SPA) measures the ability of a human sperm to penetrate a specially prepared hamster egg that has been stripped of the outer zona pellucida, allowing cross-species fertilization. This yields useful information about a sperm's ability to successfully undergo capacitation, acrosome reaction, membrane fusion with oocytes, and chromatin decondensation. A good result on SPA suggests proceeding with a trial of spontaneous conception or intrauterine insemination (IUI), whereas a poor SPA result might suggest the need for IVF with ICSI.

The acrosome reaction test measures the ability of the sperm cell to mount an effective acrosome reaction and may be useful in the setting of profound teratospermia with head predominant abnormalities where IVF is not successful. Currently, this test may be recommended in the setting of abnormal sperm head morphology or failure to fertilize oocytes in conventional IVF cycles. However, this test has been difficult to standardize, limiting its role at the present time.

Additional/Advanced Semen Testing

Antisperm Antibody Testing. Under normal anatomical circumstances, the seminiferous tubules are immunologically protected from the humoral environment as the tight junctions between the Sertoli cells form the blood-testis barrier. However, following a breech of this barrier such as after orchitis, scrotal trauma, or surgery, the immune system may be exposed to these "foreign" sperm antigens, and antisperm antibodies (ASA) may develop. The presence of sperm agglutination, especially head to head, should suggest the possibility of ASA. In addition, low sperm motility in the setting of previous injury or surgery (i.e., vasectomy), leukocytospermia, or otherwise unexplained infertility should also lower the clinician's threshold for evaluating for ASA.

Antisperm antibodies may be found in the serum and in the seminal plasma and bound to the sperm themselves. They can cause agglutination and immotility or can be spermatotoxic depending on the type of antibody. In previous reports, up to 10% of infertile men present with ASA versus only 2% of fertile men [35]. However, men can have normal semen parameters with presence of ASA as well [36]. The direct ASA test detects sperm-bound immunoglobulins, while indirect testing detects the biological activity of circulating ASA. Direct assays of sperm-bound immunoglobulins are preferred since most agree that sperm-bound antibodies are the most clinically relevant. Serum ASA testing, once widely used, has been largely discarded due to the much greater sensitivity of semen testing.

Sperm DNA Damage. Sperm DNA damage has been shown to have a positive correlation with abnormal semen parameters. [37]. Various factors and agents have been associated with sperm DNA damage including testicular cancers, tobacco use, and certain chemotherapeutic agents [27]. The etiology of sperm DNA damage at this time is thought to involve abnormal chromatin packing, elevated reactive oxygen species [27], and apoptosis [38]. There are several tests currently available to assess sperm DNA integrity by assessing strand breaks in situ [39]. The single cell gel electrophoresis assay, or comet assay, uses gel electrophoresis to assess DNA fragmentation. With the terminal deoxynucleotidyl transferase-mediated deoxyuridine triphosphate nick-end labeling (TUNEL) assay, a fluorescent-labeled nucleotide is transferred to the hydroxyl end of a broken DNA strand, and flow cytometry is used to assess DNA nicks. The sperm chromatin structure assay (SCSA) uses low pH to denature sperm DNA at the site of DNA breaks and is followed by acridine orange staining and flow cytometry to measure percentage of denatured DNA. Meta-analyses have shown that couples with sperm DNA fragmentation indices (DNI) less than 30% [40, 41] are twice as likely to achieve pregnancy using IVF. Although tests of DNA integrity are not part of the basic semen analysis, they can be useful especially in the setting of unexplained infertility but normal bulk semen parameters.

ROS Testing

Reactive oxygen species (ROS), also known as free radicals, are by-products of normal intercellular and intracellular metabolism and have been implicated in the etiology of multiple diseases across multiple organ systems. They are a necessary result of oxygen metabolism, which takes place in all healthy tissues, and are formed by the addition of unpaired electrons to the oxygen molecule through the process of reduction. The addition of an electron to molecular O_2 produces a superoxide anion radical (O_2-) that is reactive. Secondary ROS include hydroxyl radical (OH), peroxyl radical (ROO), and hydrogen peroxide (H_2O_2). ROS are critical to normal cell physiology, but excessive levels are detrimental to cell survival and function. In excess, they induce cellular damage by the oxidation of cellular and cell membrane components and cause DNA damage by modification of bases, deletions, frameshifts, and chromosomal relocations.

Oxidative stress by definition refers to the imbalance between reactive oxygen species and their scavengers, known generally as antioxidants. Antioxidants are the crux of the host defense against ROS and are formed via both enzymatic and non-enzymatic pathways. The primary enzymatic antioxidants include superoxide dismutases, catalase, and glutathione peroxidase. The superoxide dismutases convert superoxide into O_2 and H_2O_2. Catalase and glutathione peroxidase further degrade H_2O_2 into water and O_2. Glutathione is the main nonenzymatic antioxidant, and its cysteine subunit contains a sulfhydryl group which directly scavenges free radicals. Vitamins E and C are also important nonenzymatic scavengers of free radicals.

Reactive oxygen species have been shown to be critical throughout normal spermatogenesis and conception, specifically during sperm capacitation [42] and sperm-oocyte fusion [43]. Seminal fluid contains superoxide dismutase, catalase, glutathione peroxidase, and glutathione reductase. High levels of ROS are correlated with poor sperm quality and function. Spermatozoa which have been incubated with ROS overnight have increased lipid peroxidation. Further, addition of free radical scavengers like alpha tocopherol has been shown to revive sperm motility both in vitro [11] and in vivo.

Sperm are exposed to free radicals both by intrinsic production, extrinsic production in the semen, and via external and environmental sources including cigarette smoking, exposure to certain industrial compounds, and increased intrascrotal temperatures.

In normal semen, there is a low level of oxidative stress, as the free radicals necessary for certain cell signaling processes are kept in check by the antioxidants in order to avoid cellular damage. However, this balance is lost in conditions where there is either increased production of free radicals or decreased buffering capacity by available antioxidants. Leukocytes and spermatozoa are both significant sources of free radicals in the semen. Normal semen contains some white blood cells, predominantly neutrophils. Neutrophils exert their normal cytotoxic function partly by releasing high concentrations of ROS. Although the relationship is incompletely defined, leukospermia, defined as peroxidase positive leukocytes at a concentration greater than $1\times10\times6$ per mL by the WHO [21], has been associated with altered semen parameters including decreased sperm concentration, motility, and morphology [4]. Although there is a correlation between seminal leukocytes and infertility [10], some studies have failed to show an alteration of sperm parameters in the presence of leukospermia [5]. However, several studies have linked proinflammatory cytokines including IL-6, IL-8, and TNF-alpha to altered sperm function [38, 44, 45].

In addition to seminal leukocytes, spermatozoa themselves are source of ROS. As sperm mature, they extrude cytoplasm rich in reducing molecules. Abnormalities in sperm maturation lead to retention of cytoplasm and increased levels of ROS in semen. The effects of the ROS on over all sperm function may correlate with the site of ROS production, intrinsic or extrinsic to the sperm. Some authors suggest that higher levels of extrinsic ROS, such as that produced by leukospermia, have greater effects on sperm count, motility, and morphology, whereas increased intrinsic ROS production is associated with higher levels of DNA fragmentation [37].

Testing for reactive oxygen species is not a part of the standard initial evaluation of male factor infertility. However, there is increasing research being conducted in this area, and despite the lack of randomized control trials, it is becoming evident that men presenting with infertility with increased oxidative stress in the semen may benefit from antioxidant therapy [46, 47]. Additionally, infertile men with varicoceles have been shown to have elevated seminal ROS [48] with levels that correlate with varicocele grade [49], and several studies have shown that surgical varicocelectomy is correlated with decreased seminal oxidative stress, increased seminal antioxidants, and improved sperm quality [20, 50, 51].

Various direct and indirect testing modalities exist to determine the level of oxidative stress in the semen. The most commonly employed method of ROS testing is a chemiluminescence probe assay, which is used to quantify redox activities of spermatozoa [52]. Using this technique, a luminol probe (5-amino-2,3-dihydro-1,4-phthalazinedione), used to measure both intracellular and extracellular ROS, or a lucigen probe measuring superoxide radicals released extracellularly is employed. Direct assays of oxidative stress are available, but cost and practicality issues have rendered these assays tools of research with limited clinical application at this time.

Hormonal Assessment

In addition to a basic semen analysis, many patients may warrant a serum hormonal analysis at time of presentation. The goal of such an analysis is to evaluate the hypothalamic-pituitary-gonadal axis and to rule out an underlying endocrinopathy or primary testicular failure. Controversy exists as to the necessity of a hormonal evaluation in all patients presenting with infertility. However, there is a consensus that basic hormonal testing including serum follicle-stimulating hormone (FSH) and early morning serum total testosterone should be done in the setting of (1) abnormally low sperm count (<10 million/cm^3), (2) impaired sexual function, and (3) clinical findings suggestive of an endocrine abnormality such as reduced testicular volume or gynecomastia [1, 53].

The pituitary and gonadal hormones are released in a pulsatile fashion, and this rhythm is orchestrated by the hypothalamus, which receives diffuse input from multiple cortical and subcortical brain regions. The hypothalamus communicates to the anterior pituitary both via neuronal input as well as via the portal vascular system which allows direct delivery of hypothalamic hormones in high concentration to the anterior pituitary. The most important of these hypothalamic hormones is luteinizing hormone-releasing hormone (LHRH) or gonadotropin-releasing hormone (GNRH) which stimulates the secretion of luteinizing hormone (LH) and FSH. GNRH secretion is modulated by many factors and is under direct negative feedback control by circulating gonadal hormones including testosterone and inhibin.

LH, FSH, and prolactin are the primary hormones released from the anterior pituitary into the systemic circulation. LH stimulates the Leydig cells in the testes to produce testosterone, while FSH acts on the Sertoli cells of the testes and promotes development and growth of the seminiferous.

The testes are composed primarily of Leydig cells, Sertoli cells, and seminiferous tubules. The bulk of the testicular volume is comprised of seminiferous tubules and germinal elements; thus, reduced testicular size suggests impaired spermatogenesis [54]. Within the testes, Leydig cells are responsible for androgen synthesis. Testosterone, the primary circulating male androgen, is secreted in a pulsatile fashion with a regular circadian cycle peaking in the early morning. Only 2% of the serum testosterone is free in the systemic circulation with the remainder bound in roughly equal proportions to sex hormone-binding globulin (SHBG) and albumin.

Alterations in serum SHBG will increase free testosterone in the serum. SHBG levels are influenced by a number of conditions including liver and thyroid disease, medications, advanced age, and obesity. Peripherally, testosterone is reduced to dihydrotestosterone (DHT) by 5 alpha-reductase and is also converted to estradiol by aromatases.

Sertoli cells line the seminiferous tubules and are linked by tight junctions, forming the blood–testis barrier which provides an immunologically naïve environment for spermatogenesis. The Sertoli cells are under the control of FSH and produce multiple paracrine factors important in stimulating and supporting spermatogenesis. Inhibin B is released from Sertoli cells in response to FSH stimulation and is important as regulator of the HGP axis via negative feedback at the pituitary and hypothalamus. The Sertoli cells also express androgen-binding protein in response to FSH stimulation and allow for very high intraluminal testosterone levels to support spermatogenesis via paracrine mechanisms.

The most common abnormality encountered on hormonal analysis in the infertile man is an elevated serum FSH. This finding is suggestive of impaired spermatogenesis; however, the finding of elevated FSH is not always present in cases of testicular failure [55]. Abnormal preliminary screening tests should prompt a more involved endocrinologic workup consisting of total and free testosterone, prolactin, TSH, LH, and FSH. Clinical findings of headaches or visual field changes or findings of an elevated prolactin level necessitate an MRI of the sella turcica to evaluate for a potential macroadenoma of the pituitary.

Genetic Evaluation

In patients who present with azoospermia or severe oligospermia, where obstructive etiologies have been ruled out, evaluation of chromosome number and structure becomes important. A karyotype will rule out genetic conditions most commonly associated with infertility, including Klinefelter's syndrome (47, XXY), 46XX, 47XXY, and Noonan's syndrome. The chromosome structure of the Y chromosome should be assessed as well. This is done with the Y chromosome-linked microdeletion assay. Disruptions or deletions in various loci of the Y chromosome have been associated with severe defects in spermatogenesis. Early studies identified an area on the short arm of the Y chromosome critical for spermatogenesis referred to as the azoospermic factor (AZF) [56]. Subsequently, this has been divided into 3 regions: AZFa, AZFb, and AZFc [57]. Deletions in the regions of AZFa and AZFb are less common and usually associated with poor sperm retrieval rates for ART. AZFc microdeletions are the most commonly found microdeletion in azoospermic men and are associated with the most promising sperm retrieval rates [36]. Although Y chromosome microdeletions have no apparent impact on the health of the patient, the possibility of an inheritable form of infertility in male offspring via ART should prompt appropriate genetic counseling.

Expert Commentary

The purpose of this chapter was to delineate the evaluation of a man presenting with infertility with a focus on the laboratory evaluation. In the new era of the human genome project and with a better understanding of molecular biology and genetics, advances in both the diagnostic capabilities and the management options for male factor infertility are quickly advancing the field. In addition, enhancements in assisted reproductive technology are allowing many couples the opportunity to conceive when it would have been otherwise impossible. As conception is more reliant on laboratory technology, the laboratory evaluation of a man or couple presenting with infertility will remain of paramount importance.

Five-Year View

Conventional semen parameters continue to provide poor prognostic information regarding both frequency and quality of conception. Over the near term, marked research efforts will be dedicated to further elucidating sperm function. Emphasis will continue on the role of oxidative stress and sperm DNA fragmentation on subfertility. Novel research efforts in the field of metabolomics, metabolic profiling of semen, hold promise in elucidating the cause of heretofore idiopathic infertility.

Key Issues

- Infertility is the absence of conception after 12 months or regular unprotected intercourse, and male factor plays a role in up to 50% of cases.
- The initial clinical evaluation of male factor infertility should include a detailed and complete history and physical examination as well as a focused sexual history and genitourinary examination.
- Initial assessment should include a basic microscopic and macroscopic assessment of 2 separate semen analyses collected properly. Further testing should be based on the findings of the initial evaluation.
- New data on lower reference limits of semen parameters in fertile males suggests that there is a broader range of normal parameters than previously thought.
- Advanced semen testing should not be routine, but may be warranted based on the evaluation and includes antisperm antibody detection, assays of sperm DNA damage, and analysis of seminal oxidative stress and seminal antioxidant levels.
- Further testing with basic and extensive hormonal analysis as well as genetic testing may be warranted based on the initial evaluation.

- Reactive oxygen species derived from both intrinsic and extrinsic sources are being increasingly implicated in many cases of subfertility and infertility and have been shown to affect semen quality through several mechanisms including DNA fragmentation and lipid peroxidation. Antioxidant therapy as well as modification of exposures to extrinsic sources of ROS may have a role in the management of infertility.

References

1. The Optimal Evaluation of the Infertile Male: American Urological Society Best Practice Statement. American Urological Society, Education and Research Inc. 2010.
2. Said TM, Agarwal A, Sharma RK, Thomas AJ, Sikka SC. Impact of sperm morphology on DNA damage caused by oxidative stress induced by beta-nicotinamide adenine dinucleotide phosphate. Fertil Steril. 2005;83:95–103.
3. Slama R, et al. Time to pregnancy and semen parameters: a cross-sectional study among fertile couples from four European Cities. Hum Reprod. 2002;17(2):503–15.
4. Moskovtsev SI, Willis J, White J, Mullen JB. Leukocytospermia: relationship to sperm deoxyribonucleic acid integrity in patients evaluated for male factor infertility. Fertil Steril. 2007;88(3):737–40. Epub 6 Mar 2007.
5. Tomlinson MJ, Barratt CL, Cooke ID. Prospective study of leukocytes and leukocyte subpopulations in semen suggests they are not a cause of male infertility. Fertil Steril. 1993;60: 1069–75.
6. Kolettis PN, Sabanegh ES. Significant medical pathology discovered during a male infertility evaluation. J Urol. 2001;166(1):178–80.
7. Franca LR, Avelar GF, Almeida FFL. Spermatogenesis and sperm transit through the epididymis with emphasis on pigs. Theriogenology. 2005;63:300–18.
8. Mortimer D, Leslie EE, Kelly RW, Templeton AA. Morphological selection of human spermatozoa in vivo and in vitro. J Reprod Fertil. 1982;64:391–9.
9. Clermont Y, Heller C. Spermatogenesis in man: an estimate of its duration. Science. 1963;140:184–5.
10. Wolff H. The biologic significance of white blood cells in semen. Fertil Steril. 1995 Jun;63(6):1143–57. Review.
11. Verma A, Kanwar KC. Effect of vitamin E on human sperm motility and lipid peroxidation in vitro. Asian J Androl. 1999;1(3):151–4.
12. Agarwal A, Deepinder F, Cocuzza M, Short RA, Evenson DP. Effect of vaginal lubricants on sperm motility and chromatin integrity: a prospective comparative study. Fertil Steril. 2008; 89(2):375–9.
13. Kruger TF, Acosta AA, Simmons KF, et al. Predictive value of abnormal sperm morphology in in vitro fertilization. Fertil Steril. 1988;49:112–7.
14. Cendron M, Keating MA, Huff DS, et al. Cryptorchidism, orchiopexy and infertility: a critical long-term retrospective analysis. J Urol. 1989;142:559–62.
15. Charny CW. The spermatogenic potential of the undescended testis before and after treatment. J Urol. 1960;83:697.
16. Misell LM, Holochwost D, Boban D, et al. A stable isotope/mass spectrometric method for measuring the kinetics of human spermatogenesis in vivo. J Urol. 2006;175:242–6.
17. Carlsen E, et al. Effects of ejaculatory frequency and season on variations in semen quality. Fertil Steril. 2004;82(2):358–66.
18. Bjorndahl L, Kvist U. Sequence of ejaculation affects the spermatozoon as a carrier and its message. Reprod Biomed Online. 2003;7(4):440–8.

19. Cooper TG, Noonan E, von Eckardstein S, Auger J, et al. World Health Organization reference values for human semen characteristics. Hum Reprod Update. 2010;16(3):231–45.
20. Zini A, Blumenfield A, Libman J, Willis J. Beneficial effect of microsurgical varicocelectomy on human sperm DNA integrity. Hum Reprod. 2005;20:1018–21.
21. World Health Organization. World Health Organization: WHO Laboratory Manual for the Examination of Human Semen and Sperm-Cervical Mucus Interaction. 1999.
22. Jouannet P, Ducot B, Feneux D, Spira A. Male factors and the likelihood of pregnancy in infertile couples. I. Study of sperm characteristics. Int J Androl. 1988 Oct;11(5):379–94.
23. Spira A. Epidemiology of human reproduction. Hum Reprod. 1986;1:111–5.
24. Andersen AG, Jensen TK, Carlsen E, Jørgensen N, Andersson AM, Krarup T, Keiding N, Skakkebaek NE. High frequency of sub-optimal semen quality in an unselected population of young men. Hum Reprod. 2000 Feb;15(2):366–72.
25. Fedder J. Nonsperm cells in human semen: with special reference to seminal leukocytes and their possible influence on fertility. Arch Androl. 1996;36(1):41–65.
26. Sigma M, Jarow J. Male infertility. In: Wein AJ, Kavoussi LR, Novick AC, Partin AW, Peters CA, editors. Campbell-Walsh urology. 9th ed. Philadelphia: Saunders Elsevier; 2007.
27. Agarwal A, Saleh RA, Bedaiwy MA. Role of reactive oxygen species in the pathophysiology of human reproduction. Fertil Steril. 2003;79:829–43.
28. Zini A, Libman J. Sperm DNA damage: importance in the era of assisted reproduction. Curr Opin Urol. 2006;16(6):428–34.
29. Athayde KS, et al. Development of normal reference values for seminal reactive oxygen species and their correlation with leukocytes and semen parameters in a fertile population. J Androl. 2007;28(4):613–20.
30. Fredricsson B, Bjork G. Morphology of postcoital spermatozoa in the cervical secretion and its clinical significance. Fertil Steril. 1977;28:841–5.
31. Mosher WD, Pratt WF. Fecundity and infertility in the United States: incidence and trends. Fertil Steril. 1991;56:192.
32. Marks JL, McMahon R, Lipshultz LI. Predictive parameters of successful varicocele repair. J Urol. 1986;136:609–12.
33. Gandini L, Lombardo F, Paoli D, Caponecchia L, Familiari G, Verlengia C, Dondero F, Lenzi A. Study of apoptotic DNA fragmentation in human spermatozoa. Hum Reprod. 2000;15(4): 830–9.
34. Lee JD, Kamiguchi Y, Yanagimachi R. Analysis of chromosome constitution of human spermatozoa with normal and aberrant head morphologies after injection into mouse oocytes. Hum Reprod. 1996 Sep;11(9):1942–6.
35. Guzick DS, Overstreet JW, Factor-Litvak P, Brazil CK, Nakajima ST, Coutifaris C, Carson SA, Cisneros P, Steinkampf MP, Hill JA, Xu D, Vogel DL, National Cooperative Reproductive Medicine Network. Sperm morphology, motility, and concentration in fertile and infertile men. N Engl J Med. 2001;345(19):1388–93.
36. Oates RD, Silber S, Brown LG, Page DC. Clinical characterization of 42 oligospermic or azoospermic men with microdeletion of the AZFc region of the Y chromosome, and of 18 children conceived via ICSI. Hum Reprod. 2002;17(11):2813–24.
37. Agarwal A, Said TM. Role of sperm chromatin abnormalities and DNA damage in male infertility. Hum Reprod Update. 2003;9(4):331–45.
38. Sanocka D, et al. Male genital tract inflammation: The role of selected interleukins in regulation of pro-oxidant and antioxidant enzymatic substances in seminal plasma. J Androl. 2003; 24:448–55.
39. Evenson DP, Wixon R. Clinical aspects of sperm DNA fragmentation detection and male infertility. Theriogenology. 2006;65:979–91.
40. Evenson DP, Larson KL, Jost LK. Sperm chromatin structure assay: Its clinical use for detecting sperm DNA fragmentation in male infertility and comparisons with other techniques. J Androl. 2002;23:25–43.

41. Li Z, Wang L, Cai J, Huang H. Correlation of sperm DNA damage with IVF and ICSI outcomes: a systematic review and meta-analysis. J Assist Reprod Genet. 2006;23(9–10):367–76. Epub 4 Oct 2006.
42. Griveau JF, Grizard G, Boucher D, Le Lannou D. Influence of oxygen tension on function of isolated spermatozoa from ejaculates of oligozoospermic patients and normozoospermic fertile donors. Hum Reprod. 1998;13(11):3108–13.
43. O'Flaherty C, de Lamirande E, Gagnon C. Positive role of reactive oxygen species in mammalian sperm capacitation: triggering and modulation of phosphorylation events. Free Radic Biol Med. 2006;41(4):528–40.
44. Camejo MI, Segnini A, Proverbio F. Intgerleukin-6 in seminal plasma of infertile men, and lipid peroxidation in their sperm. Arch Androl. 2001;47:97–101.
45. Martinez P, Proverbio F, Camejo MI. Sperm lipid peroxidation and pro-inflammatory cytokines. Asian J Androl. 2007;9:102–7.
46. Silver EW, et al. Effect of antioxidant intake on sperm chromatin stability in healthy non-smoking men. J Androl. 2005;26:550–6.
47. Keskes-Ammar L, Feki-Chakroun N, Rebai T, et al. Sperm oxidative stress and the effect of an oral vitamin E and selenium supplement on semen quality in infertile men. Arch Androl. 2003;49: 83–94.
48. Köksal IT, Tefekli A, Usta M, Erol H, Abbasoglu S, Kadioglu A. The role of reactive oxygen species in testicular dysfunction associated with varicocele. BJU Int. 2000 Sep;86(4):549–52.
49. Allamaneni SS, Naughton CK, Sharma RK, Thomas Jr AJ, Agarwal A. Increased seminal reactive oxygen species levels in patients with varicoceles correlate with varicocele grade but not with testis size. Fertil Steril. 2004;82(6):1684–6.
50. Mostafa T, et al. Varicocelectomy reduces reactive oxygen species levels and increases antioxidant activity of seminal plasma from infertile men with varicocele. Int J Androl. 2001;24: 261–5.
51. Evers JLH, Collins JA. Assessment of efficacy of varicocele repair for male subfertility: A systematic review. Lancet. 2003;361: 1849–52.
52. Baker MA, Aitken RJ. Reactive oxygen species in spermatozoa: methods for monitoring and significance for the origins of genetic disease and infertility. Reprod Biol Endocrinol. 2005;3:67.
53. Report on optimal evaluation of the infertile male. AUA Best Practice Policy and ASRM Practice Committee Report, Volume 1, 2001. http://www.auanet.org. Accessed 20 Dec 2009.
54. Lipshultz LI, Corriere Jr JN. Progressive testicular atrophy in the varicocele patient. J Urol. 1977 Feb;117(2):175–6.
55. Turek PJ, Kim M, Gilbaugh 3rd JH, Lipshultz LI. The clinical characteristics of 82 patients with Sertoli cell-only testis histology. Fertil Steril. 1995;64(6):1197–200.
56. Tiepolo L, Zuffardi O. Localization of factors controlling spermatogenesis in the nonfluorescent portion of the human Y chromosome long arm. Hum Genet. 1976;34:119–24.
57. Vogt PH. Human chromosome deletions in Yq11, AZF candidate genes and male infertility: history and update. Mol Hum Reprod. 1998;4(8):739–44.

Further Reading

Griveau JF, Renard P, Le Lannou D. Superoxide anion production by human spermatozoa as a part of the ionophore-induced acrosome reaction process. Int J Androl. 199;18(2):67–74.
Kefer JC, Agarwal A, Sabanegh EC. Role of antioxidants in the treatment of male infertility. Int J Urol. 2009;16:449–57.
Kutteh WH, Chao CH, Ritter JO, et al. Vaginal lubricants of the infertile couple: effect on sperm activity. Int J Fertil Menopausal Stud. 1996;41:400–4.

Lampiao F, du Plessis SS. TNF-alpha and IL-6 affect human sperm function by elevating nitric oxide production. Reprod Biomed Online. 2008;17(5):628–31.

Liu DY, Baker HW. Morphology of spermatozoa bound to the zona pellucida of human oocytes that failed to fertilize in vitro. J Reprod Fertil. 1992;94:71–84.

McLachlan RI, et al. Semen analysis: its place in modern reproductive medical practice. Pathology. 2003;35(1):25–33.

Munuce MJ, Berta CL, Pauluzzi F, Caille AM. Relationship between antisperm antibodies, sperm movement, and semen quality. Urol Int. 2000;65(4):200–3.

Sakkas D, Mariethoz E, Manicardi G, Bizzaro D, Bianchi PG, Bianchi U. Origin of DNA damage in ejaculated human spermatozoa. Rev Reprod. 1999;4(1):31–7.

Shekarriz M, Sharma RK, Thomas Jr AJ, Agarwal A. Positive myeloperoxidase staining (Endtz test) as an indicator of excessive reactive oxygen species formation in semen. J Assist Reprod Genet. 1995;12(2):70–4.

Simmons FA. Human infertility. New Engl J Med. 1956;255:1140.

Thonneau P, Marchand S, Tallec A, et al. Incidence and main causes of infertility in a resident population (1,850,000) of three French regions (1988–1989). Hum Reprod. 1991;6:811–6.

Tur-Kaspa I, Maor Y, Levran D, et al. How often should infertile men have intercourse to achieve conception? Fert Steril. 1994;62(2):370–5.

Wilcox AJ, Weinberg CR, Baird DD. Timing of sexual intercourse in relation to ovulation. Effects on the probability of conception, survival of the pregnancy, and sex of the baby. New Engl J Med. 1995;333(23):1517–21.

World Health Organization, Department of Reproductive Health and Research. WHO Laboratory Manual for the Examination and Processing of Human Semen, 5th edn. 2010.

Chapter 3
Epidemiological Considerations in Male Infertility

Mark A. Faasse and Craig S. Niederberger

This chapter primarily aims to discuss the epidemiologic relationship between infertility and male reproductive potential. It will focus in detail on the accuracy and diagnostic value of semen studies. Controversial reports of declining sperm counts during the twentieth century will also be addressed, followed by a review of trends in health-care resource utilization and cost analysis models pertinent to the management of male infertility.

The subject of this textbook, antioxidant therapy for male infertility, has an epidemiologic basis in the understanding that reactive oxygen species (ROS) contribute to sperm damage and are present in higher levels in the semen of infertile men [1–4]. It may be surprising for some to encounter an epidemiologic approach to male infertility in the modern era, given the increasing availability and use of assisted reproductive technology (ART) [5]. Indeed, the relative ease of surgical sperm retrieval in cases of azoospermia and severe oligozoospermia has seemingly rendered comprehensive evaluation and treatment of infertile men less relevant. Even though such an evaluation may identify one or more modifiable risk factors for infertility (as well as potentially serious underlying or coexisting illnesses and genetic abnormalities), the outcome of pathology-directed treatment is always uncertain and may not be realized until several additional months or years have elapsed.

However, risk and uncertainty are also attendant to the use of ART. Recent cost-effectiveness studies have demonstrated that a straight-to-ART approach is less

M.A. Faasse, MD (✉)
Department of Urology, University of Illinois at Chicago, 840 South Wood Street,
M/C 955, Chicago, IL 60616, USA
e-mail: mfaasse@sbcglobal.net

C.S. Niederberger, MD, FACS
Department of Urology, University of Illinois at Chicago College of Medicine and
Department of Bioengineering, University of Illinois at Chicago College of Engineering,
Chicago, IL 60616, USA
e-mail: craignied@gmail.com

S.J. Parekattil and A. Agarwal (eds.), *Antioxidants in Male Infertility: A Guide for Clinicians and Researchers*, © Springer Science+Business Media New York 2013

efficient than pathology-directed treatment in many situations involving male infertility. Therefore, renewed emphasis is being placed on the paradigm of intervention aimed at correction of modifiable male risk factors [6].

Epidemiology of Infertility

It is important to distinguish reproductive potential, or capacity, from actual reproductive performance, or outcome [7, 8]. Infertility is ultimately defined by a reproductive *outcome* (i.e., childlessness). By contrast, "male infertility" is a diagnosis of relative impairment in male reproductive *potential*. Before discussing male infertility in more detail, we will review the epidemiology of infertility in general.

Incidence and Prevalence of Infertility in Developed Countries

Childlessness within long-standing marriage has been observed to occur in roughly 10% of couples in developed countries [9]. This figure represents a measure of reproductive outcomes, but it does not exclude couples who remain voluntarily childless or do not have regular intercourse during the fertile phase of the female's menstrual cycle. In such couples, reproductive potential may never be fully tested [5].

In order to capture the concept of impairment in reproductive potential within the definition of infertility, the World Health Organization (WHO) has specified infertility as "no conception after at least 12 months of unprotected intercourse" [10]. By this criterion, the lifetime *incidence* of unwanted infertility is approximately 15% among couples in Western countries [11]. Two thirds of these cases are primary, i.e., in couples who have never previously conceived, while one third are secondary [9].

It is not uncommon to see infertility defined by other durations of time, such as 2 or 5 years. Also, while the outcome of interest in the WHO's definition is conception, others prefer to regard infertility as the absence of live birth [8]. This distinction is important, since 10–25% of recognized pregnancies end in miscarriage [12].

The annual *prevalence* of infertility among married US women aged 15–44 years was 7.4% in 2002, down from 11.2% in 1965, and 8.5% in 1982 [13]. This trend may reflect improvements in reproductive potential, perhaps through better awareness of ideal timing for intercourse, which may be attributable to at-home ovulation tests. However, other factors could also be involved, such as more couples utilizing infertility treatment prior to reaching the 12-month threshold necessary for inclusion in the rate's numerator. Declining marriage rates among lower socioeconomic classes may also be disproportionately removing women at greater risk of infertility from the denominator [13]. A popular misconception is that infertility is synonymous with, or virtually approximates, sterility [7]. In fact, only 3–5% of couples are sterile [9, 14].

Table 3.1 Prevalence of infertility of 5 years duration in various regions of the developing world and the prevalence of infertility of 12 months duration in the USA

	Primary or secondary infertility (%)	Primary infertility (%)	Secondary infertility (%)
Sub-Saharan Africa	30.0	2.6	27.5
Near East/North Africa	20.4	2.8	17.6
South Central Asia	28.3	2.6	25.8
Southeast Asia	23.5	1.9	21.6
Latin America/Caribbean	16.0	2.8	13.2
USA	7.4	3.0	4.4

Adapted from [15], with permission. US data were reported in [13]

Infertility in the Developing World

According to the WHO, more than 25% of married women in developing countries were experiencing primary or secondary infertility of at least 5 years duration in 2002 [15]. In contrast to Western societies, the vast majority of infertility in developing countries is secondary (Table 3.1). Sexually transmitted infections and postpartum complications are the key factors contributing to this disparity [16]. The WHO found no evidence of an association between the prevalence of HIV infection and infertility.

The rate of childlessness in developing countries among sexually experienced women who are beyond childbearing age is approximately 3% [15]. This figure is comparable to the estimated prevalence of sterility in Western societies.

High cost represents an important barrier to the accessibility of most infertility treatment, and specifically ART, in the developing world [16]. Therefore, further identification of avoidable gonadotoxins, as well as clarification of the role of less-expensive therapies, would be especially welcome [17].

Reproduction—a Matter of Chance: The Natural History of Infertility

Reproduction has been described as "a matter of chance depending on the subtle balance between success or failure of complex, mostly poorly understood, sequential processes that may lead to a pregnancy and eventually to the birth of a healthy child" [14]. Failure of a couple to reproduce is a unique medical problem in that it occurs *between* rather than *within* individuals [8].

Individuals' reproductive potential is a continuous, as opposed to dichotomous, variable. It reflects the influence of many factors, including age. Reproductive potential declines in members of both sexes over 30 years old, but female age has the most profound effect on the likelihood of conception [18, 19].

Table 3.2 Cumulative spontaneous pregnancy rates of couples in five hypothetical categories of reproductive potential

	MFR (%)	Cumulative pregnancy rate after: 6 months (%)	12 months (%)	24 months (%)	60 months (%)
Highest fecundability	60	100	–	–	
Average fecundability	20	74	93	100	
Below-average fecundability	5	26	46	71	95
Severely impaired fecundability	1	6	11	21	45
Sterile	0	0	0	0	0

MFR monthly fecundity rate; cumulative pregnancy rate $= 1 - (1 - \mathrm{MFR})^{\text{\# of months}}$
From [20], with permission of Elsevier

Table 3.3 Hypothetical model of the proportion of couples with varying degrees of reproductive potential in the residual population, dependent on the duration of infertility

	MFR (%)	Composition of residual nonpregnant couples after: 0 months (%)	6 months (%)	12 months (%)	24 months (%)	60 months (%)
Highest fecundability	60	3	–	–	–	–
Average fecundability	20	79	58	30	–	–
Below-average fecundability	5	10	21	30	30	8
Severely impaired fecundability	1	5	13	24	40	44
Sterile	0	3	8	16	30	48

MFR monthly fecundity rate
From [20], with permission of Elsevier

Since a couple's reproductive capacity is the composite of its individual members' reproductive potentials, it, too, is a continuous variable. Impairment of a male's reproductive potential may be compensated for—or compounded—by that of his female partner, and vice versa. This concept is illustrated by the fact that artificial insemination with donor semen is more often successful in partners of azoospermic men than in partners of men with oligozoospermia [20].

Couples' monthly, or cycle-wise, likelihood of conception falls along a spectrum of probability. This is referred to as fecundability, or monthly fecundity rate (MFR). The average MFR for human couples having regular, unprotected intercourse is approximately 20%, and the overall distribution of human MFRs is believed to range from 0 to 60% [21, 22]. The variable likelihood of pregnancy at 6, 12, 24, and 60 months has been calculated for couples with different MFRs (Table 3.2). Based on these values, a hypothetical model has been constructed of the proportion of couples with varying degrees of reproductive potential (MFR) among residual nonpregnant couples after specified durations of infertility (Table 3.3) [23].

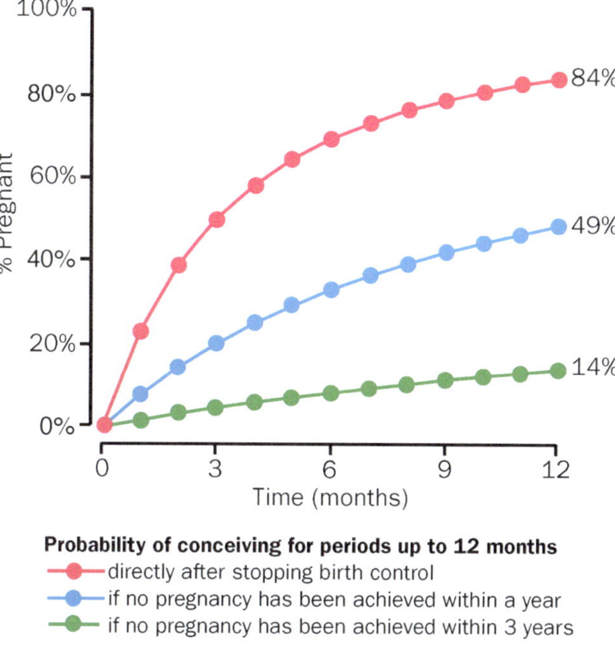

Fig. 3.1 Cumulative probability of conception in couples having unprotected intercourse (from [14], with permission)

Table 3.2 demonstrates that couples with average fecundability have a better than 90% chance of conceiving within 12 months. However, 30% of couples who do not conceive within 12 months are still of average reproductive potential (see Table 3.3). Population-based studies have found that couples who are infertile after 12 months retain a roughly 50% likelihood of achieving unassisted pregnancy by 24 months [24]. Thereafter, the odds of conception decline precipitously, as illustrated in Fig. 3.1. The proportion of couples that are sterile increases with the duration of infertility.

An obvious but nevertheless critically important factor in determining reproductive potential is the timing of sexual intercourse relative to ovulation (Fig. 3.2) [25]. In a cohort of 340 German couples who received natural family planning education intended to improve their timing of intercourse, the monthly probability of achieving pregnancy averaged 38%, markedly higher than the average human MFR of 20% [26].

Diagnostic Accuracy and Utility of Semen Studies

Male infertility is diagnosed in approximately 50% of couples presenting for evaluation of infertility [11]. Basic semen analysis remains the most widely utilized laboratory study for this purpose. However, the limitations of semen analysis should be clearly understood.

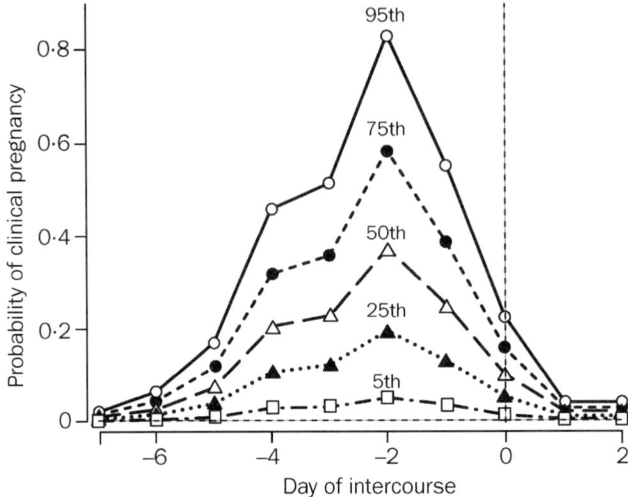

Fig. 3.2 Probability of clinical pregnancy after intercourse on a particular day relative to ovulation (day 0) for couples at specified percentiles of the population distribution of reproductive potential (from [20], with permission of Elsevier; adapted from [25], with permission of Oxford University Press)

The parameters usually assessed by semen analysis include ejaculate volume, sperm concentration (density), sperm motility, and sperm morphology. From the ejaculate volume, concentration, and percentage of motile sperm, the total sperm count and total motile count are calculated. Semen pH, viscosity, white blood cell concentration, and the degree of sperm agglutination may also be reported [27].

More specialized studies that are undertaken on a case-by-case basis include evaluation of sperm viability, antisperm antibodies, and functional assays, such as assessment of sperm–cervical mucus interaction, capacitation, and sperm penetration of a zona-free hamster oocyte [28]. Relatively recent developments have included the introduction of tests for seminal ROS levels and sperm DNA fragmentation [29, 30].

Relationship Between Semen Parameters and Male Infertility

Semen analysis definitively confirms male factor infertility in men who are found to have semen characteristics at the negative extremes, i.e., azoospermia, nonmotile sperm, or the severest cases of teratozoospermia. However, only a small fraction of men who present for evaluation of infertility have such findings [11]. The present section explores the relationship between male infertility and the entire spectrum of semen quality.

Table 3.4 WHO reference values for analysis of semen parameters

	1992	1999	2010
Ejaculate volume (mL)	≥ 2.0	≥ 2.0	≥ 1.5
Sperm concentration (10^6/mL)	≥ 20	≥ 20	≥ 15
Total sperm count (10^6/ejaculate)	≥ 40	≥ 40	≥ 39
Sperm motility (% motile)	≥ 50 (a + b)[a]	≥ 50 (a + b)	≥ 40 (a + b + c)
Sperm morphology (% normal)	≥ 30	≥ 14[b]	≥ 4
Sperm viability/vitality (% live)	≥ 75	≥ 75	≥ 58
White blood cells (10^6/mL)	<1.0	<1.0	<1.0

From [31], with permission

[a]Motility is graded as follows: a = rapid progressive motility (>25 μm/s); b = slow/sluggish progressive motility (5–25 μm/s); c = nonprogressive motility; d = immotility

[b]Kruger (Tygerberg) strict criteria were adopted by the WHO in 1999

Since 1980, the WHO has published reference values for human semen parameters. These values have been changed periodically (Table 3.4) [31]. As of 2010, they represent the fifth percentile in the distribution of semen parameters from a population of men with proven fertility [32]. They provide no information regarding the distribution of semen parameters in men who are infertile.

Although the WHO criteria are commonly used as thresholds for designation of male infertility, the diagnostic picture in a clinical setting is considerably more complex. This is because of substantial overlap between the distributions of semen characteristics in empirically fertile men and those with infertility whose female partners have had a normal fertility evaluation (Fig. 3.3).

Basic performance measures of a test such as semen analysis include calculation of its sensitivity and specificity. These concepts are illustrated in Tables 3.5 and 3.6. If a sperm concentration below 15 million/mL is the criterion for a "positive" result (i.e., diagnosis of male infertility), then men who are actually fertile will be correctly classified 95% of the time. In other words, the threshold of 15 million/mL has a specificity of 95%. However, 85% of infertile men also have sperm concentrations above 15 million/mL, so the sensitivity of the test at this threshold is only 15% [33]. Many men with impaired reproductive potential will not be recognized as such.

If we assume that 50% of couples presenting for an evaluation of infertility have a contributing male factor, then the predictive value of a positive result (i.e., its likelihood of being correct) would be 75%. The predictive value of a negative, or normal, result would be only 53% (see Table 3.6).

Of course, diagnostic thresholds can be changed. If they are increased, sensitivity improves, but there is a reciprocal decline in specificity, and vice versa. One way to assess the diagnostic accuracy of a test across all thresholds is by a receiver operating characteristic (ROC) curve [28, 34]. ROC curves are constructed by plotting the probability of detecting true positives (sensitivity) against that of detecting false positives (1 − specificity) at each threshold.

The total area under the ROC curve (AUC) for a particular test represents its overall discriminatory capability. A perfect test has an AUC of 1.0, while a test is useless if the likelihood of a true positive matches that of a false positive at every

Fig. 3.3 Frequency histograms depicting the percentage of men from fertile (*shaded bars*) and infertile (*unshaded bars*) couples with sperm concentration (**a**), sperm motility (**b**), and sperm morphology (**c**) within specified ranges. Data were obtained from 696 fertile men and 765 men from infertile couples, whose female partners had an unrevealing fertility evaluation (from [33], Copyright 2001, Massachusetts Medical Society. All rights reserved)

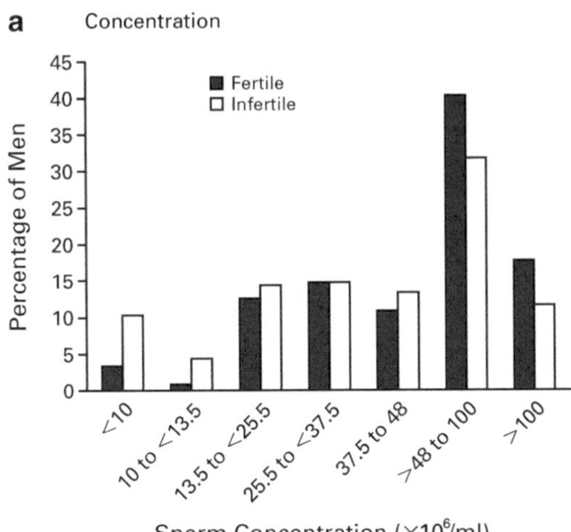

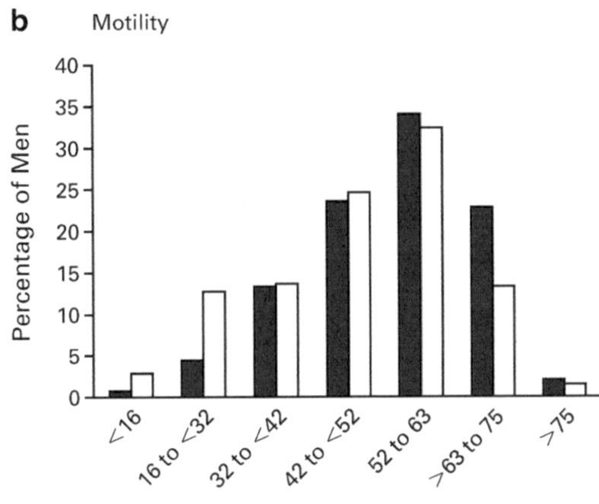

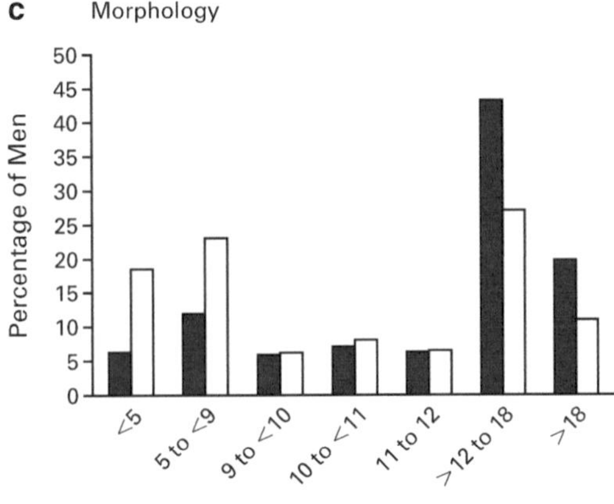

Table 3.5 2 × 2 Table depicting actual fertility status vs. test results using the 2010 WHO reference value for sperm concentration as a threshold for diagnosis of male infertility, in a hypothetical population of 200 men presenting for evaluation of infertility

		Actual fertility status	
		Infertile	Fertile
Test results	Infertile	15 (TP)	5 (FP)
	Fertile	85 (FN)	95 (TN)

TP true positives, *FP* false positives, *FN* false negatives, *TN* true negatives

Table 3.6 Accuracy metrics based on Table 3.5, using the 2010 WHO reference value for sperm concentration (15 million/mL) as a threshold for diagnosis of male infertility

Accuracy metric	Formula for calculation	Result (%)
Sensitivity	TP/(TP + FN)	15
Specificity	TN/(TN + FP)	95
Positive predictive value	TP/(TP + FP)	75
Negative predictive value	TN/(TN + FN)	53
Classification accuracy	(TP + TN)/N	55

TP true positives, *FP* false positives, *FN* false negatives, *TN* true negatives; *N* = total number

threshold, resulting in the no-discrimination line from (0, 0) to (1, 1) and an AUC of 0.5. The amount by which a test's ROC curve diverges from this line—and by extension, to which its AUC exceeds 0.5—is the degree to which it is diagnostically helpful. An AUC that exceeds 0.9 is considered excellent, while an AUC of less than 0.7 is poor.

Figure 3.4 represents an example of an ROC curve generated from MacLeod's data on sperm concentration in fertile and infertile men [35]. Its AUC is only 0.59, indicating that the overall accuracy of sperm concentration for diagnosis of male infertility just narrowly exceeds that of random chance. In Guzick and colleagues' series, which was depicted in Fig. 3.3, the AUC for sperm density, motility, and morphology were 0.60, 0.59, and 0.66, respectively [36].

The ROC curve alone does not provide information regarding the likelihood that a specific patient's positive or negative test result is correct. This probability is dependent both on test performance and the prevalence of disease in the relevant population. As previously illustrated, a diagnosis of male infertility based on sperm concentration below 15 million/mL may be correct 75% of the time in the population of males from infertile couples. False-positive results for infertility are relatively rare in this population. By comparison, if semen analysis were performed on men in the general population (e.g., to assess sperm donors with no prior reproductive history), its positive predictive value would be considerably less, on account of a much lower prevalence of male infertility.

Four studies smaller than that of Guzick and colleagues have reported higher AUCs for sperm density, motility, and morphology, as described in Table 3.7 [37–40]. In general, motility and morphology demonstrated greater discriminatory capability than sperm concentration. Although the authors of these studies reported

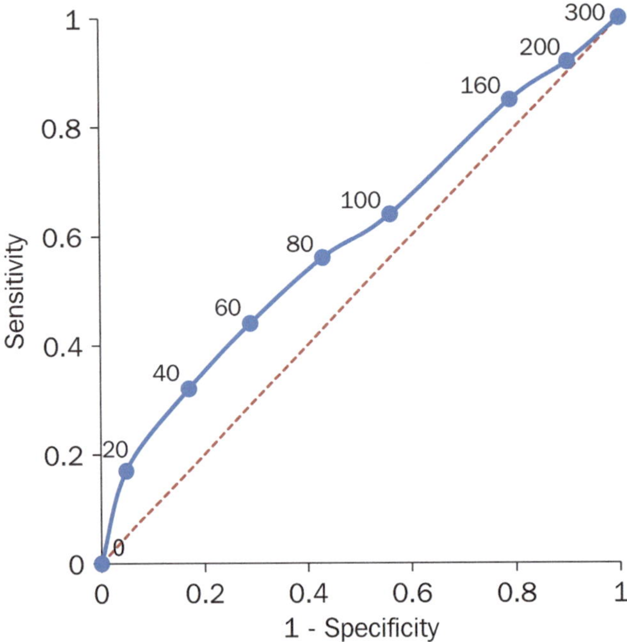

Fig. 3.4 Receiver operating characteristic (ROC) curve analysis of sperm concentration for diagnosis of male infertility at specified thresholds (data from [35]). The no-discrimination line is shown in *red* (from [36], with permission of Elsevier)

"optimal thresholds" for discrimination of fertile and infertile men, some of these thresholds have been criticized for having an unacceptably low positive predictive value in the setting of an infertile population [41].

Guzick and colleagues took a different approach to selecting diagnostic thresholds, using classification and regression tree (CART) analysis to determine *two* thresholds for each parameter that define the upper and lower boundaries of an indeterminate range lying between the fertile and infertile ranges (see Table 3.7). Unfortunately, a large number of men presenting for infertility evaluation fall into the indeterminate range, leaving unanswered the question of whether they warrant intervention for modifiable risk factors. The odds of male infertility multiply if more than one semen parameter is within the infertile range [33].

Do Semen Parameters Prospectively Predict Fertility and Assisted Reproductive Technique Outcomes?

Only a handful of studies have attempted to prospectively identify variables associated with male reproductive potential. One such project included 200 couples, some of whom had had prior pregnancies [42]. After discontinuing contraception, the

Table 3.7 Reported areas under the ROC curve for various seminal characteristics

Population		AUC density	AUC motility	AUC morphology (strict)
MacLeod [35][a]	1,000 fertile; 800 infertile[b] (ages NR)	0.59	NR	NR
Guzick et al. [33][a]	696 fertile (avg age, 33.5 ± 5.0); 765 infertile (avg age, 34.7 ± 4.9)	0.60 (13.5, 48)	0.59 (32, 63)	0.66 (9, 11)
Ombelet et al. [37]	144 fertile; 143 infertile (ages NR)	0.69 (34)	0.61 (45)	0.78 (10)
Gunalp et al. [38]	61 fertile (avg age, 29.9); 62 infertile (avg age, 31.3)	0.56 (34)	0.71 (42)	0.70 (12)
Menkveld et al. [39]	107 fertile (avg age, 33.8 ± 4.3); 103 infertile[b] (avg age, 33.7 ± 3.9)	NR	0.79 (45)	0.78 (4)
Jedrzejczak et al. [40]	113 fertile (avg age, 31 ± 4.7); 109 infertile (avg age, 32.2 ± 4.1)	0.80 (45–50)	0.91 (24)	0.82 (11)

AUC area under the ROC curve, *NR* not reported; ages of study populations are reported as mean ± SD; values in parentheses are the "optimal thresholds" identified by the respective studies for discrimination of fertile from infertile men—see text for additional details
[a]For data from these studies, the ROC curve was plotted and AUC was reported by Niederberger [36]
[b]These studies did not specifically report female partners as having had a negative fertility evaluation

couples were followed for up to 12 months. Seventy-eight percent conceived during the study period, and both sperm motility and morphology were significantly associated with fertility. The difference in sperm concentration between fertile and infertile couples remained statistically insignificant.

Bonde and colleagues investigated 430 Danish couples between 20 and 35 years old who had never previously been or tried to become pregnant, following them for up to six menstrual cycles after discontinuation of contraception [43]. Sixty percent of couples became pregnant. The probability of conception increased up to a threshold sperm concentration of 40 million/mL, but there was no additional likelihood of pregnancy at higher sperm densities (Fig. 3.5). This finding has led some reproductive specialists to argue that the appropriate threshold of sperm concentration for diagnosis of male infertility should be 40 instead of 15 million/mL [44]. A change of this sort, however, would also increase the number of false-positive diagnoses, prompting unnecessary evaluation and treatment.

Leushuis and colleagues have published an incisive review of prediction models in reproductive medicine, including several that use one or more semen characteristics to predict conception by infertile couples [45]. One such model, which has been externally validated in a population excluding men with total motile sperm counts of less than three million, takes account of sperm motility as well as characteristics of the female partner and the duration of the couple's infertility; it is available online at www.freya.nl/probability.php [46]. Another model utilizes inputs of sperm concentration, motility, morphology, and hypoosmotic swelling to assess the likelihood of

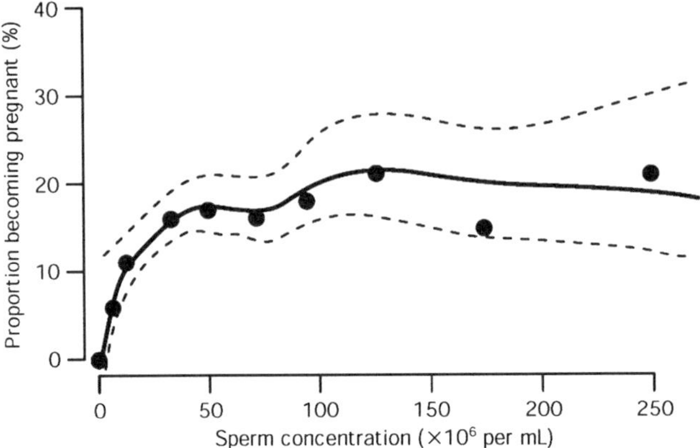

Fig. 3.5 Probability of pregnancy per menstrual cycle relative to sperm concentration (from [43], with permission of Elsevier)

pregnancy, with a reported accuracy greater than 85% [40]. Of note, however, the AUCs for each variable in this study substantially exceeded those published in the other reports described in Table 3.7, and the predictive model has yet to be validated.

Sperm quality also affects ART outcomes, at least to some degree. Several investigations have demonstrated a positive correlation between semen characteristics, including ROS levels, and in vitro fertilization/intracytoplasmic sperm injection (IVF/ICSI) success rates, yet there was no apparent association with clinical pregnancy rates [47, 48]. Studies of intrauterine insemination (IUI), by contrast, have shown a correlation between successful outcomes and sperm concentration, motility, and morphology [41, 49–51].

Novel Assays for Diagnosis of Male Infertility

Andrologists often lament the lack of more accurate studies for the diagnosis of male infertility. Several tests are currently in various stages of development, including genomic, proteomic, glycomic, lipidomic, and metabolomic analyses [52, 53]. Testing for seminal ROS levels was found to have an AUC of 0.82 in a study of 105 patients [54]. Further evaluation in a larger cohort of patients is necessary.

Are Sperm Counts Declining?

One of the most controversial issues in reproductive medicine during the past 20 years has been a purported decline in semen quality during the twentieth century. In 1992, a widely publicized meta-analysis of 61 studies appeared to demonstrate a worldwide decrease in average sperm concentration from 113 million/mL in 1940 to 66 million/mL in 1990 [55]. This report was echoed by additional publications, raising the question of whether exposure to environmental toxins, such as estrogenic compounds like diethylstilboestrol (DES), was adversely affecting testicular function [56, 57].

Important methodological shortcomings have since been identified in Carlsen and colleagues' analysis, as well as in the quality of many studies that were included in their review [58, 59]. Geographical differences were found to be the source of much of the variance in sperm density [60]. All studies included in the review from before 1970 were performed in the USA; however, since US studies generally reported higher sperm concentrations than those conducted elsewhere, the review was biased toward an apparent decline in sperm concentration by inclusion of international studies post-1970.

In subsequent investigations, Fisch and colleagues found no evidence of a decline in sperm density in the USA [61, 62]. They did identify substantial differences between the average sperm counts of men from different states. A review of worldwide studies also did not reveal a global decline in semen quality, although more limited, locoregional trends could not be excluded [58].

Health-Care Resource Utilization for Male Infertility

Medical intervention for male infertility may take the form of outpatient care, surgical procedures, and ART. The Urologic Diseases in America (UDA) Project, which published its first report in 2007, has facilitated a better understanding of the scope of health-care resource utilization for male infertility in the USA.

Office Visits and Ambulatory Surgery Cases

According to data from the National Ambulatory Medical Care Survey (NAMCS), which are summarized in the UDA Project's report, the average number of physician office visits for male infertility in the USA exceeded 150,000 annually between 1992 and 2000, with little variability [63]. However, there was a 24% decline in ambulatory surgery cases for male infertility from 1994 to 2002. Reasons for this trend are unclear but may include preferential use of ART.

Age-wise, the greatest utilization of health-care services for male infertility was among men 25–34 years old. Varicocele was the most commonly identified diagnostic code, accounting for 53% of office visits and 67% of ambulatory surgeries.

Other data from the NAMCS demonstrate substantial regional variation in resource utilization for male infertility. Men living in the Northeast USA had a rate of ambulatory surgery visits associated with a diagnosis of infertility of 104 per 100,000, while those in the Midwest, South, and West had rates of just 72, 50, and 29 per 100,000, respectively. The explanation for this variability is probably multifactorial, reflecting a combination of patient demand and availability of services.

Assisted Reproductive Technology

In 2007, 142,435 ART cycles were performed, an increase of 60% since 1998 [64]; and 43,412 live births resulted from these cycles, representing a cumulative success rate of 30.5%. A total of 18.5% of couples who had one or more ART cycles in 2007 carried a diagnosis of male factor infertility. Their overall likelihood of live birth per ART cycle was 35.8%, with a strongly inverse correlation of success to maternal age.

Sixty-three percent of ART procedures in 2007 involved ICSI, compared to 54% in 2000 [65]. Surprisingly, although ICSI was originally developed specifically to overcome severe oligozoospermia or azoospermia, a diagnosis of male infertility was recorded for only 48% of couples undergoing ICSI.

Cost of Treatment for Male Infertility

The overall economic burden of health care for male infertility is difficult to estimate with precision. While expenditures for office and ambulatory surgery visits were reported by the NAMCS to be $17 million in 2000, this figure does not account for IVF/ICSI or out-of-pocket expenditures [63]. If the assumed cost per ART cycle is $15,000, then expenditures on ART alone for male infertility exceeded $650 million in 2007, given the percentage of ART procedures involving ICSI that were associated with a diagnosis of male factor infertility.

Cost Analysis Models for Management of Male Infertility

When a male risk factor for infertility is identified, the couple is often faced with the choice of using ART or having pathology-directed treatment. Evaluating the economic efficiency of these alternatives is the domain of cost analysis.

Cost analysis is only meaningful with respect to treatments that have previously been demonstrated to be effective. Our intention in this chapter is not to review the studies that have established the effectiveness of the interventions discussed here—or, in some cases, the controversies surrounding them. Rather, our focus is limited to a brief introduction to cost analysis studies as they pertain to male infertility.

Two types of cost analysis are utilized in reproductive medicine: cost-minimization analysis and cost-effectiveness analysis. The first, cost-minimization analysis, is also known as cost identification. It involves assessment (and comparison) of the costs associated with particular treatments. Direct and/or indirect costs may be taken into account—direct costs being health-care expenditures and indirect costs being "downstream" burdens such as transportation expenses, lost wages, etc. In well-conducted economic analyses, future costs should be appropriately discounted to present values by a factor of 3–5% per year.

When the outcomes of alternative interventions are not equivalent, cost-effectiveness analysis is useful to compare them, as it involves not only identifying the costs that accrue but also expressing them relative to the probability of a particular result (e.g., dollars per pregnancy or live birth). Decision analysis, such as Markov modeling, is the most common technique employed for this purpose in the field of male infertility. Details of relevant methodology are covered in *Methods for the Economic Evaluation of Health Care Programmes* [66].

Comparison of cost-effectiveness has been applied to several management options that may be encountered in male reproductive medicine, including varicocele treatment vs. immediate ART (with or without surgical sperm retrieval), vasectomy reversal vs. ART, and hormonal therapy vs. ART for hypogonadotropic hypogonadism. Pathology-directed intervention has almost invariably been found to be more cost-effective than a straight-to-ART approach [67, 68]. One exception is when a varicocele is present in the setting of nonobstructive azoospermia; in this situation, microsurgical testicular sperm extraction (TESE) for ICSI is more cost-effective than varicocelectomy [69].

Every cost-effectiveness analysis in the arena of male infertility is sensitive to assumptions about treatment costs, success and complication rates, and the subsequent management of couples for whom first-line intervention is unsuccessful [70, 71]. Precise characterization of the clinical scenario(s) is very important and should be considered when determining the generalizability of results. For instance, the age of the female partner has a significant influence on the relative cost-effectiveness of vasectomy reversal and ART [72].

Expert Commentary

This chapter examined a number of issues that are commonly misunderstood and/or misrepresented with respect to the epidemiology of infertility, in general, and male infertility, in particular. First, infertility should not be confused with sterility—or even below-average fecundability. Approximately 10% of couples with average reproductive potential will not conceive within 12 months of unprotected intercourse and are therefore designated as infertile. Such couples may comprise a substantial proportion of those who present for evaluation of infertility (see Table 3.3). Their odds of spontaneous, unassisted conception remain high.

From a clinical standpoint, it would be ideal to accurately identify men with below-average reproductive potential. However, while semen analysis is the most common test employed for this purpose, its utility is limited by substantial overlap between the distributions of semen characteristics in empirically fertile and infertile men. Using relatively low diagnostic thresholds, such as the 2010 WHO reference values, carries the advantage of high specificity and perhaps a relatively decent positive predictive value in the setting of an infertility clinic; unfortunately, the negative predictive value only narrowly exceeds that of a coin flip.

The diagnostic inaccuracy of semen analysis is a fundamental problem for several additional reasons. From an epidemiologic perspective, the absence of a gold standard test for male infertility means that we have, at best, an uncertain grasp of its actual prevalence, let alone its association with putative risk factors, such as varicocele, cryptorchidism, sexually transmitted infections, etc. Moreover, if the true prevalence of male infertility is unclear, so, too, is the predictive value of tests employed for its diagnosis.

Finally, there is the question of how to counsel infertile men whose semen parameters exceed diagnostic thresholds. Given the poor predictive value of these "negative" results, should we advise consideration of further evaluation and treatment for modifiable risk factors identified in these individuals? An affirmative response to this query carries the risk of unnecessary treatment and costs, while the alternative may deprive some couples of an improvement in reproductive potential that facilitates natural conception, allows the use of IUI instead of IVF, or increases the odds of successful IVF/ICSI [73]. Well-designed studies to address this question are necessary.

Five-Year View

An indisputable need exists for more accurate diagnostic tests in the field of male infertility. Promising data have been published for analyses of seminal ROS levels and sperm DNA integrity, and the development of these assays is contributing to the advancement of an epidemiologic approach to the management of male factor infertility. Further improvements in understanding of the pathophysiology of male infertility will hopefully give rise to additional and more cost-effective diagnostic and treatment options as well.

Of course, rigorous validation of diagnostic tests in this arena is fraught with challenges, none greater than trying to establish males' actual reproductive potential. Time-to-pregnancy outcomes would seem to be best suited for this purpose, but numerous factors conspire against their reliability, including the play of chance, temporal fluctuations in semen parameters, confounding influences of the female partner's fecundability, and misattributed paternity.

Multivariate models, including those discussed in this chapter, may eventually prove to be valuable for diagnosis of male infertility and construction of nomograms to predict natural conception and live birth [74]. In theory, this would permit a more precise utilization of semen analysis and other test results as "continuous function parameters" that reflect a particular likelihood of male infertility, rather than as dichotomous variables with arbitrary thresholds [75]. This strategy would be analogous to the contemporary use of serum prostate-specific antigen (PSA) testing for prediction of an individual's risk of biopsy-detectable prostate cancer and would similarly permit "individualized decision making" regarding management options [76].

Key Issues

- There is a 15% lifetime incidence of infertility among couples in Western countries; only 3–5% of couples are sterile.
- If the timing of sexual intercourse relative to ovulation is deliberately controlled, the monthly probability of pregnancy may approach 40%; however, the human average for monthly fecundity is 20%.
- Couples who are infertile after 12 months retain a roughly 50% chance of natural conception within the following year. These odds are lower if either partner is over 30 years old; female age, in particular, has a profound effect on fecundability.
- The absence of a gold standard test for male infertility is a fundamental problem, preventing an accurate understanding of its epidemiology and of the predictive value of tests employed for its diagnosis.
- WHO reference values for semen parameters represent the fifth percentile in men with proven fertility; however, there are many infertile men whose semen quality exceeds these thresholds. Basic semen analysis does not capture all of the variables relevant to male reproductive potential.
- Sperm concentration correlates with the probability of conception up to a density of 40 million/mL, but there is no additional likelihood of pregnancy at higher sperm densities.
- Purported declines in semen quality during the twentieth century appear to be an artifact of bias from geographical differences in sperm counts.
- Economic analyses suggest that pathology-directed treatment of male infertility is generally more cost-effective than proceeding directly to ART. Further studies are necessary to clarify which patients will benefit from evaluation and treatment of modifiable risk factors.

Acknowledgments The author would like to thank Kelli M. Mulder-Westrate and Ranya N. Sweis for critically reviewing several drafts of this chapter and offering helpful advice. Jonathan L. Faasse and Kristin M. Faasse provided valuable assistance with the figures.

References

1. Tremellen K. Oxidative stress and male infertility—a clinical perspective. Hum Reprod Update. 2008;14:243–58.
2. Sharma RK, Said T, Agarwal A. Sperm DNA damage and its clinical relevance in assessing reproductive outcome. Asian J Androl. 2004;6:139–48.
3. Athayde KS, Cocuzza M, Agarwal A, et al. Development of normal reference values for seminal reactive oxygen species and their correlation with leukocytes and semen parameters in a fertile population. J Androl. 2007;28:613–20.
4. Agarwal A, Sharma RK, Nallella KP, Thomas AJ, Alvarez JG, Sikka SC. Reactive oxygen species as an independent marker of male factor infertility. Fertil Steril. 2006;86:878–85.
5. Lumley J. Epidemiological approaches to infertility. Reprod Fertil Dev. 1998;10:17–21.
6. Alukal JP, Lipshultz LI. Why treat the male in the era of assisted reproduction? Semin Reprod Med. 2009;27:109–14.

7. Habbema JDF, Collins J, Leridon H, Evers JLH, Lunenfeld B, te Velde ER. Towards less confusing terminology in reproductive medicine: a proposal. Hum Reprod. 2004;19:1497–501.
8. Davies MJ, De Lacey SL, Norman RJ. Towards less confusing terminology in reproductive medicine: clarifying medical ambiguities to the benefit of all. Hum Reprod. 2005;20:2669–71.
9. Greenhall E, Vessey M. The prevalence of subfertility: a review of the current confusion and a report of two new studies. Fertil Steril. 1990;54:978–83.
10. Rowe PJ, Comhaire FH, Hargreave TB, Mahmoud AMA. WHO manual for the standardized investigation, diagnosis and management of the infertile male. New York, NY: Cambridge University Press; 2000.
11. Sigman M, Jarow JP. Male infertility. In: Wein AJ, Kavoussi LR, et al., editors. Campbell-Walsh urology. 9th ed. Philadelphia, PA: Saunders Elsevier; 2007. p. 609–53.
12. Simpson JL, Jauniaux ERM. Pregnancy loss. In: Gabbe SG, Niebyl JR, Simpson JL, editors. Obstetrics: normal and problem pregnancies. 5th ed. Philadelphia, PA: Churchill Livingstone Elsevier; 2007. p. 628–49.
13. Stephen EH, Chandra A. Declining estimates of infertility in the United States: 1982–2002. Fertil Steril. 2006;86:516–23.
14. te Velde ER, Eijkemans R, Habbema HDF. Variation in couple fecundity and time to pregnancy, an essential concept in human reproduction. Lancet. 2000;355:1928–9.
15. Rutstein SO, Shah IH. Infecundity, infertility, and childlessness in developing countries. DHS Comparative Reports No. 9. Calverton, MD: ORC Macro and the World Health Organization; 2004.
16. Lunenfeld B, van Steirteghem A. Infertility in the third millennium: implications for the individual, family and society: condensed meeting report from the Bertarelli Foundation's Second Global Conference. Hum Reprod Update. 2004;10:317–26.
17. Kefer JC, Agarwal A, Sabanegh E. Role of antioxidants in the treatment of male infertility. Int J Urol. 2009;16:449–57.
18. van Noord-Zaadstra BM, Looman CWN, Alsbach H, Habbema JDF, te Velde ER, Karbaat J. Delaying childbearing: effect of age on fecundity and outcome of pregnancy. BMJ. 1991; 302:1361–5.
19. Ford WCL, North K, Taylor H, Farrow A, Hull MGR, Golding J. Increasing paternal age is associated with delayed conception in a large population of fertile couples: evidence for declining fecundity in older men. The ALSPAC Study Team. Hum Reprod. 2000;15: 1703.
20. Evers JLH. Female subfertility. Lancet. 2002;350:151–9.
21. Spira A. Epidemiology of human reproduction. Hum Reprod. 1986;1:111–5.
22. Leridon H, Spira A. Problems in measuring the effectiveness of infertility therapy. Fertil Steril. 1984;41:580–6.
23. Evers JL, te Velde ER. Vruchtbaarheidsstoornissen. In: Heineman MJ, Bleker OP, Evers JL, Heintz AP, editors. Obstetrie en Gynaecologie, de voortplanting van de mens. Maarssen: Elsevier Science; 2001. p. 435–71.
24. Bongaarts J. A method for estimation of fecundability. Demography. 1975;12:645–60.
25. Dunson DB, Colombo B, Baird DD. Changes with age in the level and duration of fertility in the menstrual cycle. Hum Reprod. 2002;17:1399–403.
26. Gnoth C, Godehardt D, Godehardt E, Frank-Herrmann PF, Freundl G. Time to pregnancy: results of the German prospective study and impact on the management of infertility. Hum Reprod. 2003;188: 1959–66.
27. Sharlip ID, Jarow JP, Belker AM, et al. Best practice policies for male infertility. Fertil Steril. 2002;77:873–82.
28. Muller CH. Rationale, interpretation, validation, and uses of sperm function tests. J Androl. 2000;21:10–30.
29. Kobayashi H, Gil-Guzman E, Mahran AM, et al. Quality control of reactive oxygen species measurement by luminol-dependent chemiluminescence assay. J Androl. 2001;22:568–74.
30. Barratt CLR, Aitken RJ, Björndahl L, et al. Sperm DNA: organization, protection and vulnerability: from basic science to clinical applications—a position report. Hum Reprod. 2010; 25:824–38.

31. Menkveld R. Clinical significance of the low normal sperm morphology value as proposed in the fifth edition of the WHO Laboratory Manual for the Examination and Processing of Human Semen. Asian J Androl. 2010;12:47–58.
32. Cooper TG, Noonan E, von Eckardstein S, et al. World Health Organization reference values for human semen characteristics. Hum Reprod Update. 2010;16:231–45.
33. Guzick DS, Overstreet JW, Factor-Litvak P, et al.; for the National Cooperative Reproductive Medicine Network. Sperm morphology, motility, and concentration in fertile and infertile men. NEJM. 2001; 345:1388–93.
34. Zweig MH, Campbell G. Receiver-operating characteristic (ROC) plots: a fundamental evaluation tool in clinical medicine. Clin Chem. 1993;39:561–77.
35. MacLeod J. Semen quality in one thousand men of known fertility and in eight hundred cases of infertile marriage. Fertil Steril. 1951;2:115–39.
36. Niederberger CS. Understanding the epidemiology of fertility treatments. Urol Clin North Am. 2002;29:829–40.
37. Ombelet W, Bosmans E, Janssen M, et al. Semen parameters in a fertile versus subfertile population: a need for change in the interpretation of semen testing. Hum Reprod. 1997; 12:987–93.
38. Gunalp S, Onculoglu C, Gurgan T, Kruger TF, Lombard CJ. A study of semen parameters with emphasis on sperm morphology in a fertile population: an attempt to develop clinical thresholds. Hum Reprod. 2001;16:110–4.
39. Menkveld R, Wong WY, Lombard CJ, et al. Semen parameters, including WHO and strict criteria morphology, in a fertile and subfertile population: an effort towards standardization of in-vivo thresholds. Hum Reprod. 2001;16:1165–71.
40. Jedrzejczak P, Taszarek-Hauke G, Hauke J, Pawelczyk L, Duleba AJ. Prediction of spontaneous conception based on semen parameters. Int J Androl. 2008;31:499–507.
41. van der Merwe FH, Kruger TF, Oehninger SC, Lombard CJ. The use of semen parameters to identify the subfertile male in the general population. Gynecol Obstet Invest. 2005;59:86–91.
42. Zinaman MJ, Brown CC, Selevan SG, Clegg ED. Semen quality and human fertility: a prospective study with healthy couples. J Androl. 2000;21:145–53.
43. Bonde JPE, Ernst E, Jensen TK, et al. Relation between semen quality and fertility: a population-based study of 430 first-pregnancy planners. Lancet. 1998;352:1172–7.
44. Skakkebaek N. Normal reference ranges for semen quality and their relations to fecundity. Asian J Androl. 2010;12:95–8.
45. Leushuis E, van der Steeg JW, Steures P, et al. Prediction models in reproductive medicine: a critical appraisal. Hum Reprod Update. 2009;15:537–52.
46. van der Steeg JW, Steures P, Eijkemans MJC, et al. Pregnancy is predictable: a large-scale prospective external validation of the prediction of spontaneous pregnancy in subfertile couples. Hum Reprod. 2007;22:536–42.
47. Zorn B, Vidmar G, Meden-Vrtovec H. Seminal reactive oxygen species as predictors of fertilization, embryo quality and pregnancy rates after conventional in vitro fertilization and intracytoplasmic sperm injection. Int J Androl. 2003;26:279–85.
48. Mercan R, Lanzendorf SE, Mayer J, Nassar A, Muasher SJ, Oehninger S. The outcome of clinical pregnancies following intracytoplasmic sperm injection is not affected by semen quality. Andrologia. 1998;30:91–5.
49. Ombelet W, Deblaere K, Bosmans E, et al. Semen quality and intrauterine insemination. Reprod Biomed Online. 2003;7:485–92.
50. Allamaneni SS, Bandaranayake I, Agarwal A. Use of semen quality scores to predict pregnancy rates in couples undergoing intrauterine insemination with donor sperm. Fertil Steril. 2004;82:606–11.
51. Shibahara H, Obara H, Ayustawati, et al. Prediction of pregnancy by intrauterine insemination using CASA estimates and strict criteria in patients with male factor infertility. Int J Androl. 2004; 27:63–8.
52. Aitken RJ. Whither must spermatozoa wander? The future of laboratory seminology. Asian J Androl. 2010;12:99–103.

53. Deepinder F, Chowdary HT, Agarwal A. Role of metabolomic analysis of biomarkers in the management of male infertility. Expert Rev Mol Diagn. 2007;7:351–8.
54. Desai N, Sharma R, Makker K, Sabanegh E, Agarwal A. Physiologic and pathologic levels of reactive oxygen species in neat semen of infertile men. Fertil Steril. 2009;92:1626–31.
55. Carlsen E, Giwercman A, Keiding N, Skakkebaek NE. Evidence for decreasing quality of semen during past 50 years. BMJ. 1992;305:609–13.
56. de Kretser DM. Declining sperm counts: environmental chemicals may be to blame. BMJ. 1996;312:457–8.
57. Sharpe RM, Skakkebaek NE. Are oestrogens involved in falling sperm counts and disorders of the male reproductive tract? Lancet. 1993;341:1392–5.
58. Fisch H. Declining worldwide sperm counts: disproving a myth. Urol Clin N Am. 2008; 35:137–46.
59. Sherins RJ. Are semen quality and male fertility changing? NEJM. 1995;332:327–8.
60. Fisch H, Goluboff ET. Geographic variations in sperm counts: a potential cause of bias in studies of semen quality. Fertil Steril. 1996;65:1044–6.
61. Fisch H, Goluboff ET, Olson JH, Feldshuh J, Broder SJ, Barad DH. Semen analyses in 1,283 men from the United States over a 25-year period: no decline in quality. Fertil Steril. 1996;65:1009–14.
62. Saidi JA, Chang DT, Goluboff ET, Bagiella E, Olsen G, Fisch H. Declining sperm counts in the United States? A critical review. J Urol. 1999;161:460–2.
63. Niederberger CS, Joyce GF, Wise M, Meacham RB. Male infertility. In: Litwin MS, Saigal CS, editors. Urologic diseases in America. US Department of Health and Human Services, Public Health Service, National Institutes of Health, National Institute of Diabetes and Digestive and Kidney Diseases. Washington, DC: U.S. Government Printing Office; 2007, NIH Publication No. 07-5512. p. 461–81.
64. Centers for Disease Control and Prevention (CDC), American Society for Reproductive Medicine, Society for Assisted Reproductive Technology. 2007 assisted reproductive technology success rates: national summary and fertility clinic reports. Atlanta: U.S. Department of Health and Human Services, Centers for Disease Control and Prevention; 2009.
65. Wright VC, Schieve LA, Reynolds MA, Jeng G. Assisted reproductive technology surveillance—United States, 2000. MMWR Surveill Summ. 2003;52(No. SS-9):1–16.
66. Drummond MF, Schulpher MJ, Torrance GW, O'Brien BJ, Stoddart GL. Methods for the economic evaluation of health care programmes. 3rd ed. New York, NY: Oxford University Press; 2005. p. 277–322.
67. Shin D, Honig SC. Economics of treatments for male infertility. Urol Clin N Am. 2002; 29:841–53.
68. Robb P, Sandlow JI. Cost-effectiveness of vasectomy reversal. Urol Clin N Am. 2009;36:391–6.
69. Lee R, Li PS, Goldstein M, Schattman G, Schlegel PN. A decision analysis of treatments for nonobstructive azoospermia associated with varicocele. Fertil Steril. 2009;92:188–96.
70. Penson DF, Paltiel AD, Krumholz HM, Palter S. The cost-effectiveness of treatment for varicocele related infertility. J Urol. 2002;168: 2490–4.
71. Meng MV, Greene KL, Turek PJ. Surgery or assisted reproduction? A decision analysis of treatment costs in male infertility. J Urol. 2005;174:1926–31.
72. Hsieh MH, Meng MV, Turek PJ. Markov modeling of vasectomy reversal and ART for infertility: how do obstructive interval and female partner age influence cost effectiveness? Fertil Steril. 2007;88:840–6.
73. Esteves SC, Oliveira FV, Bertolla RP. Clinical outcome of intracytoplasmic sperm injection in infertile men with treated and untreated clinical varicocele. J Urol. 2010;184:1442–6.
74. Boyd JC. Defining laboratory reference values and decision limits: populations, intervals, and interpretations. Asian J Androl. 2010;12:83–90.
75. Niederberger C. Responses to semen analysis CART report. J Androl. 2003;24:329–31.
76. Thompson IM, Ankerst DP, Etzioni R, Wang T. It's time to abandon an upper limit of normal for prostate specific antigen: assessing the risk of prostate cancer. J Urol. 2008;180:1218–22.

Part II
Oxidants and Antioxidants

Chapter 4
Physiological Role of Reactive Oxygen Species in Sperm Function: A Review

Aaron Thompson, Ashok Agarwal, and Stefan S. du Plessis

Introduction

Mammalian spermatozoa were the first cells reported to produce reactive oxygen species (ROS). The pathophysiological effects of ROS on sperm function have been well studied since the discovery of their toxic effects on sperm motility by McLeod [1]. The study of ROS has since focused on the concept of oxidative stress (OS). Antioxidants scavenge and negate the detrimental effects of ROS, but when overwhelmed because of high ROS or low antioxidant levels, they are unable to control the high degree of ROS-induced damage, resulting in OS [2]. OS can damage proteins, carbohydrates, nucleic acids, and lipids [3, 4]. Spermatozoa are uniquely susceptible to OS because they have limited cell repair systems [5] and antioxidant defenses due to a low cytoplasmic volume. Furthermore, spermatozoa are especially susceptible to lipid peroxidation (LPO) because of the uniquely high content of poly-unsaturated fatty acids (PUFA) present in their plasma membrane. LPO may result in membrane permeabilization, causing an efflux of ATP necessary for flagellar movement [6, 7]. OS can further affect sperm function by impairing the viability, motility, and fertilization potential of spermatozoa [8–11]. Conversely, Aitken et al. [12] was the first study to suggest that ROS are involved in normal sperm function. Since, the study of the physiological levels of ROS in sperm function has led to a general acknowledgment that ROS act as intracellular signaling molecules essential to many physiologic processes, including maturation, hyperactivation, capacitation, the acrosome reaction (AR), and sperm-oocyte fusion. A better understanding

A. Thompson • A. Agarwal (✉)
Cleveland Clinic, Center for Reproductive Medicine, Glickman Urological
and Kidney Institute, 9500 Euclid Avenue, Cleveland, OH 44195, USA
e-mail: agarwaa@ccf.org

S.S. du Plessis
Medical Physiology, Stellenbosch University, Tygerberg, South Africa

S.J. Parekattil and A. Agarwal (eds.), *Antioxidants in Male Infertility: A Guide
for Clinicians and Researchers,* © Springer Science+Business Media New York 2013

of physiological mechanisms of ROS in human spermatozoa can lead to an improved etiological understanding of male reproductive pathology. This review will focus on the beneficial role and known molecular mechanisms of ROS-essential processes, with a specific focus on human spermatozoa.

Endogenous ROS Production by Sperm

The term ROS encompasses a large group of molecules, including free radicals (superoxide, $O_2^{-\bullet}$; hydroxyl, $OH^{\bullet}$; peroxyl, $ROO^{\bullet}$), peroxides (hydrogen peroxide, H_2O_2), and various oxygen derivatives (singlet oxygen, $^{-1}O_2$; hypochlorous acid, $HOCl$) (Table 4.1). Often synonymous with ROS are reactive nitrogen species (RNS), including nitric oxide ($NO^{\bullet}$), nitrogen dioxide ($NO_2^{\bullet}$), and peroxynitrate ($ONOO^-$) (Table 4.2). A free radical is defined as any species/molecule that can exist independently and contains one or more unpaired electrons [2]. Diatomic oxygen, in its natural state, is a free radical containing two unpaired electrons, but the electronic arrangement of these two electrons—parallel spin states—makes oxygen quite inert in reactions with non-radical species [2, 13].

The $O_2^{-\bullet}$ radical is the primary free radical generated by respiring cells. It is produced in a monovalent reduction of oxygen via the addition of a single electron [13, 14]. In spermatozoa, two main sources of $O_2^{-\bullet}$ production exist, an NADH-dependent oxido-reductase (diaphorase) in the inner mitochondrial membrane

Table 4.1 Reactive oxygen species and (abbreviated) chemical formulas

Radical ROS		Non-radical ROS	
Superoxide	$O_2^{-\bullet}$	Hydrogen peroxide	H_2O_2
Hydroxyl	$OH^{\bullet}$	Hypochloric acid	$HOCl$
Thyl	$RS^{-\bullet}$	Lipid peroxide	$LOOH$
Peroxyl	$RO_2^{\bullet}$	Ozone	O_3
Lipid peroxyl	$LOO^{\bullet}$	Singlet oxygen	$^{-1}O_2$

Table 4.2 Reactive nitrogen species and (abbreviated) chemical formulas

RNS		RNS	
Nitric oxide	$NO^{\bullet}$	Nitryl chloride	NO_2Cl
Peroxynitrate	$ONOO^-$	Nitrogen dioxide	$NO_2^{\bullet}$
Peroxynitrous acid	$ONOOH$	Dinitrogen trioxide	N_2O_3
Nitroxyl anion	NO^-	Nitrous acid	HNO_2
Nitrosyl cation	NO^+		

and an NAD(P)H oxidase in the plasma membrane. It has long been known that $O_2^{-\bullet}$ is a normal by-product of oxidative phosphorylation [15]. Specifically, $O_2^{-\bullet}$ is formed between complexes I and III in the electron transport chain (ETC) (reviewed by Aitken and Clarkson [9] and Koppers et al. [16]). In between these two complexes an electron may add to an intracellular oxygen atom to produce $O_2^{-\bullet}$ [17, 18].

It was commonly hypothesized, based on the oxidative burst of neutrophils, that there existed a membrane-bound source of extracellular $O_2^{-\bullet}$ in mammalian spermatozoa [9, 19, 20]. Several later experiments showed results consistent with the presence of an NAD(P)H oxidase in spermatozoa [19, 21–27], the enzyme determined to be responsible for ROS production in leukocytes, although evidence of its existence was only recently identified by polymer chain reaction analysis [18, 28].

Although the $O_2^{-\bullet}$ radical is relatively unreactive [13], in the presence of H^+ it undergoes either spontaneous or enzyme-catalyzed dismutation into H_2O_2, a more reactive, membrane permeable molecule (Halliwell and Cross 1989). The conversion of $O_2^{-\bullet}$ into H_2O_2 is catalyzed by superoxide dismutase (SOD), an enzyme found within the cytoplasm of spermatozoa as well as the epididymis and seminal plasma [7, 29]. H_2O_2 has been established as the major initiator of peroxidative damage in the plasma membrane of spermatozoa [5, 30]. H_2O_2 can be scavenged by the enzymatic oxidants glutathione peroxidase or catalase, catalyzing the dismutation of H_2O_2 into water and oxygen. Different glutathione peroxidases (Gpx) are present within spermatozoa [31], whereas concentrations of catalase are only significant in the seminal plasma [29].

Endogenous RNS Production by Sperm

The primary RNS species in human spermatozoa is $NO^\bullet$. Its production is catalyzed by the enzyme nitric oxide synthase (NOS) in a redox-reaction between L-arginine (Arg) and oxygen, initiated by NADPH, with L-citrulline formed as a by-product. $NO^\bullet$ reacts with $O_2^{-\bullet}$ to form $ONOO^-$, a highly toxic species. The reaction of $O_2^{-\bullet}$ with $NO^\bullet$ is three times faster than the reaction of $O_2^{-\bullet}$ with SOD [32]. Thus the presence of $NO^\bullet$ may contribute to OS. Paradoxically, both high and low concentrations of $NO^\bullet$ may result in significant detriment to sperm function through the production of $ONOO^-$. In arginine-depleted cells, NOS have been shown to synthesize more $O_2^{-\bullet}$ [2, 33] (Halliwell and Cross 1998), which because of its short half-life is generally the limiting reactant in the formation of $ONOO^-$. Appropriate $NO^\bullet$ concentration has beneficial effects; it has been demonstrated to act in signal transduction pathways involved in the motility, capacitation, and the AR of spermatozoa [34, 35]. Despite these benefits, the majority of studies focus specifically on the effects of ROS on sperm function, and for this reason, $NO^\bullet$ is mentioned only briefly in the remaining sections. For greater information about the effects of $NO^\bullet$, see the reviews by Herrero and Gagnon [35] as well as Sikka [32].

Seminal Values of ROS and Fertility

The upper critical value for ROS levels in semen samples of normozoospermic men varies between studies. Das et al. [10] determined the upper threshold to be $(0.075$–$0.1)\times10^6$ counted photons per minute (cpm)/10 million cells when measured via chemiluminescence and a luminol probe. When subjects were separated into two groups, including those below and those above this threshold value, the group with higher ROS levels exhibited a lower clinical pregnancy rate (47.6 % vs. 17.6 %) [10]. In addition, in subjects with proven fertility, all 17 subjects displayed levels of ROS below this upper threshold [10], indicating that this critical value correlates with a significant difference in fertility potential.

A later study by Desai et al. [36] determined that, in estimation of positive fertility potential, a better specificity (82 %), sensitivity (78 %), and the highest accuracy (80 %) were obtained when a cutoff value of 0.0185×10^6 cpm/20×10^6 sperm was employed in comparison with several other values, including that found by Das et al. [10]. Patients divided into two groups via this cutoff value showed significant differences in concentration, motility, and viability. The use of this critical value should provide a means to select patients for antioxidant treatment as a method to improve semen parameters.

A Brief Overview of the Pathology of Oxidative Stress and Spermatozoa

Over the last 40 years, testicular dysgenesis syndrome (TDS)—the term generally applied to the overall degeneration of male reproductive health—has been evidenced as a global phenomenon. A meta-analysis by Carlsen et al. [37] reported a significant reduction in sperm concentrations of fertile men between 1940 and 1990, in which 1990 sperm concentrations were only 58.4 % of those recorded in 1940 (66×10^6/mL vs. 113×10^6/mL). As suggested by these authors and progressed by subsequent studies, this universal trend points to a common etiology, specifically related to the production of excess ROS [14, 38].

The link between OS and male infertility has been under intense scrutiny. Several statistics indicate that elevated levels of ROS are found in up to 25 % of semen samples of infertile men and up to 81 % of patients with spinal cord injury [39–41]. Male patients diagnosed with varicocele, leukocytospermia, idiopathic infertility, and spinal injuries all have been associated with elevated levels of ROS [9, 11, 41–45]. The presence of high ROS levels in seminal plasma may cause male infertility by initiating premature hyperactivation of spermatozoa. In such a case, the nonprogressive motility associated with hyperactivation may prevent coordinated movement from the cervical mucus to the oviduct [46]. In addition, premature hyperactivation may be related to early development of capacitation and the inopportune induction of the AR [47].

ROS levels vary considerably between patients [9, 39] and pathological levels of ROS are more likely due to increased production of ROS rather than decreased antioxidant capacity of spermatozoa or seminal plasma [40]. Abnormal spermatozoa [39] and leukocyte contamination [48] may be responsible for the excess production of ROS. In contrast, decreased total antioxidant capacity (TAC) of the seminal plasma has been associated with male infertility [49].

The macro-effects of OS include a decrease in sperm motility [3, 8, 39, 50] (De Lamirande and Gagnon 2002), viability [8, 51], percent normal morphology [52], as well as impairment of hyperactivation [53], capacitation [27], AR [13, 53], and sperm-oocyte fusion [10, 12, 54].

The molecular effects of ROS in sperm pathology have been well studied. The generation of toxic lipid peroxides in the plasma membrane [3, 6, 13, 14] and damage to nuclear DNA [10, 55], mitochondrial DNA [4, 56], and amino acids [14] have all been observed. The specific effect of ROS on nuclear DNA is due to an increase in DNA fragmentation, base-pair modifications, chromatin cross-linking, and chromosomal microdeletions [14, 38, 55]. Decreased energy availability is responsible for the observed loss in sperm motility [50], largely through LPO and mtDNA mutations. If one of the 13 genes for the ETC harbored in the mitochondria is damaged, not only could ATP production decrease, but intracellular ROS production may increase [4]. In addition, oxidation of an essential thiol group of glyceraldehydes-3-phosphate dehydrogenase (GAPDH), a glycolytic enzyme, or loss of adenine and pyridine nucleotides because of LPO, may be responsible for the decreased motility [6, 57].

Physiological Roles of ROS

At low concentrations, ROS have been shown to exhibit positive effects on spermatozoa during maturation, hyperactivation, capacitation, the AR, and sperm-oocyte fusion. The species responsible for the beneficial effects in specific physiologic processes—either $O_2^{-\bullet}$ or H_2O_2—is controversial. Studies using spermatozoa from different mammalian species have conflicting results, driving some researchers to conclude that species-specific differences exist [20]. The specific focus of this review will be on human spermatozoa but will also include studies from various mammalian species when appropriate.

Maturation

During transit and storage in the epididymis, spermatozoa undergo membrane, nuclear, and enzyme-related remodeling, including the release, attachment, and rearrangement of surface proteins [17, 29, 52]. These changes include the assembly of the signal transduction machinery that is necessary for the potential of spermatozoa to undergo hyperactivation and capacitation [26] and constitute maturation.

ROS are necessary for proper chromatin packing in the maturation of mammalian spermatozoa, which exhibit characteristic chromatin stability, the process of which is regulated via redox processes [18]. Responsible for the unique stability is the extensive inter- and intra-molecular disulfide bonds between cysteine residues of protamines. Protamines are small, nuclear proteins that replace histones during spermiogenesis. The oxidation of thiol groups on protamines occurs during the journey of spermatozoa from the caput to caudal epididymis [58]. This process likely occurs in the caudal epididymis, where the sperm are stored prior to ejaculation. As shown by Aitken et al. [26], a spontaneous luminol-peroxidase signal—indicating the presence of H_2O_2 or $O_2^{-\bullet}$—was unique to mature spermatozoa in the caudal epididymis. Although there are relatively few cysteine residues in human protamines ($8\ pmol/10^6$ sperm), the majority of thiol groups are in the oxidized form as disulfide bonds. Rousseaux and Rousseaux-Prevost [59] stated that only 1.5 % of the cysteine groups in human protamines were in the reduced form, suggesting that the majority of the thiol groups were occupied as disulfide bonds. ROS may act as oxidizing agents in this process, thereby facilitating the formation of disulfide bonds, increasing chromatin stability, and protecting DNA from physical or chemical damage [59]. Because spermatozoa possess minimal repair mechanisms [5], further chromatin condensation is a necessary protective process. Ironically, in this way, ROS may actually protect spermatozoa from future damage induced by OS.

In a similar manner, peroxides have been implicated in the proper formation of the "mitochondrial capsule," the protective coat surrounding mitochondria that confers protection from proteolytic degradation [60]. It is proposed that during spermatogenesis peroxides may oxidize the free, active phospholipid hydroperoxide glutathione peroxidase (PHGPx) enzyme, forming an intermediate that reacts with a protein thiol group to form a selenadisulfide bond. The result is an active mitochondrial capsule made of a complex protein network characteristically high in disulfide bonds. Mitochondria necessitate such protection because they are essential to cell metabolism, mediate apoptosis and ROS production. Damage to any of the above may result in impaired function [4].

Recent studies on the effects of oral antioxidant therapy for male infertility have shown an improved DNA integrity and reduced ROS production as a result of daily antioxidant consumption over a 3-month period [61], but problems with unusual decondensation of sperm DNA have been reported [62]. The hypothesis is that high antioxidant levels may interfere with the oxidative conditions necessary for proper formation of inter- and intra-molecular disulfide bonds, resulting in improper DNA compaction and paternal DNA decondensation.

ROS as Signal Transducers

Results from numerous studies suggest that ROS enhances hyperactivation, capacitation, and the AR via an intermediate effect [5, 17, 22, 24, 63]. This has been suggested based on the small size, short half-life, and ubiquitous nature of ROS [22]. The exact mechanism in/by which ROS stimulate these processes is thought to occur via redox regulation of cysteine residues. These thiol groups exist either in reduced (S—H) or oxidized (S—S) forms and are a reversible method to modify enzyme activity [64, 65]. The common mechanism involved in these processes is as follows (1) ROS activate adenyl cyclase (AC); (2) AC stimulates the production of cyclic AMP (cAMP) and increases intracellular concentration of cAMP; (3) cAMP signals downstream protein kinase A (PKA) molecules; (4) PKA acts on a variety of substrates depending on the maturational state of the spermatozoa and process involved.

Motility and Hyperactivation

Hyperactivation is an incompletely understood process in the maturation of spermatozoa and is considered to be a subset capacitation. Normally spermatozoa exhibit low amplitude flagellar movement, and low, linear velocity. In the hyperactivated state, spermatozoa exhibit high amplitude, asymmetric flagellar movement, pronounced lateral head displacement, and nonlinear trajectory [66, 67] that allows the sperm to penetrate the cumulus cells and zona pellucida surrounding the oocyte upon the completion of the AR [20, 68] (reviewed by Suarez [69]). In this way, hyperactivation is a necessary component for successful fertilization, although it is not necessary to undergo the AR. In addition, hyperactive motility may facilitate progressive movement through the oviduct by preventing stagnation in this tissue, adding another potential benefit to sperm function [69]. The biochemistry of hyperactivation is poorly understood, but as mentioned above, does involve a rise in cAMP activity and pH [65], increased generation of ROS [42], an initial influx of bicarbonate ions [20], and an increase in intracellular calcium (Ca^{2+}) concentrations [38, 69].

It is known that ROS affect sperm motility and SOD plays a significant role in prevention of this process [5, 70]. Hyperactivation may be the result of an increase in intracellular ATP, the cellular energy source [69, 71]. Extracellular $O_2^{-\bullet}$ is deemed nearly essential to hyperactivation in human spermatozoa because the presence of SOD, and not catalase, reduced the percentage of spermatozoa exhibiting hyperactivity in a variety of media, including Ham's F-10, Ham's + xanthine + xanthine-oxidase (X + XO), fetal cord serum (FCS), and fetal cord serum ultrafiltrate (FCSU) [47, 72, 73]. The inhibition of hyperactivation in FCS, a known biological inducer of hyperactivation and capacitation, suggests the activity of $O_2^{-\bullet}$ in this biological fluid [72, 73]. This study demonstrated that $O_2^{-\bullet}$, not H_2O_2, was the main species responsible for the enhanced hyperactivity exhibited by spermatozoa. This hypothesis was strengthened by subsequent experiments.

Kobayashi et al. [70] determined that SOD activity had a significant positive correlation with the number of motile spermatozoa. In slight contrast, a significant ($P < 0.002$) positive correlation between reduced SOD-like activity and percent sperm exhibiting hyperactivity has been shown [47]. Again, in another study [73], a significantly different level of hyperactivation was observed in media containing $O_2^{-\bullet}$ (X + XO + catalase; 15.4 ± 1.6 %) compared to the control medium of Ham's F-10 (5.4 ± 0.6 %). These studies firmly evaluated the role of ROS in

Table 4.3 Experimental results summary for the effect of ROS on hyperactivation

Study author(s)	Variable	Effect on hyperactivation
Aitken et al. [22]	H_2O_2 (50 µM)	No effect
De Lamirande and Gagnon [72]	SOD	–
	X + XO + catalase	+
De Lamirande and Gagnon [73]	X + XO + catalase	+
	X + XO + catalase + SOD	–
	X + XO	–
De Lamirande and Gagnon [47]	SOD	–
Griveau et al. [74]	H_2O_2 (25 µM)	+
	Catalase ($\geq$500 U/mL)	–
Griveau et al. [75]	SOD	No effect
Oehninger et al. [53]	H_2O_2 (10, 50 µM)	–

hyperactivation of human spermatozoa and suggest that $O_2^{-\bullet}$ is the key species involved in ROS-induced hyperactivation.

A later study by Griveau et al. [74] found results that differ from those found by De Lamirande and Gagnon [47, 72, 73], the latter having found that H_2O_2 was detrimental to hyperactivation. Griveau et al. [74] reported that the presence of 500 U/mL catalase significantly inhibited hyperactivation (by 43 %) compared to the control. In addition, a concentration of 25 µM H_2O_2 significantly enhanced hyperactivation ($P<0.005$). As suggested by Griveau et al. [74], the discrepancy may be explained by the differences in hyperactivation criteria. The two variables compared were curvilinear velocity (VCL), the total distance traveled divided by the total time the cell was tracked, and linearity, the ratio of the straight-line distance to the actual track distance. In the study by De Lamirande and Gagnon [72], spermatozoa exhibiting a VCL > 80 µm/s and linearity <6.6 were deemed to be hyperactivated. Whereas Griveau et al. [74] used more selective criteria: only those spermatozoa with a VCL > 100 µm/s and linearity <4.5 were considered to be hyperactivated. Griveau et al. [74] argue that the discrepancy in results is due to differences in hyperactivity criteria. These two studies suggest that H_2O_2 may positively affect hyperactivation at low concentrations, but noted that the beneficial role of $O_2^{-\bullet}$ is more easily observed.

Additional studies of human spermatozoa have differed from those previously discussed. Aitken et al. [22] observed that the exogenous addition of H_2O_2 to spermatozoa had no significant effect on motility and Oehninger et al. [53] found an inverse relationship between these two variables. These studies provide evidence that the impact of H_2O_2 on hyperactivation—and potentially other processes as well—is concentration specific. The use of 50 and 100 µM H_2O_2 by Aitken et al. [22] and the 10, 50 µM, and greater concentrations used by Oehninger et al. [53] both bypassed the optimally beneficial concentration (25 µM) determined by Griveau et al. [74]. Therefore the difference in concentrations employed by different studies may be a reasonable explanation for the discrepancy in observed results.

Taken together, these studies indicate that ROS can positively affect the process of hyperactivation in spermatozoa (Table 4.3). Specifically, $O_2^{-\bullet}$ seems to be the major contributor to the positive effect, but the effect of H_2O_2 is ambiguous depending on the concentration, likely due to the fine balance between peroxidative damage and functional activation. For the biochemistry of hyperactivation, please refer to the section on capacitation to follow below.

Capacitation

Capacitation is the general priming of the spermatozoa for fertilization and includes the process of hyperactivation. Capacitation is a relatively poorly understood process of final maturation that spermatozoa undergo in the female genital tract post-ejaculation. It is hypothesized that the process selects only mature spermatozoa to reach the oocyte via the benefits of hyperactive motility and an increased responsiveness to chemotactic signaling [76]. The molecular effects include a Ca^{2+} and HCO_3^- influx, cholesterol efflux, and an increase in cAMP activity, ROS generation, pH, protein phosphorylation (Ser/Thr and Tyr), and membrane hyperpolarization [20, 77]. There are few in vitro techniques to definitively distinguish between capacitated and non-capacitated spermatozoa; a common methodology is to assess the ability of spermatozoa to undergo the AR. In capacitated spermatozoa, the AR can be induced by the Ca^{2+} ionophore A23187, lysophosphatidylcholine (LPC), solubilized zona pellucida, and more recently discovered, progesterone (Tables 4.4 and 4.5). Biochemical assays exist to evaluate changes in cell surface molecules; most notable is the use of chlortetracycline (CTC) as a staining reagent [20].

The majority of studies to date on both human and other mammalian spermatozoa indicate that H_2O_2 is responsible for the activation of capacitation. Similar study designs have been implemented in order to determine whether H_2O_2 enhances capacitation or the AR, because as noted above, induction of the AR evaluates capacitation status but alone does not distinguish between the specific effects on the two processes. The addition of SOD or catalase to the incubation media either initially (time zero) or directly before the AR assesses whether ROS impact capacitation or AR [74, 75]. Use of ionophore A23187, which acts as a membrane Ca^{2+} transporter to activate the AR, showed that the addition of 25 µM H_2O_2 to the incubation medium significantly increased the AR [74]. To assess whether the effect was on capacitation or the AR, spermatozoa were exposed to catalase at various times of incubation. Catalase added initially to the incubation medium decreased the AR in relation to both the control (no catalase) and late-addition catalase (5 h 45 min) groups, indicating that H_2O_2 affects the long-term process of capacitation rather than the quick AR.

Similar studies performed by De Lamirande and Gagnon [72, 73] indicated that $O_2^{-\bullet}$ is also involved in the process of capacitation. The significantly higher levels of LPC-induced AR observed in the presence of X + XO + catalase and FCSU were unaffected when SOD was added 5 min before the addition of LPC. This suggests that SOD had no effect on the initiation of AR induced by LPC, but rather affected capacitation. This study provides evidence for the role of $O_2^{-\bullet}$, in capacitation, but not the AR.

Table 4.4 Experimental results summary for the effect of ROS on sperm capacitation

Study author(s)	Subject(s)	Measurement method	Variable	Effect on capacitation
Bize et al. [78]	Hamster	Glucose oxidase (H_2O_2)–AR	Catalase	–
		Epinephrine–AR	Catalase (10 µg/mL)	–
			SOD (50 µg/mL)	No effect
De Lamirande and Gagnon [72, 73]	Human	LPC–AR	Catalase	No effect
			SOD	–
Griveau et al. [74]	Human	A23187–AR	H_2O_2 (25 µM)	+
			Catalase	–
Griveau et al. [75]	Human	A23187–AR	SOD	–
Aitken et al. [22]	Human	A23187–AR	Catalase	–
			SOD (0.1 mg/mL)	No effect
Zini et al. [34]	Human	Diethylamine/spermine-NONOate (NO·)	Catalase	–
			SOD	No sig. effect
Leclerc et al. [24]	Human	Tyr phosphorylation	GO, H_2O_2	+
			Catalase	–
			SOD	–
Aitken et al. [79, 80]	Human	Tyr phosphorylation	NADPH ($O_2^{-·}$)	+
			NADPH + catalase	–
		Spontaneous/induced P-tyr	2-Mercaptoethanol	–
O'Flaherty et al. (1997, 1999) [81]	Bull	LPC–AR	SOD	–
Lewis and Aitken[25]	Rat	Tyrosine phosphorylation	H_2O_2	+
Zheng and Zhang (2001)	Human	Spontaneous–AR, LPC–AR, cAMP	SOD	–
Baumber et al. [82]	Horse	Progesterone–AR	X – XO, NADPH	+
			X – XO + Cat or SOD	–
Rivlin et al. [27]	Bull	Tyr phosphorylation	Catalase	–
			H_2O_2	+
Roy and Atreja [83]	Buffalo	LPC–AR, Tyr phosphorylation	X + XO, X + XO + Cat	+
			SOD/Cat + heparin	–

Many of the methods involve the induction of the acrosome reaction and are denoted "substance-AR."

Table 4.5 Experimental results summary for ROS and the effects on the acrosome reaction (AR)

Study author(s)	AR-induction method	Variable	Effect on AR
Aitken et al. [79]	Progesterone	Catalase	–
		SOD	No effect
Griveau et al. [75]	A23187	SOD	–
	Spontaneous	$O_2^{-\bullet}$ + catalase	No effect
Leclerc et al. [24]	A23187, progesterone, rhuZP3	Catalase	–
	A23187	SOD	No effect
De Lamirande et al. [84]	A23187, LPC, Ffu, FCSu	Catalase (0.2 mg/mL)	–
		SOD (0.1 mg/mL)	–
	H_2O_2	H_2O_2 (50 µM)	+

Harmonious results have been obtained in bovine spermatozoa using the same LPC-induced AR technique [81].

Although the aforementioned study showed that $O_2^{-\bullet}$ was responsible for enhanced capacitation in spermatozoa, later studies have strengthened the position that H_2O_2 is the primary initiator of capacitation [22, 27, 78]. The use of ionophore A23187 to induce the AR in spermatozoa incubated for 3 h in either SOD or catalase showed that incubation with catalase significantly decreased the percent of sperm undergoing the AR; SOD had no significant effect on the AR [22]. In addition, as capacitation is associated with an increase in tyrosine phosphorylation, the amount and banding pattern of tyrosine phosphorylation via addition of exogenous H_2O_2 was similar to that observed in the endogenous production of ROS, indicating that H_2O_2 produced endogenously is responsible for the enhanced capacitation. A more recent study by Rivlin et al. [27] showed similar results: catalase decreased and H_2O_2 increased tyrosine phosphorylation in dose-dependent manners, thereby solidifying the involvement of H_2O_2 in the process of capacitation. Of note is the involvement of NO, which is present in the female genital tract, in capacitation. NO may initiate the AR, the effects of which are likely achieved through a complex mechanism involving H_2O_2, as catalase prevented the capacitation of human spermatozoa in vitro [34].

The results of the above studies indicate that ROS can positively enhance capacitation in human spermatozoa, but diverge over the specific ROS involved. The two methods used to induce the AR, either with ionophore A23187 or LPC, may differ in the exact way in which they stimulate the AR [84]. Therefore, $O_2^{-\bullet}$ and H_2O_2 may stimulate different molecules in the biochemical pathway, and depending on the method used to induce the AR, the specific ROS involved may therefore differ (Table 4.4). Several studies have confirmed the lack of molecular specificity in the activation of capacitation and tyrosine phosphorylation, as both SOD and catalase have been shown to negate the positive effect exogenously induced capacitation and hyperactivation [83, 84]. Overall, despite the mixed results, H_2O_2 is recognized to be more centrally involved in the regulation of tyrosine phosphorylation [30, 79].

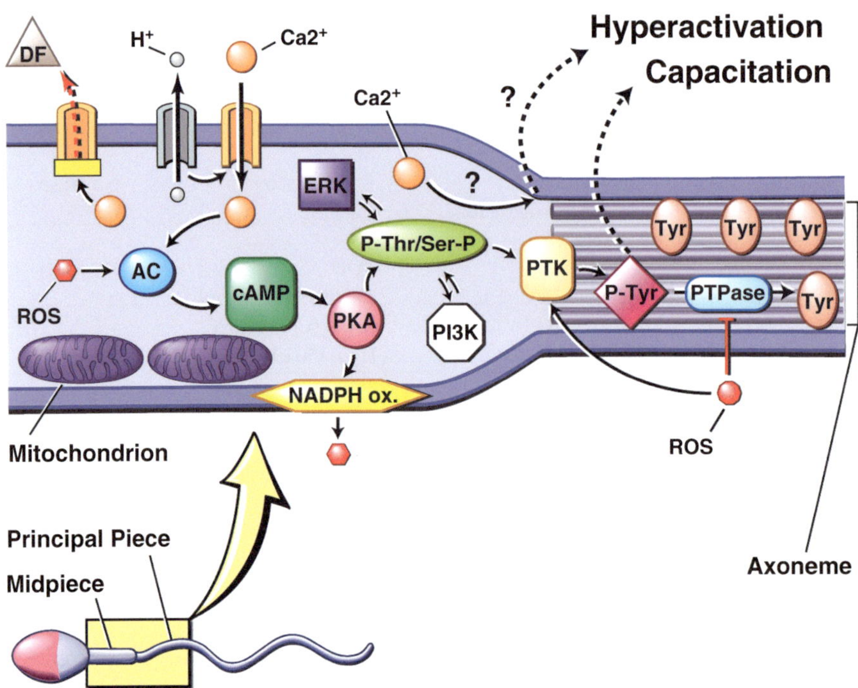

Fig. 4.1 Biochemical pathway proposed to regulate sperm capacitation and hyperactivation. The process is initiated by an influx of Ca^{2+} and HCO_3^-, possibly caused by the inactivation of an ATP-dependent Ca^{2+} regulatory channel (PMCA) and alkalization of the cytosol. Both Ca^{2+} and ROS, specifically $O_2^{-\bullet}$, activate adenylate cyclase (AC), which produces cyclic adenosine monophosphate (cAMP). cAMP activates downstream protein kinase A (PKA). PKA triggers a membrane-bound NADPH oxidase to stimulate greater ROS production. In addition, PKA triggers phosphorylation of Ser and Tyr residues that, in addition to other interconnected pathways, lead to the activation of protein tyrosine kinase (PTK). PTK phosphorylates tyrosine residues of the fibrous sheath surrounding the axoneme, the cytoskeletal component of the flagellum. ROS, specifically hydrogen peroxide, increases the amount of tyrosine phosphorylation by promoting PTK activity and inhibiting phosphotyrosine phosphatase (PTPase) activity, which normally de-phosphorylates Tyr residues. The enhanced tyrosine phosphorylation observed in capacitation is the last known step in the process, but intermediate steps or other (in)direct methods may be involved

The exact biochemistry of capacitation is still not completely understood. The process has been shown to be associated with several changes, included in these are: a cholesterol efflux from the plasma membrane, increases in free intracellular Ca^{2+}, HCO_3^-, cAMP, pH, actin polymerization, ROS production, and tyrosine phosphorylation in the proteins of the fibrous sheath and midpiece [20, 24, 27, 65, 66, 85]. ROS have been shown to increase tyrosine phosphorylation by both activation of tyrosine kinases and inhibition of phosphotyrosine phosphatases (PTPase) via oxidation of cysteine residues [20, 24] (Fig. 4.1). Recent studies have suggested that $O_2^{-\bullet}$ stimulates AC [23, 25], while H_2O_2 directly acts on kinases and phosphatases to induce capacitation [25]. AC produces cAMP, which has been shown to increase intracellular $O_2^{-\bullet}$ formation and suggests a free Ca^{2+}-dependent positive feedback loop [12, 86]. The increase in cAMP is ROS-dependent [80] (De Lamirande and O'Flaherty 2008). cAMP stimulates PKA, a necessary component for capacitation [65]. PKA acts on a variety of substrates to induce tyrosine phosphorylation, which primarily occurs in the principal piece of the flagellum and the midpiece [85], although also present at the apical piece of the plasma membrane [30]. Phosphorylation of tyrosine residues of A kinase anchoring proteins (AKAPs), structural proteins that bind PKA substrates and other signaling enzymes to the cytoskeleton, may regulate the process of hyperactivation [77]. In addition, tyrosine phosphorylation may positively affect the induction of the AR via two plasma membrane proteins (35 and 46 kDa) that when phosphorylated were shown to increase binding affinity to the ZP in boar sperm [87].

Several different biochemical pathways are implicated in the capacitation of human spermatozoa, including the PKA-dependent pathway, ERK pathway, and the PI3K axis. Cross-talk, or the interconnectivity between these pathways, has been proposed to tightly regulate tyrosine phosphorylation and capacitation to provide timely activation of spermatozoa fertilizing potential [65]. Tyrosine phosphorylation is often used as a measurement of capacitation progress because the capacity to undergo the AR in response to a variety of stimuli is dependent on the amount of tyrosine phosphorylation [79]. Even so, tyrosine phosphorylation may not be the final step in capacitation, for the reason that different effects on tyrosine phosphorylation and capacitation have been observed under certain conditions, including free intracellular Ca^{2+} concentration [86], nonspecific protein tyrosine phosphatase (PTPase) inhibitors [24], and extracellular Ca^{2+} concentration [30].

Acrosome Reaction

The AR is the release of proteolytic enzymes, mainly acrosin and hyaluronase, to degrade the zona pellucida of the oocyte. Once degraded, hyperactive motility propels the spermatozoa into the perivitelline space, at which point the spermatozoa may eventually fuse with the oocyte [3, 20]. The process is initiated by a chemotactic signal transferred from the ZP3 ligand of the oocyte to the spermatozoa plasma membrane [88].

The biochemistry of capacitation and the AR overlap in many respects. In both capacitation and the AR, ROS have been found to be involved in the phosphorylation of the same tyrosine proteins [84]. The AR is a short, irreversible process (5–15 min) associated with a respiratory burst (rapid extracellular $O_2^{-\bullet}$ production) that increases tyrosine phosphorylation of specific proteins [75, 84]. $O_2^{-\bullet}$ produced via this NADPH oxidase may dismutate into H_2O_2, and these two ROS members, at low concentrations, may have a positive effect on the AR [13, 30, 65]. NO has also been reported to increase the percentage of sperm undergoing the AR [35]. Once again, results regarding the specific ROS are conflicting. The majority of studies note the positive

Acrosome Reaction

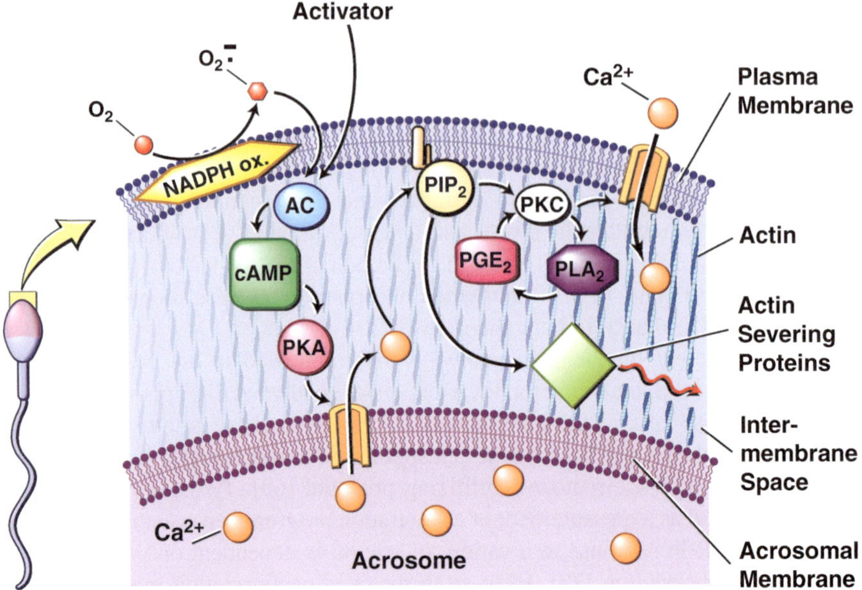

Fig. 4.2 Biochemical pathway proposed to regulate the acrosome reaction (AR). Induction of the AR can occur by physiological and nonphysiological activators, including the zona pellucida (ZP), progesterone, or ROS. Subsequent release of Ca^{2+} from the acrosomal calcium store generated during capacitation causes the cleavage of phosphatidylinosital-4,5-biphosphate (PIP$_2$), which forms diacylglycerol (DAG) and inosital triphosphate (IP3). The latter activates actin severing proteins, which leads to the fusion of the acrosomal and plasma membranes and eventual acrosomal exocytosis. DAG later activates PKC, causing a second, greater influx of Ca^{2+} and activation of PLA$_2$. The release of large amounts of membrane fatty acids increases the fluidity of the plasma membrane necessary for later fusion with the oocyte

effect of H_2O_2 and the negative effect of catalase (Table 4.5), thus suggesting that H_2O_2 is the major species responsible for the positive effect on the AR.

Keeping with the theme, ROS act as signal transducers in the AR. Elevated production of ROS may occur upon interaction with the cumulus oophorus [89], thereby enhancing the signal for exocytosis initiated by either progesterone or the zona pellucida. As mentioned, the AR is activated in response to one of many stimuli. In vivo, binding of the zona pellucida and perhaps some effect via progesterone on capacitated spermatozoa initiates this process and is associated with an influx of extracellular Ca^{2+} into the cytosol [79]. In vitro studies indicate that ROS can induce this Ca^{2+} influx [74, 86], likely by activating an upstream AC, which signals downstream molecules and initiates the biochemical cascade associated with the AR (Fig. 4.2). The biochemistry of this process has been well reviewed [88] in its specific relation to ROS [30]. Implicated in this complex process and downstream of ROS signals is the formation of lysophospholipids, specifically LPC, a fusogenic phospholipid implicated in the AR. The details of lysophospholipid formation are discussed below.

Sperm-Oocyte Fusion

The fusion event near the end of the spermatozoa's long journey through the female genital tract occurs after the degradation of the zona pellucida upon acrosomal exocytosis. The high PUFA content in the sperm plasma membrane assures some fluidity for fusion if other factors are absent. The zona-free hamster oocyte penetration test, in which the zona pellucida—normally representing a physical barrier—is removed from the oocyte, is the most common technique to measure the effects of manipulated variables on sperm-oocyte fusion.

A correlation exists between enhanced ROS levels and increased sperm-oocyte fusion [13, 30]. High rates of sperm-oocyte fusion are correlated with increased expression of phosphorylated tyrosine proteins [30], suggesting that sperm-oocyte fusion is correlated with the events of capacitation and the AR. Both H_2O_2 and $O_2^{-\bullet}$ contribute to the increase in fertilization rates, as shown by several studies from the same group [22, 30, 79]. These studies showed that the addition of catalase or SOD significantly decreased fusogenicity, whereas the addition of H_2O_2 or $O_2^{-\bullet}$ significantly increased fusogenicity (Table 4.6).

Simply put, ROS are thought to increase membrane fluidity via two mechanisms (1) de-esterification of membrane phospholipids and (2) activation of phospholipase A_2 (PLA_2). Results supporting this correlation have been witnessed in erythrocyte membranes by electron paramagnetic resonance (EPR) spectroscopy [90]. Both of these hypothesized mechanisms occur during the AR and result in an increase in free fatty acids; those de-esterified carbon chains cleaved from the triglycerol backbone of the phospholipid. Despite the proposition of the first hypothesis [75], experimental evidence for the direct de-esterification of membrane phospholipids is lacking.

The second mechanism involves greater biochemical complexity, but in brief, both $O_2^{-\bullet}$ and H_2O_2 may activate PLA_2 [91], an enzyme that removes a fatty acid

Table 4.6 Experimental results summary for ROS and the effects on sperm-oocyte fusion

Study author(s)	Variable	Effect on sperm-oocyte fusion
Aitken [30] and Aitken et al. [22, 30, 79, 80]	NADPH ($O_2^{-\bullet}$)	+
	H_2O_2	+
	Catalase	−
	Progesterone	+
	Progesterone + SOD	No effect
	Progesterone + catalase	−
	ZP3 + catalase	−
	SOD	−

from the phospholipid triglycerol backbone. Evidence supporting this hypothesis showed that the addition of XO caused a burst in $O_2^{-\bullet}$ production that correlated with a significant increase in arachidonic acid formation [92], which can be inhibited by SOD [75]. An increase in arachidonic acid release was observed upon H_2O_2 addition to murine astrocytes (mouse neural cells) and was largely blocked by both PLA_2 and protein kinase C (PKC) inhibitors [93].

Activation of PLA_2 is associated with an inhibition of phosphotyrosine phosphatases (PTPases), a general class of enzymes that dephosphorylate molecules, and in the case of PLA_2, inactivate it. Therefore, because ROS are proposed to inhibit PTPases, they may enhance PLA_2 activity [94]. In an additional pathway, ROS may cause protein tyrosine kinase (PTK) to activate PKC, which consequently phosphorylates and activates PLA_2 [88, 93, 95]. The formation of lysophospholipids and release of phospholipid fatty acids by PLA_2 increases membrane fluidity. LPC has also been implicated in the AR. In this way, lysophospholipids, and indirectly ROS, increase membrane fluidity, a necessary component for successful sperm-oocyte fusion [75, 94].

Expert Commentary

The purpose of this article was to provide a well-organized discussion of the topic of ROS and sperm physiology, a difficult feat given the disorganization of information available. In addition, there has been a general trend by researchers to focus on the direct effects of ROS, the pathological. It is our goal to refocus the study of ROS and sperm away from the individual patient and his AOX status, chromatin integrity, etc. and direct it towards finding a cure for OS-induced fertility as a whole through the study of ROS physiology. At the moment there exists little standardization in the definition of abnormal levels of ROS, AOX, and other markers of sperm integrity. As such, it is the hope that through a better understanding of the physiology we will be able to more precisely define and determine the etiology of the pathology.

Conclusion

ROS have been shown to have both positive and negative effects on the different maturation and fertilization processes of the spermatozoa. Despite the emphasis on the pathological role of ROS in OS, ROS serve an essential function in successful fertilization. In these processes, ROS act in signal transduction of biochemical cascades, likely through the redox-regulation of thiol groups. The activation of AC and cAMP triggers downstream molecules and enhances the efficacy of many maturation processes. Beneficial effects have been observed in the condensation of sperm DNA, formation of the mitochondrial capsule, and activation of the many complex processes that occur post-ejaculation. Current evidence suggests that the primary ROS involved in each process differs. $O_2^{-\bullet}$ has a more significant role in hyperactivation, but H_2O_2 has a greater role in capacitation and the AR. A greater comprehension of physiological roles of ROS, specifically their actions in vivo, is still lacking. It is of upmost importance to understand the physiological mechanisms regulating human sperm function, for there is growing evidence that male reproductive health is declining at an astonishing rate. It is only upon thorough understanding of the physiological that we can prevent, treat, and cure the pathological.

Five-Year View

Researchers are attempting to identify more of the common elements of OS-induced infertility. A comprehensive analysis of possible causes is underway and includes studies on: a variety of AOX (Gpx, taurine, alpha-tocopherol, etc.); creatine kinase activity and mitochondrial membrane potential as predictors of sperm quality; environmental factors (phthalates, cell phone radiation, etc.) as possible factors in the widespread deterioration of sperm quality.

Key Issues

- The major enzymatic antioxidants of past study are SOD and catalase, although the role of the lesser studied Gpx is likely significant.
- The most influential ROS are superoxide and hydrogen peroxide. Nitric oxide, despite its well-known role in the cardiovascular system, is less significant because it probably acts through the two ROS above
- Physiological roles of ROS include:

  - Maturation: protamine packaging and formation of the mitochondrial capsule
  - Hyperactivation: the initiation of uncoordinated motility in the uterus and fallopian tube
  - Capacitation: completion of maturation processes necessary for the acrosome reaction (AR)
  - Acrosome reaction: enhancement/induction of exocytosis
  - Sperm-oocyte fusion: enhancement of membrane fluidity necessary for fusion events

References

1. McLeod J. The role of oxygen in the metabolism and motility of human spermatozoa. Am J Physiol. 1943;138:512–8.
2. Halliwell B, Cross CE. Oxygen-derived species: their relation to human disease and environmental stress. Environ Health Perspect. 1992;102 Suppl 10:5–12.
3. Agarwal A, Saleh RA, Bedaiwy MA. Role of reactive oxygen species in the pathophysiology of human reproduction. Fertil Steril. 2003;79(4):829–43.

4. Venkatesh S, Deecaraman M, Kumar R, Shamsi MB, Dada R. Role of reactive oxygen species in the pathogenesis of mitochondrial DNA (mtDNA) mutations in male infertility. Indian J Med Res. 2009;129:127–37.
5. De Lamirande E, Gagnon C. Reactive oxygen species and human spermatozoa - I. Effects on the motility of intact spermatozoa and on sperm axonemes. J Androl. 1992;13(5):368–78.
6. Alvarez JG, Storey BT. Assessment of cell damage caused by spontaneous lipid peroxidation in rabbit spermatozoa. Biol Reprod. 1984;30:323–31.
7. Storey BT. Biochemistry of the induction and prevention of lipoperoxidative damage in human spermatozoa. Mol Hum Reprod. 1997;3(3):203–13.
8. Jones R, Mann T, Sherins R. Peroxidative breakdown of phospholipids in human spermatozoa, spermicidal properties of fatty acid peroxides, and protective action of seminal plasma. Fertil Steril. 1979;31:531–7.
9. Aitken JR, Clarkson JS. Cellular basis of defective sperm function and its association with the genesis of reactive oxygen species by human spermatozoa. J Reprod Fertil. 1987;81:459–69.
10. Das S, Chattopadhyay R, Jana SK, et al. Cut-off value of reactive oxygen species for predicting semen quality and fertilization outcome. Syst Biol Reprod Med. 2008;54:47–54.
11. Tremellen K. Oxidative stress and male infertility – a clinical perspective. Hum Reprod Update. 2008;14(3):243–58.
12. Aitken J, Clarkson JS, Fishel J. Generation of reactive oxygen species, lipid peroxidation, and human sperm function. Biol Reprod. 1989;40:183–97.
13. Griveau JF, Lannou DL. Reactive oxygen species and human spermatozoa: physiology and pathology. Int J Androl. 1997;20:61–9.
14. Agarwal A, Prabakaran SA. Mechanism, measurement, and prevention of oxidative stress in male reproductive physiology. Indian J Exp Biol. 2005;43:963–74.
15. Turrens JF, Boveris A. Generation of superoxide anion by the NADH dehydrogenase of bovine heart mitochondria. Biochem J. 1980;191:421–7.
16. Koppers AJ, De Luliis GN, Finnie JM, McLaughlin EA, Aitken RJ. Significance of mitochondrial reactive oxygen species in the generation of oxidative stress in spermatozoa. J Clin Endocrinol Metab. 2008;93:3199–207.
17. Ford WCL. Regulation of sperm function by reactive oxygen species. Hum Reprod Update. 2004;10(5):387–99.
18. Sabeur K, Ball B. Characterization of NADPH oxidase 5 in equine testis and spermatozoa. Soc Reprod Fertil. 2007;134:263–70.
19. Plante M, De Lamirande E, Gagnon C. Reactive oxygen species released by activated neutrophils, but not by deficient spermatozoa, are sufficient to affect normal motility. Fertil Steril. 1994;62:387–93.
20. De Lamirande E, Leclerc P, Gagnon C. Capacitation as a regulatory event that primes spermatozoa for the acrosome reaction and fertilization. Mol Hum Reprod. 1997;3(3):175–94.
21. Gavella M, Lipovac V. NADH-dependent oxidoreductase (diaphorase) activity and isozyme pattern of sperm in infertile men. Arch Androl. 1992;28:135.
22. Aitken RJ, Paterson M, Fisher H, Buckingham DW, Duin MV. Redox regulation of tyrosine phosphorylation in human spermatozoa and its role in the control of human sperm function. J Cell Sci. 1995;108:2017–25.
23. Zhang H, Zheng R-L. Promotion of human sperm capacitation by superoxide anion. Free Radic Res. 1996;24(4):261–8.
24. Leclerc P, de Lamirande E, Gagnon C. Regulation of protein-tyrosine phosphorylation and human sperm capacitation by reactive oxygen derivatives. Free Radic Biol Med. 1997; 22(4):643–56.
25. Lewis B, Aitken RJ. A redox-regulated tyrosine phosphorylation cascade in rat spermatozoa. J Androl. 2001;22(4):611–22.
26. Aitken RJ, Ryan AL, Baker MA, McLaughlin EA. Redox acitivity associated with the maturation and capacitation of mammalian spermatozoa. Free Radic Biol Med. 2004;36(8):994–1010.
27. Rivlin J, Mendel J, Rubinstein S, Etkovitz N, Breitbart H. Role of hydrogen peroxide in sperm capacitation and acrosome reaction. Biol Reprod. 2004;70:518–22.

28. Banfi B, Molnar G, Maturana A, et al. A Ca^{2+}-activated NADPH oxidase in testis, spleen, and lymph nodes. J Biol Chem. 2001;276(40):37594.

29. Vernet P, Aitken RJ, Drevet JR. Antioxidant strategies in the epididymis. Mol Cell Endocrinol. 2004;216:31–9.

30. Aitken JR. Molecular mechanisms regulating human sperm function. Mol Hum Reprod. 1997;3(3):169–73.

31. Godeas C, Tramer F, Micali F, Soranzo M, Sandri G, Panfili E. Distribution and possible novel role of phospholipid hydroperoxide glutathione peroxidase in rat epididymal spermatozoa. Biol Reprod. 1997;57:1502–8.

32. Sikka SC. Relative impact of oxidative stress on male reproductive function. Curr Med Chem. 2001;8:851–62.

33. Rosselli M, Keller PJ, Dubey RK. Role of nitric oxide in the biology, physiology and pathophysiology of reproduction. Hum Reprod Update. 1998;4(1):3–24.

34. Zini A, De Lamirande E, Gagnon C. Low levels of nitric oxide promote human sperm capacitation in vitro. J Androl. 1995;16(5):424–31.

35. Herrero MB, Gagnon C. Nitric oxide: a novel mediator of sperm function. J Androl. 2001;22(3):349–56.

36. Desai N, Sharma R, Makker K, Sabanegh E, Agarwal A. Physiologic and pathologic levels of reactive oxygen species in neat semen of infertile men. Fertil Steril. 2008;92:1626–31.

37. Carlsen E, Giwercman A, Keiding N, Skakkebaek NE. Evidence for decreasing quality of semen during past 50 years. BMJ. 1992;305:609–13.

38. Aitken JR. The Amoroso lecture: the human spermatozoon – a cell in crisis? J Reprod Fertil. 1999;115:1–7.

39. Iwasaki A, Gagnon C. Formation of reactive oxygen species in spermatozoa of infertile patients. Fertil Steril. 1992;57:409–16.

40. Zini A, De Lamirande E, Gagnon C. Reactive oxygen species in semen of infertile patients: levels of superoxide dismutase- and catalase-like activities in seminal plasma and spermatozoa. Int J Androl. 1993;16:183–8.

41. De Lamirande E, Leduc BE, Iwasaki A, Hassouna M, Gagnon C. Increased reactive oxygen species formation in semen of patients with spinal cord injury. Fertil Steril. 1995;63:637–42.

42. De Lamirande E, Gagnon C. Capacitation-associated production of superoxide anion by human spermatozoa. Free Radic Biol Med. 1995;18(3):487–95.

43. Padron OF, Brackett NL, Sharma RK, Lynne CM, Thomas Jr AJ, Agarwal A. Seminal reactive oxygen species and sperm motility and morphology in men with spinal cord injury. Fertil Steril. 1997;67(6):1115–20.

44. Agarwal A, Said TM. Oxidative stress, DNA damage and apoptosis in male infertility: a clinical approach. BJU Int. 2005;95:503–7.

45. Deepinder F, Cocuzza M, Agarwal A. Should seminal oxidative stress measurement be offered routinely to men presenting for infertility evaluation? Endocrine Pract. 2008;14(4):484–91.

46. Shalgi R, Smith TT, Yanagimachi R. A quantitative comparison of the passage of capacitated and uncapacitated hamster spermatozoa through the uterotubal junction. Biol Reprod. 1992;46:419–24.

47. De Lamirande E, Gagnon C. Human sperm hyperactivation in whole semen and its association with low superoxide scavenging capacity in seminal plasma. Fertil Steril. 1993;59(6):1291–5.

48. Aitken J, West K, Buckingham DW. Leukocytic infiltration into the human ejaculate and its association with semen quality, oxidative stress, and sperm function. J Androl. 1994; 15(4):343–52.

49. Pasqualotto FF, Sharma RK, Kobayashi H, Nelson Jr DR, Thomas AJ, Agarwal A. Oxidative stress in normospermic men undergoing infertility evaluation. J Androl. 2001;22(2):316–22.

50. De Lamirande E, Gagnon C. Reactive oxygen species and human spermatozoa II. Depletion of adenosine triphosphate plays an important role in the inhibition of sperm motility. J Androl. 1992;13(5):379–86.

51. Mahfouz RZ, du Plessis SS, Aziz N, Sharma R, Sabanegh E, Agarwal A. Sperm viability, apoptosis, and intracellular reactive oxygen species levels in human spermatozoa before and after induction of oxidative stress. Fertil Steril. 2010;93(3): 814–21.

52. Gil-Guzman E, Ollero M, Lopez MC, et al. Differential production of reactive oxygen species by subsets of human spermatozoa at different stages of maturation. Hum Reprod Update. 2001;16(9):1922–39.
53. Oehninger S, Blackmore P, Mahony M, Hodgen G. Effects of hydrogen peroxide on human spermatozoa. J Assist Reprod Genet. 1995;12(1):41–7.
54. Aitken J, Harkiss D, Buckingham DW. Relationship between iron-catalyzed lipid peroxidation potential and human sperm function. J Reprod Fertil. 1993;98:257–65.
55. Cocuzza M, Sikka SC, Athayde KS, Agarwal A. Clinical relevance of oxidative stress and sperm chromatin damge in male infertility: an evidence based analysis. Int Braz J Urol. 2007;33:603–21.
56. Kumar R, Venkatesh S, Kumar M, et al. Oxidative stress and sperm mitochondrial DNA mutation in idiopathic oligoasthenozoospermic men. Indian J Biochem Biophys. 2009;46(2):172–7.
57. Rao B, Soufir JC, Martin M, David G. Lipid peroxidation in human spermatozoa as related to midpiece abnormalities and motility. Gamete Res. 1989;24:127–34.
58. Saowaros W, Panyim S. The formation of disulfide bonds in human protamines during sperm maturation. Experientia. 1978;35(2):191–2.
59. Rousseaux J, Rousseaux-Prevost R. Molecular localization of free thiols in human sperm chromatin. Biol Reprod. 1995;52:1066–72.
60. Roveri A, Ursini F, Flohe L, Maiorino M. PHGPx and spermatogenesis. Biofactors. 2001; 14:213–22.
61. Tunc O, Thompson J, Tremellen K. Improvement in sperm DNA quality using an oral antioxidant therapy. Reprod Biomed Online. 2009;18(6):761–8.
62. Menezo Y. Antioxidants to reduce sperm DNA fragmentation: an unexpected adverse effect. Reprod Biomed Online. 2007;14(4):418–21.
63. De Lamirande E, O'Flaherty C. Sperm activation: role of reactive oxygen species and kinases. Biochim Biophys Acta. 2008;1784:106–15.
64. De Lamirande E, Gagnon C. Redox control of changes in protein sulfhydryl levels during human sperm capacitation. Free Radic Biol Med. 2003;35(10):1271–85.
65. O'Flaherty C, Lamirande ED, Gagnon C. Positive role of reactive oxygen species in mammalian sperm capacitation: triggering and modulation of phosphorylation events. Free Radic Biol Med. 2006;41:528–40.
66. Baldi E, Luconi M, Bonaccorsi L, Muratori M, Forti G. Intracellular events and signaling pathways involved in sperm acquisition of fertilizing capacity and acrosome reaction. Front Biosci. 2000;5:110–23.
67. Burkman LJ. Discrimination between nonhyperactivated and classical hyperactivated motility patterns in human spermatozoa. Fertil Steril. 1991;55(2):363–71.
68. Aitken J, Fisher H. Reactive oxygen species generation and human spemeratozoa: the balance of benefit and risk. Bioessays. 1994;16(4):259–67.
69. Suarez SS. Control of hyperactivation in sperm. Hum Reprod Update. 2008;14(6):647–57.
70. Kobayashi T, Miyazaki T, Natori M, Nozawa S. Protective role of superoxide dismutase in human sperm motility: superoxide dismutase activity and lipid peroxide in human seminal plasma and spermatozoa. Hum Reprod. 1991;6(7):987–91.
71. Williams AC, Ford CL. The role of glucose in supporting motility and capacitation in human spermatozoa. J Androl. 2001;22(4):680–95.
72. De Lamirande E, Gagnon C. Human sperm hyperactivation and capacitation as parts of an oxidative process. Free Radic Biol Med. 1993;14:157–66.
73. De Lamirande E, Gagnon C. A positive role for the superoxide anion in triggering hyperactivation and capacitation of human spermatozoa. Int J Androl. 1993;16:21–5.
74. Griveau JF, Renard P, Le Lannou D. An in vitro promoting role for hydrogen peroxide in human sperm capacitation. Int J Androl. 1994;17:300–7.
75. Griveau J, Renard P, Le Lannou D. Superoxide anion production by human spermatozoa as a part of the ionophore-induced acrosome reaction process. Int J Androl. 1995;18(2):67–74.
76. Eisenbach M. Mammalian sperm chemotaxis and its association with capacitation. Dev Genet. 1999;25:87–94.

77. Visconti PE, Westbrook VA, Chertihin O, Demarco I, Sleight S, Diekman AB. Novel signaling pathways involved in sperm acquisition of fertilizing capacity. J Reprod Immunol. 2002; 53:133–50.
78. Bize I, Santander G, Cabello P, Driscoll D, Sharpe C. Hydrogen peroxide is invovled in hamster sperm capacitation in vitro. Biol Reprod. 1991;44:398–403.
79. Aitken RJ, Buckingham DW, Harkiss D, Paterson M, Fisher H, Irvine DS. The extragenomic action of progesterone on human spermatozoa is influenced by redox regulated changes in tyrosine phosphorylation during capacitation. Mol Cell Endocrinol. 1996;117:83–93.
80. Aitken RJ, Harkiss D, Knox W, Paterson M, Irvine DS. A novel signal transduction cascade in capacitating human spermatozoa characterised by a redox-regulated, cAMP-mediated induction of tyrosine phosphorylation. J Cell Sci. 1998;111:645–56.
81. O'Flaherty C, Beorlegui N, Beconi MT. Participation of superoxide anion in the capacitation of cryopreserved bovine sperm. Int J Androl. 2003;26:109–14.
82. Baumber J, Sabeur K, Vo A, Ball BA. Reactive oxygen species promote tryosine phosphorylation and capacitation in equine spermatozoa. Theriogenology. 2003;60:1239–47.
83. Roy SC, Atreja SK. Effect of reactive oxygen species on capacitation and associated protein tyrosine phosphorylation in buffalo (*Bubalus bubalis*) spermatozoa. Anim Reprod Sci. 2008;107:68–84.
84. De Lamirande E, Tsai C, Harakat A, Gagnon C. Involvement of reactive oxygen species in human sperm acrosome reaction induced by A23187, lysophosphatidylcholine, and biological fluid ultrafiltrates. J Androl. 1998;19(5):585–94.
85. Aitken RJ, Nixon B, Lin M, Koppers AJ, Lee YH, Baker MA. Proteomic changes in mammalian spermatozoa during epididymal maturation. Asian J Androl. 2007;9:554–64.
86. Leclerc P, De Lamirande E, Gagnon C. Interaction between Ca^{2+}, cyclic $3',5'$ adenosine monophosphate, the superoxide anion, and tyrosine phosphorylation pathways in the regulation of human sperm capacitation. J Androl. 1998;19(4):434–43.
87. Flesch F, Wijnand E, Lest CVD, Colenbrander B, Golde LV, Gadella B. Capacitation dependent activation of tyrosine phosphorylation generates two sperm head plasma membrane proteins with high primary binding affinity for the zona pellucida. Mol Reprod Dev. 2001;60:107–15.
88. Breitbart H, Spungin B. The biochemistry of the acrosome reaction. Mol Hum Reprod. 1997;3(3):195–202.
89. Tanghe S, Soom AV, Mehrzad J, Maes D, Duchateau L, Kruif AD. Cumulus contributions during bovine fertiliation in vitro. Theriogenology. 2003;60:135–49.
90. Rosen GM, Barber MJ, Rauckman EJ. Disruption of erythrocyte membranal organization by superoxide. J Biol Chem. 1983;258(4):2225–8.
91. Sawada M, Carlson JC. Rapid plasma membrane changes in superoxide radical formation, fluidity, and phospholipase A_2 activity in the Corpus Luteum of the rat during induction of luteolysis. Endocrinology. 1991;128(6):2992–8.
92. Wu X, Sawada M, Carlson J. Stimulation of phospholipase A_2 by xanthine oxidase in the rat Corpus Luteum. Biol Reprod. 1992;47:1053–8.
93. Xu J, Yu S, Sun AY, Sun GY. Oxidant-mediated AA release from astrocytes involves $cPLA_2$ and $iPLA_2$. Free Radic Biol Med. 2003;34(12):1531–43.
94. Goldman R, Ferber E, Zort U. Reactive oxygen species are involved in the activation of cellular phospholipase A_2. Fed Eur Biochem Soc. 1992;309(2):190–2.
95. Zor U, Ferber E, Gergely P, Szucs K, Dombradi V, Goldman R. Reactive oxygen species mediate phorbol ester-regulated tyrosine phosphorylation and phospholipase A_2 activation: potentiation by vanadate. Biochem J. 1993;295:879–88.

Chapter 5
Molecular Mechanisms of Antioxidants in Male Infertility

Kathleen Hwang and Dolores J. Lamb

The failure to conceive within 1 year occurs in approximately 15% of couples [1], and approximately 50% of problems related to conception is either caused entirely by the male or is a combined problem with the male and his partner. Male infertility continues to be a clinical challenge of increasing significance. While the etiology of suboptimal semen quality is currently not completely understood, oxidative stress has demonstrated ability to affect fertility [2, 3]. Oxidative stress is induced by reactive oxygen species (ROS). ROS in the form of superoxide anion, hydrogen peroxide, and hydroxyl radical are formed as a by-product of oxygen metabolism. The presence of excess ROS can cause oxidative damage to lipids, proteins, and DNA [4–6]. Spermatozoa, like any other aerobic cell, are constantly trying to maintain that fine balance [7]. Abnormal ROS formation is found in up to 40% of infertile patients [8], with some reports suggesting an inverse relationship between seminal ROS levels and spontaneous pregnancy outcomes of infertile couples [9]. Many studies have attempted to define the relationship between seminal ROS and IVF [10, 11] but have met with conflicting results. Nevertheless, a growing body of knowledge on ROS and fertility makes testing for oxidants in the semen an important part of the infertile male evaluation.

K. Hwang, MD (✉)
Department of Surgery (Urology), Brown University,
2 Dudley Street, Ste 175, Providence, RI 02905, USA
e-mail: Kathleen_hwang@brown.edu

D.J. Lamb, PhD
Scott Department of Urology, Baylor College of Medicine,
One Baylor Plaza, N730, Houston, TX 77030, USA
e-mail: dlamb@bcm.edu

S.J. Parekattil and A. Agarwal (eds.), *Antioxidants in Male Infertility: A Guide for Clinicians and Researchers*, © Springer Science+Business Media New York 2013

Reactive Oxygen Species and Antioxidants

ROS are formed via several mechanisms but essentially are products of normal cellular metabolism. Most of the energy generated in the body is produced by the enzymatically controlled reaction of oxygen with hydrogen in oxidative phosphorylation occurring within the mitochondria [12]. Free radicals are formed during the enzymatic reduction of oxygen to produce energy [13]. A free radical is an oxygen molecule containing one or more unpaired electrons, which makes this structure highly susceptible to radical formation. The primary form of ROS, superoxide anion radical, is formed with the addition of one electron to dioxygen. Secondary ROS include the hydroxyl radical, peroxyl radical, and hydrogen peroxide. Furthermore, there is another class of free radicals derived from nitrogen, which includes nitrous oxide, peroxynitrile, nitroxyl anion, and peroxy-nitrous acid.

Oxidative stress occurs when the production of ROS overwhelms the natural antioxidant defense mechanisms leading to cellular damage. Cellular damage occurs when the free radicals donate their unpaired electron onto nearby cellular structures. To prevent cellular damage by excessive production of ROS, enzymatic and nonenzymatic antioxidant pathways scavenge surplus ROS and allow a balance to be achieved. Oxidative stress leads to the activation of transcription factors and signaling pathways, partly through the activation of the innate immune response. Such activation leads to the release of cytokines and chemokines.

These cytokines are synthesized and secreted on demand, for example, during an infection. Cytokines are also involved in gonadal and sperm function. A multitude of cytokines have been shown to be present in human semen, such as TGF-α [14] and TNF-α [15]. Various cytokines have demonstrated the ability to decrease spermatozoan motility as well as increase the generation of ROS in semen [16, 17].

Antioxidant Pathways

Fortunately, the human body has developed several antioxidant strategies to protect itself from ROS damage. These mechanisms allow for normal oxidative metabolism to occur without damaging cells while still allowing for normal cellular responses such as destruction of infectious pathogens [13]. Superoxide dismutase (SOD) and catalase are enzymatic metal-containing antioxidants, which inactivate the superoxide anion and peroxide radicals, converting them into oxygen and water. Glutathione peroxidase also participates in the reduction of hydrogen peroxide using glutathione as an electron donor.

Nonenzymatic antioxidants present within semen include vitamins E and C, glutathione, flavenoids, and albumin [18]. The majority of these participants primarily act by directly neutralizing free radical activity chemically. Several researchers have reported a significant reduction in nonenzymatic activity in seminal plasma of infertile men [19–21]. Under normal conditions, these antioxidants act to maintain this delicate balance to achieve an overall low level of oxidative stress in the semen.

Vitamin E is a major chain-breaking antioxidant and acts by trapping organic free radicals and/or deactivating excited oxygen molecules to prevent tissue damage. It specifically acts as a peroxyl and alkoxyl radical scavenger in lipid environments and thus prevents lipid peroxidation in lipoproteins and particularly membranes [22]. Similarly, vitamin C has powerful antioxidant capabilities as it neutralizes hydroxyl, superoxide, and hydrogen peroxide radicals and prevents sperm agglutination [22]. As a water-soluble antioxidant, it has also been shown to recycle oxidized vitamin E.

Sources of Reactive Oxygen Species

Oxidative stress and its role in the origins of male infertility was first established in 1943, when MacLeod demonstrated that catalase could support the motility of human spermatozoa incubated under aerobic conditions [23]. This observation then prompted him to suggest that sperm must produce hydrogen peroxide during normal oxidative metabolism. Human spermatozoa are capable of generating low levels ROS associated with the positive physiological event of sperm capacitation necessary for fertility.

During spermatogenesis, a low-level production of free radicals by sperm plays a necessary role in preparation for capacitation. Hydrogen peroxide stimulates the acrosome reaction, sperm hyperactivation [24], and tyrosine phosphorylation [25], leading to binding to the zona pellucida. Cytoplasm is normally extruded from the spermatozoa prior to release of the germinal epithelium. This cytoplasmic residue is a source of high levels of the enzyme glucose-6-phosphate dehydrogenase, which generates nicotinamide adenine dinucleotide phosphate (NADPH). NADPH then generates ROS via NADPH oxidase within the sperm membrane [26, 27].

The two main sources of free radicals within semen are leukocytes and sperm. The rate of production of ROS by leukocytes is reported to be 1,000 times higher than that of spermatozoa at capacitation [28]. This finding seems to implicate leukocytes as the likely dominant producer of seminal ROS; however, further evidence suggests that oxidative stress and consequent sperm injury is as much related to location as well as concentration. To better characterize seminal ROS production, the sources are separated into intrinsic (sperm) and extrinsic (leukocytes). Henkel et al. suggested that there is a stronger relationship for intrinsic ROS production as the more important variable in terms of fertility potential with increased levels of DNA fragmentation [29].

Although several studies have attempted to characterize the relationship between the presence of leukocytes in semen and male infertility, it still remains incompletely defined. Leukocytospermia has long been associated with decreased sperm concentration, motility, and morphology and defective fertilization; however, these clinical, epidemiological, and experimental studies have reported inconsistent results [30–32], leaving this relationship still controversial.

Lifestyle

Despite the fact that smoking is a lifestyle hazard for both the active and passive smoker, almost one-third of Americans between the ages of 18 and 24 smoke, and the number continues to rise [33]. While much is known of the carcinogenic properties of tobacco and its resultant effects on organs such as lung and bladder, the impact on fertility still remains less defined. Numerous studies, however, have established the fact that toxins in cigarette smoke reach the male reproductive system and their effects are mainly due to their direct interaction with the components of seminal fluid [34]. This interaction has led to a greater presence of ROS and increased leukocytes and rounds cells, as well as a higher frequency of DNA fragmentation in comparison to nonsmokers [35–37]. In smokers, either male or female, there was noted to be a significant delay of over 6 months in natural conception in comparison to nonsmokers [38].

Nicotine and its metabolites are present in the spermatozoa of smokers, and furthermore, these toxicants are found in embryos resulting from in vitro fertilization cycles with male smokers [39]. Cigarette smoking results in a 48% increase in seminal leukocyte concentration [37], and smokers have decreased levels of seminal plasma antioxidants such as vitamin E and vitamin C, placing their sperm at additional risk for oxidative damage [40, 41].

Ethanol is one of the most abused substances worldwide. It has been shown to have deleterious effects at all levels of the male reproductive system. Excessive alcohol consumption causes an increase in systemic oxidative stress as ethanol stimulates the production of ROS, confounded by the antioxidant-deficient diets that most alcohol abusers maintain [42, 43]. However, despite the demonstrated link, there has been no study to date that has examined the direct link between alcohol intake and sperm oxidative damage.

Environmental

Phthalates are among the most widely used man-made chemicals released into the environment over the last several decades. They are primarily used as plasticizers in the manufacture of flexible vinyl, which is found in medical devices, toys, floor and wall coverings, personal care products, and food packaging. Ubiquitous use of phthalates results in exposure mainly through dietary consumption, dermal absorption, or inhalation and has been linked with impaired spermatogenesis and increased sperm DNA damage [44, 45]. Lee et al. reported an increase in the generation of ROS within the testis after oral administration of phthalate esters to rats, leading to a concomitant decrease in antioxidant levels and subsequent impaired spermatogenesis [46].

Furthermore, several environmental pesticides [47, 48] as well as heavy metal exposure [49] have been linked with testicular oxidative stress and subsequent sperm oxidative damage. Patients employed in industries with high levels of exposure risks should be counseled to take aggressive precautionary measures to avoid future contact as well as be tested for heavy metals.

Infection/Inflammation

The invasion of microorganisms into tissue results in a natural defense mechanism which includes the oxidative burst of leukocytes and macrophages [50]. Mazzilli et al. demonstrated significantly elevated superoxide anion generation in patients with sperm cultures positive for aerobic bacteria compared with fertile controls [51]. Men prone to genitourinary infection, such as paraplegics, have been found to have high degrees of sperm oxidative pathology [52] and were negatively correlated with sperm motility and independent of the method of ejaculation [53]. *Chlamydial* infections, current or past, have also been linked with an increase in oxidative damage to sperm [54].

Up to 50% of men at some point in their lives will experience prostatitis, and chronic nonbacterial prostatitis will account for in excess of 90% of all cases [55]. It is reported that an adverse autoimmune response to seminal or prostate antigens is responsible for the pathology leading to an increase in proinflammatory cytokines and activated ROS [56, 57]. These antigens will stimulate a release of T lymphocytes followed by a subsequent liberation of cytokines such as TNF-α, IFN-γ, and IL-1β that stimulates chemotaxis and activation of further leukocytes leading to the resultant oxidative stress [56]. Hence, it is not so surprising that many studies link chronic nonbacterial prostatitis with a reduction in sperm density, motility, and morphology [58, 59].

Testicular

Oxidative stress is now believed to be the principal underlying pathology linking varicoceles with male infertility [60–62]. Clinical varicoceles are one of the most common causes of male infertility. There is a strong correlation between the increase in varicocele-related ROS production and subsequent reduction in sperm DNA integrity when assessed by terminal deoxynucleotidyl transferase dUTP nick end labeling (TUNEL) [62]. Several researchers have also proposed that oxidative stress plays a significant role for infertility following vasectomy reversal. Many believe that vasectomy disrupts the normal blood–testis barrier, leading to a loss of immune integrity and activation of immune responses [63]. Multiple studies have demonstrated an increase in seminal leukocytes, proinflammatory cytokines, and free radical production following vasectomy reversal [64, 65].

Cryptorchidism has been established as a common cause for male factor infertility wherein the primary pathology is hypospermatogenesis due to deficient maturation of gonocytes [66]. It has also recently been reported that men with cryptorchidism surgically treated with orchidopexy early in life still have markedly elevated sperm ROS production and DNA fragmentation compared with fertile controls [67].

Prolonged periods of ischemia followed by spontaneous or surgical restoration of blood flow results in an influx of leukocytes into both testicles [68] and a subsequent increase in generation of free radicals [69]. The annual incidence of torsion of the spermatic cord is 1 in 4,000 males and has been long recognized as a cause of male infertility. This ischemic-reperfusion injury model leads to necrosis of the germinal cells with resulting subfertility or infertility.

Molecular Defects

Experimental evidence is emerging that ROS are involved in several fundamental mechanisms of sperm physiology. However, at present, the precise mechanisms are still not completely defined and still under investigation. Nonetheless, there has been convincing data reported in animal models that may highlight specific potential molecular relationships.

Mitochondria

Mitochondria are responsible for the generation of the majority of adenosine triphosphate (ATP) and are crucial as human cells rely on ATP for growth, differentiation, cellular homeostasis, and several physiological functions. They also serve as an important source of ROS within most mammalian cells [70]. Spermatozoa have mitochondria uniquely located around the midpiece to be precisely at the site of maximal energy requirement. Mitochondrial DNA (mtDNA) accumulates polymorphisms and mutations about 10–17 times faster than nuclear DNA [71]. Several studies have reported that human cells harboring mutated mtDNA have lower respiratory function and show increased production of superoxide anions, hydroxyl radicals, and hydrogen peroxide [72, 73].

Another investigator reported a correlation between ROS and mitochondria in apoptosis, where high levels of ROS were found to disrupt the inner and outer mitochondrial membrane resulting in a release of cytochrome C [74]. Cytochrome C protein activates the caspases and induces apoptosis, which was also noted to be higher in infertile men with elevated levels of ROS. A recent study in mice carrying different proportions of pathogenic mtDNA showed respiratory chain defects that lead to meiotic arrest during spermatogenesis and subsequent oligospermia, asthenospermia, and teratospermia [75]. An increased number of mtDNA mutations may also lead to abnormal sperm morphology and ultrastructural defects [76].

DNA Damage

Cells are constantly being exposed to environmental and endogenous stressors, such as alkylating agents, ROS, and other active metabolites that are capable of causing DNA damage. During replication and repair, lesions induced by these toxic compounds can produce alternate nucleotides, potentially leading to permanent alterations in genetic material. Fortunately, there are intrinsic repair mechanisms in place such as base excision repair (BER). Although DNA polymerase β is known to be the main polymerase in the BER pathway, there are multiple other DNA polymerases that participate in this process as well.

Braithwaite et al. [77] recently examined the interrelationship between these enzymes in mammalian cells and their effect on oxidative stress-induced mutagenesis. They focused in on DNA polymerase β and DNA polymerase λ and were able to generate double knockout mouse embryonic fibroblast cell lines. These cell lines were examined for sensitivity to 3 DNA-damaging agents: an alkylating agent, hydrogen peroxide, and a thymidine analog. The double knockout cell lines demonstrated a hypersensitivity to hydrogen peroxide in comparison to wild-type mice indicating significant roles of DNA polymerases β and λ in protection of these cells against toxic agents, particularly hydrogen peroxide.

OGG1 and MYH are two major enzymes involved in mammalian oxidative DNA damage repair, most commonly preventing G to T mutations [78, 79]. Xie et al. [80] examined the roles of MYH and OGG1 in the protection against oxidative stress. They generated double knockout mice and developed embryonic fibroblast cell lines and examined their phenotypes associated with oxidative stress. The cells were exposed to hydrogen peroxide, *cis*-platinum, and γ-irradiation. The cells had significantly increased sensitivity to hydrogen peroxide exposure. Their findings that having both these deficiencies contribute to centrosome amplification and multinuclear formation, suggesting that *myh* and *ogg1* are likely required for normal cell cycle progression and cell division under oxidative stress.

Impact on Semen Quality

The structure of the sperm membrane is unique as it contains large amounts of unsaturated fatty acids rendering them particularly vulnerable to oxidative stress. These unsaturated fatty acids provide fluidity necessary for membrane fusion events; however, these molecules also make them more susceptible to free radical attack. Seminal fluid is an important source of antioxidants and is key in protecting spermatozoa from oxidative injury [81, 82]. SOD, catalase, glutathione peroxidase, vitamin E, and vitamin C are all contained in seminal fluid. This is particularly important as spermatozoa, unlike most cells, have little cytoplasmic fluid and subsequently contain only minimal amounts of the critical ROS scavenging enzymes and pathways, leaving them virtually no capacity for protein synthesis and little antioxidant capacity [81].

Table 5.1 Linking oxidative stress and male infertility

Author	Year	n	Findings
Athayde et al. [83]	2007	47	Infertile men with significantly ↑ levels of ROS compared to fertile controls
Mostafa et al. [41]	2006	68	Infertile men with significantly ↓ levels of protective antioxidants in semen compared to fertile controls
Twigg et al. [18]	1998	0	In vitro generation of ROS associated with evidence of sperm peroxidation, ↓ motility
Saleh et al. [61]	2003	92	Seminal ROS in infertile men correlated with ↓ motility and ↑ sperm membrane oxidation
Keskes-Ammar et al. [107]	2003	54	Antioxidant treatment may improve sperm motility
Twigg et al. [18]	1998	0	In vitro generation of ROS associated with ↑ in sperm DNA damage
Henkel et al. [29]	2005	63	Infertile men with seminal ROS is correlated with ↑ in sperm DNA damage
Greco et al. [108]	2005	64	Antioxidant treatment in infertile men may improve sperm DNA quality
Tremellen et al. [110]	2007	60	The use of antioxidant supplements by infertile men may ↑ partner's chances of spontaneous or IVF assisted pregnancy

Elevated levels of ROS have been detected in the semen of 25% of infertile men [8, 81, 83] (Table 5.1). These elevated levels of ROS have been correlated with sperm DNA damage, although no ROS threshold above which sperm DNA damage is detected has been established [61, 84, 85]. DNA damage in male germline cells is associated with poor fertilization rates following IVF, defective preimplantation embryonic development, and high rates of miscarriage. Several studies have demonstrated that ROS can induce sperm DNA damage in vitro, supporting that ROS may play a role in the etiology of sperm DNA damage in infertile men [18, 86]. There has also been evidence to suggest that ROS generation has a central role in the pathophysiology of age-related decrease in male fertility (reviewed in Desai et al. [87]). Several studies have also evaluated the relationship between semen antioxidant levels and sperm DNA damage and have reported conflicting results.

Increased ROS levels have also been associated with decreased sperm motility [88–90]. Proposed mechanisms by which ROS reduces sperm motility is by decreasing axonemal protein phosphorylation as well as lipid peroxidation [91]. The ability to revive sperm motility both in vivo and in vitro with antioxidants, such as vitamin E, confirms the evidence that lipid peroxidation is a major cause of motility loss in spermatozoa [92].

Detection of Oxidative Stress in Male Infertility

There are various methods to identify seminal ROS; however, the most common method is via the indirect chemiluminescence assay. These tests have been designed to quantify the level of oxidative stress in men undergoing evaluation for infertility with the goal of deriving a therapeutic plan to decrease oxidative stress levels and improve overall sperm quality. The chemiluminescence assay utilizes a luminometer to measure chemical reactions between ROS found in human semen and a chemiluminescent probe, such as luminol or lucigenin. Luminol is an uncharged particle that is cell membrane permeable and therefore can react extracellularly and intracellularly with hydrogen peroxide, hydroxyl anions, and superoxide anions. In contrast, lucigenin is a positively charged particle that is membrane impermeable and reacts with superoxide anions in the extracellular space [93]; therefore, luminol is used more commonly because of its ability to measure extracellular as well as intracellular levels of ROS.

Leukocyte contamination in the semen has been shown to negatively impact fertility [31]. Leukocytes have been shown to be responsible for a significant proportion of ROS activity in the semen [32, 94]; therefore, these assays should be coupled with selective leukocyte removal strategies if pyospermia is present [95]. Not doing so would lead to a falsely elevated ROS value. Other factors that may spuriously increase ROS results include repeated centrifugation of the sample and the use of certain oxidase-containing buffers for sample preparation [96, 97]. In contrast, prolonged time from preparation to analysis of the sample can artificially decrease the ROS identifiable in the semen [98]. For this reason, it is recommended that testing be performed within an hour of sperm preparation [99]. Finally, poor liquefaction of the sample can interfere with the normal oxidative process resulting in a falsely lower ROS value [97].

Management of Oxidative Stress in Male Infertility

As our clinical understanding of the impact of oxidative stress on male fertility expands, the natural desire to define and provide more effective therapeutic options for these patients also increases. Primarily, treatment should be aimed at identification and amelioration of any underlying cause before implementing any antioxidant treatment. While many trials have been performed to address this exact situation, many of these studies are difficult to interpret. However, the low cost and toxicity range of the majority of these antioxidant therapies offers a huge appeal for both patients and clinicians.

Lifestyle Modifications

Lifestyle choices such as smoking, poor diet, alcohol abuse, obesity, and even exposure to environmental toxins have all been linked with oxidative stress. First and foremost, patients should be counseled on making positive lifestyle changes such as a diet high in fruits and vegetables, and a reduction or cessation in smoking and alcohol intake. However, there have been conflicting results in the literature regarding the benefits of dietary supplements or individual vitamins [100, 101]. Patients exposed to occupational or environmental toxins should be counseled and reeducated on proper ventilation and use of personal protective equipment at work.

Treatment of Infection/Inflammation

Chlamydia and *Ureaplasma* infections within the semen and male accessory glands have been definitively linked to an increase in oxidative stress [51, 54]. Antibiotics can effectively treat both of these pathogens, and recent studies have confirmed the ability of appropriate antibiotic treatment to improve sperm quality by reducing sperm oxidative stress [102, 103]. Men with either *Chlamydia* or *Ureaplasma* were randomized to receive no treatment vs. antibiotic treatment for 3 months. The antibiotic-treated group demonstrated a significant reduction in seminal leukocyte and ROS production compared with the controls. They further exhibited an improvement in sperm motility and natural conception [103].

Nonsteroidal anti-inflammatory (NSAID) drugs may also reduce free radical production by seminal leukocytes. Gambera et al. reported that a 1-month course of a COX-2 inhibitor was able to significantly improve sperm motility, morphology, and viability while reducing the sperm leukocyte count [104].

Antioxidant Supplementation

Oral antioxidant supplements have been reported to augment the scavenging capacity of seminal plasma thereby reducing levels of ROS within the semen. The oral antioxidants vitamin E, vitamin C, β-carotene, and acetyl-cysteine are all potent scavengers of ROS and have all been shown to reduce seminal ROS levels [105]. A randomized control study evaluated 3 months of vitamin E treatment with placebo, confirming this reduction in seminal ROS levels [106]. Keskes-Ammar et al. randomized 54 men to either vitamin E and selenium or vitamin B for 3 months, examining the semen for quantitative levels of MDA, a lipid peroxidation marker. While less than half of the patients completed the study, results revealed that vitamin E and selenium supplementation produced a significant decrease in MDA concentrations with improved sperm quality in comparison to vitamin B [107]. Most recently, a well-designed prospective, randomized controlled trial of 2 months treatment with vitamin C and vitamin E demonstrated a very significant reduction in percent of DNA-fragmented spermatozoa [108]; however, no differences in basic sperm parameters were noted.

While many studies have shown significant improvements in sperm motility with antioxidant supplementation [107, 109, 110], other authors have not found any changes in semen parameters nor any pregnancies initiated during this period in prospective randomized trials [111]. Although these data seemingly conflict, it is difficult to directly compare the results due to varying study design. While the data supporting improvements in sperm quality with antioxidant treatment is more established, the ability of these changes to translate into improved chances of pregnancy is less clear. Nevertheless, the majority of the studies provide persuasive evidence to support the efficacy of antioxidants, particularly the vitamins, on improving overall sperm quality.

Varicocele

Several studies have concluded that surgical treatment of a varicocele is highly effective and can reduce seminal ROS levels and improve sperm DNA integrity [112, 113]. Using the Cochrane Menstrual Disorders and Subfertility Group register, Evers et al. performed a meta-analysis which did not show any benefit [114]. However, the most recent meta-analysis examining the effect of varicocele repair on spontaneous conception by Marmar et al. noted that men undergoing varicocelectomy demonstrated lower oxidative stress and a significant benefit in spontaneous conception in comparison to the control group [115].

Key Issues

Over the past decade, there has been an expanding body of evidence that now supports a role for oxidative stress as a significant cause of male infertility, as well as refining the relationship between the two. Despite our increased understanding of the role of ROS on male fertility, many questions still remain unanswered. Well-designed randomized controlled trials will be required to truly assess the potential of these antioxidants alone or in combination to be able to derive consistent clinical guidelines of therapy. Nonetheless, the evaluation of oxidative stress in male infertility patients should be routine in clinical practice.

Acknowledgments This study was supported in part by the 1K12DK083014 Multidisciplinary K12 Urology Research Career Development Program at Baylor to D.J.L. and K.H. from the National Institute of Kidney and Digestive Diseases.

References

1. Thonneau P, Marchand S, Tallec A, et al. Incidence and main causes of infertility in a resident population (1,850,000) of three French regions (1988–1989). Hum Reprod. Jul 1991; 6(6):811–6.
2. Aitken RJ. A free radical theory of male infertility. Reprod Fertil Dev. 1994;6(1):19–23. discussion 23–14.

3. Vine MF. Smoking and male reproduction: a review. Int J Androl. Dec 1996;19(6):323–37.
4. Aitken RJ, Baker MA, Sawyer D. Oxidative stress in the male germ line and its role in the aetiology of male infertility and genetic disease. Reprod Biomed Online. 2003;7(1):65–70.
5. Griveau JF, Le Lannou D. Reactive oxygen species and human spermatozoa: physiology and pathology. Int J Androl. 1997;20(2):61–9.
6. Henkel R, Hajimohammad M, Stalf T, et al. Influence of deoxyribonucleic acid damage on fertilization and pregnancy. Fertil Steril. 2004;81(4):965–72.
7. Sies H. Strategies of antioxidant defense. Eur J Biochem. 1993;215(2):213–9.
8. Iwasaki A, Gagnon C. Formation of reactive oxygen species in spermatozoa of infertile patients. Fertil Steril. 1992;57(2):409–16.
9. Aitken RJ, Irvine DS, Wu FC. Prospective analysis of sperm-oocyte fusion and reactive oxygen species generation as criteria for the diagnosis of infertility. Am J Obstet Gynecol. 1991;164(2):542–51.
10. Sukcharoen N, Keith J, Irvine DS, Aitken RJ. Prediction of the in-vitro fertilization (IVF) potential of human spermatozoa using sperm function tests: the effect of the delay between testing and IVF. Hum Reprod. 1996;11(5):1030–4.
11. Hammadeh ME, Radwan M, Al-Hasani S, et al. Comparison of reactive oxygen species concentration in seminal plasma and semen parameters in partners of pregnant and non-pregnant patients after IVF/ICSI. Reprod Biomed Online. 2006;13(5):696–706.
12. Tremellen K. Oxidative stress and male infertility–a clinical perspective. Hum Reprod Update. 2008;14(3):243–58.
13. Valko M, Leibfritz D, Moncol J, Cronin MT, Mazur M, Telser J. Free radicals and antioxidants in normal physiological functions and human disease. Int J Biochem Cell Biol. 2007;39(1):44–84.
14. Yie SM, Lobb DK, Clark DA, Younglai EV. Identification of a transforming growth factor alpha-like molecule in human seminal plasma. Fertil Steril. 1994;61(1):129–35.
15. Hussenet F, Dousset B, Cordonnier JL, et al. Tumour necrosis factor alpha and interleukin 2 in normal and infected human seminal fluid. Hum Reprod. 1993;8(3):409–11.
16. Fedder J, Ellerman-Eriksen S. Effect of cytokines on sperm motility and ionophore-stimulated acrosome reaction. Arch Androl. 1995;35(3):173–85.
17. Rajasekaran M, Hellstrom WJ, Naz RK, Sikka SC. Oxidative stress and interleukins in seminal plasma during leukocytospermia. Fertil Steril. 1995;64(1):166–71.
18. Twigg J, Fulton N, Gomez E, Irvine DS, Aitken RJ. Analysis of the impact of intracellular reactive oxygen species generation on the structural and functional integrity of human spermatozoa: lipid peroxidation, DNA fragmentation and effectiveness of antioxidants. Hum Reprod. 1998;13(6):1429–36.
19. Song GJ, Norkus EP, Lewis V. Relationship between seminal ascorbic acid and sperm DNA integrity in infertile men. Int J Androl. 2006;29(6):569–75.
20. Lewis SE, Sterling ES, Young IS, Thompson W. Comparison of individual antioxidants of sperm and seminal plasma in fertile and infertile men. Fertil Steril. 1997;67(1):142–7.
21. Fraga CG, Motchnik PA, Shigenaga MK, Helbock HJ, Jacob RA, Ames BN. Ascorbic acid protects against endogenous oxidative DNA damage in human sperm. Proc Natl Acad Sci USA. 1991;88(24):11003–6.
22. Agarwal A, Nallella KP, Allamaneni SS, Said TM. Role of antioxidants in treatment of male infertility: an overview of the literature. Reprod Biomed Online. 2004;8(6):616–27.
23. MacLeod J. The role of oxygen metabolism and motility of human spermatozoa. Am J Physiol. 1943;138:512–8.
24. de Lamirande E, Gagnon C. Human sperm hyperactivation and capacitation as parts of an oxidative process. Free Radic Biol Med. 1993;14(2):157–66.
25. Aitken RJ, Buckingham DW, Brindle J, Gomez E, Baker HW, Irvine DS. Analysis of sperm movement in relation to the oxidative stress created by leukocytes in washed sperm preparations and seminal plasma. Hum Reprod. 1995;10(8):2061–71.

26. Fisher HM, Aitken RJ. Comparative analysis of the ability of precursor germ cells and epididymal spermatozoa to generate reactive oxygen metabolites. J Exp Zool. 1997; 277(5):390–400.
27. Said TM, Agarwal A, Sharma RK, Thomas Jr AJ, Sikka SC. Impact of sperm morphology on DNA damage caused by oxidative stress induced by beta-nicotinamide adenine dinucleotide phosphate. Fertil Steril. 2005;83(1):95–103.
28. Plante M, de Lamirande E, Gagnon C. Reactive oxygen species released by activated neutrophils, but not by deficient spermatozoa, are sufficient to affect normal sperm motility. Fertil Steril. 1994;62(2):387–93.
29. Henkel R, Kierspel E, Stalf T, et al. Effect of reactive oxygen species produced by spermatozoa and leukocytes on sperm functions in non-leukocytospermic patients. Fertil Steril. 2005;83(3):635–42.
30. Moskovtsev SI, Willis J, White J, Mullen JB. Leukocytospermia: relationship to sperm deoxyribonucleic acid integrity in patients evaluated for male factor infertility. Fertil Steril. 2007;88(3):737–40.
31. Wolff H. The biologic significance of white blood cells in semen. Fertil Steril. 1995; 63(6):1143–57.
32. Saleh RA, Agarwal A, Kandirali E, et al. Leukocytospermia is associated with increased reactive oxygen species production by human spermatozoa. Fertil Steril. 2002; 78(6):1215–24.
33. Orleans CT. Increasing the demand for and use of effective smoking-cessation treatments reaping the full health benefits of tobacco-control science and policy gains–in our lifetime. Am J Prev Med. 2007;33(6 Suppl):S340–348.
34. Kulikauskas V, Blaustein D, Ablin RJ. Cigarette smoking and its possible effects on sperm. Fertil Steril. 1985;44(4):526–8.
35. Sepaniak S, Forges T, Fontaine B, et al. Negative impact of cigarette smoking on male fertility: from spermatozoa to the offspring. J Gynecol Obstet Biol Reprod (Paris). 2004; 33(5):384–90.
36. Trummer H, Habermann H, Haas J, Pummer K. The impact of cigarette smoking on human semen parameters and hormones. Hum Reprod. 2002;17(6):1554–9.
37. Saleh RA, Agarwal A, Sharma RK, Nelson DR, Thomas Jr AJ. Effect of cigarette smoking on levels of seminal oxidative stress in infertile men: a prospective study. Fertil Steril. 2002;78(3):491–9.
38. Hull MG, North K, Taylor H, Farrow A, Ford WC. Delayed conception and active and passive smoking. The Avon Longitudinal Study of Pregnancy and Childhood Study Team. Fertil Steril. 2000;74(4):725–33.
39. Zenzes MT, Puy LA, Bielecki R, Reed TE. Detection of benzo[a]pyrene diol epoxide-DNA adducts in embryos from smoking couples: evidence for transmission by spermatozoa. Mol Hum Reprod. 1999;5(2):125–31.
40. Fraga CG, Motchnik PA, Wyrobek AJ, Rempel DM, Ames BN. Smoking and low antioxidant levels increase oxidative damage to sperm DNA. Mutat Res. 1996;351(2):199–203.
41. Mostafa T, Tawadrous G, Roaia MM, Amer MK, Kader RA, Aziz A. Effect of smoking on seminal plasma ascorbic acid in infertile and fertile males. Andrologia. 2006;38(6):221–4.
42. Villalta J, Ballesca JL, Nicolas JM, Martinez de Osaba MJ, Antunez E, Pimentel C. Testicular function in asymptomatic chronic alcoholics: relation to ethanol intake. Alcohol Clin Exp Res. 1997;21(1):128–33.
43. Wu D, Cederbaum AI. Alcohol, oxidative stress, and free radical damage. Alcohol Res Health. 2003;27(4):277–84.
44. Hauser R, Meeker JD, Singh NP, et al. DNA damage in human sperm is related to urinary levels of phthalate monoester and oxidative metabolites. Hum Reprod. 2007;22(3):688–95.
45. Duty SM, Silva MJ, Barr DB, et al. Phthalate exposure and human semen parameters. Epidemiology. 2003;14(3):269–77.

46. Lee E, Ahn MY, Kim HJ, et al. Effect of di(*n*-butyl) phthalate on testicular oxidative damage and antioxidant enzymes in hyperthyroid rats. Environ Toxicol. 2007;22(3):245–55.
47. Chitra KC, Sujatha R, Latchoumycandane C, Mathur PP. Effect of lindane on antioxidant enzymes in epididymis and epididymal sperm of adult rats. Asian J Androl. 2001;3(3):205–8.
48. Latchoumycandane C, Chitra KC, Mathur PP. 2,3,7,8-Tetrachlorodibenzo- p-dioxin (TCDD) induces oxidative stress in the epididymis and epididymal sperm of adult rats. Arch Toxicol. 2003;77(5):280–4.
49. Hsu PC, Guo YL. Antioxidant nutrients and lead toxicity. Toxicology. 2002;180(1):33–44.
50. Roos D. The involvement of oxygen radicals in microbicidal mechanisms of leukocytes and macrophages. Klin Wochenschr. 1991;69(21–23):975–80.
51. Mazzilli F, Rossi T, Marchesini M, Ronconi C, Dondero F. Superoxide anion in human semen related to seminal parameters and clinical aspects. Fertil Steril. 1994;62(4):862–8.
52. Brackett NL, Ibrahim E, Grotas JA, Aballa TC, Lynne CM. Higher sperm DNA damage in semen from men with spinal cord injuries compared with controls. J Androl. 2008;29(1):93–9. discussion 100–101.
53. Padron OF, Brackett NL, Sharma RK, Lynne CM, Thomas Jr AJ, Agarwal A. Seminal reactive oxygen species and sperm motility and morphology in men with spinal cord injury. Fertil Steril. 1997;67(6):1115–20.
54. Segnini A, Camejo MI, Proverbio F. Chlamydia trachomatis and sperm lipid peroxidation in infertile men. Asian J Androl. 2003;5(1):47–9.
55. Schaeffer AJ. Epidemiology and demographics of prostatitis. Andrologia. 2003;35(5):252–7.
56. Motrich RD, Maccioni M, Molina R, et al. Reduced semen quality in chronic prostatitis patients that have cellular autoimmune response to prostate antigens. Hum Reprod. 2005;20(9):2567–72.
57. Batstone GR, Doble A, Gaston JS. Autoimmune T cell responses to seminal plasma in chronic pelvic pain syndrome (CPPS). Clin Exp Immunol. 2002;128(2):302–7.
58. Henkel R, Ludwig M, Schuppe HC, Diemer T, Schill WB, Weidner W. Chronic pelvic pain syndrome/chronic prostatitis affect the acrosome reaction in human spermatozoa. World J Urol. 2006;24(1):39–44.
59. Krieger JN, Berger RE, Ross SO, Rothman I, Muller CH. Seminal fluid findings in men with nonbacterial prostatitis and prostatodynia. J Androl. 1996;17(3):310–8.
60. Barbieri ER, Hidalgo ME, Venegas A, Smith R, Lissi EA. Varicocele-associated decrease in antioxidant defenses. J Androl. 1999;20(6):713–7.
61. Saleh RA, Agarwal A, Nada EA, et al. Negative effects of increased sperm DNA damage in relation to seminal oxidative stress in men with idiopathic and male factor infertility. Fertil Steril. 2003;79 Suppl 3:1597–605.
62. Smith R, Kaune H, Parodi D, et al. Increased sperm DNA damage in patients with varicocele: relationship with seminal oxidative stress. Hum Reprod. 2006;21(4):986–93.
63. Filippini A, Riccioli A, Padula F, et al. Control and impairment of immune privilege in the testis and in semen. Hum Reprod Update. 2001;7(5):444–9.
64. Kolettis PN, Sharma RK, Pasqualotto FF, Nelson D, Thomas Jr AJ, Agarwal A. Effect of seminal oxidative stress on fertility after vasectomy reversal. Fertil Steril. 1999; 71(2):249–55.
65. Shapiro RH, Muller CH, Chen G, Berger RE. Vasectomy reversal associated with increased reactive oxygen species production by seminal fluid leukocytes and sperm. J Urol. 1998;160(4):1341–6.
66. Huff DS, Hadziselimovic F, Snyder III HM, Blyth B, Duckett JW. Early postnatal testicular maldevelopment in cryptorchidism. J Urol Aug. 1991;146(2 (Pt 2)):624–6.
67. Smith R, Kaune H, Parodi D, et al. Extent of sperm DNA damage in spermatozoa from men examined for infertility. Relationship with oxidative stress. Rev Med Chil. 2007;135(3): 279–86.
68. Turner TT, Bang HJ, Lysiak JL. The molecular pathology of experimental testicular torsion suggests adjunct therapy to surgical repair. J Urol. 2004;172(6 Pt 2):2574–8.

69. Filho DW, Torres MA, Bordin AL, Crezcynski-Pasa TB, Boveris A. Spermatic cord torsion, reactive oxygen and nitrogen species and ischemia-reperfusion injury. Mol Aspects Med. 2004;25(1–2):199–210.
70. Balaban RS, Nemoto S, Finkel T. Mitochondria, oxidants, and aging. Cell. 2005;120(4): 483–95.
71. Bogenhagen DF. Repair of mtDNA in vertebrates. Am J Hum Genet. 1999;64(5):1276–81.
72. Liu CY, Lee CF, Hong CH, Wei YH. Mitochondrial DNA mutation and depletion increase the susceptibility of human cells to apoptosis. Ann N Y Acad Sci. 2004;1011:133–45.
73. Taylor RW, Turnbull DM. Mitochondrial DNA mutations in human disease. Nat Rev Genet. 2005;6(5):389–402.
74. Wang X, Sharma RK, Gupta A, et al. Alterations in mitochondria membrane potential and oxidative stress in infertile men: a prospective observational study. Fertil Steril. 2003;80 Suppl 2:844–50.
75. Nakada K, Sato A, Yoshida K, et al. Mitochondria-related male infertility. Proc Natl Acad Sci USA. 2006;103(41):15148–53.
76. Shamsi MB, Kumar R, Bhatt A, et al. Mitochondrial DNA Mutations in etiopathogenesis of male infertility. Indian J Urol. 2008;24(2):150–4.
77. Braithwaite EK, Kedar PS, Stumpo DJ, et al. DNA polymerases beta and lambda mediate overlapping and independent roles in base excision repair in mouse embryonic fibroblasts. PLoS One. 2010;5(8):e12229.
78. Yang H, Clendenin WM, Wong D, et al. Enhanced activity of adenine-DNA glycosylase (Myh) by apurinic/apyrimidinic endonuclease (Ape1) in mammalian base excision repair of an A/GO mismatch. Nucleic Acids Res. 2001;29(3):743–52.
79. Slupska MM, Luther WM, Chiang JH, Yang H, Miller JH. Functional expression of hMYH, a human homolog of the Escherichia coli MutY protein. J Bacteriol. 1999;181(19):6210–3.
80. Xie Y, Yang H, Miller JH, et al. Cells deficient in oxidative DNA damage repair genes Myh and Ogg1 are sensitive to oxidants with increased G2/M arrest and multinucleation. Carcinogenesis. 2008;29(4):722–8.
81. Zini A, de Lamirande E, Gagnon C. Reactive oxygen species in semen of infertile patients: levels of superoxide dismutase- and catalase-like activities in seminal plasma and spermatozoa. Int J Androl. 1993;16(3):183–8.
82. Jeulin C, Soufir JC, Weber P, Laval-Martin D, Calvayrac R. Catalase activity in human spermatozoa and seminal plasma. Gamete Res. 1989;24(2):185–96.
83. Athayde KS, Cocuzza M, Agarwal A, et al. Development of normal reference values for seminal reactive oxygen species and their correlation with leukocytes and semen parameters in a fertile population. J Androl. 2007;28(4):613–20.
84. Barroso G, Morshedi M, Oehninger S. Analysis of DNA fragmentation, plasma membrane translocation of phosphatidylserine and oxidative stress in human spermatozoa. Hum Reprod. 2000;15(6):1338–44.
85. Irvine DS, Twigg JP, Gordon EL, Fulton N, Milne PA, Aitken RJ. DNA integrity in human spermatozoa: relationships with semen quality. J Androl. 2000;21(1):33–44.
86. Sawyer DE, Mercer BG, Wiklendt AM, Aitken RJ. Quantitative analysis of gene-specific DNA damage in human spermatozoa. Mutat Res. 2003;529(1–2):21–34.
87. Desai N, Sabanegh Jr E, Kim T, Agarwal A. Free radical theory of aging: implications in male infertility. Urology. 2010;75(1):14–9.
88. Lenzi A, Lombardo F, Gandini L, Alfano P, Dondero F. Computer assisted sperm motility analysis at the moment of induced pregnancy during gonadotropin treatment for hypogonadotropic hypogonadism. J Endocrinol Invest. 1993;16(9):683–6.
89. Agarwal A, Ikemoto I, Loughlin KR. Relationship of sperm parameters with levels of reactive oxygen species in semen specimens. J Urol. 1994;152(1):107–10.
90. Armstrong JS, Rajasekaran M, Chamulitrat W, Gatti P, Hellstrom WJ, Sikka SC. Characterization of reactive oxygen species induced effects on human spermatozoa movement and energy metabolism. Free Radic Biol Med. 1999;26(7–8):869–80.

 91. Agarwal A, Makker K, Sharma R. Clinical relevance of oxidative stress in male factor infertility: an update. Am J Reprod Immunol. 2008;59(1):2–11.
 92. Suleiman SA, Ali ME, Zaki ZM, el-Malik EM, Nasr MA. Lipid peroxidation and human sperm motility: protective role of vitaminE. J Androl. 1996;17(5):530–7.
 93. McKinney KA, Lewis SE, Thompson W. Reactive oxygen species generation in human sperm: luminol and lucigenin chemiluminescence probes. Arch Androl. 1996;36(2):119–25.
 94. Aitken RJ, West KM. Analysis of the relationship between reactive oxygen species production and leucocyte infiltration in fractions of human semen separated on Percoll gradients. Int J Androl. 1990;13(6):433–51.
 95. Aitken RJ, Buckingham DW, West K, Brindle J. On the use of paramagnetic beads and ferrofluids to assess and eliminate the leukocytic contribution to oxygen radical generation by human sperm suspensions. Am J Reprod Immunol. 1996;35(6):541–51.
 96. Shekarriz M, DeWire DM, Thomas Jr AJ, Agarwal A. A method of human semen centrifugation to minimize the iatrogenic sperm injuries caused by reactive oxygen species. Eur Urol. 1995;28(1):31–5.
 97. Aitken RJ, Baker MA, O'Bryan M. Shedding light on chemiluminescence: the application of chemiluminescence in diagnostic andrology. J Androl. 2004;25(4):455–65.
 98. Aitken RJ, Clarkson JS. Cellular basis of defective sperm function and its association with the genesis of reactive oxygen species by human spermatozoa. J Reprod Fertil. 1987; 81(2):459–69.
 99. Kobayashi H, Gil-Guzman E, Mahran AM, et al. Quality control of reactive oxygen species measurement by luminol-dependent chemiluminescence assay. J Androl. 2001;22(4): 568–74.
100. Piomboni P, Gambera L, Serafini F, Campanella G, Morgante G, De Leo V. Sperm quality improvement after natural anti-oxidant treatment of asthenoteratospermic men with leukocytospermia. Asian J Androl. 2008;10(2):201–6.
101. Silver EW, Eskenazi B, Evenson DP, Block G, Young S, Wyrobek AJ. Effect of antioxidant intake on sperm chromatin stability in healthy nonsmoking men. J Androl. 2005; 26(4):550–6.
102. Omu AE, Al-Othman S, Mohamad AS, Al-Kaluwby NM, Fernandes S. Antibiotic therapy for seminal infection. Effect on antioxidant activity and T-helper cytokines. J Reprod Med. 1998;43(10):857–64.
103. Vicari E. Effectiveness and limits of antimicrobial treatment on seminal leukocyte concentration and related reactive oxygen species production in patients with male accessory gland infection. Hum Reprod. 2000;15(12):2536–44.
104. Gambera L, Serafini F, Morgante G, Focarelli R, De Leo V, Piomboni P. Sperm quality and pregnancy rate after COX-2 inhibitor therapy of infertile males with abacterial leukocytospermia. Hum Reprod. 2007;22(4):1047–51.
105. Comhaire FH, Christophe AB, Zalata AA, Dhooge WS, Mahmoud AM, Depuydt CE. The effects of combined conventional treatment, oral antioxidants and essential fatty acids on sperm biology in subfertile men. Prostaglandins Leukot Essent Fatty Acids. 2000;63(3): 159–65.
106. Kessopoulou E, Powers HJ, Sharma KK, et al. A double-blind randomized placebo cross-over controlled trial using the antioxidant vitamin E to treat reactive oxygen species associated male infertility. Fertil Steril. 1995;64(4):825–31.
107. Keskes-Ammar L, Feki-Chakroun N, Rebai T, et al. Sperm oxidative stress and the effect of an oral vitamin E and selenium supplement on semen quality in infertile men. Arch Androl. 2003;49(2):83–94.
108. Greco E, Iacobelli M, Rienzi L, Ubaldi F, Ferrero S, Tesarik J. Reduction of the incidence of sperm DNA fragmentation by oral antioxidant treatment. J Androl. 2005;26(3):349–53.
109. Lenzi A, Sgro P, Salacone P, et al. A placebo-controlled double-blind randomized trial of the use of combined l-carnitine and l-acetyl-carnitine treatment in men with asthenozoospermia. Fertil Steril. 2004;81(6):1578–84.

110. Tremellen K, Miari G, Froiland D, Thompson J. A randomised control trial examining the effect of an antioxidant (Menevit) on pregnancy outcome during IVF-ICSI treatment. Aust N Z J Obstet Gynaecol. 2007;47(3):216–21.
111. Rolf C, Cooper TG, Yeung CH, Nieschlag E. Antioxidant treatment of patients with astheno-zoospermia or moderate oligoasthenozoospermia with high-dose vitamin C and vitamin E: a randomized, placebo-controlled, double-blind study. Hum Reprod. 1999;14(4):1028–33.
112. Zini A, Blumenfeld A, Libman J, Willis J. Beneficial effect of microsurgical varicocelectomy on human sperm DNA integrity. Hum Reprod. 2005;20(4):1018–21.
113. Werthman P, Wixon R, Kasperson K, Evenson DP. Significant decrease in sperm deoxyribo-nucleic acid fragmentation after varicocelectomy. Fertil Steril. 2008;90(5):1800–4.
114. Evers JL, Collins JA. Assessment of efficacy of varicocele repair for male subfertility: a systematic review. Lancet. 2003;361(9372):1849–52.
115. Marmar JL, Agarwal A, Prabakaran S, et al. Reassessing the value of varicocelectomy as a treatment for male subfertility with a new meta-analysis. Fertil Steril. 2007;88(3):639–48.

Chapter 6
Oxidative Stress

Fanuel Lampiao, C.J. Opperman, Ashok Agarwal, and Stefan S. du Plessis

The idea that free radicals are produced by spermatozoa was first proposed by Macleod in 1943 [1]. While evaluating the influence of oxygen tension on sperm cell motility, he observed that the addition of the catalase enzyme to sperm incubation medium significantly reduced their motility loss. Macleod concluded in this pioneering study that hydrogen peroxide (H_2O_2) must be produced by spermatozoa during oxygen metabolism, thereby setting the trend for future research along these lines. However, it was not until 1979 that Jones and colleagues resolved the underlying mechanism behind free radicals and their ability to reduce sperm motility. They reported a decrease in the flexibility of sperm membranes due to reactive oxygen species (ROS)-induced peroxidation [1].

Nearly 70 years after the discovery of Macleod, interest is turning toward free radicals as the origin of male infertility with 1 in every 20 male individuals being infertile and accounting for half of all cases of couple infertility in the general population [2]. It is no surprise that ROS-mediated sperm cell damage is accountable in up to 30–80% of these cases as the foremost contributing pathological factor of male infertility [3]. A free radical is defined as a molecule that has one or more unpaired electrons with the capability to oxidize biomolecules [4]. Leukocytes (extrinsic ROS) and spermatozoa (intrinsic ROS) are the foundation to the production of free radicals within semen [5], not excluding external origins of oxidative tension. Free radicals can attack the deoxyribose backbone of spermatozoa directly or damage its pyrimidine and purine basis [3]. Alternatively, caspase enzymatic

F. Lampiao, PhD (✉) • C.J. Opperman, BSc • S.S. du Plessis, PhD, MBA
Department of Medical Physiology, Faculty of Health Sciences, Stellenbosch University, 19063, Tygerberg, Western Cape 7505, South Africa
e-mail: flampiao@medcol.mw; ssdp@sun.ac.za

A. Agarwal, PhD
Center for Reproductive Medicine, Glickman Urological and Kidney Institute, Cleveland Clinic Foundation, 9500 Euclid Avenue, Desk A19, Cleveland, OH 44195, USA
e-mail: agarwaa@ccf.org

S.J. Parekattil and A. Agarwal (eds.), *Antioxidants in Male Infertility: A Guide for Clinicians and Researchers*, © Springer Science+Business Media New York 2013

degradation of DNA is subsequent to the initiation of ROS-mediated apoptosis [6]. Furthermore, the large amount of membrane polyunsaturated fatty acids (PUFAs) within spermatozoa makes them vulnerable to free radicals. On the other hand, the value of physiological ROS levels in the functioning of spermatozoa during the stimulation of capacitation, hyperactivation, and the acrosome reaction cannot be overlooked [7]. Therefore, the body has developed several defense mechanisms which are focused on oxidant scavenging to protect itself from the detrimental effect of ROS damage. These include enzymes such as superoxide dismutase (SOD) [8, 9] and glutathione peroxidase (GPX) [10, 11] as well as nonenzymatic molecules, for instance, ascorbic acid (vitamin C) and alpha-tocopherol (vitamin E) within the semen [12, 13]. For this reason, oxidative stress is only achieved when the balance is shifted toward the production of ROS and when its overwhelming effect on antioxidant defense mechanisms becomes prominent.

A new diagnostic era is on the horizon, with over 30 advanced direct and indirect screening assays available to assess oxidative stress. Promising as it might seem, routine testing is still shortcoming due to cost contributing factors, complexity dilemmas, and the lack of a standardized routine [14]. Nonetheless, management of oxidative stress-related male infertility is focused on the identification of underlying pathology prior to antioxidant treatment. If areas such as lifestyle modifications or lessening the burden of environmental exposures would still be attractive to pharmaceutical companies from a business perspective in the long run when compared to conventional medical supplementation regimens or possible surgery remains debatable. Finally, this overview chapter will provide the reader with the biochemistry, etiology and management of oxidative stress in male infertility. Moreover, it is hoped that the importance of free radicals in spermatogenesis is realized and further exploring into this field stimulated.

Oxidative Stress: Etiology and the Oxygen Paradox

Aerobic metabolism is associated with the production of free radical molecules. These prooxidant molecules are formed throughout the controlled enzymatic reduction of oxygen within the mitochondria during oxidative phosphorylation [11]. A free radical is defined as a molecule that has one or more unpaired electrons in its molecular or atomic orbital. Therefore, this highly reactive group of chemical molecules has the potential to significantly contribute in the oxidation of biomolecules such as amino acids in proteins and lipids in membranes, while seeking to alleviate their unpaired electron state [4, 15]. The superoxide anion radical ($O_2{}^{\cdot-}$), the primary form of ROS, is formed following the addition of an electron to dioxygen (O_2). However, this molecule can then be indirectly as well as directly (metal catalyzed, enzymatic) converted to secondary ROS (Fig. 6.1b), such as H_2O_2, the peroxyl radical ($ROO^{\cdot}$), and the hydroxyl radical ($^{\cdot}OH$). Interestingly, not all ROS are considered to be free radicals despite the fact that the terms are used in a common interchangeable manner [16]. For example, H_2O_2 does not contain unpaired electrons and therefore

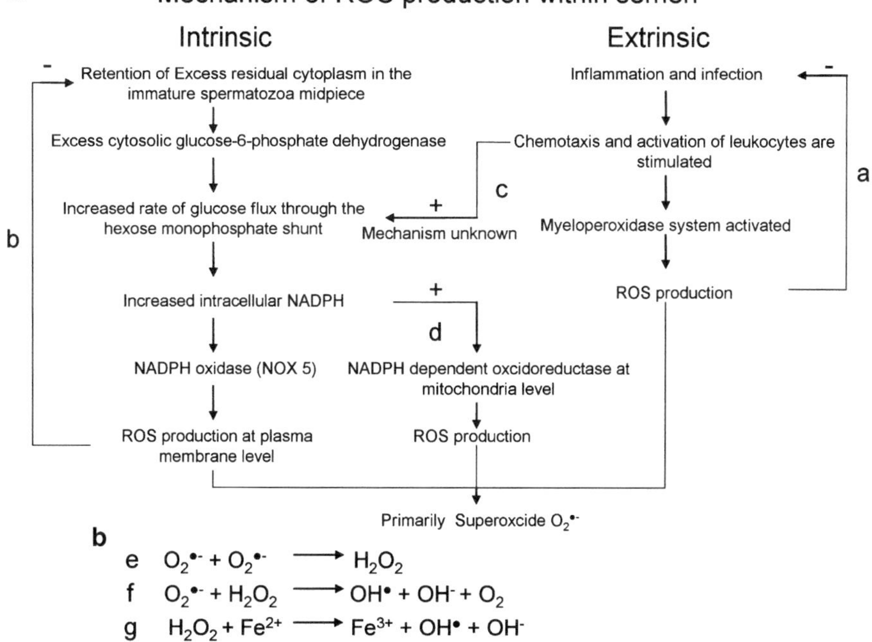

Fig. 6.1 Free radicals and their production. (**a**) Free radicals (superoxide) can be produced within the sperm cell or via leukocytes in the semen, not excluding external systemic and local genital tract sources (a, b—negative feedback; c, d—positive feedback). (**b**) Superoxide, the primary form of reactive oxygen species, is converted directly (metal catalyzed, enzymatic) and indirectly to secondary (e–g) reactive oxygen species

Table 6.1 Reactive oxygen species consist of radical and none radical oxygen derivatives

Radicals		Nonradicals	
Lipid peroxyl	$LOO^•$	Lipid peroxide	$LOOH$
Thyl	$RS^•$	Ozone	O_3
Peroxyl	$RO_2^•$	Singlet oxygen	$^{-1}O_2$
Nitric oxide	$NO^•$	Hydrogen peroxide	H_2O_2
Superoxide	$O_2^{•-}$	Hypochloric acid	$HOCl$
Hydroxyl	$OH^•$	Peroxynitrite	$ONOO^-$

by definition is not a free radical (Table 6.1). Still, it is an addition to the ROS family since it has been derived from the metabolism of oxygen. Additionally, there is a subclass of ROS molecules derived from nitrogen. They are known as the reactive nitrogen species (RNS) and embrace a free radical nature. Some of the most common RNS are listed in Table 6.2 [17].

Leukocytes (extrinsic ROS production) and spermatozoa (intrinsic ROS production) form the two cornerstones in the production of free radicals within semen [5]. Neutrophils form the bulk of leukocytes in semen and are predominantly

Table 6.2 Summary of various reactive nitrogen species, also considered as a subclass of reactive oxygen species

Peroxynitrite	$OONO^-$	Nitrous acid	HNO_2
Peroxynitrous acid	$OONOH$	Dinitrogen trioxide	N_2O_3
Nitryl chloride	NO_2Cl	Nitrogen dioxide	$NO_2^{\cdot}$
Nitrous oxide	$NO^{\cdot}$	Nitroxyl cation	NO^+
Nitroxyl anion	NO^-		

Table 6.3 Sperm and seminal plasma are well equipped with a collection of both enzymatic and nonenzymatic antioxidant defenses

Antioxidant	Mechanism	References
Enzyme		
Superoxide dismutase (SOD)	Inactivates superoxide radicals by converting it into oxygen	[8, 9]
Catalase	Inactivates hydrogen peroxide by converting it into water	[52, 53]
Glutathione peroxidase (GPX 1–5)	Responsible for the reduction of hydrogen peroxide through the utilizing of glutathione as an electron donor	[10, 11]
Nonenzyme		
Ascorbic acid (vitamin C)	All of these antioxidants within the semen act according to the chemical principle of directly neutralizing free radicals. Additional mechanisms of protection are provided by albumin and prostasomes. Albumin can be oxidized itself, thereby intercepting free radicals. Alternatively, prostasomes (extracellular organelles secreted by the prostate) have been reported to fuse leukocytes and influence their ROS production	[12, 13]
Alpha-tocopherol (vitamin E)		
Urate		
Prostasomes		
Albumin		
Carnitine		
Carotenoids		
Flavonoids		

responsible for destroying pathogens by means of ROS production (Fig. 6.1a). A definite correlation between oxidative stress and the presence of elevated leukocyte numbers has been established [18]. It is important to remember throughout this chapter that oxidative stress only occurs when the production of free radicals overwhelms antioxidant defenses, which can ultimately lead to sperm cell damage. For this reason, spermatozoa and seminal plasma contain a selection of protective antioxidant mechanisms (Table 6.3). Nonetheless, no distinct relationship has been described between male infertility and leukocytes thus far [19]. The importance of leukocyte activation in ROS production cannot be overlooked. Several studies have reported elevated levels of proinflammatory cytokines within seminal plasma prior to the production of large ROS amounts. These molecules include tumor necrosis factor-alpha, interleukin-8 [20], and interleukin-6 [21]. Sperm isolation and quantification techniques have not only revealed ROS production by sperm cells but also the motive behind excessive ROS output in teratozoospermia (less than the reference value for morphology) during impaired spermatogenesis. In morphologically normal spermatozoa, cytoplasm deposits in the midpiece are extruded to allow for cell elongation and condensation to occur during spermatogenesis. Furthermore, these cytoplasm deposits contain large amounts of the glucose-6-phosphate dehydrogenase enzyme which is responsible for the rate of glucose flux in the cell and the intracellular production of beta-nicotinamide adenine dinucleotide phosphate (NADPH). As a result, ROS is generated from NADPH via intermembrane-located NADPH oxidase [11]. Teratozoospermia is characterized by large amounts of cytoplasm, and therefore, higher levels of ROS is expected when these specimens are compared to normozoospermic spermatozoa. In addition, a calcium-dependent NADPH oxidase called NOX 5 has been reported in sperm. It appears to be quite distinct from the NADPH oxidase enzyme located in leukocytes. Still, expression of the NOX 5 in infertile men is unknown [3]. An interesting observation is that leukocytes are the predominant producer of ROS during spermatozoa capacitation and per cell basis. However, intrinsic production of ROS within close proximity to the sperm cell's DNA formulates a more important variable in terms of oxidative stress infertility [4].

Table 6.4 shows the origin of well-established external causes for potential oxidative stress in the male reproductive tract. A number of articles have addressed the impact of lifestyle modifications on seminal ROS levels as well as the correlation with sperm DNA damage and infertility. Alcohol has been reported to stimulate the production of ROS. Moreover, studies have shown that excessive alcohol consumers tend to be malnourished and have a diet with insufficient antioxidants [22]. A recent study reported that a person who smoked had a 48% increase in testicular leukocyte levels, accompanied by a 107% increase in seminal ROS concentration [23]. Furthermore, smokers tend to have decreased concentrations of natural antioxidants such as vitamins C and E in their seminal plasma [24], implying an additional risk for infertility. Studies confirm a link between high-antioxidant intake and an increase in motile sperm percentages as well as decreased sperm DNA damage [25]. Although, it is more likely that individual antioxidant levels within the semen reflects the biological effects before diet supplementary intake more accurately since different food preparation techniques and sources can vastly influence antioxidant levels. Unsurprisingly, fertile men with low levels of oxidative stress will not require the same amount of protection from antioxidants to maintain their DNA integrity. Therefore, insufficient antioxidants in men with a low oxidative stress risk may not lead to sperm DNA damage per se.

It is no surprise that extreme exercise activities lead to the production of large amounts of ROS following increased aerobic muscle metabolism [26]. Similarly, obesity provokes oxidative stress as cytokines are released from adipose tissue during proinflammatory reactions which leads to an increase in leukocytes [27]. What is more is that heating of the testicles due to the accumulation of groin region adipose tissue has shown to result in reduced sperm quality [28]. Several studies have reported a direct link between age and sperm DNA damage in both fertile as well as infertile men. In addition, systemic oxidative stress seems to increase with age [29], making oxidative stress a most likely candidate for the underlying sperm pathology in older infertile men. Finally, psychological stress has been concurrent with low sperm quality due to an increase in ROS production and reduced antioxidant defenses [30].

Table 6.4 Established causes of sperm oxidative stress potentially leading to male factor infertility

Origin of oxidative stress	References
Lifestyle	
Smoking	[24]
Insufficient diet	[25]
Psychological stress	[30]
Obesity	[27]
Alcohol	[22]
Age-related	[29]
Environmental	
Pollution	[35]
Heavy metals	[36]
Heat	[26, 28]
Plasticizers	[31]
Pesticides	[33]
Herbicides	[34]
Infection	
Systemic infection	[41–44]
Genitourinary tract	[39]
Autoimmune	
Chronic prostatitis	[45–47]
Vasectomy	[48]
Torsion	[3, 59]
Testicular	[56, 57]
Idiopathic	[49, 50]
Iatrogenic	
Medications	[54]
Centrifugation, cryopreservation	[3, 51]
Chronic disease	
Hemoglobinopathies	[63]
Diabetes	[64, 65]
Chronic kidney disease	[60–62]
Hyperhomocysteinemia	[66]

Numerous environmental pollutants have been linked with oxidative stress. Increased sperm DNA damage and impaired spermatogenesis have been reported in cases of phthalates absorption. Phthalates are chemicals used in personal care products and plastic food packaging [31]. Sulfur dioxide, a frequently used preservative [32], pesticides such as methoxychlor [33], and the herbicide dioxin TCDD [34] have resulted in the production of ROS during laboratory animal trials. While airborne pollutants such as diesel have the potential to increase infertility [35], exposure to heavy metals (lead, cadmium) is conclusively associated with testicular oxidative stress [36].

Male infertility might not be treated by addressing bacterial infections as a first-line therapy, but recent studies have provoked interest into this alternative treatment approach. It has been estimated that up to 50% of men will experience prostatitis [37]. The bacteria responsible for this infection can be sexually transmitted or acquired from a local urinary tract infection [38]. The recurrent entering of these pathogens into the genital tract results in an acute inflammatory response, with an influx of leukocytes and a subsequent increase in ROS production. High levels of oxidative sperm pathology have been confirmed in individuals with an elevated tendency for genitourinary tract infections, such as paraplegics [39]. Oxidative damage to sperm cells can also be linked to viral infections which include the herpes simplex virus. The DNA of this virus is found to be present in the semen of between 14% and 50% of infertile men. In addition, its presence is associated with an increase in IgM antibodies and the rate of leukocytospermia production [40]. Despite the fact that no study has directly linked chronic systemic infections with sperm oxidative stress, it remains unlikely that the male reproductive tract will be spared from these infectious diseases, which include human immunodeficiency virus [41], hepatitis B and C [42], tuberculosis [43], and malaria [44].

Chronic prostatitis of nonbacterial infectious nature affects 10% of all men [37] and has been associated with elevated levels of oxidative tension in semen [45]. An autoimmune response to prostate and seminal antigens is reported to cause a proinflammatory reaction with an increase in leukocytes [46]. Although the exact nature of this reaction is unknown, it is believed to be the result of a polymorphism linked to Th-2 cytokine interleukin-10. The production of T lymphocytes reactive against the above antigens might be due to the lack of Th-2 cytokines, shifting the balance toward the Th-1 cytokines in the immune system. Chemotaxis and activation of leukocytes are stimulated as a result of cytokines (such as tumor necrosis factor-alpha, interleukin-1-beta and interferon-gamma) liberated in response to the T lymphocytes [47]. A clinical example of this is when the blood–testis barrier is disrupted following vasectomy. Consequently, immune defense against spermatozoa is lost, leading to significant oxidative stress and infertility after vasectomy reversal [48].

Compelling results have shown that morphologically abnormal sperm cells tend to yield higher levels of ROS production and portray a lower capacity of antioxidant protection [49]. In addition, teratozoospermia is commonly observed in one of every three infertile men. For that reason, oxidative stress is frequently exhibited in the male population with idiopathic infertility. This principal association of elevated seminal ROS levels and decreased antioxidant values has also been made amongst idiopathic infertile men presenting with normozoospermia, the reason for this however is still ambiguous [50].

Sperm oxidative stress can also be augmented during assisted reproductive techniques. At some point during intrauterine insemination and similar assisted reproductive technologies, semen is separated from the seminal plasma by means of techniques that involve centrifugation. This exacerbates ROS production within the sperm cells, while removing the sperm from their antioxidant environment [3]. Cryopreservation, a commonly used technique, also increases the likelihood of an oxidative assault on sperm cells [51]. Resent chemotherapeutic agent studies on animal models have revealed a link with oxidative stress. The administration of cyclophosphamide has indicated a decrease in testicular catalase [52, 53] and an increase in testicular malondialdehyde levels, implying the presence of oxidative stress [54]. Also, commonly used household medications, such as aspirin and paracetamol, tend to elevate cytochrome P450 activity, thereby enhancing the production of free radicals [55].

It has become widely accepted that oxidative stress forms the foundation to the pathology when linking male infertility to testicular varicocele [56]. This phenomenon of increased ROS production in the presence of a varicocele is strongly correlated with the reduction in sperm DNA integrity [57]. Cryptorchidism also contributes to male infertility. Hypospermatogenesis is the primary pathology in this condition due to insufficient maturation of gonocytes to spermatogonia type A. Interestingly, men treated with orchidopexy still show a significant increase in male infertility due to DNA fragmentation and ROS production when compared to control groups [58]. Ischemia reperfusion injury in the contralateral and torted testis during torsion of the spermatic cord has been recognized in male infertility. It is no surprise that oxidative stress is generally accepted to be the underlying cause to the pathology, even when the torsion is unilateral. Spontaneous or surgical restoration of blood flow during a long-standing ischemia period leads to an influx of leukocytes in their activated form to both testes. A subsequent increase in free radicals follows with necrosis of germinal cells. Ultimately, oxidative stress results in infertility or subfertility [59].

Oxidative stress and chronic inflammation are both highly prevalent in cases of end-stage renal and chronic kidney disease [60]. In addition, patients with no evident sign of immune rejection of their graft and stable renal function following renal transplantation also reveal high levels of oxidative stress [61]. Interestingly, a constant state of oxidative stress and chronic inflammation persists after the reversal of uremia following hemodialysis [62]. Beta-thalassemia major, a hemoglobinopathy, is associated with high levels of systemic oxidative stress. Furthermore, this oxidative stress also involves sperm with iron overload forming the most likely cause due to multiple blood transfusions [63]. Diabetic men also show a tendency to produce sperm that has higher DNA fragmentation when compared to their counterparts [64]. Many of the complications of diabetes mellitus are due to an underlying oxidative pathology; therefore, it is probable that oxidative stress is responsible for sperm DNA fragmentation in these individuals as supported by recent studies [65, 66].

Physiological Importance of Reactive Oxygen Species in Normal Spermatozoa Function

Even though oxidative stress is associated with detrimental sperm function, at physiological levels, ROS play a vital role in the regulation of normal sperm function [67]. Physiological levels of ROS have been reported to act as crucial intracellular signaling molecules during the process sperm capacitation. Capacitation is the course of action whereby spermatozoa gain the ability to respond to signals presented by the oocyte–cumulus complex and initiate the cascade of cellular interactions that necessitate fertilization. Although numerous hypotheses have been developed, the precise nature of capacitation is still obscure. Changes associated with sperm capacitation include an increase in respiration and subsequent changes in the motility pattern, called hyperactivation, which is characterized by pronounced flagellar movements and a marked lateral excursion of sperm head in a nonlinear trajectory [68], removal of cholesterol from the plasma membrane, destabilization of the sperm membrane, an increase in intracellular pH and calcium levels, activation of second messenger systems and removal of zinc [69].

The most important change in sperm after capacitation is its ability to undergo the acrosome reaction in response to the *zona pellucida* protein 3 (ZP3), progesterone, and calcium ionophore [70]. Capacitation is also associated with changes in sperm plasma membrane fluidity, intracellular changes in ionic concentration, and sperm cell metabolism [71]. ROS such as O_2^- and H_2O_2 have been reported to play a role in the initiation of the processes capacitation and acrosome reaction [71].

Superoxide anion radical plays an important role during maturation of spermatozoa [72] and in the control of sperm function through the redox regulation of tyrosine phosphorylation [73]. Superoxide has been shown to promote the capacitation of human spermatozoa [74], and there is a superoxide surge in the capacitated spermatozoa during the process [75]. It has been reported that (1) exogenously generated superoxide through the xanthine/xanthine oxidase system induced hyperactivation and capacitation, (2) capacitating sperm produced elevated concentrations of superoxide over prolonged periods of time, and (3) removal of this ROS by SOD prevented hyperactivation and capacitation [76]. H_2O_2 was also shown to promote capacitation of human spermatozoa [77]. The mechanisms and targets of action of H_2O_2 are still unknown.

Nitric oxide (NO) is a free radical synthesized in vivo during the conversion of L-arginine to L-citrulline by the enzyme nitric oxide synthase (NOS). Recent reports suggested the expression of NOS in mouse and human spermatozoa [78]. NO appears to be involved in sperm hyperactivation [79] and *zona pellucida* binding [80]. However, the role of endogenous NO in human sperm capacitation still remains to be elucidated.

Pathological Effects of Oxidative Stress on Spermatozoa and Their Functional Capacity

The lipid composition of plasma membranes of mammalian spermatozoa is markedly different from those of mammalian somatic cells. They have very high levels of phospholipids, sterols, saturated fatty acids, and PUFAs. Therefore, spermatozoa are particularly susceptible to damage induced by excessive ROS release and subsequent development of oxidative stress [81]. Lipids are major substances responsible for the fluidity of membrane lipid bilayers and changes in composition of plasma membranes of spermatozoa from their epididymal maturation to their capacitation in the female reproductive tract. They are also involved as intermediates in cell fusion [82]. Lipid peroxidation of sperm plasma membranes is considered to be the key mechanism of ROS-induced sperm damage leading to infertility. As illustrated in Fig. 6.2, oxidative stress affects spermatozoa function by inducing apoptosis, membrane lipid peroxidation, and DNA fragmentation.

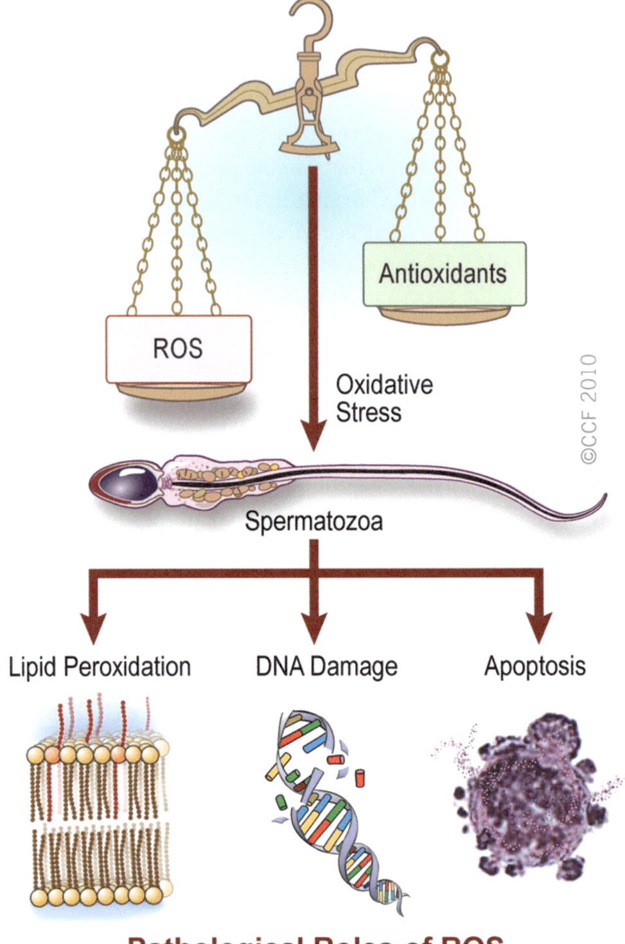

Fig. 6.2 An imbalance between reactive oxygen species (ROS) and antioxidants can lead to the development of oxidative stress which can have detrimental effects on human spermatozoa and sperm function

DNA Damage

Two factors protect the sperm DNA from an oxidative insult: (1) the characteristic tight packaging of the DNA and (2) the antioxidants present in the seminal plasma [83]. Studies in which spermatozoa was exposed to artificially produced ROS resulted in a significant increase in DNA damage in the form of modification of all bases, production of base-free sites, deletions, frameshifts, DNA cross-links, and chromosomal arrangements [84]. Oxidative stress has also been correlated with high frequencies of single and double DNA strand breaks [83].

Apoptosis

Apoptosis is a process of programmed cell death. It is a physiological phenomenon characterized by cellular morphological and biochemical alterations that cause a cell to commit suicide [85]. It is genetically determined and takes place to help discard cells that have an altered function or no function at all [86]. In the male reproductive system, apoptosis may be responsible for controlling the overproduction of male gametes [87]. Apoptosis appears to be strictly regulated by extrinsic and intrinsic factors and can be triggered by a wide variety of stimuli. Examples of extrinsic stimuli that are potentially important in testicular apoptosis are irradiation, chemotherapy, and toxin exposure [88]. Apoptosis-inducing genes such as p53, Bax, and Fas and apoptosis-suppressing genes such as Bcl-2 and c-kit play a prominent role in the genetic control of apoptosis [89]. Spontaneous germ cell apoptosis has been shown in spermatogonia, spermatocytes, and spermatids in the testis of normal men and in patients with nonobstructive azoospermia [90]. Ejaculated spermatozoa have also been shown to demonstrate changes consistent with apoptosis [88]. It has been shown that the levels of apoptosis in mature spermatozoa were significantly correlated with levels of seminal ROS [90]. It was also found that caspase 3 and caspase 9 levels, from infertile patients, were significantly higher in ejaculated spermatozoa when compared to normal healthy sperm donors. In addition, levels of seminal ROS were positively correlated with levels of caspase 3 and caspase 9. This caspase gene family encodes a set of proteases responsible for carrying out programmed cell death [90].

Lipid Peroxidation

Peroxidation of PUFAs in sperm cell membranes is an autocatalytic, self-propagating reaction [91] which can give rise to cell dysfunction associated with loss of membrane function and integrity. It is divided into two steps: initiation and propagation [92]. Initiation is the removal of the hydrogen atom from an unsaturated fatty acid. The second step, propagation, is the formation of a lipid alkyl radical followed by its rapid reaction with oxygen to form a lipid peroxyl radical. The peroxyl radical is capable of removing a hydrogen atom from an unsaturated fatty acid resulting in the formation of a lipid radical and lipid hydroperoxide [91]. Since the alkyl and peroxyl radicals are regenerated, the cycle of propagation could continue indefinitely or end when one of the substrates is consumed or terminated in the radical–radical reaction.

Preventive Measures, Antioxidants, and the Clinical Relevance Thereof in Male Infertility

There are a lot of preventive measures that people can take to minimize the detrimental effects of oxidative stress on the reproductive function. Lifestyle behaviors such as smoking, poor diet, alcohol abuse, obesity, or psychological stress have been implicated in increasing OS. Minimizing lifestyle triggers of oxidative stress mentioned above is therefore one way of preventing or minimizing the harmful effects of oxidative stress on the reproductive function.

It is well established that exposure to heat, pollution, and toxins (heavy metals and organic solvents) leads to an increase in OS. Avoiding activities which may heat the scrotum such as long hot water baths and saunas could help to minimize OS. Use of proper protective equipment at work places that reduces men's exposure to chemicals and vapors linked with oxidative stress is also one way of minimizing OS.

Antioxidants are the main defense mechanisms against oxidative stress induced by free radicals. Antioxidants can be preventive or scavenging. Preventive antioxidants such as metal chelators and metal-binding proteins block formation of new free radicals, whereas scavenging antioxidants remove free radicals that are already formed. Metal chelators such as transferrin, lactoferrin, and ceruloplasmin which are found in sperm plasma membrane protect spermatozoa from lipid peroxidation caused by transition metals such as iron [93]. In vitro supplementation of metal chelators such as DL-penicillamine, 2,3-dimercaptopropan-1 sulfonate and meso-2,3-dimercapto-succinimic acid showed enhancement of sperm quality during assisted reproductive technique [94].

Dietary antioxidants form an essential part of the human antioxidant defense system. These antioxidants are obtained from fruits and vegetables as well as daily dietary supplements. Oxidative stress could also be limited by using chain-breaking antioxidants such as vitamin E and vitamin C taken as drug supplements. Vitamin C has been reported to be a very potent chain-breaking antioxidant and is present in the extracellular fluid. It is capable of neutralizing hydroxyl, superoxide, and H_2O_2 radicals [95].

Vitamin E is also a chain-breaking antioxidant present within the cell membrane. It neutralizes H_2O_2 and protects the plasma membrane from lipid peroxidation. Studies have shown that vitamin E treatment directly reduced seminal ROS levels [96]. Carotenoids such as beta-carotene and lycopene have also been reported to be very potent antioxidants [97]. Beta-carotene protects the plasma membrane against lipid peroxidation. Lycopene is found in abundance in tomatoes and has been shown to be twice as potent as beta-carotene and ten times more potent than vitamin E in scavenging singlet oxygen and inhibiting lipid peroxidation in serum plasma [98].

Expert Commentary

Oxygen toxicity is an inherent challenge to cells which live under aerobic conditions including the spermatozoa. OS can be defined as the imbalance between prooxidative and antioxidative molecules in a biological system which arises as a consequence of excessive production of free radicals and impaired antioxidant defense mechanisms. The increase in oxidative damage to sperm membranes, proteins, and DNA is associated with defective sperm function. A variety of defensive mechanisms encompassing antioxidant enzymes are involved in biological systems. A balance between the benefits and risks from free radicals and antioxidants appears to be necessary for the survival and normal functioning of spermatozoa. The use of antioxidant supplements has been greatly advocated. However, the positive effects of antioxidants are still debatable. Resolving the various factors that lead to the generation of ROS is very crucial because such data will help design methods for both the treatment and prevention of pathologies involving oxidative stress in the male reproductive system.

Five-Year View

An expanding body of evidence supports a role of oxidative stress as a significant cause of male infertility. Treatment that would minimize oxidative stress in the male reproductive system is therefore highly recommended. Antioxidant supplements have now been shown in randomized placebo controlled studies to protect sperm from oxidative-related DNA damage. It may, therefore, be the right time to consider using antioxidants in all infertile men exhibiting OS. Most importantly, these antioxidants should be offered in combination with changes in lifestyle such as avoiding toxins (cigarette smoke, pollutants, heavy metals) and excessive heat.

Key Issues

- Oxidative stress occurs when antioxidant levels are overwhelmed by free radicals.
- Oxidative stress is one of the major causes of male infertility.
- Examples of free radicals that contribute to oxidative stress in human reproduction are ROS (e.g., superoxide, H_2O_2, hydroxyl radicals, etc.) and RNS (e.g., nitric oxide, peroxynitrite, etc.).
- ROS are beneficial to spermatozoa function at low physiological concentrations.
- High ROS levels cause sperm DNA damage, apoptosis, and lipid peroxidation.
- Antioxidants protect spermatozoa from OS-induced insult.

References

1. Jones R, Mann T, Sherins R. Peroxidative breakdown of phospholipids in human spermatozoa, spermicidal properties of fatty acid peroxides, and protective action of seminal plasma. Fertil Steril. 1979;31(5):531–7.
2. McLachlan RI, de Kretser DM. Male infertility: the case for continued research. Med J Aust. 2001;174(3):116–7.
3. Tremellen K. Oxidative stress and male infertility—a clinical perspective. Hum Reprod Update. 2008;14(3):243–58.
4. Agarwal A, Prabakaran S, Allamaneni S. What an andrologist/urologist should know about free radicals and why. Urology. 2006;67(1):2–8.
5. Garrido N, Meseguer M, Simon C, Pellicer A, Remohi J. Pro-oxidative and anti-oxidative imbalance in human semen and its relation with male fertility. Asian J Androl. 2004;6(1):59–65.
6. Wang X, Sharma RK, Sikka SC, Thomas Jr AJ, Falcone T, Agarwal A. Oxidative stress is associated with increased apoptosis leading to spermatozoa DNA damage in patients with male factor infertility. Fertil Steril. 2003;80(3):531–5.
7. de Lamirande E, Gagnon C. Human sperm hyperactivation and capacitation as parts of an oxidative process. Free Radic Biol Med. 1993;14(2):157–66.
8. Zini A, de Lamirande E, Gagnon C. Reactive oxygen species in semen of infertile patients: levels of superoxide dismutase- and catalase-like activities in seminal plasma and spermatozoa. Int J Androl. 1993;16(3):183–8.
9. Kobayashi T, Miyazaki T, Natori M, Nozawa S. Protective role of superoxide dismutase in human sperm motility: superoxide dismutase activity and lipid peroxide in human seminal plasma and spermatozoa. Hum Reprod. 1991;6(7):987–91.
10. Vernet P, Aitken RJ, Drevet JR. Antioxidant strategies in the epididymis. Mol Cell Endocrinol. 2004;216(1–2):31–9.
11. Williams AC, Ford WC. Functional significance of the pentose phosphate pathway and glutathione reductase in the antioxidant defenses of human sperm. Biol Reprod. 2004;71(4):1309–16.
12. Twigg J, Fulton N, Gomez E, Irvine DS, Aitken RJ. Analysis of the impact of intracellular reactive oxygen species generation on the structural and functional integrity of human spermatozoa: lipid peroxidation, DNA fragmentation and effectiveness of antioxidants. Hum Reprod. 1998;13(6):1429–36.
13. Saez F, Motta C, Boucher D, Grizard G. Antioxidant capacity of prostasomes in human semen. Mol Hum Reprod. 1998;4(7):667–72.
14. Ochsendorf FR. Infections in the male genital tract and reactive oxygen species. Hum Reprod Update. 1999;5(5):399–420.
15. Agarwal A, Gupta S, Sharma RK. Role of oxidative stress in female reproduction. Reprod Biol Endocrinol. 2005;3:28.
16. Cheesman MJ, Baer BR, Zheng YM, Gillam EM, Rettie AE. Rabbit CYP4B1 engineered for high-level expression in *Escherichia coli*: ligand stabilization and processing of the N-terminus and heme prosthetic group. Arch Biochem Biophys. 2003;416(1):17–24.
17. Agarwal A, Prabakaran SA. Mechanism, measurement, and prevention of oxidative stress in male reproductive physiology. Indian J Exp Biol. 2005;43(11):963–74.
18. Sharma RK, Pasqualotto AE, Nelson DR, Thomas Jr AJ, Agarwal A. Relationship between seminal white blood cell counts and oxidative stress in men treated at an infertility clinic. J Androl. 2001;22(4):575–83.
19. Rodin DM, Larone D, Goldstein M. Relationship between semen cultures, leukospermia, and semen analysis in men undergoing fertility evaluation. Fertil Steril. 2003;79 Suppl 3:1555–8.
20. Martinez P, Proverbio F, Camejo MI. Sperm lipid peroxidation and pro-inflammatory cytokines. Asian J Androl. 2007;9(1):102–7.

21. Nandipati KC, Pasqualotto FF, Thomas Jr AJ, Agarwal A. Relationship of interleukin-6 with semen characteristics and oxidative stress in vasectomy reversal patients. Andrologia. 2005;37(4):131–4.
22. Koch OR, Pani G, Borrello S, et al. Oxidative stress and antioxidant defenses in ethanol-induced cell injury. Mol Aspects Med. 2004;25(1–2):191–8.
23. Saleh RA, Agarwal A, Sharma RK, Nelson DR, Thomas Jr AJ. Effect of cigarette smoking on levels of seminal oxidative stress in infertile men: a prospective study. Fertil Steril. 2002;78(3):491–9.
24. Mostafa T, Tawadrous G, Roaia MM, Amer MK, Kader RA, Aziz A. Effect of smoking on seminal plasma ascorbic acid in infertile and fertile males. Andrologia. 2006;38(6):221–4.
25. Song GJ, Norkus EP, Lewis V. Relationship between seminal ascorbic acid and sperm DNA integrity in infertile men. Int J Androl. 2006;29(6):569–75.
26. Peake JM, Suzuki K, Coombes JS. The influence of antioxidant supplementation on markers of inflammation and the relationship to oxidative stress after exercise. J Nutr Biochem. 2007;18(6):357–71.
27. Singer G, Granger DN. Inflammatory responses underlying the microvascular dysfunction associated with obesity and insulin resistance. Microcirculation. 2007;14(4–5):375–87.
28. Perez-Crespo M, Pintado B, Gutierrez-Adan A. Scrotal heat stress effects on sperm viability, sperm DNA integrity, and the offspring sex ratio in mice. Mol Reprod Dev. 2008;75(1):40–7.
29. Junqueira VB, Barros SB, Chan SS, et al. Aging and oxidative stress. Mol Aspects Med. 2004;25(1–2):5–16.
30. Eskiocak S, Gozen AS, Taskiran A, Kilic AS, Eskiocak M, Gulen S. Effect of psychological stress on the L-arginine-nitric oxide pathway and semen quality. Braz J Med Biol Res. 2006;39(5):581–8.
31. Hauser R, Meeker JD, Singh NP, et al. DNA damage in human sperm is related to urinary levels of phthalate monoester and oxidative metabolites. Hum Reprod. 2007;22(3):688–95.
32. Meng Z, Bai W. Oxidation damage of sulfur dioxide on testicles of mice. Environ Res. 2004;96(3):298–304.
33. Latchoumycandane C, Mathur PP. Induction of oxidative stress in the rat testis after short-term exposure to the organochlorine pesticide methoxychlor. Arch Toxicol. 2002;76(12):692–8.
34. Latchoumycandane C, Chitra KC, Mathur PP. 2, 3, 7, 8-tetrachlorodibenzo-p-dioxin (TCDD) induces oxidative stress in the epididymis and epididymal sperm of adult rats. Arch Toxicol. 2003;77(5):280–4.
35. Alaghmand M, Blough NV. Source-dependent variation in hydroxyl radical production by airborne particulate matter. Environ Sci Technol. 2007;41(7):2364–70.
36. Acharya UR, Acharya S, Mishra M. Lead acetate induced cytotoxicity in male germinal cells of Swiss mice. Ind Health. 2003;41(3):291–4.
37. Schaeffer AJ. Epidemiology and demographics of prostatitis. Andrologia. 2003;35(5):252–7.
38. Fraczek M, Sanocka D, Kamieniczna M, Kurpisz M. Proinflammatory cytokines as an intermediate factor enhancing lipid sperm membrane peroxidation in in vitro conditions. J Androl. 2008;29(1):85–92.
39. Brackett NL, Ibrahim E, Grotas JA, Aballa TC, Lynne CM. Higher sperm DNA damage in semen from men with spinal cord injuries compared with controls. J Androl. 2008;29(1):93–9. discussion 100-101.
40. Krause W, Bohring C, Gueth A, Horster S, Krisp A, Skrzypek J. Cellular and biochemical markers in semen indicating male accessory gland inflammation. Andrologia. 2003;35(5):279–82.
41. Umapathy E, Simbini T, Chipata T, Mbizvo M. Sperm characteristics and accessory sex gland functions in HIV-infected men. Arch Androl. 2001;46(2):153–8.
42. Vicari E, Arcoria D, Di Mauro C, Noto R, Noto Z, La Vignera S. Sperm output in patients with primary infertility and hepatitis B or C virus; negative influence of HBV infection during concomitant varicocele. Minerva Med. 2006;97(1):65–77.
43. Srinivasan S, Jenita X, Kalaiselvi P, Muthu V, Chandrasekar D, Varalakshmi P. Salubrious effect of vitamin E supplementation on renal stone forming risk factors in urogenital tuberculosis patients. Ren Fail. 2004;26(2):135–40.

44. Guha M, Kumar S, Choubey V, Maity P, Bandyopadhyay U. Apoptosis in liver during malaria: role of oxidative stress and implication of mitochondrial pathway. FASEB J. 2006;20(8): 1224–6.
45. Potts JM, Pasqualotto FF. Seminal oxidative stress in patients with chronic prostatitis. Andrologia. 2003;35(5):304–8.
46. Motrich RD, Maccioni M, Riera CM, Rivero VE. Autoimmune prostatitis: state of the art. Scand J Immunol. 2007;66(2–3):217–27.
47. Motrich RD, Maccioni M, Molina R, et al. Presence of INF gamma-secreting lymphocytes specific to prostate antigens in a group of chronic prostatitis patients. Clin Immunol. 2005; 116(2):149–57.
48. Filippini A, Riccioli A, Padula F, et al. Control and impairment of immune privilege in the testis and in semen. Hum Reprod Update. 2001;7(5):444–9.
49. Said TM, Agarwal A, Sharma RK, Thomas Jr AJ, Sikka SC. Impact of sperm morphology on DNA damage caused by oxidative stress induced by beta-nicotinamide adenine dinucleotide phosphate. Fertil Steril. 2005;83(1):95–103.
50. Kumanov P, Nandipati K, Tomova A, Agarwal A. Inhibin B is a better marker of spermatogenesis than other hormones in the evaluation of male factor infertility. Fertil Steril. 2006; 86(2):332–8.
51. Watson PF. The causes of reduced fertility with cryopreserved semen. Anim Reprod Sci. 2000;60–61:481–92.
52. Zini A, Garrels K, Phang D. Antioxidant activity in the semen of fertile and infertile men. Urology. 2000;55(6):922–6.
53. Sanocka D, Miesel R, Jedrzejczak P, Chelmonska-Soyta AC, Kurpisz M. Effect of reactive oxygen species and the activity of antioxidant systems on human semen; association with male infertility. Int J Androl. 1997;20(5):255–64.
54. Das UB, Mallick M, Debnath JM, Ghosh D. Protective effect of ascorbic acid on cyclophosphamide-induced testicular gametogenic and androgenic disorders in male rats. Asian J Androl. 2002;4(3):201–7.
55. Agarwal A, Said TM. Oxidative stress, DNA damage and apoptosis in male infertility: a clinical approach. BJU Int. 2005;95(4):503–7.
56. Ishikawa T, Kondo Y, Yamaguchi K, Sakamoto Y, Fujisawa M. Effect of varicocelectomy on patients with unobstructive azoospermia and severe oligospermia. BJU Int. 2008;101(2): 216–8.
57. Chen SS, Huang WJ, Chang LS, Wei YH. 8-hydroxy-2′-deoxyguanosine in leukocyte DNA of spermatic vein as a biomarker of oxidative stress in patients with varicocele. J Urol. 2004;172(4 Pt 1):1418–21.
58. Smith R, Kaune H, Parodi D, et al. Extent of sperm DNA damage in spermatozoa from men examined for infertility. Relationship with oxidative stress. Rev Med Chil. 2007;135(3): 279–86.
59. Filho DW, Torres MA, Bordin AL, Crezcynski-Pasa TB, Boveris A. Spermatic cord torsion, reactive oxygen and nitrogen species and ischemia-reperfusion injury. Mol Aspects Med. 2004;25(1–2):199–210.
60. Oberg BP, McMenamin E, Lucas FL, et al. Increased prevalence of oxidant stress and inflammation in patients with moderate to severe chronic kidney disease. Kidney Int. 2004;65(3): 1009–16.
61. Moreno JM, Ruiz MC, Ruiz N, et al. Modulation factors of oxidative status in stable renal transplantation. Transplant Proc. 2005;37(3):1428–30.
62. Danielski M, Ikizler TA, McMonagle E, et al. Linkage of hypoalbuminemia, inflammation, and oxidative stress in patients receiving maintenance hemodialysis therapy. Am J Kidney Dis. 2003;42(2):286–94.
63. Carpino A, Tarantino P, Rago V, De Sanctis V, Siciliano L. Antioxidant capacity in seminal plasma of transfusion-dependent beta-thalassemic patients. Exp Clin Endocrinol Diabetes. 2004;112(3):131–4.

64. Agbaje IM, Rogers DA, McVicar CM, et al. Insulin dependent diabetes mellitus: implications for male reproductive function. Hum Reprod. 2007;22(7):1871–7.
65. Shrilatha B, Muralidhara. Early oxidative stress in testis and epididymal sperm in streptozotocin-induced diabetic mice: its progression and genotoxic consequences. Reprod Toxicol. 2007; 23(4):578–87.
66. Sonmez M, Yuce A, Turk G. The protective effects of melatonin and vitamin E on antioxidant enzyme activities and epididymal sperm characteristics of homocysteine treated male rats. Reprod Toxicol. 2007;23(2):226–31.
67. Aitken RJ, Harkiss D, Knox W, Peterson M, Irvine DS. A novel signal transduction cascade in capacitating human spermatozoa characterized by a redox-regulated cAMP-mediated induction of tyrosine phosphorylation. J Cell Sci. 1998;111:645–56.
68. Ehrenwald E, Parks JE, Foote RH. Bovine oviductal fluid components and their potential role in sperm cholesterol efflux. Mol Reprod Dev. 1990;25:195–204.
69. Andrews JC, Bavister BD. Capacitation of hamster spermatozoa with the divalent cation chelators D-penicillamine, L-histidine and L-cysteine in a protein free culture medium. Gamete Res. 1989;23:159–70.
70. Russel JH, Hale AH, Inbar D, Fisen HN. Loss of reactivity of BAL B/c myeloma tumor with allogeneic and syngeneic cytotoxic T lymphocytes. Eur J Immunol. 1978;8:640–5.
71. Yamaguchi R. Mammalian fertilization. In: Knobil E, Neill J, editors. Physiology of reproduction. New York: Raven; 1994. p. 189–317.
72. Kumar GP, Laloraya MM. Superoxide radical and superoxide dismutase activity changes in maturing mammalian spermatozoa. Andrologia. 1991;23:171–5.
73. Aitken RJ, Buckingham DW, Brindles J, Gomez E, Baker HW, Irvine DS. Analysis of sperm movement in relation to the oxidative stress created by leukocytes in washed sperm preparations and seminal plasma. Hum Reprod. 1995;10:2061–71.
74. Zhang H, Zheng RL. Promotion of human sperm capacitation by superoxide anion. Free Radic Res. 1996;24:261–7.
75. Purohit SB, Laloraya M, Kumar GP. Acrosome reaction inducers impose alterations in repulsive strain and hydration barrier in human sperm membrane. Biochem Mol Bio Int. 1998;45:227–35.
76. de Lamirande E, Gagnon C. Impact of reactive oxygen species on spermatozoa: a balancing act between beneficial and detrimental effects. Hum Reprod. 1995;10:15–21.
77. Griveau JF, Renard P, Lannou D. An *in vitro* promoting role for hydrogen peroxide in human sperm capacitation. Int J Androl. 1994;17:300–7.
78. Lewis SEM, Boyle PM, Mc Kinney KA. Total antioxidant capacity of seminal plasma is different in fertile and infertile men. Fertil Steril. 1996;64:863–9.
79. Herrero MB, Cebral E, Boquet M, Viggiano JM, Vitullo A, Ginenno MA. Effect of nitric oxide on mouse sperm hyperactivation. Acta Physiol Pharmacol Ther Latinoam. 1994;44:65–9.
80. Sengoku K, Tamate K, Yoshida T, Takaoka Y, Miyamoto T, Ishikawa M. Effects of low concentrations of nitric oxide on zona pellucida binding ability of human spermatozoa. Fertil Steril. 1998;69:522–7.
81. Alvarez JG, Storey BT. Differential incorporation of fatty acids into and peroxidative loss of fatty acids from phospholipids of human spermatozoa. Mol Reprod Dev. 1995;42:334–46.
82. Yeagle PL. Lipids and lipid-intermediate structures in the fusion of biological membranes. Curr Top Membr. 1994;4:197–214.
83. Twigg J, Irvine DS, Aitken RJ. Oxidative damage to DNA in human spermatozoa does not prelude pronucleus formation at intracytoplasmic sperm injection. Hum Reprod. 1998;103: 1864–71.
84. Duru NK, Morshedi M, Oehninger S. Effects of hydrogen peroxide on DNA and plasma membrane integrity of human spermatozoa. Fertil Steril. 2000;74:1200–7.
85. Vaux DL, Flavell RA. Apoptosis genes and autoimmunity. Curr Opin Immunol. 2000; 12:719–24.
86. Vaux DL, Korsmeyer SJ. Cell death in development. Cell. 1999;96:245–54.

87. Sakkas D, Mariethoz E, Manicardi G, Bizzaro D, Bianchi P, Bianchi U. Origin of DNA damage in ejaculated human spermatozoa. Rev Reprod. 1999;4:31–7.
88. Lee J, Richburg JH, Younkin SC, Boekelbeide K. The Fas system is a key regulator of germ cell apoptosis in the testis. Endocrinology. 1997;138:2081–8.
89. Sinha HAP, Swerdloff RS. Hormonal and genetic control of germ cell apoptosis in the testis. Rev Reprod. 1999;4:38–47.
90. Agarwal A, Saleh R, Bedaiwy MA. Role of reactive oxygen species in the pathophysiology of human reproduction. Fertil Steril. 2003;79:829–43.
91. Halliwell B. How to characterize a biological antioxidant. Free Radic Res Commun. 1990;9:1–32.
92. Aitken RJ, Fisher H. Reactive oxygen species generation and human spermatozoa: the balance of benefit and risk. Bioassays. 1994;16:259–67.
93. Sanocka D, Kurpisz M. Reactive oxygen species and sperm cells. Reprod Biol Endocrinol. 2004;2:12.
94. Henkel RR, Schill B. Sperm preparation for ART. Reprod Biol Endocrinol. 2003;1:108.
95. Agarwal A, Nallella KP, Allamaneni SS, Said TM. Role of antioxidants in treatment of male infertility: an overview of the literature. Reprod Biomed Online. 2004;8:616–27.
96. Comhaire FH, Christophe AB, Zalata AA, Dhooge WS, Mahmoud AM, Depuydt CE. The effects of combined conventional treatment, oral antioxidants and essential fatty acids on sperm biology in subfertile men. Prostaglandins Leukot Essent Fatty Acids. 2000;63:159–65.
97. Gupta NP, Kumar R. Lycopene therapy in idiopathic male infertility—a preliminary report. Int Urol Nephrol. 2002;34:369–72.
98. Di Mascio P, Kaiser S, Sies H. Lycopene as the most efficient biological carotenoid singlet oxygen quencher. Arch Biochem Biophys. 1989;274:532–8.

Chapter 7
Loss of Intracellular Antioxidant Enzyme Activity During Sperm Cryopreservation: Effects on Sperm Function After Thawing

Juan G. Alvarez

Despite many advances in cryopreservation methodology [1, 2], one of the main reported detrimental effects of cryopreservation on human spermatozoa is a marked reduction in sperm motility [3–5]. The primary cause of cellular damage during cryopreservation is the formation of intracellular ice [6, 7]. Whenever cells, or culture media, are cooled below their freezing point, water is removed from the solution in the form of ice. The concentration of solutes remaining in the unfrozen fraction increases, thereby both depressing the freezing point [8] and increasing the osmotic pressure of the remaining solution. Hence, biological systems freeze progressively over a wide temperature range, during which the solute becomes gradually more concentrated as the temperature falls [8]. This leads to irreversible rupturing of plasma and nuclear membranes and disturbance of cellular organelles. The nucleus has generally been considered to be a stable constituent of the cell. However, recent studies have suggested that this is not the case and that inappropriate chromatin condensation can occur [9, 10] with freezing. Cryoprotectants such as glycerol or propanediol can be added to cells to reduce freezing damage by lowering the salt concentrations and increasing the unfrozen water fraction, thereby reducing osmotic stress. They can also insert into phospholipid membranes to reduce the likelihood of fracture [7]. Further cellular damage may be caused during the thawing process as the ice melts or recrystallizes. Slow thawing is most likely to induce injury, as it allows time for consolidation of microscopic ice crystals into larger forms which are known to be damaging [11]. The production and dissolution of ice is associated with the actual rate of freezing and thawing. Slow freezing and gradual dehydration may accommodate cell survival, whereas rapid freezing and thawing is more likely to result in cell death [6].

J.G. Alvarez, MD, PhD (✉)
Centro de Infertilidad Masculina Androgen, C/Fernando Macias,
8, 1C, La Coruña 15005, Spain

Harvard Medical School, Boston, USA
e-mail: jalvarez@androgen.es

S.J. Parekattil and A. Agarwal (eds.), *Antioxidants in Male Infertility: A Guide for Clinicians and Researchers*, © Springer Science+Business Media New York 2013

Increase in Oxygen Radical Production After Cryopreservation

It has been previously reported that the production of oxygen radicals, and of superoxide anion in particular, increases during thawing of cryopreserved ejaculated sperm [12]. According to these authors, motility loss during thawing of cryopreserved sperm appears to be related, at least in part, to oxidation of reduced glutathione [12]. Recently, several groups have reported the effect of cryopreservation on sperm DNA integrity [13–17]. It has been shown that during cryopreservation, and more specifically during thawing, sperm are exposed to high levels of oxygen radicals [12, 18] due, at least in part, to a slow recovery of antioxidant enzyme activity after freezing [19]. This may help explain why membrane damage occurs during thawing [18].

Ejaculated sperm are composed of discrete subsets of spermatozoa, which can be isolated by density-gradient centrifugation. It has been previously shown that these subsets differ in their degree of maturation [20]. Cells isolated in the lowest density layer include immature germ cells, leukocytes, and immature or defective sperm with proximal cytoplasmic retention and abnormal head morphology. Spermatozoa isolated in this fraction had the highest content of docosahexaenoic acid (DHA) and sterols [20, 21] and produced the highest levels of reactive oxygen species (ROS) [21, 22]. ROS production was highest in immature sperm from males displaying abnormal semen parameters [22]. The fact that immature and defective sperm produce the highest levels of ROS and have the highest content of DHA, the primary target of ROS-induced lipoperoxidative damage explains, at least in part, the high levels of malondialdehyde observed in spermatozoa from teratozoospermic samples [23].

However, peroxidative damage in sperm not only depends on ROS production and DHA levels but also on sperm antioxidant defenses. Mammalian sperm have been reported to contain antioxidant enzyme defenses against ROS-induced damage [24–26]. These defenses include superoxide dismutase (SOD), glutathione peroxidase/reductase, and low-molecular substances [27, 28]. SOD, in particular, and glutathione peroxidase/reductase activity have been reported in sperm of several mammalian species including human [24–26, 29–31]. SOD may be the most important antioxidant factor in semen [32], and its stoichiometric relationship to DHA content, the main substrate of lipid peroxidation in sperm, will ultimately determine the susceptibility of a given sperm sample to oxidative damage. High levels of this enzyme have been associated with impaired sperm function [33]. In addition, it has been previously reported that cryopreservation increases the rate of lipid peroxidation and that this might be related, at least in part, to the loss of antioxidant enzyme activity [34]. Therefore, the increase in oxygen radical production after cryopreservation could be due to two main mechanisms: (a) a decrease in antioxidant activity, mainly in antioxidant enzyme activity or (b) an increase in the actual generation of oxygen radicals. Since oxygen radical export to the extracellular medium by mature spermatozoa is very low and relatively constant between samples from different males [20, 22] and intracellular oxygen radical production, defined as V_{int} [25, 35], is metabolized to a large extent by enzymes such as glutathione peroxidase and SOD, we can safely conclude that oxygen radical production by mature spermatozoa at constant temperature and oxygen concentration mainly depends on antioxidant enzyme activity.

Loss of Intracellular Enzyme Antioxidant Activity

It has been recently reported that motility recovery after cryopreservation can be increased by increasing thawing temperature. Sperm thawing at 40°C resulted in a 23.1% increase in sperm motility recovery compared to 37°C [19]. This finding was observed after cryopreservation of either liquefied raw semen samples or their corresponding 90% gradient fractions, known to contain spermatozoa of the highest functional quality [36]. Therefore, based on the above, it has been proposed that the increase in oxygen radical production observed after thawing would be due to damage of sperm SOD leading to partial loss of its enzyme activity. If that were the case, we should observe an increase in membrane and DNA damage after thawing. One potential explanation for the observed increase in motility recovery following thawing at 40°C would be a faster rate of recovery of sperm enzyme antioxidant activity. During thawing, there are two competing processes that determine the degree of cell damage: (a) the magnitude of oxygen radical production and (b) the rate of recovery of enzyme antioxidant activity. The higher the temperature, the faster the recovery of enzyme antioxidant activity and, therefore, at 40°C sperm will be able to neutralize more efficiently than at 37°C the increase in oxygen radical production reported during thawing [12]. However, since sperm viability, acrosomal status, DNA integrity, and sperm survival were similar at 37°C vs. 40°C, the type of cell damage prevented by a faster rate of recovery of antioxidant enzyme activity might be related to ATP production/utilization in the axoneme. That is, rather than affecting the recovery of enzyme antioxidant activity at the level of the membrane and/or nuclear compartments, it would affect antioxidant enzyme activity localized in the highly compact axonemal compartment, virtually devoid of cytoplasm. Although there were no statistically significant differences in ATP content in sperm from the 90% gradient pellet following thawing at 37°C vs. 40°C, a higher ATP content was found in samples with a motility recovery higher than 50%. Since ATP steady-state levels represent the balance between biosynthesis and consumption, it cannot be ruled out that thawing at 40°C might have an effect in increasing the ATP utilization in the axoneme by preventing more efficiently oxygen radical-induced damage to key components of the axoneme. This damage could be reversible in the first stage and become irreversible thereafter [25]. However, since long-term motility, as measured by the sperm survival test, acrosomal integrity, and DNA integrity, was not significantly different following thawing at 40°C vs. 37°C, this suggests that the beneficial effect of increasing thawing temperature only affects antioxidant enzyme activity from the axonemal compartment and not from the membrane or nuclear compartments. Therefore, the results of the study of Calamera et al., related to the effects of thawing of cryopreserved human sperm at 40°C compared to other temperatures, suggest that cryopreservation results in the loss of antioxidant enzyme activity. This damage could be reversed, at least in part, in the axonemal compartment by increasing thawing temperature. The fact that motility loss, as measured by the sperm survival test (an indicator of damage to the membrane compartment), and DNA integrity, as measured by the TUNEL test (an indicator of damage to the nuclear compartment), were not significantly different after thawing at 40°C vs. 37°C, suggests that perhaps the recovery of enzyme antioxidant activity in the axonemal compartment after thawing is slower compared to the membrane and nuclear compartments and that damage to antioxidant enzymes in the axoneme may actually occur during thawing and is mediated by oxygen radicals [19]. Previous studies have already reported the occurrence of SOD inactivation by oxygen radicals [24, 25].

Enzyme Antioxidant Activity, Rate of Lipid Peroxidation, and Sperm Damage

There is general agreement that motility loss during aerobic incubation at 37°C is significantly higher in fresh compared to cryopreserved spermatozoa. Since antioxidant enzymes, namely SOD, play a central role in protecting mammalian sperm against lipid peroxidation and motility loss during aerobic incubation, we can safely conclude that cryopreservation results in the loss of antioxidant enzyme activity. Loss of sperm motility due to lipid peroxidation during incubation becomes apparent after several hours of incubation and is mainly determined by the activation energy of lipid peroxidation reactions which requires of several hours to result in phospholipid breakdown, loss of membrane permeability, and loss of ATP leading to motility loss [25]. Assuming that mature sperm have an equivalent content of DHA and produce similar levels of oxygen radicals, the constitutive content of antioxidant enzyme activity in sperm is going to determine the rate of lipid peroxidation and the motile life span of sperm. Thus, sperm samples with a higher content of antioxidant enzyme activity would have a higher motile life span than samples with a lower content of antioxidant enzyme activity. At the same time, since motility loss of a given sperm sample does not take place in all sperm at the same time but it occurs in a stepwise fashion, it can also be concluded that, under similar conditions of DHA content and oxygen radical production, the motile life span of each individual sperm cell would be mainly determined by its antioxidant enzyme activity. At the same time, since membrane damage induced by oxygen radicals depends, for the most part, on the activation energy of lipid peroxidation which requires several hours of incubation at 37°C to be observed via motility loss, it can be postulated that oxygen radical-induced DNA damage occurring after cryopreservation should be observed earlier since the activation energy of DNA damage is much lower than that of lipid peroxidation. And this is precisely what it is observed in vitro after sperm cryopreservation. Massive DNA damage in cryopreserved mature sperm from the 80% gradient pellet can be observed as early as 2.5 h of incubation at 37°C after

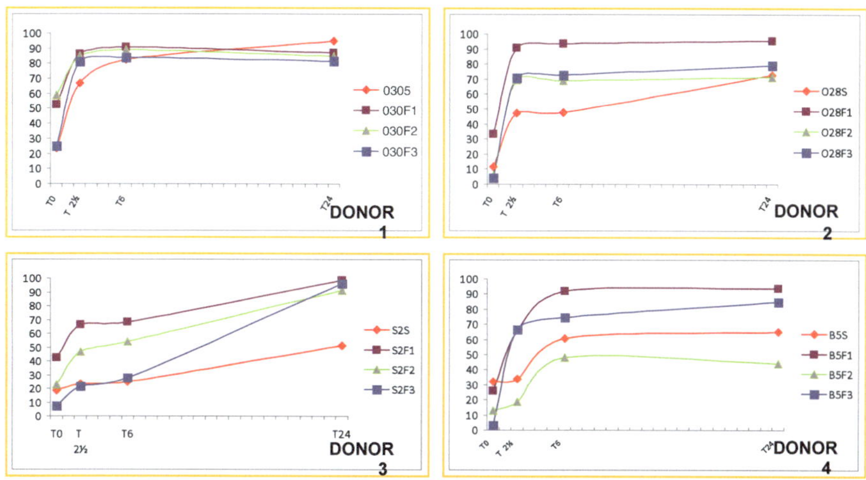

Fig. 7.1 Dynamics of sperm DNA fragmentation following incubation of subsets of cryopreserved human spermatozoa. A total of four semen samples were obtained from four fertile sperm donors and processed for density-gradient centrifugation using a 40/80% SpermFilter® gradient (Cryos International, Denmark). Following centrifugation, sperm from the seminal plasma/40% (F1) and 40/80% (F2) interfaces and from the 80% pellet (F3), were aspirated, transferred to test tubes, and washed with SpermWash® medium (Cryos International, Denmark). Aliquots of the resulting fractions and of the raw semen sample (S) were mixed 1:1, v/v with CryoProtec medium (Nidacon, Sweden), placed under liquid nitrogen vapors for 15 min, and finally immersed in liquid nitrogen. After cryopreservation, aliquots of the samples were thawed at 37°C for 5 min and incubated during 2.5, 6, and 24 h at 37°C. The percentage of sperm with DNA damage (DFI) was assessed using the Halosperm test (Halotech-DNA, Madrid) and the type of DNA strand damage using the two-dimensional COMET test

thawing [37], while 80% motility loss is not observed until about 24 h of aerobic incubation [19, 37]. As shown in Fig. 7.1, DNA damage after 2.5 h incubation at 37°C of thawed mature sperm from the 80% pellet isolated from samples obtained from fertile sperm donors reaches DFI values of 70–80%. Interestingly, in the sample from donor 3, the DFI value observed after 2.5 h of incubation was 20%, a value significantly lower than that observed in the other three samples. The same applies to the cryopreserved raw semen sample aliquot of sample 4. This certainly may be related to higher levels of antioxidant enzyme activity. Concerning the mechanism of DNA damage as shown in Fig. 7.2, all the DNA damage observed during incubation of thawed spermatozoa is oxidative in nature. All spermatozoa expressing DNA fragmentation, as measured by the SCD-Halosperm test (left panels), are positive for nucleotide damage of the 8-oxoguanine type (right panels) and indicator of oxidative damage. The same applies to the samples from the other donors. If we ask the question: why the remaining 20–30% spermatozoa still maintain intact their DNA after 2.5 h of incubation? Are these sperm better equipped with antioxidant enzyme activity? This is a question that is certainly amenable to experimental testing by looking at DNA integrity and SOD and/or GPx activity in the same sperm cell. Sperm cells with intact DNA should have a higher content and activity of SOD and/or GPx than sperm cells with damaged DNA.

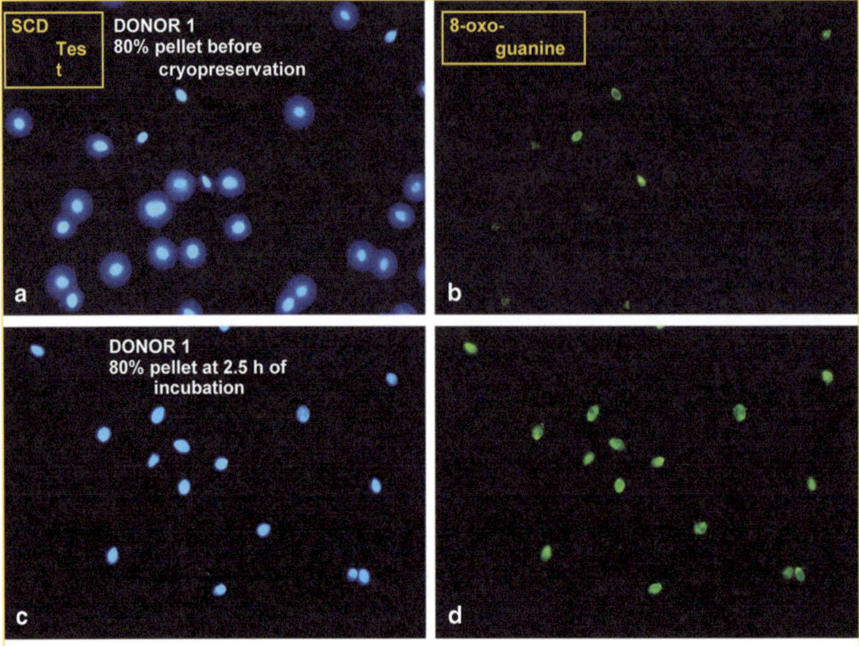

Fig. 7.2 Correlation between DNA fragmentation and DNA oxidation during incubation of cryo-preserved sperm after thawing. Aliquots of testicular and ejaculated sperm obtained from the same patient were analyzed for sperm DNA fragmentation and 8-oxoguanine content using the Halosperm test (Halotech-DNA, Madrid) and the OxyDNA assay kit (Calbiochem, Barcelona, Spain), respectively

Another important conclusion that can be drawn from the results of the study of the effects of cryopreservation of subsets of human sperm on DNA integrity is that related to the occurrence of intracellular vs. extracellular oxygen radical-mediated DNA damage during thawing. As shown in Fig. 7.1, the DFI value in semen from donor 2 is significantly lower than that observed in sperm from fraction 3. Since antioxidant enzymes in the extracellular medium, i.e., seminal plasma, do not have access to the intracellular compartment, it can be concluded that the DNA damage observed in semen depends mainly on the levels of oxygen radicals exported to the extracellular medium by immature sperm, while the DNA damage observed in mature sperm from fraction 3 depends mainly on the intracellular levels of oxygen radicals that normally would be metabolized by antioxidant enzymes. If constitutive intracellular SOD and/or GPx content is lower, the steady-state levels of oxygen radicals would be higher and also DNA damage. Antioxidant enzyme activity in seminal plasma would suppress oxygen radical-mediated DNA damage going from the extracellular to the intracellular compartment, while intracellular antioxidant enzyme activity in washed or mature sperm (devoid of seminal plasma) would suppress DNA damage mediated by intracellular oxygen radical levels. Therefore, the protective effect of semen is most likely determined by the presence of antioxidant enzyme activity in seminal plasma, e.g., SOD and GPx. The contribution of low-molecular-weight antioxidants in seminal plasma to this protective effect can be largely excluded, since these antioxidants are membrane permeable and would also have access to the intracellular compartment [27] thus preventing intracellular oxidative damage. Therefore, antioxidant enzyme activity in seminal plasma from samples 2 and 3 should be higher than that in sample 1. Since the dynamics of motility loss during incubation of cryopreserved sperm after thawing should mimic the dynamics of sperm DNA damage, although with a lower rate, this model would also predict that motility recovery following cryopreservation of raw semen may not always correlate with motility recovery after cryopreservation of mature sperm from the 80% gradient pellet obtained from the same semen sample, e.g., IUI-ready samples. That is, some samples may have higher motility recovery and lower DNA damage after semen than after cryopreservation of mature sperm from the gradient pellet and vice versa.

Therefore, sperm motility recovery, acrosomal status, and DNA integrity after cryopreservation are going to be mainly determined by the sperm content and activity of antioxidant enzymes. Sperm with a higher overall level of antioxidant enzyme activity would have a higher probability of maintaining the plasma and acrosomal membranes and the DNA intact and have a higher fertilizing ability. With regard to the sperm fertilizing ability, it should be pointed out that since sperm capacitation at 37°C may take up to 2–3 h and that sperm penetration in conventional IVF may take up to 1 h, based on these preliminary results, oocyte insemination by conventional IVF should not be recommended when using cryopreserved sperm since incubation of sperm at 37°C during 3–4 h may result in extensive DNA damage. ICSI should be used in these cases.

Sperm Enzyme Antioxidant Activity and Donor Selection

Based on the above, it can be concluded that the constitutive antioxidant enzyme content of spermatozoa should determine the motility recovery and the acrosomal and DNA integrity of cryopreserved human spermatozoa after thawing. Previous studies have shown that SOD [24] and GPx [26] play a central role in protecting mammalian spermatozoa against motility loss caused by spontaneous lipid peroxidation. SOD or GPx activity in ejaculated spermatozoa, mainly in mature sperm, should be a useful marker of sperm resistance to cryopreservation, for the selection of donor sperm samples that better withstand cryopreservation and, ultimately, for the selection of sperm to be used in in vitro fertilization. Should SOD and GPx from the paternal genome play a relevant role in embryo viability, it would be of paramount importance in preventing oxidative stress in the embryo. It is well known the beneficial effect of the use of low oxygen tension during embryo culture in preventing embryo fragmentation and improving embryo viability during long culture and IVF outcome [38–40]. It has been reported that low SOD activity in the embryo is associated with neural tube defects under high steady-state levels of oxidative stress [41].

Therefore, SOD and GPx activity may not only be important in donor selection for donor sperm cryopreservation but also for sperm selection for ICSI. Selection and microinjection of spermatozoa with higher SOD activity may result in higher embryo quality. However, SOD and GPx (and possibly catalase) activities should be stoichiometrically balanced to have a net antioxidant effect. That is, if SOD activity is exceedingly high compared to GPx activity, the high levels of H_2O_2 produced by the dismutation of the superoxide anion by SOD may not be hydrolyzed by GPx resulting in oxidative damage [26]. This explains why oxidative stress in immature spermatozoa from the lower-density layers of the gradient is higher than that in mature sperm from the 90% gradient pellet, because SOD levels (and also DHA content) are much higher in mature sperm [22]. Whether SOD and/or GPx content in spermatozoa is correlated with SOD and/or GPx content in somatic cells remains to be investigated.

Envoy

Sperm function and viability after cryopreservation appears to be determined to a great extent by the preservation of the activity of their antioxidant enzyme defenses. SOD and glutathione peroxidase are the main antioxidant enzymes present in mammalian sperm and play a central role in protecting sperm against oxidative damage. It has been shown that the motile life span and fertilizing ability of sperm in in vivo and in vitro is mainly determined by the rate of lipid peroxidation. This rate is governed by oxygen concentration in the extracellular medium, membrane-bound DHA content, and intracellular antioxidant enzyme activity. Therefore, under physiological conditions, the rate-limiting factor that determines the life span and function of sperm is the antioxidant enzyme activity. This activity not only may vary between samples from different males or even within a given male but also between individual sperm cells in a given sample. The in vitro and in vivo motile life span of mature sperm within a sample is not the same. Motility loss takes place in a stepwise fashion. That is, some sperm cells lose their motility before others and vice versa, and some sperm cells maintain their motility longer than others. Since, under these conditions, oxygen concentration and sperm DHA content are comparable [20, 21], the rate-limiting factor would be intracellular antioxidant enzyme activity. Therefore, antioxidant enzyme activity in a given sample, ΦSOD_T, could be considered the sum of the individual antioxidant enzyme activity of each sperm cell: $\Phi SOD_T = \Sigma[(\Phi SOD_1) + (\Phi SOD_2) + (\Phi SOD_3) + \ldots + (\Phi SOD_n)]$. There is evidence that during cryopreservation antioxidant enzymes may be damaged. This may be related to structural damage during the freezing process due to damage during thawing or both. Physical damage during freezing is considered irreversible and, therefore, not recoverable, while damage during thawing may be, at least in part, reversible. These are the conclusions that can be drawn from the effect of thawing temperature on sperm motility [19]. According to the results of this study, motility recovery following thawing at 40°C is significantly higher than at 37°C.

Given the high levels of oxygen radicals produced intracellularly by sperm cells, defined as V_{int} [25, 30], which are normally metabolized by antioxidant enzymes, should oxygen radical production be recovered at a faster rate than antioxidant enzyme activity, during thawing the sperm cell would be exposed to supraphysiological levels of oxygen radicals leading to sperm damage. It is postulated that thawing at 40°C accelerates antioxidant enzyme activity recovery and, therefore, reduces oxidative injury to the sperm cell. However, the higher recovery of sperm motility observed after thawing at 40°C is not related to a reduction in membrane damage. Sperm viability at 40°C was identical to that observed at 37°C [19]. This is why in the study of Calamera et al., it was concluded that the reversible effect of motility loss observed was related to the production/utilization of ATP in the axoneme [19]. Should antioxidant enzyme activity in the axonemal compartment be recovered at a slower rate than that associated with the membrane compartment, the resulting damage should be preferentially observed in those axonemal components responsible for the production/utilization of ATP, a key factor that determines sperm motility. Once these components are damaged, motility loss can no longer be recovered. The main axonemal components that may be vulnerable to oxidative damage during thawing would be glycolytic enzymes, ATPase, and the microtubules. On the other hand, damage of antioxidant enzymes during thawing will have a delayed effect on membrane damage since the activation energy of lipid peroxidation reactions and phospholipid breakdown requires several hours for membrane damage to occur leading to ATP and motility loss. This explains, at least in part, why long-term motility following incubation is much higher in fresh than in cryopreserved sperm. Finally, since antioxidant enzyme activity may vary between samples, selection of sperm samples with higher antioxidant enzyme activity may result in better motility recovery after cryopreservation. Furthermore, microinjection of spermatozoa with higher antioxidant enzyme activity may result in higher embryo quality.

Key Issues

- The production of oxygen radicals, and of superoxide anion in particular, increases during thawing of cryopreserved ejaculated sperm.
- It has been recently reported that motility recovery after cryopreservation can be increased by increasing thawing temperature.
- There is general agreement that motility loss during aerobic incubation at 37°C is significantly higher in fresh compared to cryopreserved spermatozoa.
- The protective effect of semen is most likely determined by the presence of antioxidant enzyme activity in seminal plasma.
- Sperm motility recovery, acrosomal status, and DNA integrity after cryopreservation are going to be mainly determined by the sperm content and activity of antioxidant enzymes.
- Sperm function and viability after cryopreservation appears to be determined to a great extent by the preservation of the activity of their antioxidant enzyme defenses.

References

1. Centola GM, Raubertas RF, Mattox JH. Cryopreservation of human semen: comparison of cryopreservation, sources of variability, and prediction of post-thaw survival. J Androl. 1992;13:283–8.
2. Agarwal A, Tolentine MV, Sidhu Jr RS, et al. Effect of cryopreservation on semen quality in patients with testicular cancer. Urology. 1995;46:382–6.
3. Critzer JK, Huse-Benda AR, Aaker DV, et al. Cryopreservation of human spermatozoa. III. The effects of cryoprotectants on motility. Fertil Steril. 1988;50:314–20.
4. Englert Y, Delvigne A, Vekemans M, et al. Is fresh or frozen semen to be used in in vitro fertilization with donor sperm. Fertil Steril. 1989;5:661–4.
5. Yoshida H, Hoshiai H, Fukaya T, et al. Fertilizability of fresh and frozen human spermatozoa. Assist Reprod Technol Androl. 1990;1:164–72.
6. Muldrew K, McGann LE. Mechanisms of intracellular ice formation. Bio J. 1990;57:525–33.
7. Watson PF. Recent developments and concepts in cryopreservation of spermatozoa and the assessment of their post-thaw function. Reprod Fertil Dev. 1995;7:871–91.
8. Brotherton J. Cryopreservation of human semen. Arch Androl. 1990;25:181–95.
9. Royere D, Hamamah S, Nicolle JC, et al. Freezing and thawing alter chromatin stability of ejaculated human spermatozoa: fluorescence acridine orange staining and fuelgen DNA cytophotometric studies. Gamete Res. 1988;21:51–7.
10. Royere D, Hamamah S, Nicolle JC, Lansac J. Chromatin alterations induced by freeze-thawing influence the fertilizing ability of human sperm. Int J Androl. 1991;14:328–32.
11. Mazur P, Rall WF, Rigopoulos N. Relative contribution of the fraction of unfrozen water and of salt concentration to the survival of slowly frozen human erythrocytes. Biophys J. 1981;36:653–75.
12. Chatterjee S, Gagnon C. Production of reactive oxygen species by spermatozoa undergoing cooling, freezing, and thawing. Mol Reprod Dev. 2001;59:451–8.
13. Kalthur G, Adiga SK, Upadhya D, Rao S, Kumar P. Effect of cryopreservation on DNA integrity in patients with teratozoospermia. Fertil Steril. 2008;89:1723–7.
14. Zribi N, Chakroun NF, El Euch H, Gargouri J, Bahloul A, Keskes LA. Effects of cryopreservation on human sperm deoxyribonucleic acid integrity. Fertil Steril. 2010;93:159–66.
15. Gandini L, Lombardo F, Lenzi A, Spanò M, Dondero F. Cryopreservation and sperm DNA integrity. Cell Tissue Bank. 2006;7:91–8.
16. Gosalvez J, Cortes-Gutierez E, Lopez-Fernandez C, Fernandez JL, Caballero P, Nunez R. Sperm deoxyribonucleic acid fragmentation dynamics in fertile donors. Fertil Steril. 2009 Jul;92(1):170–3.
17. Toro E, Fernández S, Colomar A, Casanovas A, Alvarez JG, López-Teijón M, Velilla E. Processing of semen can result in increased sperm DNA fragmentation. Fertil Steril. 2009;92:2109–12.
18. Aitken RJ. Free radicals, lipid peroxidation and sperm function. Reprod Fertil Dev. 1995;7:659–68.
19. Calamera JC, Buffone MG, Doncel GF, Brugo-Olmedo S, de Vicentis S, Calamera MM, Storey BT, Alvarez JG. Effect of thawing temperature on the motility recovery of cryopreserved human spermatozoa. Fertil Steril. 2010;93:789–94.
20. Ollero M, Powers RD, Alvarez JG. Variation of docosahexaenoic acid content in subsets of human spermatozoa at different stages of maturation: implications for sperm lipoperoxidative damage. Mol Reprod Dev. 2000;55:326–34.
21. Ollero M, Gil-Guzman E, Lopez MC, Sharma RK, Agarwal A, Larson K, Evenson D, Thomas Jr AJ, Alvarez JG. Characterization of subsets of human spermatozoa at different stages of maturation: implications in the diagnosis and treatment of male infertility. Hum Reprod. 2001;16:1912–21.

22. Gil-Guzman E, Ollero M, Lopez MC, Sharma RK, Alvarez JG, Thomas AJ, Agarwal A. Differential production of reactive oxygen species by subsets of human spermatozoa at different stage of maturation. Hum Reprod. 2001;16:1022–30.
23. Jones R, Mann T, Sherings RJ. Adverse effects of peroxidized lipid on human spermatozoa. Proc R Soc Lond B Biol Sci. 1978;201:413–7.
24. Alvarez JG, Storey BT. Role of superoxide dismutase in protecting rabbit spermatozoa from O2 toxicity due to lipid peroxidation. Biol Reprod. 1983;28:1129–36.
25. Alvarez JG, Storey BT. Assessment of cell damage caused by spontaneous lipid peroxidation in rabbit spermatozoa. Biol Reprod. 1984;30:323–32.
26. Alvarez JG, Storey BT. Role of glutathione peroxidise in protecting mammalian spermatozoa from loss of motility caused by spontaneous lipid peroxidation. Gamete Res. 1989;23:77–90.
27. Alvarez JG, Storey BT. Taurine, hypotaurine, epinephrine and albumin inhibit lipid peroxidation in rabbit spermatozoa and protect against loss of motility. Biol Reprod. 1983;29:548–55.
28. Kovalski NN, de Lamirande E, Gagnon C. Reactive oxygen species generated by human neutrophils inhibit sperm motility: protective effect of seminal plasma and scavengers. Fertil Steril. 1992;58:809–15.
29. Li TK. The glutathione and thiol content of mammalian spermatozoa and seminal plasma. Biol Reprod. 1975;12:641–6.
30. Menella MRF, Jones R. Properties of spermatozoal superoxide dismutase and lack of involvement of superoxides in metals ion-catalyzed lipid peroxidation reactions in semen. Biochem J. 1980;191:289–97.
31. Alvarez JG, Touchstone JC, Blasco L, Storey BT. Spontaneous lipid peroxidation and production of hydrogen peroxide and superoxide in human spermatozoa. Superoxide dismutase as major enzyme protectant against oxygen toxicity. J Androl. 1987;8:338–48.
32. Gavella M, Lipovac V, Vucic M, Rocic B. Relationship of sperm superoxide dismutase-like activity with other sperm-specific enzymes' and experimentally induced lipid peroxidation in infertile men. Andrologia. 1996;28:223–9.
33. Aitken RJ, Buckingham DW, Carreras A, Irvine DS. Superoxide dismutase in human sperm suspensions: relationship with cellular composition, oxidative stress, and sperm function. Free Radic Biol Med. 1996;21:495–504.
34. Alvarez JG, Storey BT. Evidence for increased lipid peroxidative damage and loss of superoxide dismutase activity as a mode of sublethal cryodamage to human sperm during cryopreservation. J Androl. 1992;13:232–41.
35. Holland MK, Alvarez JG, Storey BT. Production of superoxide and activity of superoxide dismutase in rabbit epididymal spermatozoa. Biol Reprod. 1982;27:1109–18.
36. Buffone MG, Doncel GF, Marín Briggiler CI, Vazquez-Levin MH, Calamera JC. Human sperm subpopulations: relationship between functional quality and protein tyrosine phosphorylation. Hum Reprod. 2004;19:139–46.
37. Alvarez et al. Dynamics of DNA fragmentation after thawing of subsets of cryopreserved human spermatozoa. Annual Meeting of the Spanish Fertility Society. Valencia, Spain; 2010.
38. Bahçeci M, Ciray HN, Karagenc L, Uluğ U, Bener F. Effect of oxygen concentration during the incubation of embryos of women undergoing ICSI and embryo transfer: a prospective randomized study. Reprod Biomed Online. 2005;11:438–43.
39. Meintjes M, Chantilis SJ, Douglas JD, et al. A controlled randomized trial evaluating the effect of lowered incubator oxygen tension on live births in a predominantly blastocyst transfer program. Hum Reprod. 2009;24:300–7.
40. Kovačič B, Sajko MC, Vlaisavljević V. A prospective, randomized trial on the effect of atmospheric versus reduced oxygen concentration on the outcome of intracytoplasmic sperm injection cycles. Fertil Steril. 2010;94:511–9.
41. Weksler-Zangen S, Yaffe P, Ornoy A. Reduced SOD activity and increase neural tube defects in embryos of the sensitive but not of the resistant Cohen diabetic rats cultured under aerobic conditions. Birth Defects Res A Clin Mol Teratol. 2003;67:429–37.

Further Reading

Aitken RJ. Evaluation of human sperm function. Br Med Bull. 1990;46:654–74.

Alvarez JG, Storey BT. Differential incorporation of fatty acids into and peroxidative loss of fatty acids from phospholipids of human spermatozoa. Mol Reprod Dev. 1995;42:334–46.

Calamera JC, Brugo S, Vilar O. Relation between motility and adenosinetriphosphate (ATP) in human spermatozoa. Andrologia. 1982;14:239–41.

Calamera JC, Doncel GF, Olmedo SB, Kolm P, Acosta AA. "Modified sperm stress test: a simple assay that predicts sperm-related abnormal in-vitro fertilization. Hum Reprod. 1998;13: 2484–8.

Gravance CG, Vishwanath R, Pitt C, Garner DL, Casey PJ. Effects of cryopreservation on bull sperm head morphometry. J Androl. 1998;19:704–9.

Jones R, Mann T, Sherins R. Peroxidative breakdown of phospholipids in human spermatozoa, spermicidal properties of fatty acid peroxides, and protective action of seminal plasma. Fertil Steril. 1979;31:531–7.

Part III
Causes of Male Infertility

Chapter 8
Infection in Infertility

Ralf Henkel

Despite global overpopulation, human infertility is a growing concern since it is declining in both developed and developing countries [1, 2]. Reasons for this remarkable decline are manifold and include socio-economic changes [2], changes in lifestyle with higher prevalence of obesity [3, 4] or environmental pollution [5]. In general, data on the prevalence of infertility, i.e. the inability of a sexually active, non-contracepting couple to achieve pregnancy within 1 year's time [6], vary considerably between 3% and 25%, of which 15% seek for medical assistance [7, 8]. Infertility is a couple problem as both men and women contribute more or less equally, with prevalence reported for male infertility between 30 and 50% [9]. Approximately 7% of all men are confronted with fertility problems during their reproductive lifetime, thus making male infertility a problem, which has an even higher prevalence than diabetes mellitus with an overall estimate of 2.8% in the year 2000 and 4.4% in 2030, and which is considered a common disease [10, 11].

Potentially correctable causes of male infertility are genital tract infections [12], which play a major role in male infertility. Infections and inflammations are not only seriously affecting spermatogenesis and sperm transit during ejaculation as can be seen in clinical findings in cases of oligozoospermia (decreased number of sperm), asthenozoospermia (decreased sperm motility) or azoospermia (absence of sperm in the ejaculate) [13, 14], but are also the cause of dysfunctional male accessory glands [12] and significantly impaired sperm functions [15, 16]. These changes can be triggered in various ways, namely direct action of the pathogens on spermatozoa and sperm functions [17] or indirectly by inducing inflammatory processes in the seminal tract by activating leukocytes [18]. In non-selected cases, the prevalence of male genital tract infection-related infertility varies between 10 and 20% and amounts to up to 35% in a large study comprising more than 4,000 patients

R. Henkel, BEd, PhD (✉)
Department of Medical Biosciences, University of the Western Cape, X17,
Bellville, 7535, South Africa
e-mail: rhenkel@uwc.ac.za

S.J. Parekattil and A. Agarwal (eds.), *Antioxidants in Male Infertility: A Guide for Clinicians and Researchers*, © Springer Science+Business Media New York 2013

consulting for infertility [19]. It also appears that bacterial infections have a more detrimental effect in fertility-compromised patients than in fertile men [20], indicating that the impact of such bacterial genital tract infections may have to be differentiated.

Pathogens Causing Male Genital Tract Infections

Male urogenital tract infections can be classified according to the kind of microorganism causing the infection and the location, namely the testis (orchitis), epididymis (epididymitis), prostate (prostatitis) or urethra (urethritis). The most prevalent pathogens are *Chlamydia trachomatis*, *Ureaplasma urealyticum*, *Neisseria gonorrhoeae*, *Mycoplasma hominis*, *Mycoplasma genitalium* or *Escherichia coli*. While the first pathogens are sexually transmitted, *E. coli* is regarded as the most common cause of non-sexually transmitted urogenital tract infection, particularly of epididymo-orchitis or prostatitis where it is the cause of 65–80% of the cases [21]. Furthermore, viral infections like mumps virus, human papillomavirus (HPV), herpes simplex virus (HSV) and particularly human immunodeficiency virus (HIV) have also been associated with increased seminal leukocyte concentrations [22]. The latter virus can infect the testes and male sex accessory glands [23].

C. trachomatis

C. trachomatis is a gram-negative bacterium that is worldwide one of the most frequently sexually transmitted bacterial pathogens, accounting for an estimated 92 million new urogenital infections per year [24]. This number may be underestimated because of the high asymptomatic nature of the pathogen, with approximately 70–80% of women and up to 50% of men infected having no symptoms [25]. Reportedly, in symptomatic men, the prevalence of infections varies from 4 to 10% [26]. Another report found a prevalence of up to 35.9% in men and 38% in women [27]. Since a high number of chlamydial infections remain undiagnosed, the pathogen can even be transferred to the newborn during delivery accounting for 25–50% of conjunctivitis and 10–20% of pneumonia in newborns, thus posing a health risk on the offspring as well as enormous costs for diagnosis and treatment on countries' health systems. For the United States, these costs estimate to $2.2 million for each 500 cases [25].

In men, *C. trachomatis* has been associated with prostatitis, epididymitis and urethritis. The bacterium has been detected in the testis including Leydig cells [28], the prostate [29] and even epididymis and seminal vesicles [30]. Apart from the lesions triggered by the infection and the implications and acute inflammation can cause in the male genital tract, reports on the influence of chlamydial infections on male fertility are inconsistent. While some authors [31, 32] found no significant association, most others have shown a direct negative influence of the chlamydial infection on male fertility [29, 33, 34]. *In vitro* studies by Hosseinzadeh et al. [35–37] even indicate that the pathogen directly causes changes in sperm proteins and premature cell death induced by lipopolysaccharides secreted by Chlamydiae. These discrepancies in findings may be due to the fact that in numerous cases, chlamydial infections are accompanied by other microbial infections making a clear association of infertility with the chlamydial infection difficult [38]. Furthermore, the various detection methods for the pathogen in asymptomatic cases appear challenging, and especially the sensitivity and specificity of serological markers were regarded as problematic [25]. For that reason, recent studies suggest PCR amplification of bacterial rDNA in semen as this approach seems to be promising especially to identify asymptomatic patients [39, 40].

Mycoplasms

Mycoplasms and ureaplasms belong to the family of *Mycoplasmataceae*, which are widely distributed in vertebrate species. They are the smallest bacteria replicating in culture and are lacking a cell wall [41, 42]. Five species colonize the male urogenital tract and may contaminate the semen during ejaculation, namely *U. urealyticum, U. parvum, M. hominis, M. genitalium* and *M. fermentans*, of which only the first four are pathogenic.

U. urealyticum

Among other disorders, *U. urealyticum* is reported to cause non-gonococcal urethritis, pelvic inflammatory disease or infertility [12, 43]. In the past, the association between ureaplasma infections and male infertility was discussed controversially [44, 45]. In a recent large study including 346 selected subjects, Wang et al. [46] showed that ureaplasma infections cause higher seminal viscosity, decreased sperm concentrations, and lower pH. Although this study could not find any further effect on other sperm parameters, Potts et al. [45] found significantly increased seminal reactive oxygen species (ROS) levels, and Reichart et al. [47] higher levels of sperm DNA damage. These discrepancies might be due to the fact that *U. urealyticum* shows a distinct energy metabolism-dependent effect on sperm activity [48]. According to this theory, sperm motility is impaired by the bacterium at low pH since it competes with sperm mitochondrial energy production. On the other hand, at higher pH, sperm motility will even be enhanced as ureaplasma stimulates glycolysis.

The prevalence of male genital ureaplasma infections among infertile men varies considerably from 10 to 40% [49], most probably as a result of different diagnostic methods used in various studies and different population groups examined. Like in patients with chlamydial infections, detection of *U. urealyticum* and mycoplasms is particularly problematic in asymptomatic patients because these patients may shed fewer colony-forming units (CFU; organisms) to be detected in a standard culture assay. Therefore, PCR should be the diagnostic method of choice [50].

M. hominis, M. genitalium

Although the direct impact of these two bacteria on male fertility was debated in earlier years, recent reports associate *M. hominis* and *M. genitalium* with genitourinary infections [51, 52]. Frequencies of infection are with 10.8% for *M. hominis* and 5% for *M. genitalium*, respectively, reportedly lower than for other pathogens [53]. Both species can attach to and penetrate human sperm plasma membrane [54, 55], which might have a significant long-term impact on male fertility as well as on the onset of pregnancy and the health of the offspring. While the first may contribute to the distribution of the bacterium to the female to cause cervicitis and endometritis [56] or an alteration of the plasma membrane affecting acrosome reaction [57], the latter might particularly be caused by the sperm DNA damage triggered by the infection [33].

N. gonorrhoeae

These gram-negative, immotile cocci are growing in pairs (diplococci) and cause the most common infectious disease in men leading to urethritis, prostatitis and epididymitis which in turn may impair male fertility. These bacteria have pili on their surface, which facilitate attachment to other cells [58]. In sperm, an asialoglycoprotein receptor has been identified that recognizes and binds lipopolysaccharides in gonococcal membranes [59]. Since chlamydial lipopolysaccharides can cause death of human sperm by inducing apoptosis [60], it is conceivable that Neisseria lipopolysaccharides might also induce such reactions. Yet, this has not been shown thus far.

Even though its incidence has been declining in Western countries during the past decades, 150–400 new infections per 100,000 are still recorded in Europe per year [58]. Presumably due to socio-economic and behavioural factors, these numbers are much higher in Third World and developing countries, with highest numbers in Sub-Saharan Africa and South and Southeast Asia [61].

E. coli

E. coli is a gram-negative bacterium that belongs to the family of *Enterobacteriaceae* and is responsible for most urogenital tract and male accessory gland infections with up to 80% of the bacterial prostatitis [12, 62]. In contrast to other uropathogens like

Enterococcus or *Staphylococcus saprophyticus*, *E. coli* has significant direct negative effects on sperm motility [63]. An in vitro study by Köhn et al. [57] revealed that this microbe can even negatively affect sperm functions like acrosome reaction. This might be due to morphological alterations, particularly on the acrosome and flagellum, seen after exposure of human sperm to the pathogen [64]. Due to the direct interaction of bacterial pili with the sperm plasma membrane [65], *E. coli* is interfering with sperm motility [66]. A recent study [67] demonstrated two mechanisms by which *E. coli* affects spermatozoa, the described direct interaction and by action of soluble factors that induce apoptosis and a breakdown in the mitochondrial membrane potential. Potential candidate substances causing these cellular reactions might be α-hemolysin and Shiga-like toxin as these have already been associated with sperm motility loss [68] and apoptosis in Hep-2 cells [69], respectively.

Viruses

A number of viruses are also able to infect all parts of the male genital system, namely the testes (e.g. mumps virus, HIV-1), epididymis (e.g. Coxsackie virus), seminal vesicle (e.g. cytomegalovirus [CMV]), prostate (e.g. HPV, HSV, HIV-1) and the semen (e.g. HSV, HPV, HIV) [70]. In a recent study including 241 asymptomatic patients attending an infertility clinic for semen analysis, viral DNA was detected in 45 patients; CMV (8.7%), HPV (4.5%), HHV-6 (3.7%), HSV (3.6%), Epstein–Barr virus (0.4%) and hepatitis B virus (0.0%) [71].

While for some of the viral infections like HSV or HIV-1 are associated with poor semen and sperm quality [22, 72], this could not be confirmed for CMV and human herpesvirus type 6 (HHV6) [71]. Thus, the latter viruses appear not to cause male infertility. However, in patients with viral infections affecting male fertility, leukocytospermia ($>1 \times 10^6$ leukocytes/ml ejaculate) is strongly associated with the infection as well as with elevated levels of inflammatory markers like PMN-elastase or interleukins [71].

A matter of concern is the high number of globally more than 65 million people infected with HIV, out of which a growing number of HIV-positive people are seeking for assisted reproduction to have children without infecting the partner or the offspring. Since a few years, some IVF centres started treating infected couples and received acceptable pregnancy rates; the worst in couples where both partners were infected [73]. In these patients, not only the risk of vertical transmission from a seropositive mother to her unborn child has to be dealt with but also the fact that semen is a vector of viral propagation and sperm can bind and incorporate the virus via a CD4-independent receptor and/or the HIV co-receptor CCR5 [74, 75]. Despite it is generally accepted that motile sperm are not productively infected by HIV, sperm can carry viral particles deriving from the testis or epididymis [76, 77]. In view of the fact that seminal leukocytes shed different viral strains than those in the blood [78], the question rises whether infected leukocytes and free virions contaminating the semen are of different origin, and an infected testis might represent a special reservoir for the virus as this area is resistant to antiviral drugs due to the blood–testis barrier [77]. Therefore, special care must be taken when separating sperm for assisted reproduction, particularly for ICSI.

Male Genital Tract Infections

Orchitis

As per definition by the European Association of Urology, the term *orchitis* describes an inflammatory lesion of the testicle, which is associated with a leukocytic exudate inside and outside the seminiferous tubules, resulting in tubular damage [13]. The condition can be a reason for spermatogenic arrest and testicular atrophy leading to low seminal sperm concentration and poor sperm quality [13, 79]. An acute infectious orchitis is characterized by an abrupt onset of severe pain with visible swelling of the affected testicle as well as of the inguinal lymph nodes and can be accompanied by fever. Further symptoms are similar to those of testicular torsion and can include hematuria and blood in the ejaculate. Subacute and chronic inflammatory conditions, however, often remain asymptomatic [80]. Yet, an orchitis may lead to intratesticular obstruction, which is the case in about 15% of obstructive azoospermia [13].

In contrast, non-infectious inflammations of the testis may occur in patients with testicular seminoma where predominantly CD8-positive T-lymphocytes infiltrate the tumour tissue, and macrophages are found in the fibrovascular septae and at the periphery [14]. Such infiltration of activated T-lymphocytes into testicular tissue is also indicative of a significant disturbance of the local immunoregulation [81]. Thus, due to an impaired blood–testis barrier, these inflammatory cells overcome the testicular immunosuppressive mechanisms and the formation of anti-sperm autoantibodies under such conditions would be conceivable, particularly in cases of prolonged inflammatory processes as is in chronic orchitis [82]. On the other hand, except for a few cases with positive titres for autoantibodies in patients with a mumps history, only little evidence is available for this relationship [83, 84].

As reported in a large study, the prevalence of an isolated orchitis is with 0.42% among testicular pathologies relatively low [85]. However, due to retrograde ascending infectious lesions, a "non-specific" orchitis triggered by *Pneumococcus* sp., *Salmonella* sp., *Klebsiella* sp. or *Haemophilus influenza* is in most cases associated with an epididymitis as epididymo-orchitis. The close vicinity of the different compartments as well as the ascending nature of the infections makes a distinction between inflammations, i.e. isolated epididymitis vs. epididymo-orchitis, very difficult in the clinical routine [82].

Sexually transmitted bacteria like *C. trachomatis* and *N. gonorrhoeae* are the cause of the acute infection in men younger than 35 years, while *E. coli* is the predominant trigger in older men [14]. On the other hand, an orchitis can also occur after hematogenous dissemination of pathogens like the Coxsackie B or the mumps virus [13] as a complication of a systemic viral infection. For instance, the mumps virus may affect the tests (mumps orchitis) in 20–30% [86] and lead to infertility in 13% of the cases with unilateral and in 30–87% in patients with bilateral orchitis [87, 88]. However, clinicians should realize that an epididymo-orchitis can also develop secondary to the mumps infection, even in the absence of a parotitis [89]. While bacterial infections as described above cause a 'non-specific' orchitis, *Mycobacterium tuberculosis*, *M. leprae*, *Treponema pallidum* or *Brucella* sp. may cause a 'specific', predominantly granulomatous orchitis [13].

Epididymitis

Epididymitis, an inflammation of the epididymis, is a painful, feverish, almost unilateral condition with tender swelling of epididymis and scrotum. Based on the duration of the symptoms, epididymitis may be sub-classified as acute, subacute and chronic. In the latter, symptoms are present for more than 6 weeks. In cases of acute infectious epididymitis, an involvement of the testicle due to ascending canalicular bacterial infections can represent a complication which may occur in up to 60% of affected patients as epididymo-orchitis [90]. Although up to 35% of patients consulting for fertility problems present with male genital tract infections [19, 91], data on the prevalence of epididymitis/epididymo-orchitis vary considerably from 0.29% of all consultations [92] to 20% of all urologic admissions in an US Army setup [93].

As for orchitis, *C. trachomatis* and *N. gonorrhoeae* are the most common cause of epididymitis in sexually active men younger than 35 years. In contrast, Gram-negative *Enterobacteriaceae*, of which *E. coli* is the predominant pathogen, are aetiologically responsible for the disease in older men [12, 90], which are also particularly at risk of having urethral strictures, bladder neck obstruction or benign prostate hyperplasia (BPH) resulting in increased voiding pressure to empty the bladder resulting in a reflux of contaminated urine into the excurrent genital ducts and subsequent infection [94].

Potential risk factors for epididymitis include sexual activity, strenuous activities like lifting heavy goods, bicycle and motorbike riding or extended periods of sitting at job or travelling [95]. Even traumatic events such as accidents or scrotal traumas and iatrogenic injury to the epididymis during surgeries can be a cause of epididymitis.

Major problems for male fertility may arise particularly in patients with epididymitis as this disease appears to have a greater influence on semen quality and male fertility than an infection/inflammation of the prostate or seminal vesicle [96]. In addition, in quite a number of patients, the diagnosis of chronic epididymitis is extremely difficult as these patients do not feel discomfort and their health is not compromised [82]. Due to a *silent* nature of the infection/inflammation, epididymitis will only be diagnosed once these patients appear in an andrological clinic consulting for infertility. Eventually, inflammatory lesions of the epididymis can result in dysfunction of the organ and ultimately in obstructive azoospermia, which is the most common cause for this condition [13].

In patients with an acute epididymitis, a semen analysis is not recommended [13]. In cases of chronic epididymitis, semen parameters may be dramatically affected with lower sperm count, motility and seminal α-glucosidase. In contrary, many patients can present with leukocytospermia, i.e. leukocyte count of more than 1×10^6/ml [97], elevated seminal levels of polymorphonuclear granulocyte elastase and atypically stained sperm flagella [82].

Prostatitis

Despite the numbers of urological consultations for prostatitis outnumbered those for benign prostate hyperplasia or prostate cancer [98], prostatitis has been called "the third most important disease of the prostate gland" [99]. Epidemiological studies revealed an estimated prevalence of 4–11% for prostatitis, which then represents the most common urological diagnosis in men younger than 50 years [100]. A large study with more than 600 men included suggests that only about 5–10% of these cases are of bacterial origin [101]. Yet, more recently, Bjerklund Johansen et al. [102] and Nickel et al. [103] showed that only about 50% of all patients with chronic prostatitis (bacterial and abacterial) respond positively to antibiotic treatment.

According to the classification system suggested by Drach et al. [104], prostatitis was divided into four clinical syndromes, namely acute, chronic bacterial and chronic abacterial prostatitis, and prostatodynia. Considering that this system was never validated and left clinicians confused about diagnostic and therapeutic strategies, particularly since many cases without infection have pathogenic processes outside the prostate, the National Institutes of Health (NIH) introduced a new system classifying prostatitis [105, 106] (Table 8.1). Even though many clinicians diagnose "prostatitis," it rather represents diverse clinical symptoms ranging from acute bacterial infection to chronic pelvic pain and should actually be referred to as "prostatitis syndrome" as patients present with a variety of urogenital, perineal and perianal complaints [99, 107].

Considering the various problems around understanding prostatitis and its diagnosis [108], particularly chronic bacterial prostatitis, it is obvious that the diagnosis of an acute infection does not pose a problem for urologists. The symptoms for the acute bacterial prostatitis are quite clear; the patients are presenting with an urosepsis, fever, obstructive voiding symptoms and local pelvic pain [109]. In about 80% of acute bacterial prostatitis, *E. coli* can be identified as pathogen, while *Pseudomonas aeruginosa*, *Klebsiella* or Enterococci are the cause in the remaining patients [110]. Nevertheless, there are major concerns differentiating the category II from category III prostatitis. Many of these patients have a history of recurrent urinary tract infections and are asymptomatic in non-infectious intervals. If the bacterial culture is positive for an established uropathogen like *E. coli* or *Klebsiella* sp., the diagnosis is unproblematic [105] (Table 8.2). However, the classic classification scheme might fail in cases where enterococci or anaerobes are identified in prostate specimens.

Table 8.1 NIH classification and definition of the categories of prostatitis

NIH classification		Definition
Category I	Acute bacterial prostatitis	Acute infection of the prostate gland
Category II	Chronic bacterial prostatitis	Recurrent infection of the prostate
Category III	Chronic abacterial prostatitis/ CPPS	No demonstrable infection
Category IIIA	Inflammatory CPPS	White blood cells in semen/EPS/voided bladder urine-3 (VB-3 or postprostatic massage)
Category IIIB	Non-inflammatory CPPS	No white blood cells in semen/EPS/VB-3
Category IV	Asymptomatic inflammatory prostatitis	No subjective symptoms detected either by prostate biopsy or the presence of white blood cells in EPS/semen during evaluation for other disorders

Table 8.2 Uropathogens causing chronic prostatitis

Established pathogens	Potential pathogens
Escherichia coli	*Staphylococcus saprophyticus*
Klebsiella pneumonia	*Staphylococcus aureus*
Proteus mirabilis	*Staphylococcus epidermidis*
Pseudomonas aeruginosa	*Mycoplasma genitalium*
Enterococcus faecalis	*Ureaplasma urealyticum*
Chlamydia trachomatis	

Data from Nickel JC, Moon T. Chronic bacterial prostatitis: an evolving clinical enigma. Urology. 2005;66:2–8

Even more so in patients who had initially positive cultures but are negative at the time of recurrent symptoms. Apparently, in these cases, the detection is false negative because the bacterial colonization of the prostate can be veiled as bacteria can form microcolonies or aggregates, which are surrounded by a thick protective layer [105, 111].

Urethritis

Urethritis is the infectious or non-infectious inflammation of the urethra. While non-infectious causes include injuries through traumas, masturbation, manipulation by the patient or medical treatments, acute infectious urethritis may be caused by known sexually transmitted uropathogens like *C. trachomatis*, *Mycoplasms* or *N. gonorrhoea* with incidences of 15–26%, 10–21% and 0.4–18%, respectively. In addition, among the not sexually transmitted pathogens, Enterobacteriaceae and staphylococci are causing the disease with frequencies between 20 and 31% [112]. Chronic urethritis is a rare condition, which is why the prevalence is not known [113].

The clinical symptoms of an acute urethritis vary considerably. While some patients present with distinct urethral discharge and dysuria, others are symptom-free or only show some pus prior to the first voiding of urine in the morning, which may be occur in 5–10% of the patients [12]. As can be seen for the symptoms, clinical findings also vary from inflammatory stickiness, redness and swelling at the glans penis or the urethral orifice to the absence of any clinical sign. Normally, the infection remains localized to the urethra. However, ascension of gonococci may occur in about 1% of the infected patients causing epididymitis [112].

The impact of urethritis on male fertility is debatable, particularly since the inflammatory discharge present in the anterior urethra makes an ejaculate analysis impossible as the pus contaminates the ejaculate [114] and both direct effect of bacteria [16, 37, 67, 115] and leukocytes [116, 117] demonstrated detrimental effects on sperm functions. On the other hand, obstruction due to urethral stricture or as a result of lesions in the area of the seminal colliculus may result in ejaculatory disturbances [13].

Male Accessory Gland Infection

According to definition, the male accessory glands comprise the prostate, seminal vesicles and the Cowper's glands (bulbourethral glands). However, in many publications, the term *male accessory gland infection* (MAGI) describes the clinical symptoms of the inflammation as a result of canalicularily ascending infections of the male accessory glands including the deferent duct and the epididymis via the urethra as "prostate-seminal vesiculitis," "epididymo-prostato-vesiculitis," or "male adnexitis" as long as urethritis or a urinary tract infection has been excluded [118]. Considering that in MAGI these organs are commonly inflamed, clear distinctions between prostatitis, epididymitis and glandulitis vesiculitis cannot be made [58]. General symptoms of MAGI are leukocytospermia (more than 10^6 peroxidase-positive leukocytes/ml), elevated seminal levels of polymorphonuclear granulocyte elastase ($\geq$230 ng/ml), C3c complement ($\geq$0.01 mg/ml), ROS and cytokines [118–120].

As a result of the leukocyte infiltration due to the infection as well as the elevated concentrations of pro-inflammatory cytokines like interleukin-6 (IL-6), IL-8 or tumour necrosis factor-α (TNF-α) into the genital system, sperm functions may be compromised by directly affecting sperm function and intensifying the level of oxidative stress, respectively [117, 121, 122]. As a result of the inflammatory processes in the male accessory glands, their secretory function may be impaired, consequently resulting in decreased seminal concentrations of citric acid, fructose, α-glucosidase, phosphatase and zinc [58, 123, 124].

In addition, there are concerns that patients presenting with MAGI are at a higher risk of developing sperm autoantibodies due to the inflammatory processes compromising the immune barrier [125, 126]. Furthermore, like in orchitis or epididymitis, stenosis or obstruction of the excurrent ducts may occur.

Consequences of Infections on Sperm Fertilizing Capacity

Apart from the specific effects on male fertility described above, male genital tract infections and inflammations cause general reactions that also negatively affect sperm fertilizing capacity by compromising specific sperm functions. In the light of spermatozoa being the most polarized cells in the body, the male germ cell has to maintain its extreme polarization, for which one of the most important prerequisites is a highly fluid plasma membrane. Therefore, sperm cells contain an extraordinary high amount of polyunsaturated fatty acids (PUFA), particularly docosahexaenoic acid, which has 6 double bonds in its molecule [127]. Since most sperm functions are dependent on membrane functionality, this high content of PUFA is also essential for normal sperm function and respective disturbances result in a loss of sperm function.

As a result of an urogenital tract infection, activated leukocytes infiltrate the infected organs releasing high amounts of ROS and cytokines such as IL-6, IL-8 or TNF-α as inflammatory mediators [128, 129]. Both ROS and cytokines have been shown to be associated not only with the impairment of sperm functions like motility but also to DNA damage and infertility by induction and stimulation of membrane lipid peroxidation through oxidative stress [120, 130–133]. By way of this mechanism, male genital tract infections/inflammations do not only damage sperm DNA and reduce sperm count and seminal volume but also impair sperm functions like motility, acrosome reaction or acrosin activity [57, 117, 134–138].

Treatment of Infections

Generally, the first choice of treatment of male genital tract infections has to be antibiotic in order to eradicate pathogenic microorganisms, normalize inflammatory parameters, prevent transmission to the female partner and decrease the risk of potential complications [12]. Considering that many urogenital tract infections are sexually transmitted, however, simultaneous treatment of the partner has to be considered, particularly in *C. trachomatis* infections. While standardized recommendations only exist for the treatment of acute bacterial epididymitis, epididymo-orchitis and specific granulomatous orchitis [13, 139], guidelines for the treatment of chronic infections and inflammations of the male genital tract have not been drawn up yet and are rather empirical and only few uncontrolled studies are available [13, 90]. For mumps orchitis, the systemic treatment with α-2β-interferon may be considered to prevent testicular atrophy and azoospermia [140].

The very same is true for acute bacterial and chronic bacterial prostatitis. While an antibiotic treatment for these conditions is mandatory, the benefit for patients with inflammatory chronic pelvic pain syndrome is questionable [102]. Still, treatment of the prostatitis syndrome with antibiotics poses the major problem of the penetrability of the agents into the prostate and its secretions, and only a few modern antibiotics like fluoroquinolones have the chemical properties to enter these compartments well [141, 142].

In order to alleviate the inflammatory lesions, therapy with both corticosteroids and non-steroidal antiphlogistic substances has shown considerable positive effects on semen quality in terms of sperm and leukocyte count and sperm motility [143–145]. Furthermore, antioxidative therapies with vitamins and/or antioxidant supplementations to reduce the oxidative stress caused by leukocytes and defective spermatozoa are currently highly debated [146, 147]. Although several studies with various antioxidants alone or in combination have shown a significant reduction in seminal ROS levels [148–150] and improvement in sperm count and motility [151–153], other studies found the opposite [154, 155]. Therefore, notwithstanding the indubitable positive effects of an antioxidative supplementation for general health purposes, no definite recommendation can be made at this point in time with regard to the treatment of male genital tract infections. Most probably, it is not only the administration of singular antioxidative substances that causes the beneficial effects but the combination of different antioxidants at very specific concentrations.

Expert Commentary

The purpose of this chapter was to discuss the contribution of male genital tract infections/inflammations to male infertility. Considering that many of these male genital tract infections are sexually transmitted, the knowledge of its impact on the female partner as well as treatment of the couple is mandatory. Moreover, as there is still a lack of knowledge about the impact of such infections on sperm functions, this chapter is dealing with impaired sperm functions as a result of the infection/inflammation. Since many patients suffer from asymptomatic, the so-called 'silent' infections, it is essential for the clinician to identify these conditions and also to urge the patients to continue with the treatment long enough. Appropriate treatment is particularly a problem in prostatitis as only few drugs penetrate the prostate and its secretions sufficiently. Therefore, this chapter was also to give an up-to-date overview on the impact of different male genital tract infections/inflammations on sperm functions and various treatment options.

Five-Year View

Although our knowledge on male genital tract infections and its impact on male fertility increased during recent years, there is still a lack of knowledge particularly regarding the impact of the infection/inflammation on sperm functions, and the following topics will have to be addressed in future studies:
- The impact of the infection/inflammation on male germ cell's DNA.
- Currently, the seminal leukocyte concentration is under debate and several authors argue that the WHO's cut-off value of leukocytospermia is too high.

Therefore, clarity has to be provided for clinicians in order to properly diagnose male genital tract infections.

- Since the diagnosis, particularly of asymptomatic patients, constitutes a problem in the clinic, new test system including PCR has to be introduced into the diagnostic set-ups.
- Special care has to be taken when handling with or performing assisted reproduction with sperm deriving from HIV-positive subjects, and further investigations have to be carried out in order to clarify the possibility of transmission of the virus.
- Development of new antibiotics that penetrate more easily into the male genital tract system.

Key Issues

- Male infertility is a major issue of concern as it affects more people during their lifetime as a common disease, diabetes mellitus.
- Among these infertile men, the prevalence of male genital tract infection is reportedly between 20 and 40%.
- Many pathogens, including bacteria and viruses, are sexually transmitted and require treatment of the couple.
- Among the sexually transmitted bacteria, infections with *C. trachomatis* and mycoplasms are most prevalent, while *E. coli* causes the most prevalent non-sexually transmitted male genital tract infection.
- Among the viral infections, mumps and HIV infections are the most important as mumps can cause permanent infertility due to mumps orchitis and HIV can be carried by spermatozoa from the testis or epididymis.
- Special care must be taken in assisted reproduction with HIV-positive men since an infected testis might represent a special reservoir for the virus as this area is resistant to antiviral drugs due to the blood-testis barrier.
- Male genital tract infections can be acute or asymptomatic, which represents a particular problem as patients and doctors might not recognize the disease that impairs male fertility.
- Male genital tract infections can ascent the genital tract.
- Apart from the specific complications such as obstructions causing azoospermia, male genital tract infections/inflammations may directly impair sperm fertilizing capacity by compromising specific sperm functions through ROS and interleukins.
- Generally, infections have to be treated with appropriate antibiotics. However, antiphlogistic treatment has also been proven to have positive effects on sperm count and motility.
- Despite certain positive effects, treatment with antioxidants like vitamins to alleviate the effects of ROS is still highly debated.

References

1. Lutz W, O'Neill BC, Scherbov S. Demographics. Europe's population at a turning point. Science. 2003;299:1991–2.
2. Skakkebaek NE, Jorgensen N, Main KM, et al. Is human fecundity declining? Int J Androl. 2006;29:2–11.
3. Pasquali R, Pelusi C, Genghini S, et al. Obesity and reproductive disorders in women. Hum Reprod Update. 2003;9:359–72.
4. Sallmen M, Sandler DP, Hoppin JA, et al. Reduced fertility among overweight and obese men. Epidemiology. 2006;17:520–3.
5. Foster WG, Neal MS, Han MS, et al. Environmental contaminants and human infertility: hypothesis or cause for concern? J Toxicol Environ Health B Crit Rev. 2008;11:162–76.
6. World Health Organization. Manual for the standardized investigation and diagnosis of the infertile couple. Cambridge, UK: Cambridge University; 2000.
7. Dohle GR, Colpi GM, Hargreave TB, et al. EAU guidelines on male infertility. Eur Urol. 2005;48:703–11.
8. Henkel R. ROS and sperm DNA integrity—implications of male accessory gland infections. In: Giwercman A, Tournaye H, Björndahl L, Weidner W, editors. Clinical andrology, informa healthcare. London: Parthenon Publishing, Marcel Dekker, Taylor & Francis Medical; 2010. p. 324–8.
9. Hull MG, Glazener CM, Kelly NJ, et al. Population study of causes, treatment, and outcome of infertility. Br Med J (Clin Res Ed). 1985;291:1693–7.
10. Nieschlag E, Behre HM. Andrology. Male reproductive health and dysfunction. 2nd ed. Berlin, Heidelberg, New York: Springer; 2000.
11. Wild S, Roglic G, Green A, et al. Global prevalence of diabetes: estimates for the year 2000 and projections for 2030. Diabetes Care. 2004;27:1047–53.
12. Weidner W, Krause W, Ludwig M. Relevance of male accessory gland infection for subsequent fertility with special focus on prostatitis. Hum Reprod Update. 1999;5:421–32.
13. Weidner W, Colpi GM, Hargreave TB, et al. EAU guidelines on male infertility. Eur Urol. 2002;42:313–22.
14. Schuppe HC, Meinhardt A, Allam JP, et al. Chronic orchitis: a neglected cause of male infertility? Andrologia. 2008;40:84–91.
15. Henkel R, Schill W-B. Sperm separation in patients with urogenital infections. Andrologia. 1998;30 Suppl 1:91–7.
16. Sanocka-Maciejewska D, Ciupinska M, Kurpisz M. Bacterial infection and semen quality. J Reprod Immunol. 2005;67:51–6.
17. Monga M, Roberts JA. Spermagglutination by bacteria: receptor-specific interactions. J Androl. 1994;15:151–6.
18. Eggert-Kruse W, Kiefer I, Beck C, et al. Role for tumor necrosis factor alpha (TNF-alpha) and interleukin 1-beta (IL-1beta) determination in seminal plasma during infertility investigation. Fertil Steril. 2007;87:810–23.
19. Henkel R, Maaß G, Jung A, et al. Age-related changes in seminal polymorphonuclear elastase in men with asymptomatic inflammation of the genital tract. Asian J Androl. 2007;9:299–304.
20. Moretti E, Capitani S, Figura N, et al. The presence of bacteria species in semen and sperm quality. J Assist Reprod Genet. 2009;26:47–56.
21. Pellati D, Mylonakis I, Bertoloni G, et al. Genital tract infections and infertility. Eur J Obstet Gynecol Reprod Biol. 2008;140:3–11.
22. Umapathy E, Simbini T, Chipata T, et al. Sperm characteristics and accessory sex gland functions in HIV-infected men. Arch Androl. 2001;46:153–8.
23. Le Tortorec A, Le Grand R, Denis H, et al. Infection of semen-producing organs by SIV during the acute and chronic stages of the disease. PLoS One. 2008;3:e1792.

24. World Health Organization. Global prevalence and incidence of selected sexually transmitted diseases: overview and estimates. World Health Organization: Geneva, Switzerland; 2001.
25. Gonzales GF, Munoz G, Sanchez R, et al. Update on the impact of *Chlamydia trachomatis* infection on male fertility. Andrologia. 2004;36:1–23.
26. Rietmeijer CAM, Judson FN, van Hensbroek MB, et al. Unsuspected *Chlamydia trachomatis* infection in heterosexual men attending a sexually transmitted disease clinic: evaluation of risk factors and screening methods. Sex Transm Dis. 1991;18:28–35.
27. Gdoura R, Keskes-Ammar L, Bouzid F, et al. *Chlamydia trachomatis* and male infertility in Tunisia. Eur J Contracept Reprod Health Care. 2001;6:102–7.
28. Villegas H, Pinon M, Shor V, et al. Electron microscopy of *Chlamydia trachomatis* infection of the male genital tract. Arch Androl. 1991;27:117–26.
29. Kadar A, Bucsek M, Kardos M, et al. Detection of *Chlamydia trachomatis* in chronic prostatitis by in situ hybridization (preliminary methodological report). Orv Hetil. 1995;136: 659–62.
30. Bornman MS, Ramuthaga TN, Mahomed MF, et al. Chlamydia infection in asymptomatic infertile men attending an Andrology clinic. Arch Androl. 1998;41:203–8.
31. Ruijis GJ, Kauer FM, Jager S, et al. Epidemiological aspects of chlamydial infections and tubal abnormalities in infertile couples. Eur J Obstet Gynecol Reprod Biol. 1990 Jul-Aug; 36(1–2):107–16.
32. Habermann B, Krause W. Altered sperm function or sperm antibodies are not associated with chlamydial antibodies in infertile men with leukocytospermia. J Eur Acad Dermatol Venerol. 1999;12:25–9.
33. Gallegos G, Ramos B, Santiso R, et al. Sperm DNA fragmentation in infertile men with genitourinary infection by *Chlamydia trachomatis* and *Mycoplasma*. Fertil Steril. 2008;90:328–34.
34. Mazzoli S, Cai T, Addonisio P, et al. *Chlamydia trachomatis* infection is related to poor semen quality in young prostatitis patients. Eur Urol. 2010;57(4):708–14. Epub 27 May 2009.
35. Hosseinzadeh S, Brewis IA, Pacey AA, et al. Coincubation of human spermatozoa with *Chlamydia trachomatis* in vitro causes increased tyrosine phosphorylation of sperm proteins. Infect Immun. 2000;68:4872–6.
36. Hosseinzadeh S, Brewis IA, Eley A, et al. Co-incubation of human spermatozoa with *Chlamydia trachomatis* serovar E causes premature sperm death. Hum Reprod. 2001;16: 293–9.
37. Hosseinzadeh S, Pacey AA, Eley A. Chlamydia trachomatis-induced death of human spermatozoa is caused primarily by lipopolysaccharide. J Med Microbiol. 2003;52:193–200.
38. Creighton S, Tenant-Flowers M, Taylor CB, et al. Co-infection with gonorrhoea and chlamydia: how much is there and what does it mean? Int J STD AIDS. 2003;14:109–13.
39. Witkin SS, Jeremias J, Grifo JA, et al. Detection of *Chlamydia trachomatis* in semen by the polymerase chain reaction in male members of infertile couples. Am J Obstet Gynecol. 1993;168:1457–62.
40. Kiessling AA, Desmarais BM, Yin HZ, et al. Detection and identification of bacterial DNA in semen. Fertil Steril. 2008;90:1744–56.
41. Styler M, Shapiro SS. Mollicutes (mycoplasma) in infertility. Fertil Steril. 1985;44:1–12.
42. Kilic D, Basar MM, Kaygusuz S, et al. Prevalence and treatment of Chlamydia trachomatis, Ureaplasma urealyticum, and Mycoplasma hominis in patients with non-gonococcal urethritis. Jpn J Infect Dis. 2004 Feb;57(1):17–20.
43. Schiefer HG. Microbiology of male urethroadnexitis: diagnostic procedures and criteria for aetiologic classification. Andrologia. 1998;30 Suppl 1:7–13.
44. Kjaergaard N, Kristensen B, Hansen ES, et al. Microbiology of semen specimens from males attending a fertility clinic. APMIS. 1997;105:566–70.
45. Potts JM, Sharma R, Pasqualotto F, et al. Association of *Ureaplasma urealyticum* with abnormal reactive oxygen species levels and absence of leukocytospermia. J Urol. 2000;163: 1775–8.

46. Wang Y, Liang CL, Wu JQ, et al. Do *Ureaplasma urealyticum* infections in the genital tract affect semen quality? Asian J Androl. 2006;8:562–8.
47. Reichart M, Kahane I, Bartoov B. *In vivo* and *in vitro* impairment of human and ram sperm nuclear chromatin integrity by sexually transmitted *Ureaplasma urealyticum* infection. Biol Reprod. 2000;63:1041–8.
48. Reichart M, Levi H, Kahane I, et al. Dual energy metabolism-dependent effect of Ureaplasma urealyticum infection on sperm activity. J Androl. 2001;22:404–12.
49. Cottell E, Harrison RF, McCaffrey M, et al. Are seminal fluid microorganisms of significance or merely contaminants? Fertil Steril. 2000;74:465–70.
50. Witkin SS. Immunological aspects of genital chlamydia infections. Best Pract Res Clin Obstet Gynaecol. 2002;16:865–74.
51. Deguchi T, Maeda S. *Mycoplasma genitalium*: another important pathogen of non-gonococcal urethritis. J Urol. 2002;167:210–7.
52. Andrade-Rocha FT. *Ureaplasma urealyticum* and *Mycoplasma hominis* in men attending for routine semen analysis. Prevalence, incidence by age and clinical settings, influence on sperm characteristics, relationship with the leukocyte count and clinical value. Urol Int. 2003;71:377–81.
53. Gdoura R, Kchaou W, Chaari C, et al. Ureaplasma urealyticum, Ureaplasma parvum, Mycoplasma hominis and Mycoplasma genitalium infections and semen quality of infertile men. BMC Infect Dis. 2007;7:129.
54. Taylor-Robinson D. *Mycoplasma genitalium*—an update. Int J STD AIDS. 2002;13:145–51.
55. Diaz-Garcia FJ, Herrera-Mendoza AP, Giono-Cerezo S, et al. Mycoplasma hominis attaches to and locates intracellularly in human spermatozoa. Hum Reprod. 2006;21:1591–8.
56. Cohen CR, Manhart LE, Bukusi EA, et al. Association between *Mycoplasma genitalium* and acute endometritis. Lancet. 2002;359:765–6.
57. Köhn FM, Erdmann I, Oeda T, et al. Influence of urogenital infections on sperm functions. Andrologia. 1998;30 Suppl 1:73–80.
58. Krause W. Male accessory gland infection. Andrologia. 2008;40:113–6.
59. Harvey HA, Porat N, Campbell CA, et al. Gonococcal lipooligosaccharide is a ligand for the asialoglycoprotein receptor on human sperm. Mol Microbiol. 2000;36:1059–70.
60. Eley A, Hosseinzadeh S, Hakimi H, et al. Apoptosis of ejaculated human sperm is induced by co-incubation with *Chlamydia trachomatis* lipopolysaccharide. Hum Reprod. 2005;20: 2601–7.
61. AVERT.org. STD Statistics Worldwide. http://www.avert.org/stdstatisticsworldwide.htm. Accessed 8 Apr 2010.
62. Weidner W, Jantos C, Schiefer HG, et al. Semen parameters in men with and without proven chronic prostatitis. Arch Androl. 1991;26:173–83.
63. Huwe P, Diemer T, Ludwig M, et al. Influence of different uropathogenic microorganisms on human sperm motility parameters in an in vitro experiment. Andrologia. 1998;30 Suppl 1:55–9.
64. Diemer T, Huwe P, Michelmann HW, et al. *Escherichia coli*-induced alterations of human spermatozoa. An electron microscopy analysis. Int J Androl. 2000;23:178–86.
65. Sanchez R, Villagran E, Concha M, et al. Ultrastructural analysis of the attachment sites of *Escherichia coli* to the human spermatozoon after *in vitro* migration through estrogenic cervical mucus. Int J Fert. 1989;34:363–7.
66. Diemer T, Huwe P, Ludwig M, et al. Influence of autogenous leucocytes and *Escherichia coli* on sperm motility parameters in vitro. Andrologia. 2003;35:100–5.
67. Schulz M, Sanchez R, Soto L, et al. Effect of *Escherichia coli* and its soluble factors on mitochondrial membrane potential, phosphatidylserine translocation, viability, and motility of human spermatozoa. Fertil Steril. 2010 Jul;94(2):619–23.
68. Diemer T, Ludwig M, Huwe P, et al. Influence of urogenital infection on sperm function. Curr Opin Urol. 2000;10:39–44.
69. Ching JC, Jones NL, Ceponis PJ, et al. *Escherichia coli* shiga-like toxins induce apoptosis and cleavage of poly(ADP-ribose) polymerase via in vitro activation of caspases. Infect Immun. 2002;70:4669–77.

70. Dejucq N, Jegou B. Viruses in the mammalian male genital tract and their effects on the reproductive system. Microbiol Mol Biol Rev. 2001;65:208–31.
71. Bezold G, Politch JA, Kiviat NB, et al. Prevalence of sexually transmissible pathogens in semen from asymptomatic male infertility patients with and without leukocytospermia. Fertil Steril. 2007;87:1087–97.
72. Kapranos N, Petrakou E, Anastasiadou C, et al. Detection of herpes simplex virus, cytomegalovirus, and Epstein-Barr virus in the semen of men attending an infertility clinic. Fertil Steril. 2003;79 Suppl 3:1566–70.
73. Manigart Y, Rozenberg S, Barlow P, et al. ART outcome in HIV-infected patients. Hum Reprod. 2006;21:2935–40.
74. Bandivdekar AH, Velhal SM, Raghavan VP. Identification of CD4-independent HIV receptors on spermatozoa. Am J Reprod Immunol. 2003;50:322–7.
75. Muciaccia B, Padula F, Gandini L, et al. HIV-1 chemokine co-receptor CCR5 is expressed on the surface of human spermatozoa. AIDS. 2005;19:1424–6.
76. Muciaccia B, Corallini S, Vicini E, et al. HIV-1 viral DNA is present in ejaculated abnormal spermatozoa of seropositive subjects. Hum Reprod. 2007;22:2868–78.
77. Le Tortorec A, Dejucq-Rainsford N. HIV infection of the male genital tract - consequences for sexual transmission and reproduction. Int J Androl. 2010;33:e98–e108.
78. Pillai SK, Good B, Pond SK, et al. Semen-specific genetic characteristics of human immunodeficiency virus type 1 env. J Virol. 2005;79:1734–42.
79. Diemer T, Desjardins C. Disorders of spermatogenesis. In: Knobil E, Neill JD, editors. Encyclopedia of reproduction, vol. 4. San Diego: Academic; 1999. p. 546–56.
80. Schuppe HC, Meinhardt A. Immunology of the testis and the excurrent ducts. In: Schill W-B, Comhaire F, Hargreave TB, editors. Andrology for the clinician. Heidelberg: Springer; 2006. p. 292–300.
81. Schuppe HC, Meinhardt A. Immune privilege and inflammation of the testis. Chem Immunol Allergy. 2005;88:1–14.
82. Haidl G, Allam JP, Schuppe HC. Chronic epididymitis: impact on semen parameters and therapeutic options. Andrologia. 2008;40:92–6.
83. Mazumdar S, Levine AS. Antisperm antibodies: etiology, pathogenesis, diagnosis, and treatment. Fertil Steril. 1998;70:799–810.
84. Kalaydjiev S, Dimitrova D, Nenova M, et al. Serum sperm antibodies are not elevated after mumps orchitis. Fertil Steril. 2002;77:76–82.
85. Nistal M, Paniagua R, editors. Testicular and epididymal pathology. Stuttgart, New York: Thieme; 1984.
86. Bartak V. sperm count, morphology and motility after unilateral mumps orchitis. J Reprod Fertil. 1973;32:491–3.
87. Casella R, Leibundgut B, Lehman K, et al. Mumps orchitis: Report of a mini-epidemic. J Urol. 1997;158:2158–61.
88. Behrman RE, Kliegman RM, Jenson HB, editors. Nelson textbook of pediatics. 17th ed. Philadelphia: Saunders; 2004.
89. Philip J, Selvan D, Desmond AD. Mumps orchitis in the non-immune postpubertal male: a resurgent threat to male fertility? BJU Int. 2006;97:138–41.
90. Ludwig M. Diagnosis and therapy of acute prostatitis, epididymitis and orchitis. Andrologia. 2008;40:76–80.
91. Kopa Z, Wenzel J, Papp GK, et al. Role of granulocyte elastase and interleukin-6 in the diagnosis of male genital tract inflammation. Andrologia. 2005;37:188–94.
92. Collins MM, Stafford RS, O'Leary MP, et al. How common is prostatitis? A national survey of physician visits. J Urol. 1998;159:1224–8.
93. Vordermark JS. Acute epididymitis: experience with 123 cases. Mil Med. 1985;150:27–30.
94. Chan PT, Schlegel PN. Inflammatory conditions of the male excurrent ductal system. Part II. J Androl. 2002;23:461–9.
95. Trojian TH, Lishnak TS, Heiman D. Epididymitis and orchitis: an overview. Am Fam Physician. 2009;79:583–7.

96. Comhaire F, Mahmoud A. Infection/inflammation of the accessory sex glands. In: Schill W-B, Comhaire F, Hargreave TB, editors. Andrology for the clinician. Heidelberg: Springer; 2006. p. 72–4.

97. World Health Organization. WHO Laboratory Manual for the Examination of Human Semen and Semen-Cervical Mucus Interaction. 4th ed. Cambridge, UK: Cambridge University; 1999.

98. National Kidney and Urologic Disease Advisory Board. Long-Range Plan Window on the 21st Century. United States Department of Health and Human Services, National Institutes of Health publication. (1990) No. 90-583: 20.

99. Roberts RO, Lieber MM, Bostwick DG, et al. A review of clinical and pathological prostatitis syndromes. Urology. 1997;49:809–21.

100. Nickel JC, Downey J, Hunter D, et al. Prevalence of prostatitis-like symptoms in a population based study using the National Institutes of Health chronic prostatitis symptom index. J Urol. 2001;165:842–5.

101. Brunner H, Weidner W, Schiefer H-G. Studies on the role of *Ureaplasma urealyticum* and *Mycoplasma hominis* in prostatitis. J Infect Dis. 1983;147:807–13.

102. Bjerklund Johansen TE, Grüneberg RN, Guibert J, et al. The role of antibiotics in the treatment of chronic prostatitis: a consensus statement. Eur Urol. 1998;34:457–66.

103. Nickel JC, Downey J, Johnston B, et al. Predictors of patient response to antibiotic therapy for the chronic prostatitis/chronic pelvic pain syndrome: a prospective multicenter clinical trial. J Urol. 2001;165:1539–44.

104. Drach GW, Fair WR, Meares EM, et al. Classification of benign diseases associated with prostatic pain: prostatitis or prostatodynia? J Urol. 1978;120:266.

105. Nickel JC. Prostatitis: myths and realities. Urology. 1998;51:362–6.

106. Krieger JN, Nyberg LJ, Nickel JC. NIH consensus definition and classification of prostatitis. JAMA. 1999;282:236–7.

107. Roberts RO, Lieber MM, Rhodes T, et al. Prevalence of a physician-assigned diagnosis of prostatitis: the Olmsted County Study of Urinary Symptoms and Health Status Among Men. Urology. 1998;51:578–84.

108. Nickel JC. Prostatitis: the last frontier. World J Surg. 2000;24:1197–9.

109. Nickel JC. Classification and diagnosis of prostatitis: a gold standard? Andrologia. 2003;35:160–7.

110. Lopez-Plaza I, Bostwick DG. Prostatitis. In: Bostwick DG, editor. Pathology of the prostate. New York: Churchill Livingstone; 1990. p. 15–30.

111. Nickel JC, Costerton JW, McLean RJC, et al. Bacterial biofilms: influence on the pathogenesis, diagnosis and treatment of urinary tract infections. J Antimicrob Chemother. 1994;33(Suppl A):31–41.

112. Ochsendorf F. Urethritis, Sexually Transmitted Diseases (STD), Acquired Immunodeficiency Syndrome (AIDS). In: Schill W-B, Comhaire F, Hargreave TB, editors. Andrology for the clinician. Heidelberg: Springer; 2006. p. 327–38.

113. Krieger JN, Hooton TM, Brust PJ, et al. Evaluation of chronic urethritis. Defining the role for endoscopic procedures. Arch Intern Med. 1988;148:703–7.

114. Chambers RM. The mechanism of infection in the urethra, prostate and epididymis. In: Keith LG, Berger GS, Edelmann DA, editors. Infections in reproductive health. Common infections. Lancaster: MTP; 1985. p. 283–96.

115. Urata K, Narahara H, Tanaka Y, et al. Effect of endotoxin-induced reactive oxygen species on sperm motility. Fertil Steril. 2001;76:163–6.

116. Sanocka D, Fraczek M, Jedrzejczak P, et al. Male genital tract infection: an influence of leukocytes and bacteria on semen. J Reprod Immunol. 2004;62:111–24.

117. Henkel R, Kierspel E, Stalf T, et al. Effect of reactive oxygen species produced by spermatozoa and leukocytes on sperm functions in non-leukocytospermic patients. Fertil Steril. 2005;83:635–42.

118. Schiefer HG, von Graevenitz A. Clinical microbiology. In: Schill W-B, Comhaire F, Hargreave TB, editors. Andrology for the clinician. Heidelberg: Springer; 2006. p. 401–7.

119. Depuydt CE, Bosmans E, Zalata A, et al. The relation between reactive oxygen species and cytokines in andrological patients with or without male accessory gland infection. J Androl. 1996;17:699–707.
120. Kocak I, Yenisey C, Dündar M, et al. Relationship between seminal plasma interleukin-6 and tumor necrosis factor alpha levels with semen parameters in fertile and infertile men. Urol Res. 2002;30:263–7.
121. Aitken RJ, Gordon E, Harkiss D, et al. Relative impact of oxidative stress on the functional competence and genomic integrity of human spermatozoa. Biol Reprod. 1998;59:1037–46.
122. Fraczek M, Sanocka D, Kamieniczna M, et al. Proinflammatory cytokines as an intermediate factor enhancing lipid sperm membrane peroxidation in in vitro conditions. J Androl. 2008;29:85–92.
123. Cooper TG, Weidner W, Nieschlag E. The influence of inflammation of the human male genital tract on secretion of the seminal markers alpha-glucosidase, glycerophosphocholine, carnitine, fructose and citric acid. Int J Androl. 1990;13:329–36.
124. Wolff H, Bezold G, Zebhauser M, et al. Impact of clinically silent inflammation on male genital tract organs as reflected by biochemical markers in semen. J Androl. 1991;12:331–4.
125. Munoz MG, Jeremias J, Witkin SS. The 60 kDa heat shock protein in human semen: relationship with antibodies to spermatozoa and *Chlamydia trachomatis*. Hum Reprod. 1986;11:2600–1.
126. Bohring C, Krause E, Habermann B, et al. Isolation and identification of spermatozoa membrane antigens, recognized by antisperm antibodies and their possible role in immunological infertility disease. Mol Hum Reprod. 2001;7:113–8.
127. Zalata AA, Christophe AB, Depuydt CE, et al. The fatty acid composition of phospholipids of spermatozoa from infertile patients. Mol Hum Reprod. 1998;4:111–8.
128. Plante M, de Lamirande E, Gagnon C. Reactive oxygen species released by activated neutrophils, but not by deficient spermatozoa, are sufficient to affect normal sperm motility. Fertil Steril. 1994;62:387–93.
129. Comhaire FH, Mahmoud AM, Depuydt CE, et al. Mechanisms and effects of male genital tract infection on sperm quality and fertilizing potential: the andrologist's viewpoint. Hum Reprod Update. 1999;5:393–8.
130. Aitken RJ, Clarkson JS, Fishel S. Generation of reactive oxygen species, lipid peroxidation, and human sperm function. Biol Reprod. 1989;41:183–97.
131. Henkel R, Hajimohammad M, Stalf T, et al. Influence of deoxyribonucleic acid damage on fertilization and pregnancy. Fertil Steril. 2004;81:965–72.
132. Motrich RD, Maccioni M, Molina R, et al. Reduced semen quality in chronic prostatitis patients that have cellular autoimmune response to prostate antigens. Hum Reprod. 2005;20:2567–72.
133. Martinez R, Proverbio F, Camejo MI. Sperm lipid peroxidation and pro-inflammatory cytokines. Asian J Androl. 2007;9:102–7.
134. Mortimer D. Sperm preparation techniques and iatrogenic failures of in-vitro fertilization. Hum Reprod. 1991;6:173–6.
135. Alvarez JG, Sharma RK, Ollero M, et al. Increased DNA damage in sperm from leukocytospermic semen samples as determined by the sperm chromatin structure assay. Fertil Steril. 2002;78:319–29.
136. Henkel R, Maaß G, Hajimohammad M, et al. Urogenital inflammation: changes of leucocytes and ROS. Andrologia. 2003;35:309–13.
137. Henkel R, Ludwig M, Schuppe HC, et al. Chronic pelvic pain syndrome/chronic prostatitis affect the acrosome reaction in human spermatozoa. World J Urol. 2006;24:39–44.
138. Zalata AA, Ahmed AH, Allamaneni SSR, et al. Relationship between acrosin activity of human spermatozoa and oxidative stress. Asian J Androl. 2004;6:313–8.
139. Centres for Disease Control and Prevention. Sexually transmitted diseases treatment guidelines. Morb Mortal Wkly Rep. 2006;55:35–62.
140. Yeniyol CO, Sorguc S, Minareci S, et al. Role of interferon-alpha-2B in prevention of testicular atrophy with unilateral mumps orchitis. Urology. 2000;55:931–3.

141. Naber KG, Madsen PO. Antibiotics: basic concepts. In: Nickel JC, editor. Textbook of prostatitis. Cambridge: Isis Medical Media; 1999. p. 83–94.
142. Naber KG, Weidner W. Chronic prostatitis-an infectious disease? J Antimicrob Chemother. 2000;46:157–61.
143. Hendry WF, Stedronska J, Hughes L, et al. Steroid treatment of male subfertility caused by antisperm antibodies. Lancet. 1979;2:498–501.
144. Montag M, van der Ven H, Haidl G. Recovery of ejaculated spermatozoa for intracytoplasmic sperm injection after anti-inflammatory treatment of an azoospermic patient with genital tract infection: a case report. Andrologia. 1999 May;31(3):179–81.
145. Haidl G. Management strategies for male factor infertility. Drugs. 2002;62:1741–53.
146. Tremellen K. Oxidative stress and male infertility—a clinical perspective. Hum Reprod Update. 2008;14:243–58.
147. Lanzafame FM, La Vignera S, Vicari E, et al. Oxidative stress and medical antioxidant treatment in male infertility. Reprod Biomed Online. 2009;19:638–59.
148. Comhaire FH, Christophe AB, Zalata AA, et al. The effects of combined conventional treatment, oral antioxidants and essential fatty acids on sperm biology in subfertile men. Prostaglandins Leukot Essent Fatty Acids. 2000;63:159–65.
149. Comhaire FH, El Garem Y, Mahmoud A, et al. Combined conventional/antioxidant "Astaxanthin" treatment for male infertility: a double blind, randomized trial. Asian J Androl. 2005;7:257–62.
150. Vicari E, Calogero AE. Effects of treatment with carnitines in infertile patients with prostato-vesiculo-epididymitis. Hum Reprod. 2001;16:2338–42.
151. Lenzi A, Sgro P, Salacone P, et al. A placebo-controlled double-blind randomized trial of the use of combined l-carnitine and l-acetyl-carnitine treatment in men with asthenozoospermia. Fertil Steril. 2004;81:1578–84.
152. Balercia G, Regoli F, Armeni T, et al. Placebo-controlled double-blind randomized trial on the use of l-carnitine, l-acetylcarnitine, or combined l-carnitine and l-acetylcarnitine in men with idiopathic asthenozoospermia. Fertil Steril. 2005;84:662–71.
153. Akmal M, Qadri JQ, Al-Waili NS, et al. Improvement in human semen quality after oral supplementation of vitamin C. J Med Food. 2006;9:440–2.
154. Greco E, Iacobelli M, Rienzi L, et al. Reduction of the incidence of sperm DNA fragmentation by oral antioxidant treatment. J Androl. 2005;26:349–53.
155. Menezo YJ, Hazout A, Panteix G, et al. Antioxidants to reduce sperm DNA fragmentation: an unexpected adverse effect. Reprod Biomed Online. 2007;14:418–21.

Chapter 9
Varicocele

Sandro C. Esteves

Approximately 8% of men in reproductive age seek for medical assistance for fertility-related problems. Of these, 1–10% carry conditions that compromise the reproductive potential, and varicocele accounts for 35% of the cases [1]. In a group of 2,875 infertile couples attending our tertiary center for male reproduction, a varicocele was identified in 21.9% of the male partners.

The first reports of the existence of varicose veins surrounding the testis are dated to the first century AC; however, the association of varicocele and infertility was only suspected at the end of the nineteenth century when surgical occlusion of dilated veins was shown to improve semen quality [2]. Tulloch, in 1952, was the first to report that bilateral varicocele repair in a male with azoospermia resulted in an increase in sperm concentration and in a spontaneous pregnancy [3]. In 1965, MacLeod first reported that most semen specimens obtained from infertile men with varicocele had decreased sperm count, decreased motility, and increased abnormal forms [4].

Varicocele is a condition involving the dilation of the veins of the pampiniform plexus that drain the testicles. Normally, the backward blood flow is prevented by small one-way valves. Valve abnormalities or vein compression by adjacent structures can cause vein dilation. The pathophysiology of varicocele and its impact on the male reproductive potential have been debated for the last 50 years. Varicocele is still one of the most controversial issues in the field of male infertility, especially regarding why, when, and to whom treatment should be applied. Varicocele repair is considered the treatment of choice for varicocele-associated infertility, but its effectiveness has been discussed for several years. Although the ultimate end point for the treatment of male factor infertility is a live birth, efforts to maximize the couple's fertility potential by improving testicular function should be the main

S.C. Esteves, M.D, Ph.D. (✉)
Center for Male Reproduction, ANDROFERT, Andrology & Human Reproduction Clinic,
Av. Dr. Heitor Penteado, 1464, Campinas, SP 13075-460, Brazil
e-mail: s.esteves@androfert.com.br

S.J. Parckattil and A. Agarwal (eds.), *Antioxidants in Male Infertility: A Guide for Clinicians and Researchers*, © Springer Science+Business Media New York 2013

purpose of varicocele treatment. This chapter discusses the current concepts and controversies regarding the epidemiology, pathophysiology, diagnosis, treatment, and significance of clinical and subclinical varicoceles in male infertility. It also reviews the management of varicoceles in azoospermic patients and the novel indications of varicocelectomy in the era of assisted reproductive technology (ART). A critical commentary, based on the author's 15-year experience treating infertile men with varicoceles, and a review of important publications from the last 5 years are included. Finally, a list of key issues is provided to summarize the current knowledge of varicocele-associated infertility.

Varicocele

Epidemiology

Varicoceles are identified in approximately 7% and 10–25% of prepuberal and postpuberal males, respectively [5, 6]. In older men, varicoceles can be identified in up to 43% of the individuals [7]. Prevalence of varicocele increases over time, and it is estimated that a 10% rise in incidence occurs for each decade of life. It is identified in approximately 35% of men with primary and 80% of men with secondary infertility [1, 8]. The higher frequency of varicoceles in both the elderly and in men with secondary infertility suggests that it is a progressive disease. Although the frequency of unilateral left-sided varicocele has historically been reported to be approximately 85–90%, recent data indicate that bilateral palpable varicocele may be found in more than 50% of the affected subjects [5].

An inverse relationship between the occurrence of varicocele and body mass index has been reported [9]. Also, intense physical activity (2–4 h daily, ×4–5 per week) over several years seems to worsen semen quality of men with varicoceles and abnormal semen parameters [10]. Moreover, increased incidence of varicose veins has been reported in first-degree relatives of men with varicoceles, suggesting this condition may be inherited [8].

Pathophysiology

The etiology of varicocele formation is likely to be multifactorial. The right internal spermatic vein inserts directly into the inferior vena cava at an acute angle, while the left one inserts into the left renal vein at a right angle. It is also suggested that a partial obstruction of the left spermatic vein due to the compression of the left renal vein between the aorta and the upper mesenteric artery exists (the "nutcracker" phenomenon). An increase in the hydrostatic pressure of the left spermatic vein may be transferred to the venous plexus of the spermatic cord, causing its dilation [11].

Moreover, primary insufficiency of the internal spermatic and subsequent malfunction of the external spermatic and cremasteric veins valves may lead to regression of blood [12, 13]. A fivefold increase in the hydrostatic pressure of the spermatic veins has been observed in men with varicocele as compared to controls [14]. Microscopic evaluation of the spermatic vein fragments revealed alterations in the longitudinal muscle layers and a decrease in the number of nerve elements in the vessel wall [15]. These findings suggest a defective contractile mechanism of blood transport through the pampiniform plexus that may lead to a reversal of the pressure gradient and cause a hypoxic status.

Several theories aim to explain the impact of varicoceles on testicular function, but none of them can fully elucidate the variable effect of varicocele on human spermatogenesis and male fertility [11]. Proposed mechanisms include hypoxia and stasis, testicular venous hypertension, elevated testicular temperature, and increase in spermatic vein catecholamine, leading to testicular underperfusion and increased oxidative stress [16]. It is believed that reflux of warm blood from the abdominal cavity to the varicose veins increases the scrotum temperature, but the mechanism by which temperature influences spermatogenesis is not clearly understood. Germ cell apoptosis and subsequent oligozoospermia, a common phenomenon in men with varicocele, can be attributed to increased scrotal temperature, increased intra-testicular cadmium concentration, and reduced levels of androgens [17, 18]. Increased concentration of regressed toxic metabolites inside the testicles (e.g., catecholamines from the kidney and adrenal glands) can cause chronic vasoconstriction of the intratesticular arterioles, contributing, along with impaired venous return caused by valve insufficiency, to persistent testicular underperfusion and subsequent dysfunction of the spermatic epithelium [19]. Biopsies of varicocele-affected testicles showed a decrease in E-cadherin and alpha-catenin in the Sertoli-Sertoli junction and a subsequent disruption of the blood–testis barrier that can contribute to the pathology and impairment in sperm production [20]. However, histopathologic findings typical of varicocele have not been observed [21].

Excessive oxidative stress (OS) is often seen in infertile men with varicocele [22]. High production of reactive oxygen species (ROS) in the reproductive tract impairs both the fluidity of the sperm plasma membrane and the integrity of deoxyribonucleic acid (DNA) in the sperm nucleus. Abnormal high levels of sperm DNA damage are associated with a decrease in several fertility markers including fertilization rate, embryo cleavage rate, implantation rate, pregnancy rate, and live birth rate [22]. It has been recently proposed that fertility reduction in men with varicocele results from decreased pH in the spermatozoa cytosol and seminal plasma [23]. According to this hypothesis, testicular underperfusion diminishes cell oxygen and glucose supply to the metabolically active tissues. Under conditions of low glucose supply, the flux through the pentose-phosphate pathway is markedly decreased, as well as the provision of reductants to the antioxidant system. Indeed, the drastic fall in the reduced nicotinamide adenine dinucleotide phosphate/oxidized nicotinamide adenine dinucleotide phosphate (NADPH/NADP+) ratio leads to an impairment in the tissue antioxidant capacity because glutathione regeneration is retarded. Under such pathologic circumstances, ROS production surpasses the antioxidant capacity and causes increased oxidative stress [24]. Spermatozoa are susceptible to damage by oxidative stress through ROS, especially lipid peroxidation [22], owing to the low amount of cytoplasm and abundance of polyunsaturated fatty acids in the sperm plasma membrane. Lipid peroxidation damages membrane function in sperm head and midpiece, thus altering sperm morphology and impairing motility, but it also leads to a decrease in intracellular pH, partly because of malondialdehyde-mediated reactions. Malondialdehyde, produced by the peroxidation of polyunsaturated fatty acids, reacts with spermine, a polyamine essential for sperm activity, forming Schiff bases. It results in further decrease of pH as well as in a direct impairment of spermine-dependent cellular functions. The optimum pH for ROS scavenging by the enzymatic antioxidant systems ranges between neutral and slightly alkaline, but their activity is markedly depressed in low pH. It has been observed that antioxidant enzyme activity is significantly impaired in infertile men with varicocele, and it may further diminish sperm motility [22]. This novel hypothesis adds to other proposed mechanisms for defective sperm function in men with varicocele, such as the peroxidation of the unsaturated fatty acids in the sperm plasma membrane and the impaired acrosome reaction and DNA integrity induced by ROS [24]. However, it has also been speculated that individual differences may exist; therefore, the mechanism described above may not be deterministic. If, for example, the glucose supply is less restricted or the accessory glands are particularly efficient, the accumulation of ROS and acidification of the seminal plasma could be minimized. This hypothesis may help us understand the variable effect of varicocele on male fertility.

Varicocele and Infertility

The concept that varicocele causes infertility is based on three main aspects: (a) the increased incidence of this condition among infertile men, (b) the association of varicocele with reduced semen parameters and testicular size, and (c) the improvement of semen parameters and pregnancy rates after surgical repair of clinical varicoceles.

In a large observational study involving 9,034 men, it was observed that 25.6% of men with abnormal semen analysis had varicocele. It was also noted that total sperm count and testosterone levels were lower in men with varicoceles as compared to those without varicoceles. Also, testicular size was significantly reduced at the varicocele side as compared to the contralateral one in the cases of unilateral varicoceles [25]. Surgical repair of varicocele was shown to restore testicular temperature in both animals and humans [19].

The hypothesis that varicocele can cause testicular damage was further confirmed on pubertal boys in which the reduction in the size of the ipsilateral testis was restored by surgical repair of varicocele [26]. Despite the proven association between varicocele and infertility, it is still unclear the reasons why about 2/3 of men with varicocele retain their fertility [2, 27] and why fertility potential is not always improved after surgical varicocele repair [28, 29].

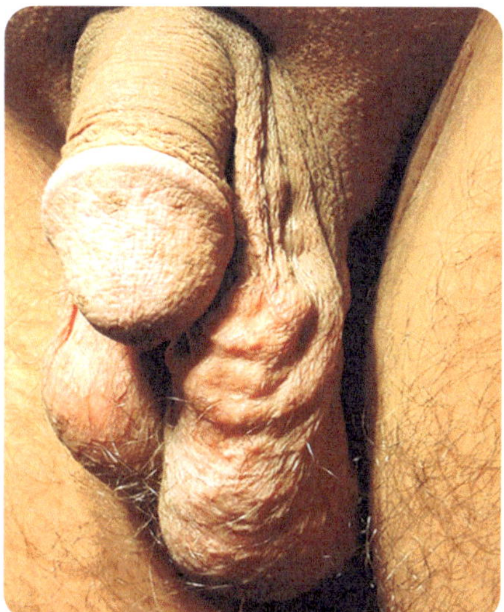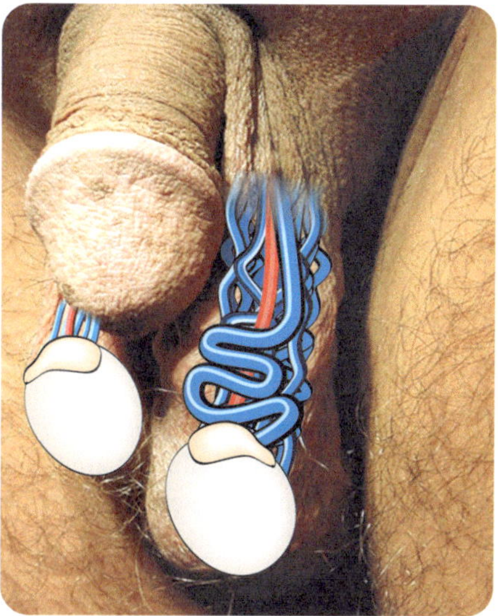

Fig. 9.1 Photograph of a large left varicocele (grade III) seen through the scrotal skin (*left*). Illustration of varicose veins on the left spermatic cord as compared to normal-sized veins on the right side (*right*)

Diagnosis

Currently, physical examination with the patient standing in a warm room is the preferred diagnostic method. Varicoceles diagnosed by this method are termed "clinical" and may be graded according to the size. It is important to ask the patient to perform a Valsalva maneuver during examination. Large varicoceles (grade III) are varicose veins seen through the scrotal skin (Fig. 9.1). Moderate (grade II) and small-sized varicoceles (grade I) are dilated veins palpable without and with the aid of the Valsalva maneuver, respectively [30]. Physical examination is limited by a sensibility and specificity of about 70% when compared to other diagnostic modalities [31, 32]. Interobserver and intraobserver variability has been observed when diagnosing varicocele. Physical examination may be inconclusive or equivocal in cases of low-grade varicocele and in men with a history of previous scrotal surgery, concomitant hydroceles, or obesity. Imaging studies may be recommended when evaluating infertile men for varicocele when physical examination is inconclusive. When a varicocele is not palpable but a retrograde blood flow is detected by other diagnostic methods such as venography, Doppler examination, ultrasonography, scintigraphy, and thermography, the varicocele is termed subclinical [32, 33].

The gold standard method to diagnose blood reflux into the veins of the pampiniform plexus is the percutaneous venography of the spermatic veins; however, it is not routinely used because of its invasiveness [32, 33]. Among the noninvasive diagnostic modalities, color Doppler ultrasound (CDU) has been shown to be the best diagnostic tool. The commonly accepted CDU criterion for varicocele (maximum vein diameter of 3 mm or greater) has a sensitivity of about 50% and specificity of 90% compared to physical examination [34]. However, a scoring system, incorporating the venous diameter, the presence of a venous plexus, and the change of flow on Valsalva maneuver, yields a sensitivity and specificity greater than 85% when compared to physical examination [34] or venography [31]. A pencil-probe Doppler (9 MHz) stethoscope is an inexpensive tool that may aid in the diagnosis of the varicocele. The patient is examined in the upright position, and a venous "rush" representing blood reflux is heard with or without the Valsalva maneuver. Although simple and easily performed in the office, Hirsht et al. demonstrated that more than 50% of men without clinical varicoceles exhibited a Valsalva-maneuver Doppler-positive reflux [35]. Despite that, Doppler examination has been advocated as a useful tool to examine the contralateral spermatic cord to determine if a subclinical varicocele exists when a clinical varicocele is found on the other side [36]. Unfortunately, none of these adjunctive diagnostic methods can differentiate between clinical and subclinical varicoceles. The significance of a positive test result using any of these adjuvant techniques in infertile men remains uncertain.

Treatment

Treatment of varicocele in infertile men aims to restore or improve testicular function. Current recommendations suggest that treatment should be offered for couples with documented infertility whose male partner has a clinically palpable varicocele and abnormal semen analysis. Additionally, an adult male presenting with palpable varicocele and abnormal semen analyses who is not currently attempting to achieve conception but has a desire for future fertility is also a candidate for varicocele repair [37]. The ideal treatment must combine low complication rates with the highest seminal improvement to either increase the chances of spontaneous conception or to optimize assisted conception outcomes.

The role of medical therapy in varicocele-related infertility is poorly understood, and well-designed studies are rare. It has been reported that the use of L-carnitine in combination with the nonsteroidal anti-inflammatory agent cinnoxicam did not improve sperm parameters in infertile men with clinical varicoceles [38]. Also, the use of clomiphene citrate in men with subclinical varicoceles showed no benefit [39]. On the other hand, kallikrein therapy for 3 months (600 units orally per day) improved sperm motility and morphology in a small group of infertile men with left-sided varicocele and asthenozoospermia [40]. Early use of menotropin in association with varicocelectomy yielded to a better improvement in sperm parameters as compared to varicocelectomy alone [41]. Recently, preliminary data from very small series have been reported on the use of vitamins and antioxidants as a medical therapy for infertile men with varicocele [42, 43]. Daily oral administration of pentoxifylline, zinc, and folic acid for 3 months was shown to improve sperm morphology in men with varicocele-associated infertility [42]. Also, a combination of

Table 9.1 Treatment options for varicocele repair in infertile men. Vein ligation sites and postoperative recurrence, hydrocele formation, and spontaneous pregnancy rates among different techniques

Technique	Internal spermatic vein ligation	External spermatic vein ligation	Recurrence rate	Hydrocele formation rate	Spontaneous pregnancy rate
Retroperitoneal high ligation (Palomo) [44, 45, 53]	Yes	No	7–35%	6–10%	25–55%
Laparoscopic [44, 49, 50, 53]	Yes	No	2–7%	0–9%	14–42%
Embolization [44, 45, 53]	Yes	No	2–24%	NR	20–40%
Macroscopic inguinal (Ivanissevich) [44]	Yes	Yes	0–37%	7%	34–39%
Microscopic inguinal or subinguinal [44, 50, 53, 54]	Yes	Yes	0–0.3%	0–1.6%	33–56%

NR not reported. Values are expressed as range

vitamins and minerals was shown to significantly improve sperm count in men with persistent oligozoospermia after varicocele embolization, although spontaneous conception rates were not increased in a 1-year follow-up period [43].

Currently, varicoceles are treated either by surgery (open with or without magnification and laparoscopy) or percutaneous embolization of the internal spermatic vein. Although techniques vary, the main concept is the occlusion of the dilated veins of the pampiniform plexus. The high retroperitoneal (Palomo), radiologic, and laparoscopic approaches are performed for internal spermatic vein ligation, while the inguinal (Ivanissevich) and subinguinal approaches also allow the ligation of the external spermatic and cremasteric veins that may contribute to the varicocele (Table 9.1). Percutaneous embolization is successfully accomplished in approximately 90% of the attempts. It is associated with faster recovery and minimal pain as compared to the standard surgical approaches, but with higher recurrence rates (Table 9.1). Embolization requires interventional radiologic expertise and has potentially serious complications such as vascular perforation, coil migration, and thrombosis of pampiniform plexus [44–47]. Nonetheless, percutaneous embolization may have a role in the treatment of persistent or recurrent varicoceles previously treated by surgery [48]. Laparoscopic varicocelectomy provides higher magnification with low incidence of hydrocele formation. However, external spermatic veins, the second cause of varicocele recurrence, cannot be ligated, leading to a recurrence rate of approximately 5% [44]. Laparoscopic approach requires extensive training, and the cost of instrumentation is high. It is more invasive than an open microsurgical approach, requiring general anesthesia and placement of a urethral catheter [49, 50]. Complications include intestinal and vascular injuries that occur in approximately 8% of the cases [44].

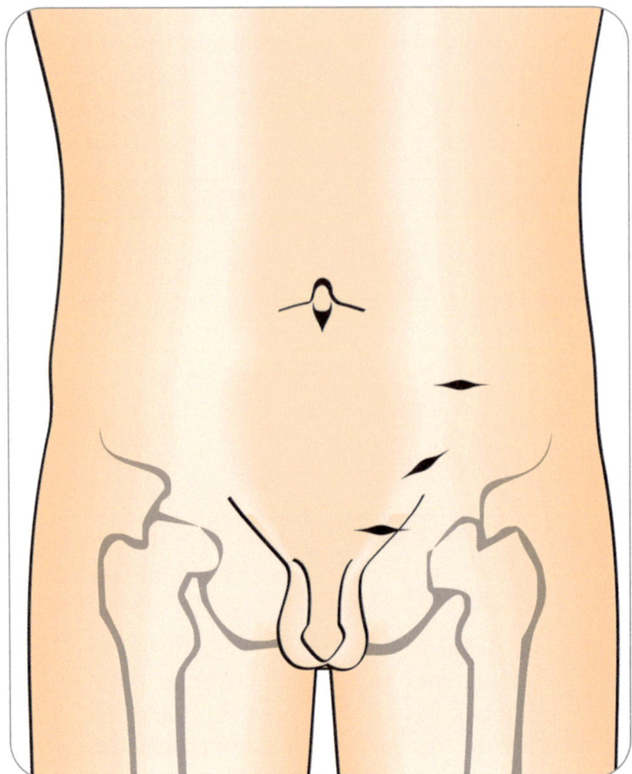

Fig. 9.2 Incision sites used for subinguinal, inguinal, and retroperitoneal open surgical varicocele repair. In the subinguinal approach, a transverse incision is made just below the level of the external inguinal ring. An oblique incision is made along the axis between the anterior superior iliac spine and the pubic tubercle for the inguinal approach. In the retroperitoneal approach, a transverse incision is made medial to the anterior superior iliac spine

Open surgical varicocele repair is often performed using a retroperitoneal, inguinal, or subinguinal approach (Fig. 9.2). High ligation of the internal spermatic vein can be easily performed via the retroperitoneal approach, but it is associated with high recurrence and hydrocele formation rates (see Table 9.1). Inguinal and subinguinal approaches offer the advantage of also allowing the ligation of the external spermatic veins. Internal and external spermatic veins can be identified via inguinal/subinguinal approaches macroscopically, but the use of magnification facilitates identification and preservation of internal spermatic artery and lymphatics, which may prevent testicular atrophy and hydrocele formation, respectively [51] (Fig. 9.3).

Microsurgical varicocelectomy can be performed via an inguinal or subinguinal approach with similar results, and reported recurrence and hydrocele formation are below 2% (Table 9.1). The main advantage of the subinguinal over the inguinal approach is that the former obviates the need to open the aponeurosis of the external

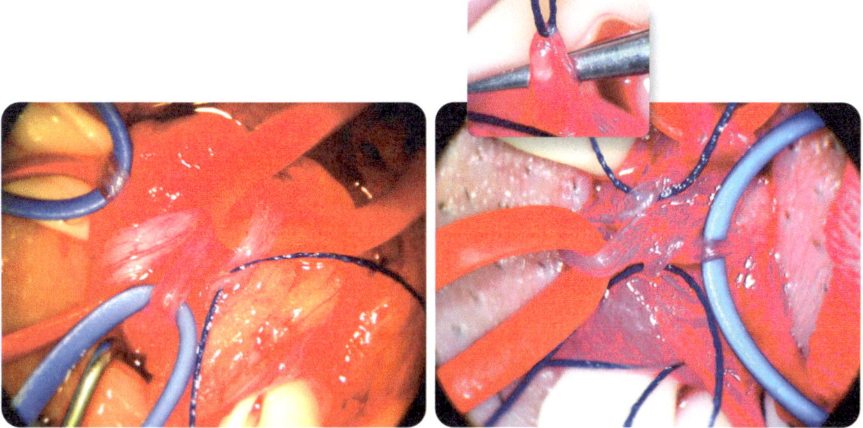

Fig. 9.3 Intraoperative photographs of the spermatic cord structures during a subinguinal micro-surgical varicocelectomy. Testicular arteries and dilated varicose veins are exposed using *blue* and *red* Vessiloops, respectively. Lymphatics are identified and exposed using *blue cotton sutures*. On the left, double testicular arteries are identified. On the right, a single testicular artery is identified, and the lymphatic channels are easily seen (also highlighted on *top right image*)

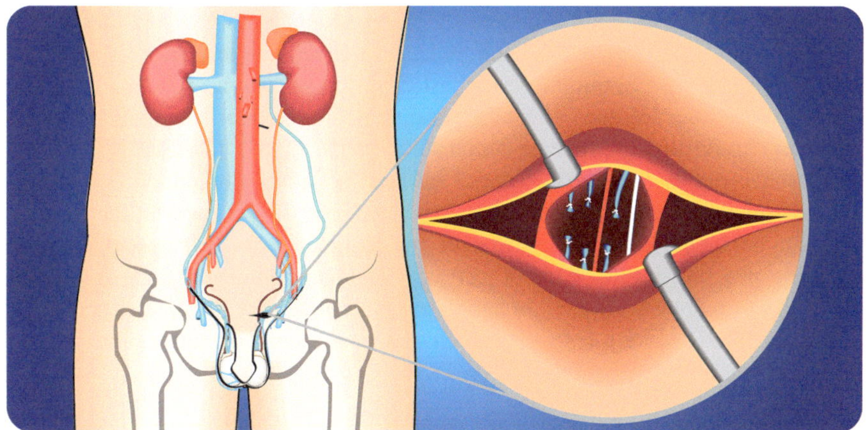

Fig. 9.4 Illustration representing a left subinguinal microsurgical varicocelectomy. A 2-cm trans-versal skin incision is made immediately below the external inguinal ring (*left*). The muscle layers and the inguinal canal are not violated. Dilated varicose veins are identified, transected, and ligated with nonabsorbable sutures. Testicular artery, lymphatic channels, and vas deferens are identified and preserved (*right*)

oblique, which usually results in more postoperative pain and a longer time before the patient can return to work (Fig. 9.4). It is believed that subinguinal microsurgical varicocelectomy requires more microsurgery skills because it is associated with a greater number of arteries and internal spermatic veins with smaller diameter as compared to the inguinal approach [44]. However, histomorphological studies were unable to find differences in number and wall thickness of spermatic cord veins and arteries between the subinguinal and inguinal levels [52].

A recent systematic review including 4,473 individuals was performed to define the best treatment modality of palpable varicocele in infertile men [44]. The authors concluded that open microsurgical inguinal or subinguinal varicocelectomy techniques resulted in higher spontaneous pregnancy rates and fewer recurrences and postoperative complications than laparoscopic, radiologic embolization, and macroscopic inguinal or retroperitoneal varicocelectomy techniques.

Overall, varicocelectomy studies report significant improvements in one or more semen parameters in approximately 65% of men [53]. The mean time for semen improvement and spontaneous pregnancy after surgery is approximately 5 and 7 months, respectively [54]. However, it is still unknown why fertility potential is not always improved after varicocelectomy. Studies evaluating predictors for successful varicocele repair would aid in the identification of the best candidates for treatment, but to date, few reports exist and results are conflicting [44, 53, 55–60]. From the existing data, it seems that infertile men either with higher preoperative semen parameters or undergoing varicocele repair for large varicoceles are more likely to show postoperative semen parameters improvement [53, 55]. It was also shown that men who achieved a postoperative total motile sperm count greater than 20 million were more likely to initiate a pregnancy either spontaneously or via intrauterine insemination [56]. On the other hand, reduced preoperative testicular volume, elevated serum FSH levels, diminished testosterone concentrations, subclinical varicocele, as well as the presence of Y chromosome microdeletions seem to be negative predictors for fertility improvement after surgery [16, 57–62]. Interestingly, a recent report suggested that advanced paternal age does not adversely influence reproductive outcomes of men with varicocele-associated infertility. However, the authors' results might be biased by the fact that the group of men with 40 years and older had a significantly higher proportion of men with secondary infertility compared to the one with younger subjects [63]. In the presence of bilateral palpable varicocele, it is recommended to perform surgery on both sides at the same operative time [64].

Subclinical Varicocele

Subclinical varicocele refers to the presence of retrograde blood flow that cannot be detected by physical examination of the spermatic cord during Valsalva maneuver, and requires adjunctive tests for diagnosis, such as Doppler examination, color Doppler ultrasound (CDUS), scrotal thermography, isotope imaging, or venography [31–35].

The role of subclinical varicocele as a cause of male infertility remains debatable. Currently, existing evidence does not support the recommendation for treating infertile men with subclinical varicocele [28, 39, 62, 65]. The management of infertile men with a unilateral clinical varicocele and a subclinical one at the contralateral side, on the other hand, may pose a different dilemma. Zheng et al. compared the efficacy of bilateral and left unilateral varicocelectomy in a group of 104 infertile men with left clinical and right subclinical varicoceles, and found that bilateral varicocelectomy had no benefit over the left clinical varicocelectomy [66]. In their study, however, a retroperitoneal approach was used for vein ligation, which was shown to be associated with high recurrence rate [44]. Elbendary et al., in a recent prospective trial, studied a group of 145 infertile men with clinical left and subclinical right varicoceles [67]. Patients were randomized to undergo either unilateral inguinal repair of clinical varicocele or bilateral repair of both clinical and subclinical ones. Although a significant improvement in sperm parameters was observed in both groups, the magnitude of change in sperm count and motility and the spontaneous pregnancy rates were significantly higher in the group of men who had bilateral varicocele repair. Their findings are in agreement with earlier studies suggesting that bilateral varicocelectomy is more effective than unilateral for such patients [68, 69]. It is also postulated that altered blood flow after unilateral clinical varicocelectomy may unmask an underlying contralateral venous anomaly that may result in a clinically manifested varicocele [36, 68].

Varicocele and Azoospermia

Nonobstructive azoospermia (NOA) comprises a spectrum of testicular histopathology resulting from various causes that include gonadotoxins, medications, genetic and congenital abnormalities, trauma, endocrine disorders, and idiopathic. Men with NOA have historically been the infertile men most difficult to treat, but since the advent of in vitro fertilization/intracytoplasmic sperm injection (IVF/ICSI) and surgical methods for testicular sperm extraction (TESE), several pregnancies have been achieved with the use of testicular sperm. However, only about 50% of men will have sperm present at the time of TESE [70].

Varicoceles are found in approximately 5% of men with azoospermia, but it is still debatable whether varicoceles can cause or contribute to azoospermia [71]. There has been a renewed interest in varicocele repair in azoospermic men resulting from the introduction of ICSI. Success rates varied and no predictors of success have been definitively identified because of the small numbers in the case series [71–78]. A recent meta-analysis examined the impact of varicocele repair to recover spermatogenesis in NOA men [79]. A total of 233 infertile men with clinical varicocele and NOA were analyzed in a mean postoperative follow-up of 13 months. Motile sperm was found on postoperative ejaculate in 39% of men. Pregnancies were achieved in approximately 26% of men with sperm in the ejaculate, 60% unassisted, and 40% with the assistance of IVF. Postoperative mean sperm density and motility were 1.6 million and 20%, respectively. Levels of serum follicle-stimulating hormone (FSH) and testosterone, testis size, patient age, varicocele grade, and surgical technique did not appear to affect outcomes, but the limited number of patients precluded conclusions. Histopathology was the only predictor of success. Postoperatively

Table 9.2 Results of varicocele repair in infertile men with clinical varicocele and nonobstructive azoospermia

Publication	Esteves and Glina [71]	Weedin et al. meta-analysis [79]
Number of patients	17	233
Mean age	34.2	30.1
Treatment technique	Subinguinal; microsurgical	Microsurgical inguinal and subinguinal; embolization
Mean FSH (mIU/mL)	14.6	Range 12.3–35.0
Bilateral repair; N (%)	11 (64.7)	151 (64.8)
Patients with motile sperm in postoperative ejaculates; N (%)	6/17 (35.3)	91/233 (39.0)
Mean postoperative sperm density; $\times 10^6$/mL	0.8 (range 0.1–1.8)	1.6 ± 1.2
Mean time to appearance of sperm in the ejaculate; months	5 (range 3–9)	NR
Outcome according to histopathology; N (%)[a] Hypospermatogenesis Maturation arrest Sertoli cell only	5/6 (83.3) 3/5 (75.0) 0/6 (0.0)	30/55 (54.5) 24/57 (42.0) 5/44 (11.4)
Relapse to azoospermia; N (%)	0 (0.0)	11 (4.6)
Spontaneous pregnancy; N (%)	1 (5.8)	14 (6.0)
Mean follow-up; months	18.9	13.3

NR not reported

[a]Patients with motile sperm in postoperative ejaculates

appearance of sperm in the ejaculates was significantly higher in patients with biopsy-proven hypospermatogenesis (HS) or maturation arrest (MA) than Sertoli cell only (odds ratio 9.4; 95% confidence interval 3.2–27.3). Combined success was 48% with HS or MA compared to 11% with SCO (Table 9.2). Unfortunately, randomized control trials are lacking, and studies included in the meta-analysis by Weedin et al. were case series lacking a control group that did not undergo varicocele repair. Although an argument can be made that a control group would remain azoospermic, it is not rare to observe that NOA men occasionally ejaculate small quantities of motile sperm despite any intervention. Therefore, one cannot exclude that the appearance of very small number of motile sperm in the ejaculates after varicocele repair may be merely coincidental. Moreover, reports including men with germinal cell aplasia who ejaculated motile sperm after varicocele repair are intriguing [78]. It is unlikely that men lacking any sperm precursor within the testicle may benefit from treatment, but the only way to investigate this relationship is to repeat the testicular biopsy after the surgical repair of varicocele. In one series [71], patients with SCO were re-biopsied 6 months after varicocele repair and testicular histopathology results remained unchanged (Table 9.2). The persistence of SCO after surgery denotes that varicocele coexisted with primary testicular failure, which of course was not affected by the surgery. However, testicular biopsy has many limitations and may not reflect the most advanced site of spermatogenesis due to the heterogeneity of sperm production within the testicle; therefore, it is still possible to retrieve sperm from men whose testicles exhibit SCO [80, 81].

Even with the improvement in spermatogenesis in up to half of the NOA patients with a favorable testicular histopathology after varicocele repair, intracytoplasmic sperm injection (ICSI) will be necessary for most couples to initiate a pregnancy [71, 79]. However, the use of motile ejaculated sperm is preferred for ICSI since their fertilizing ability is higher than that of sperm retrieved from the testis [82]. Nonetheless, continuing azoospermia after varicocele repair is still a potential problem, and sperm extraction before ICSI will be inevitable for many individuals. Results of testicular sperm extraction (TESE) for men who remain azoospermic after varicocelectomy are scarce and conflicting [83, 84]. Schlegel et al. reported sperm retrieval rates of 60% per attempt using testicular microdissection (micro-TESE) in men with NOA and varicocele, regardless of whether previous varicocelectomy had been done [83]. It is questionable, however, if the inclusion of patients with subclinical varicocele biased their results since the benefit of treating subclinical varicocele is debatable [62, 65]. On the other hand, Inci et al., also using micro-TESE, reported a 2.6-fold increase in the chances of retrieving testicular sperm for ICSI after repair of clinical varicoceles [84]. Unfortunately, testicular histopathology results were not available in their study. Therefore, it cannot be excluded that higher retrieval rates were obtained after varicocelectomy because this group was biased by patients with favorable histopathology patterns for successful sperm retrieval, such as the ones exhibiting hypospermatogenesis or maturation arrest [81, 85].

Expert Commentary

The purpose of this chapter was to discuss the current concepts and controversies of varicocele as the leading cause of male infertility. Despite of extensive investigation, approximately 4,000 peer-reviewed papers have been published on this topic, and varicocele remains one of the most debatable issues in the field of reproductive medicine. An important argument to be included in the discussion is the multifactorial origin of infertility. Several factors may interact synergistically in the same individual, and the presence of a significant condition affecting the female partner adds to the complexity of the problem. For example, many men with varicocele-associated infertility have lifestyle choices that include smoking, obesity, poor nutrition, use of gonadotoxic medication, and exposure to environmental toxins. These conditions are often associated with increased systemic or seminal oxidative stress and may have a negative synergistic effect in men with varicocele [86]. Treatment of varicocele alone in the presence of inadequate lifestyle choices is likely to solve only part of the problem. Lifestyle modifications may have an important beneficial impact on both systemic and reproductive health [87]; therefore, when considering therapeutic measures to treat varicocele-associated infertility, counseling toward lifestyle modifications should be strongly encouraged.

This strategy, along with the cause-specific treatment, is more likely to lead to a marked improvement in the male reproductive health as compared to varicocele repair alone.

The treatment of varicocele in infertile men should aim to achieve the highest improvement in the male fertility status, with lower rates of complications such as recurrence or persistence, hydrocele formation, and testicular atrophy. Increase in the spontaneous pregnancy rates after the treatment of varicocele is difficult to ascertain due to a variety of factors that include the lack of a uniform posttreatment follow-up interval and the female factor parameters, such as age and reproductive health. Therefore, the ultimate treatment goal should be the improvement in the chances of conception, either unassisted or assisted. The ideal surgical technique should aim for ligation of all internal and external spermatic and cremasteric veins, with preservation of spermatic arteries and lymphatics (see Fig. 9.3). This can only be achieved by the inguinal or subinguinal microsurgical approaches. In our practice, when a clinically palpable varicocele is identified in one side, the contralateral cord is examined using a pencil-probe Doppler (9 MHz) stethoscope to determine if a subclinical varicocele exists. If so, it is treated at the same time as the coexistent clinical varicocele. This is based on the observation that altered blood flow after varicocelectomy may unmask an underlying venous anomaly and result in clinical varicocele formation [36, 68]. Although loupe magnification may be used to facilitate the ligation of the dilated varicose veins, it is insufficient for identification of both testicular arteries and lymphatics. Using this method, we found that instillation of papaverine was needed in most cases to aid in the identification of arterial pulsations. Also, recurrence seems to be higher when loupe magnification is used in association with the inguinal or subinguinal approach to repair varicoceles (Table 9.3). An intraoperative pencil Doppler examination (9 MHz) can also be used to aid in the identification of the artery pulsations. In our hands, the subinguinal microsurgical varicocelectomy using the operating microscope is the method of choice to treat varicocele-associated infertility (Table 9.3 and Fig. 9.4). The subinguinal approach provides excellent results, and the surgical intervention can be performed in an outpatient basis using intravenous anesthesia in association with spermatic cord blockade with lidocaine [71]. Although empirical, the early use of antioxidants and vitamins is a common practice after varicocelectomy in our institution [daily use of antioxidants (vitamin C 500 mg and vitamin E 400 UI) and commercial multivitamin preparation containing minerals, β-carotene (3,500 IU), vitamin C (60 mg), vitamin E (30 UI), zinc phosphate (11 mg), selenium (55 mcg), and vitamin B complex (thiamine, riboflavin, niacin, pantothenic acid, pyridoxine, biotin, folic acid, and cyanocobalamin)].

The urologist who opts to treat varicocele using microsurgery should obtain appropriate training. It is also important to have adequate microsurgical instruments and a binocular operating microscope with foot-control zoom magnification. Microsurgical varicocelectomy, either using inguinal or subinguinal approaches, requires more skill as compared to other surgical modalities because a higher number of internal spermatic vein channels and smaller-diameter artery are seen at

Table 9.3 Results of microsurgical subinguinal varicocelectomies in a group of 485 men with varicocele and infertility

Type of magnification	Loupe	Operating microscope
Number of procedures	101	384
Male age in years; mean (range)	32.4 (24.0–63.0)	34.5 (24.0–52.0)
Varicocele side; N (%)	51 (50.4)	184 (47.9)
Unilateral	50 (49.6)	200 (52.1)
Bilateral		
Varicocele grade[a]; N (%)	14 (13.9)	73 (19.0)
Grade I	48 (47.5)	199 (51.8)
Grade II	39 (38.6)	112 (29.2)
Grade III		
Endocrine profile; mean ± SD	5.7 ± 8.8	6.1 ± 7.8
Serum FSH (mUI/mL)	523.8 ± 547.1	575.3 ± 677.2
Serum testosterone (ng/dL)		
Mean operative time; min (range)	78.6 (50–90)	89.2 (60–105)
Unilateral	101.1 (80–150)	112.9 (90–150)
Bilateral		
Number of veins ligated; mean (range)	4.8 (2–7)	6.1 (2–9)
Left side	4.2 (2–6)	5.1 (2–7)
Right side		
Vein diameter in millimeters; mean (range)	3.2 (1–6)	3.1 (1–6)
Left side	2.8 (1–4)	2.5 (1–5)
Right side		
Testicular artery identified; %	84.1[b]	97.6
Improvement in seminal parameters[c]; %	60.4	68.5
Recurrence rate; N (%)	3 (2.9)	4 (1.0)
Hydrocele formation rate; N (%)	1 (1.0)	0 (0.0)
Other complications; N (%)	2 (1.9)[d]	1 (0.2)[e]
Clinical pregnancy rate; N	85[f]	270[f]
Spontaneous; N (%)	20/69 (28.9)	58/172 (33.7)
Assisted reproduction; N (%)	4/16 (25.0)[g]	56/98 (57.1)[h]

[a]The largest varicocele grade is reported in cases of bilateral varicocele
[b]Instillation of papaverine for identification of artery pulsation was necessary in 85% of the cases
[c]≥15% improvement from baseline preoperative values in at least one of the semen parameters (sperm count, progressive motility, strict morphology), in a minimum of three postoperative semen analyses
[d]Scrotal hematoma (1 case); testicular atrophy (1 case)
[e]Scrotal hematoma
[f]Reported number of patients assessed for pregnancy
[g]Intrauterine insemination (IUI; $n = 12$); in vitro fertilization/intracytoplasmic sperm injection (IVF/ICSI; $n = 04$)
[h]IUI ($n = 18$); IVF/ICSI ($n = 80$)

the level of the inguinal canal. However, the routine use of microsurgery during varicocele repair may help the urologist to master his/her microsurgical skills, which will be of great benefit when performing more demanding and less frequent microsurgical procedures, such as vasovasostomies and vasoepididymostomies.

Five-Year Review

Infertile men with clinical varicocele have a significantly lower sperm production and quality as compared to normal controls and fertile men with varicocele [88]. Such differences are observed not only in the standard sperm parameters, such as sperm count, motility, and morphology but also in the novel functional markers for oxidative stress and DNA integrity. Seminal plasma total antioxidant capacity (TAC) and sperm mitochondrial activity are decreased [22, 89, 90], while the frequency of sperm exhibiting abnormal DNA integrity and chromatin immaturity is increased [90, 91] in ejaculates of infertile men with varicocele. Although elevation of scrotal temperature is seen in both fertile and infertile men with varicocele, increase of oxidative stress (OS) is only observed in the latter, thus indicating that a disturbance of the OS scavenging system is likely to play a major role in the pathophysiology of varicocele-associated infertility [22, 92]. Using novel noninvasive contrast imaging, it has been shown that intratesticular microcirculation perfusion, which is altered in men with clinical varicocele, affects spermatogenesis [93]. Molecular biology studies show that high cadmium content and hypoxic conditions induce overexpression of metallothionein, a metal-binding protein that protects against cell apoptosis, in internal spermatic veins of infertile men with clinical varicocele [94]. Recently, Ichioka et al. determined the distribution of antioxidant enzymes genes genotype in infertile men with varicocele. Their preliminary data suggest that genetic polymorphisms in the glutathione S-transferase T1 gene may affect individual response to varicocelectomy [95].

When clinical palpable varicocele coexists with impaired semen quality, surgical repair has been shown to be the best treatment option. Varicocele repair may partially or totally restore spermatogenesis and fertility, and it offers a better cost-effectiveness as compared to ART [96]. Recent meta-analyses demonstrated a beneficial effect of varicocelectomy on the fertility status of infertile men with clinical varicocele [88, 96–98]. Agarwal et al. examined the effect of varicocelectomy on semen parameters and demonstrated that sperm concentration increased by 9.7 million/mL (95% confidence interval [CI] 7.34–12.08, $p < 0.001$), sperm motility increased by 9.9% (95% CI 4.90–14.95, $p < 0.001$), and WHO sperm morphology increased by 3.1% (95% CI 0.72–5.60, $p = 0.01$) after varicocelectomy [88]. Ficarra et al. reviewed randomized clinical trials for varicocele repair and found a significant increase in the pregnancy rates for patients who underwent varicocele treatment (36.4%) compared to ones having no treatment (20%) [97]. Similarly, Marmar et al. reported significantly higher pregnancy rate (33%) after varicocelectomy compared to the group of patients having no surgery (15.5%) [98]. In their study, the chances of obtaining a spontaneous conception were 2.8 times higher in the varicocelectomy group as compared to the group of patients who received either no treatment or medication. Other studies demonstrated that markers of sperm function were also significantly improved after varicocele repair [99–104]. It has been reported that seminal oxidative stress may be attenuated by varicocelectomy in infertile men with varicocele, but this beneficial effect is not always associated with an improve in the conventional sperm parameters [99, 100]. Sperm DNA integrity is also increased 6 months after repair in infertile men with clinically palpable varicocele [101, 102]. Recently, Smit et al. reported a decrease in sperm DNA fragmentation after varicocelectomy and an association between DNA fragmentation index and the ability to conceive either spontaneously or via assisted reproduction [103].

Even though spontaneous pregnancy remains the litmus test for evaluating varicocele treatment success, many patients with varicocele-related infertility will require ART due to the severity of sperm abnormalities and/or the presence of a significant problem affecting the female partner. The indication of varicocele repair prior to IVF/ICSI is unusual, but in certain circumstances, varicocele treatment should be considered. Men with nonobstructive azoospermia with favorable testicular histopathology may restore sperm to the ejaculate after repair of clinical varicoceles [79]. Sperm restoration, although minimal, yields the possibility of IVF/ICSI without the need of sperm retrieval techniques (SRT). It has been shown that for patients who are still azoospermic after varicocelectomy, SRT success rates using testicular microdissection sperm extraction, and as a result the couple's chance for pregnancy, may be increased [84]. Varicocelectomy has also a potential to obviate the need for ART or to down stage the level of ART needed to bypass male factor infertility [104]. Recently, it has been shown that treatment of clinical varicoceles may also improve the outcomes of assisted reproduction in couples with varicocele-related infertility [105]. Esteves et al. studied 242 infertile men with treated and untreated clinical varicoceles who underwent intracytoplasmic sperm injection (ICSI), and found significantly higher live birth rates after ICSI in the group of men who underwent microsurgical varicocele repair before ART (46.2%) as compared to the ones undergoing ICSI in the presence of a clinical varicocele (31.4%). In their study, the chances of achieving a live birth (odds ratio = 1.87; 95% confidence interval 1.08–3.25; p = 0.03) by ICSI were increased, while the chances of miscarriage occurrence after obtaining a pregnancy by ICSI were reduced (odds ratio = 0.433; 95% confidence interval 0.22–0.84; p = 0.01) if the varicocele had been treated before assisted conception.

Key Issues

- Approximately 8% of men in reproductive age seek for medical assistance for fertility-related problems. Of these, 1–10% carries conditions that compromise the reproductive potential, and varicocele accounts for 35% of the cases.
- Epidemiology data show that approximately 35% of men with primary and 80% of men with secondary infertility have varicocele. The higher frequency of varicoceles in both the elderly and in men with secondary infertility suggests that it is a progressive disease. Bilateral varicoceles are more common than previously reported.
- Impaired drainage or pooling of blood around the testicles leading to increased scrotal temperature, hypoxia, increased testicular pressure, reflux of renal and adrenal metabolites, excessive oxidative stress, and decreased pH in the spermatozoa cytosol and seminal plasma are the leading theories to explain the detrimental effects of varicocele on spermatogenesis.

- The concept that varicocele causes infertility is based on three main aspects: (a) the increased incidence of this condition among infertile men, (b) the association of varicocele with reduced semen parameters and testicular size, and (c) the improvement of semen parameters and pregnancy rates after surgical repair of clinical varicoceles.
- Varicoceles diagnosed by physical examination, the preferred diagnostic method, are termed "clinical" and may be graded according to the size. When a varicocele is not palpable but a retrograde blood flow is detected by other diagnostic methods, the varicocele is termed subclinical. The significance of a positive test result using adjuvant diagnostic techniques in infertile men remains uncertain.
- Varicocele treatment is indicated for men with clinically palpable varicocele and abnormal semen parameters. Open microsurgical inguinal or subinguinal techniques are considered the best treatment modalities because they result in higher spontaneous pregnancy rates and fewer recurrences and postoperative complications than laparoscopic, radiologic embolization, and macroscopic inguinal or retroperitoneal varicocelectomy techniques. There are no absolute predictive factors for successful varicocele repair, and existing evidence does not support the recommendation for treating infertile men with subclinical varicocele.
- Recovery of spermatogenesis can be achieved after repair of clinical varicocele in infertile men with nonobstructive azoospermia. Testicular histopathology is predictive of success, and men with maturation arrest and hypospermatogenesis are more likely to ejaculate motile spermatozoa after surgery.
- Functional markers for oxidative stress and DNA integrity are impaired in infertile men with clinical varicocele, but may be significantly improved after varicocele repair.
- Surgical repair of varicocele increases the chance for either spontaneous or assisted conception in infertile couples whose male partner has a clinical varicocele. Also, the chance of retrieving testicular sperm for ICSI may be optimized in nonobstructive-azoospermic men with treated clinical varicocele.
- Lifestyle modifications may benefit reproductive health. When considering therapeutic measures to treat varicocele-associated infertility, counseling toward lifestyle modifications should be strongly encouraged.

Acknowledgment The author is indebted to Mrs. Fabiola Bento for her editorial assistance and text revision.

References

1. Vital and Health Statistics, series 23, no.26, CDC. http://www.cdc.gov. Accessed 10 Dec 2009.
2. Saypol DC. Varicocele. J Androl. 1981;2:61–71.
3. Tulloch WS. A consideration of sterility factors in the light of subsequent pregnancies. Edinburgh Med J. 1952;59:29–34.
4. MacLeod J. Seminal cytology in the presence of varicocele. Fertil Steril. 1965;16:735–57.

5. Akbay E, Cayan S, Doruk E, et al. The prevalence of varicocele and varicocele-related testicular atrophy in Turkish children and adolescents. BJU Int. 2000;86:490–3.
6. Callam MJ. Epidemiology of varicose veins. BJU Int. 1994;81:167–73.
7. Canales BK, Zapzalka DM, Ercole CJ, et al. Prevalence and effect of varicoceles in an elderly population. Urology. 2005;66:627–31.
8. Raman JD, Walmsley K, Goldstein M. Inheritance of varicoceles. Urology. 2005;65:1186–9.
9. Handel LN, Shetty R, Sigman M. The relationship between varicoceles and obesity. J Urol. 2006;176:2138–40.
10. Luigi L, Gentile V, Pigozzi F, et al. Physical activity as a possible aggravating factor for athletes with varicocele: impact on the semen profile. Hum Reprod. 2001;16:1180–4.
11. Nistal M, Gonzalez-Peramato P, Serrano A, et al. Physiopathology of the infertile testicle. Etiopathogenesis of varicocele. Arch Esp Urol. 2004;57:883–904.
12. Goldstein M, Eid JF. Elevation of intratesticular and scrotal skin surface temperature in men with varicocele. J Urol. 1989;142:743–5.
13. Chehval MJ, Purcell MH. Varicocelectomy: incidence of external vein involvement in the clinical varicocele. Urology. 1992;39:573–5.
14. Shafik A, Bedeir GAM. Venous tension patterns in cord veins in normal and varicocele individuals. J Urol. 1980;123:383–5.
15. Tilki D, Kilic E, Tauber R, et al. The complex structure of the smooth muscle layer of spermatic veins and its potential role in the development of varicocele testis. Eur Urol. 2007;51:1402–9.
16. Marmar JL. The pathophysiology of varicoceles in the light of current molecular and genetic information. Hum Reprod Update. 2001;7:461–72.
17. Simsek F, Turkeri L, Cevik I, et al. Role of apoptosis in testicular damage caused by varicocele. Arch Esp Urol. 1998;9:947–50.
18. Benoff S, Gilbert BR. Varicocele and male infertility: Part I. Preface. Hum Reprod Update. 2001;7:47–54.
19. Naugton DK, Nangia AK, Agarwal A. Varicocele and male infertility: Part II. Pathophysiology of varicoceles in male infertility. Hum Reprod Update. 2001;7:473–81.
20. Koksal IT, Ishak Y, Usta M, et al. Varicocele-induced testicular dysfunction may be associated with disruption of blood-testis barrier. Arch Androl. 2007;53:43–8.
21. Wang YX, Lei C, Dong SG, et al. Study of bilateral histology and meiotic analysis in men undergoing varicocele ligation. Fertil Steril. 1991;55:152–5.
22. Agarwal A, Prabakaran S, Allamaneni SS. Relationship between oxidative stress, varicocele and infertility: a meta-analysis. Reprod Biomed Online. 2006;12:630–3.
23. Kamyar Ghabili K, Shoja MM, Agutter PS, et al. Hypothesis: intracellular acidification contributes to infertility in varicocele. Fertil Steril. 2009;92:399–401.
24. Naughton CK, Nangia AK, Agarwal A. Pathophysiology of varicoceles in male infertility. Hum Reprod Update. 2001;7:473–81.
25. World Health Organization. The influence of varicocele on parameters of fertility in a large group of men presenting to infertility clinics. Fertil Steril. 1992;57:1289–93.
26. Jarow JP. Effects of varicocele on male fertility. Hum Reprod Update. 2001;7:59–64.
27. Evers JL, Collins JA. Assessment of efficacy of varicocele repair for male subfertility: a systematic review. Lancet. 2003;361:1849–52.
28. Nieschlag E, Hertle L, Fischedick A, et al. Update on treatment of varicocele: counseling as effective as occlusion of the vena spermatica. Hum Reprod. 1998;13:2147–50.
29. Redmon JB, Carey P, Pryor JL. Varicocele-the most common cause of male factor infertility? Hum Reprod Update. 2002;8:53–8.
30. Dubin R, Amelar RD. Varicocele size and results of varicocelectomy in selected subfertile men with varicocele. Fertil Steril. 1970;21:606–9.
31. Trum JW, Gubler FM, Laan R, van der Veen F. The value of palpation, varicoscreen contact thermography and colour Doppler ultrasound in the diagnosis of varicocele. Hum Reprod. 1996;11:1232–5.

32. Gat Y, Bachar GN, Zukerman Z, et al. Physical examination may miss the diagnosis of bilateral varicocele: a comparative study of 4 diagnostic modalities. J Urol. 2004;172:1414–7.
33. Geatti O, Gasparini D, Shapiro B. A comparison of scintigraphy, thermography, ultrasound and phlebography in grading of clinical varicocele. J Nucl Med. 1991;32:2092–7.
34. Chiou RK, Anderson JC, Wobig RK, et al. Color Doppler ultrasound criteria to diagnose varicoceles: correlation of a new scoring system with physical examination. Urology. 1997;50:953–6.
35. Hirsh AV, Cameron KM, Tyler JP, et al. The Doppler assessment of varicoceles and internal spermatic vein reflux in infertile men. Br J Urol. 1980;52:50–6.
36. Nagler HM, Luntz RK, Martinis FG. Varicocele. In: Lipshultz LI, Howards SS, editors. Infertility in the Male. 3rd ed. Mosby; 1997. pp. 336–359.
37. Practice Committee of the American Society for Reproductive Medicine. Report on varicocele and infertility. Fertil Steril. 2006 Nov;86(5 Suppl 1):S93–5. Review. PubMed PMID: 17055852.
38. Cavallini G, Ferraretti AP, Gianaroli L, et al. Cinnoxicam and L-carnitine/acetyl-L-carnitine treatment for idiopathic and varicocele-associated oligoasthenospermia. J Androl. 2004;25:761–70.
39. Unal D, Yeni E, Verit A, Karatas OF. Clomiphene citrate versus varicocelectomy in treatment of subclinical varicocele: a prospective randomized study. Int J Urol. 2001;8:227–30.
40. Micic S, Tilic C, Dotlic R. Kallikrein therapy of infertile men with varicocele and impaired sperm motility. Andrologia. 1990;22:179–83.
41. De Rose AF, Gallo F, Giglio M, et al. Early use of menotropin in the treatment of varicocele. Arch Ital Urol Androl. 2003;75:53–7.
42. Oliva A, Dotta A, Multigner L. Pentoxifylline and antioxidants improve sperm quality in male patients with varicocele. Fertil Steril. 2009;91(Suppl):1536–9.
43. Paradiso Galatioto G, Gravina GL, Angelozzi G, et al. May antioxidant therapy improve sperm parameters of men with persistent oligospermia after retrograde embolization for varicocele? World J Urol. 2008;26:97–102.
44. Cayan S, Shavakhabov S, Kadioglu A. Treatment of palpable varicocele review in infertile men: a meta-analysis to define the best technique. J Androl. 2009;30:33–40.
45. Shlansky-Goldberg RD, Van Arsdalen KN, Rutter CM, et al. Percutaneous varicocele embolization versus surgical ligation for the treatment of infertility: changes in seminal parameters and pregnancy outcomes. J Vasc Interv Radiol. 1997;8:759–67.
46. Bahren W, Lenz M, Porst H, et al. Side effects, complications and contraindications for percutaneous sclerotherapy of the internal spermatic vein in the treatment of idiopathic varicocele. Rofo. 1983;138:172–9.
47. Matthews RD, Roberts J, Walker WA, et al. Migration of intravascular balloon after percutaneous embolotherapy of varicocele. Urology. 1992;39:373–5.
48. Sharlip ID, Jarow JP, Belker AM, et al. Best practice policies for male infertility. Fertil Steril. 2002;77:873–82.
49. Sautter T, Sulser T, Suter S, et al. Treatment of varicocele: a prospective randomized comparison of laparoscopy versus antegrade sclerotherapy. Eur Urol. 2002;41:398–400.
50. Al-Kandari AM, Shabaan H, Ibrahim HM, et al. Comparison of outcomes of different varicocelectomy techniques: open inguinal, laparoscopic, and subinguinal microscopic varicocelectomy: a randomized clinical trial. Urology. 2007;69:417–20.
51. Hopps CV, Lemer ML, Schlegel PN, et al. Intraoperative varicocele anatomy: a microscopic study of the inguinal versus subinguinal approach. J Urol. 2003;170:2366–70.
52. Tuccar E, Yaman O, Erdemli E, et al. Histomorphological differences of spermatic cords regarding subinguinal versus inguinal levels: a cadaveric study. Urol Int. 2009;82:444–7.
53. Schlesinger MH, Wilets IF, Nagler HM. Treatment outcome after varicocelectomy. A critical analysis. Urol Clin North Am. 1994;21:517–29.
54. Colpi GM, Carmignani L, Nerva F, et al. Surgical treatment of varicocele by a subinguinal approach combined with antegrade intraoperative sclerotherapy of venous vessels. BJU Int. 2006;97:142–5.

55. Steckel J, Dicker AP, Goldstein M. Relationship between varicocele size and response to varicocelectomy. J Urol. 1993;149:769–71.
56. Matkov TG, Zenni M, Sandlow J, et al. Preoperative semen analysis as a predictor of seminal improvement following varicocelectomy. Fertil Steril. 2001;75:63–8.
57. Marks JL, McMahon R, Lipshultz LI. Predictive parameters of successful varicocele repair. J Urol. 1986;136:609–12.
58. Yoshida K, Kitahara S, Chiba K, et al. Predictive indicators of successful varicocele repair in men with infertility. Int J Fertil. 2000;45:279–84.
59. Cayan S, Lee D, Black LD, Reijo Pera RA, Turek PJ. Response to varicocelectomy in oligospermic men with and without defined genetic infertility. Urology. 2001;57:530–5.
60. Pryor JL, Kent-First M, Muallem A, et al. Microdeletions in the Y chromosome of infertile men. N Engl J Med. 1997;336:53453–9.
61. Kondo Y, Ishikawa T, Yamaguchi K, et al. Predictors of improved seminal characteristics by varicocele repair. Andrologia. 2009;41:20–3.
62. Yamamoto M, Hibi H, Hirata Y, et al. Effect of varicocelectomy on sperm parameters and pregnancy rate in patients with subclinical varicocele: a randomized prospective controlled study. J Urol. 1996;155:1636–8.
63. Zini A, Boman J, Jarvi K, et al. Varicocelectomy for infertile couples with advanced paternal age. Urology. 2008;72:109–13.
64. Libman J, Jarvi K, Lo K, Zini A. Beneficial effect of microsurgical varicocelectomy is superior for men with bilateral versus unilateral repair. J Urol. 2006;176:2602–5.
65. Kantartzi PD, Goulis ChD, Goulis GD, et al. Male infertility and varicocele: myths and reality. Hippokratia. 2007;11:99–104.
66. Zheng YQ, Gao X, Li ZJ, Yu YL, Zhang ZG, Li W. Efficacy of bilateral and left varicocelectomy in infertile men with left clinical and right subclinical varicoceles: a comparative study. Urology. 2009;73:1236–40.
67. Elbendary MA, Elbadry AM. Right subclinical varicocele: how to manage in infertile patients with clinical left varicocele? Fertil Steril. 2009;92:2050–3.
68. Dhabuwala CB, Hamid S, Moghisi KS. Clinical versus subclinical varicocele: improvement in fertility after varicocelectomy. Fertil Steril. 1992;57:854–7.
69. Amelar RD, Dubin L. Right varicocelectomy in selected infertile patients who have failed to improve after previous left varicocelectomy. Fertil Steril. 1987;47:833–7.
70. Carpi A, Sabanegh E, Mechanick J. Controversies in the management of nonobstructive azoospermia. Fertil Steril. 2009;91:963–70.
71. Esteves SC, Glina S. Recovery of spermatogenesis after microsurgical subinguinal varicocele repair in azoospermic men based on testicular histology. Int Braz J Urol. 2005;31:541–8.
72. Matthews GJ, Matthews ED, Goldstein M. Induction of spermatogenesis and achievement of pregnancy after microsurgical varicocelectomy in men with azoospermia or severe oligoasthenospermia. Fertil Steril. 1998;70:71–5.
73. Kim ED, Leibman BB, Grinblat DM, et al. Varicocele repair improves semen parameters in azoospermic men with spermatogenic failure. J Urol. 1999;162:737–40.
74. Kadioglu A, Tefekli A, Cayan S, et al. Microsurgical inguinal varicocele repair in azoospermic men. Urology. 2001;57:328–33.
75. Cayan M, Altug U. Induction of spermatogenesis by inguinal varicocele repair in azoospermic men. Arch Androl. 2004;50:145–50.
76. Poulakis V, Ferakis N, de Vries R, et al. Induction of spermatogenesis in men with azoospermia or severe oligoteratoasthenospermia after antegrade internal spermatic vein sclerotherapy for the treatment of varicocele. Asian J Androl. 2006;8:613–9.
77. Ishikawa T, Kondo Y, Yamaguchi K, et al. Effect of varicocelectomy on patients with unobstructive azoospermia and severe oligospermia. Br J Urol Int. 2007;101:216–8.
78. Lee JS, Park HJ, Seo JT. What is the indication for varicocelectomy in men with nonobstructive azoospermia? Urology. 2007;69:352–5.
79. Weedin JW, Khera M, Lipshultz LI. Varicocele Repair in Patients with Nonobstructive Azoospermia – A Meta-Analysis. J Urol. 2010 Jun;183(6):2309–15.

80. Esteves SC. Editorial comment. J Urol. 2010 Jun;183(63):2315.
81. Esteves SC, Verza Jr S, Gomes AP. Successful retrieval of testicular spermatozoa by micro-dissection (micro-TESE) in nonobstructive azoospermia is related to testicular histology. Fertil Steril. 2006;86(Suppl):354.
82. Verza Jr S, Esteves SC. Sperm defect severity rather than sperm source is associated with lower fertilization rates after intracytoplasmic sperm injection. Int Braz J Urol. 2008;34:49–56.
83. Schlegel PN, Kaufmann J. Role of varicocelectomy in men with nonobstructive azoospermia. Fertil Steril. 2004;81:1585–8.
84. Inci K, Hascicek M, Kara O, et al. Sperm retrieval and intracytoplasmic sperm injection in men with nonobstructive azoospermia, and treated and untreated varicocele. J Urol. 2009;182:1500–5.
85. Esteves SC. Editorial comment. J Urol. 2009;182:1504–5.
86. Collodel G, Capitani S, Iacoponi F, et al. Retrospective assessment of potential negative synergistic effects of varicocele and tobacco use on ultrastructural sperm morphology. Urology. 2009;74:794–9.
87. Zampieri N, Zamboni C, Ottolenghi A, et al. The role of lifestyle changing to improve the semen quality in patients with varicocele. Minerva Urol Nefrol. 2008;60:199–204.
88. Agarwal A, Deepinder F, Cocuzza M, et al. Efficacy of varicocelectomy in improving semen parameters: new meta-analytical approach. Urology. 2007;70:532–8.
89. Giulini S, Sblendorio V, Xella S, et al. Seminal plasma total antioxidant capacity and semen parameters in patients with varicocele. Reprod Biomed Online. 2009;18:617–21.
90. Blumer CG, Fariello RM, Restelli AE, et al. Sperm nuclear DNA fragmentation and mitochondrial activity in men with varicocele. Fertil Steril. 2008;90:1716–22.
91. Talebi AR, Moein MR, Tabibnejad N, et al. Effect of varicocele on chromatin condensation and DNA integrity of ejaculated spermatozoa using cytochemical tests. Andrologia. 2008;40:245–51.
92. Shiraishi K, Takihara H, Naito K. Testicular volume, scrotal temperature, and oxidative stress in fertile men with left varicocele. Fertil Steril. 2009;91 Suppl 4:1388–91.
93. Caretta N, Palego P, Schipilliti M, et al. Testicular contrast harmonic imaging to evaluate intratesticular perfusion alterations in patients with varicocele. J Urol. 2010;183:263–9.
94. Jeng SY, Wu SM, Lee JD. Cadmium accumulation and metallothionein overexpression in internal spermatic vein of patients with varicocele. Urology. 2009;73:1231–5.
95. Ichioka K, Nagahama K, Okubo K, et al. Genetic polymorphisms in glutathione S-transferase T1 affect the surgical outcome of varicocelectomies in infertile patients. Asian J Androl. 2009;11:333–41.
96. Meng MV, Greene KL, Turek PJ. Surgery or assisted reproduction? A decision analysis of treatment costs in male infertility. J Urol. 2005;174:1926–31.
97. Ficarra V, Cerruto MA, Liguori G, et al. Treatment of varicocele in subfertile men: the Cochrane Review–a contrary opinion. Eur Urol. 2006;49:258–63.
98. Marmar JL, Agarwal A, Prabaskan S, et al. Reassessing the value of varicocelectomy as a treatment for male subfertility with a new meta-analysis. Fertil Steril. 2007;88:639–48.
99. Cervellione RM, Cervato G, Zampieri N, et al. Effect of varicocelectomy on the plasma oxidative stress parameters. J Pediatr Surg. 2006;41:403–6.
100. Chen SS, Huang WJ, Chang LS, Wei YH. Attenuation of oxidative stress after varicocelectomy in subfertile patients with varicocele. J Urol. 2008;179:639–42.
101. Zini A, Blumenfeld A, Libman J, et al. Beneficial effect of microsurgical varicocelectomy on human sperm DNA integrity. Hum Reprod. 2005;20:1018–21.
102. Moskovtsev SI, Lecker I, Mullen JB, et al. Cause-specific treatment in patients with high sperm DNA damage resulted in significant DNA improvement. Syst Biol Reprod Med. 2009;55:109–15.

103. Smit M, Romijn JC, Wildhagen MF, et al. Decreased sperm DNA fragmentation after surgical varicocelectomy is associated with increased pregnancy rate. J Urol. 2010;183:270–4.
104. Cayan S, Erdemir F, Ozbey I, et al. Can varicocelectomy significantly change the way couple use assisted reproductive technologies? J Urol. 2002;167:1749–52.
105. Esteves SC, Oliveira FV, Bertolla RP. Clinical outcomes of intracytoplasmic sperm injection in infertile men with treated and untreated clinical varicocele. J Urol. 2010 Oct;184(4):1442–6.

Chapter 10
Sperm DNA Damage and Antioxidant Use: Roles in Male Fertility

Ashok Agarwal and Aspinder Singh

Introduction

Infertility is formally characterized as a state in which a couple of reproductive age desiring a child is unable to conceive following 12 months of unprotected intercourse. Infertility represents one of the most common diseases and affects between 17% and 25% of couples [1]. Of these, male factor infertility is responsible for approximately 50% of the infertility cases. With female parameters held constant, the physician and andrologist must turn to semen characteristics to decipher what are the causative agents behind male infertility. WHO standard protocol requires analysis of sperm concentration, motility, and morphology [2]. However, recent evidence implies that such parameters are not enough to fully depict the basis for male infertility and suggests that the effects of sperm DNA damage on infertility be considered [3].

With the increasing ease of artificial reproduction, factors affecting embryo viability and offspring health related to the quality of sperm used and associated integrity of DNA must be strictly analyzed. Male gametes with damaged DNA can transmit genetic defects, lead to pregnancy loss, infant mortality, birth defects, and genetic diseases in the offspring [4, 5]. Furthermore, studies report that more than 80% of the structural de novo chromosome aberrations are of paternal origin [6].

This chapter begins by reviewing the process of spermatozoal chromatin organization and DNA packaging. Next, DNA damage and the factors causing this damage shall be considered. Subsequently, recognition and detection of this DNA damage will be reviewed followed finally by the effects of this damage and clinical applications encompassing treatment options involving antioxidants.

A. Agarwal, Ph.D. (✉) • A. Singh, BS
Center for Reproductive Medicine, Glickman Urological and Kidney Institute,
Cleveland Clinic Foundation, 9500 Euclid Avenue, Desk A19, Cleveland, OH 44195, USA
e-mail: agarwaa@ccf.org

S.J. Parekattil and A. Agarwal (eds.), *Antioxidants in Male Infertility: A Guide for Clinicians and Researchers*, © Springer Science+Business Media New York 2013

How Is Spermatozoal Chromatin Organized and the DNA Packaged?

Unlike somatic cells, the packaging of sperm DNA utilizes a special procedure and also very unique proteins [7]. It is packed and coiled such that proper condensation and augmentation can be controlled in a time appropriate manner at specific stages of embryo development. Mammalian sperm chromatic can be divided into three major structural domains: the majority of sperm DNA is coiled into toroids by protamines, a smaller percent remains bound to histones, and the remaining DNA is attached to the sperm nuclear matrix at matrix attachment regions (MARs) at intervals of roughly 50 kb throughout the genome (Fig. 10.1) [8].

Protamine-bound DNA is the most condensed and therefore most protected form of sperm DNA. The tight condensation of the DNA allows for it to exist in toroids in a semicrystalline state, making it resistant to nuclease digestion. This type of DNA must first be uncoiled such that a reading frame can be exposed for protein synthesis. Protamines have large tracts of positively charged arginine residues that neutralize the negative phosphodiester backbone of the DNA. The presence of these

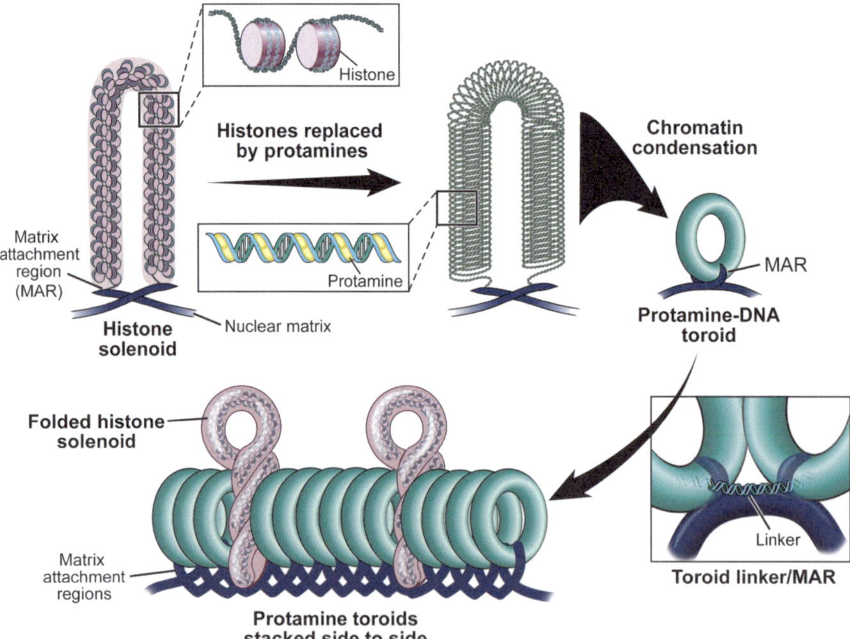

Fig. 10.1 Organization of sperm DNA. Majority of the sperm DNA is coiled into DNAse-insensitive toroids which are stacked side to side to maximize compaction. This toroid structure is held stable due to the presence of protamines which neutralize the repulsion between the phosphodiester backbone. Sperm maturation involves histone replacement via these protamines, allowing for proper transmission of paternal genetic material (adapted from [8], with permission)

arginine residues allows for the repulsion between the DNA residues and backbone to be reduced such that DNA can be packaged tighter and wound into highly compact toroids. This neutralization mimics that of divalent cations that can also cause DNA to form similar toroids with smaller amounts of DNA [8]. Furthermore, mammalian protamines contain several cysteines, which confer an increased stability on sperm chromatin by intermolecular disulfide cross-links, making sperm chromatin rich in protamines resistant to much greater mechanical disruption than somatic cells, supporting protamines' role in DNA protection [9]. Once compacted, protamine toroids are stacked side to side like a package of lifesavers (Fig. 10.1). Variations of this theme are two adjacent lines of toroids, which are aligned together with alternating toroids on the same chromatin being packaged on one line [10].

Protamine toroids are unique to mature sperm cells, and their major function is entirely for fertilization and not for embryonic development. Protamine binding causes gene expression silencing during spermiogenesis [11]. Postfertilization, the protamines are completely replaced in the first 4 h by histone proteins by the oocyte such that the paternal chromatin has increased accessibility. Ogura et al. found that when round spermatids lacking protamine condensation are used for injection into mouse oocytes, normal fertile mice developed. This therefore indicates that this level of sperm chromatin structure is sufficient for proper fertilization [12, 13].

The second largest manner of sperm DNA organization is sperm chromatin bound to histones. Depending on the mammalian species, between 2% and 15% of the sperm chromatin is bound to histones rather than protamines [14]. These histones are nonrandomly distributed throughout the sperm genome and are associated with specific genes. They are primarily found associated with gene promoter sites. Furthermore, entire functional gene families that are important for spermiogenesis and early fertilization development are preferentially associated with histones in human spermatozoa [14–16]. This correlates with the properties of DNA bound to histones. This type of association allows for a more easily accessible reading frame; however, this accessibility also makes the DNA more prone to nuclease activity. Sotolongo et al. proposed that histone-bound DNA made up the linker regions between each protamine toroid in the chromatin fiber because these were the regions that were the most nuclease sensitive [9].

Unlike protamines, which are replaced by histones provided by the oocyte postfertilization, the regions where histones are already present are not substituted. The transmission of sperm histones, and the associated chromatin structures, suggests that it is possible for the newly fertilized oocyte to inherit histone-based chromatin structural organization from the sperm [13, 17]. This also implies that any histone-based chromatin damage and malformation is also transmitted without modification.

The third and final form of sperm DNA organization is that bound to the nuclear matrix. The chromatin is organized into loop domains which are attached every 20–120 kb in length to a proteinaceous structure termed the nuclear matrix. This organizes the chromatin into functional loops of DNA that help regulate DNA replication and gene transcription [8, 18]. These MARs, no larger than 1,000 bp, occur between each protamine toroid and are termed the toroid linkers. These regions are nuclease sensitive and point to the presence of histones, which is consistent with the wide yet regular distribution of histones throughout the sperm genome

[8, 16]. The two main roles of the sperm nuclear matrix are to properly associate DNA to the nuclear matrix such that paternal pronuclear DNA can be replicated in the one-cell embryo and to function as a checkpoint for sperm DNA integrity after fertilization [8].

A study conducted by Shaman et al. utilized sperm halos to determine the role of the loop domains in fertilization and development. Sperm halos can be constructed by treating the chromatin with high salt and reducing agents, which remove the protamine condensation and histone-bound nucleosomes, leaving only the sperm nuclear matrix with its associated loop domains. The study found that these halos were able to suffi-ciently form pronuclear and allow DNA replication, yet do not support developmental progression to the blast cyst stage, suggesting the loop domain DNA organization is required for replication but is not sufficient for development [18].

Of the three types of packaging, histones and MARs are inherent to the embryo and needed for proper development. Therefore, methods to manipulate spermatozoa for ART should be developed that maintain the integrity of the sperm chromatin structure, as well as taking into consideration the integrity of the paternal DNA [8].

One final consideration that must be taken when studying sperm DNA is that of the organization of the sperm chromosome. These chromosomes are relatively homogenous in structure, with the sperm chromatin folded into hairpin-like structures with the controlees positioned near the center of the sperm cell and the telomeres of each chromosome paired and arrayed around the periphery of the sperm nucleus [19, 20]. These individual chromosomes are positioned into nonoverlapping regions within the nucleolus entitled "chromosome territories." Existence of a preferred chro-mosome territory positioning in the human spermatozoa implies that deviation from the regular localization may be possibly deleterious for proper fertilization and devel-opment [21, 22]. Determination of such sperm chromosome territories is done using 2D and 3D florescent in situ hybridization (FISH) in interphone cells.

What Is DNA Damage and What Can Cause It?

Strand Breaks

DNA damage comes in a wide array of forms. Besides cardinal damage such as point deletions or frame shifts, the main categories of DNA damage are stand breaks, base modifications, and telomere shortening via oxidation. These damages can modify the genome and lead to translational errors, ultimately affecting the viability of the embryo and health of progeny. Single-strand breaks are found at regular intervals throughout the sperm genome. These breaks may be needed to reduce the torsion stress caused by chromatin packaging. Unfortunately, the single-strand breaks often lead to double-strand breaks via the activities of topoisomerase II variants [23]. These double-strand breaks can be difficult to repair by the limited innate DNA polymerase activity in the spermatozoa.

Base Modifications

In addition to stand breaks, base modifications are the second most common form of DNA damage. These modifications come in the forms of base supplementation such as fappy G, thymidine glycols addition, or adducts and also via chemical modifications such as oxidation of guanosine sites and abasic sites [24]. Furthermore, improper residue linkage resulting in mismatched pairs, formation of intrastrand bridges, and pyridine dimerization can lead to erroneous transmission of genetic data [24, 25].

Telomere Shortening

Finally, reactive oxygen species insult can yield mitochondrial dysfunction which leads to telomere attrition [26]. Liu et al. found that when mitochondrial function was disrupted in one-cell zygotes, cascade events led to a significant increase in measurements of reactive oxygen species which negatively correlated with embryo survival in a time-dependent manner [26].

Mitochondrial dysfunction was accompanied by telomere shortening, telomere loss, and chromosome fusion, leading to development arrest [26]. This halted developmental progress, thereby leading to apoptosis. However, they discovered that the antioxidant *N*-acetylcysteine scavenges ROS, forms cysteine by deacetylation, and increases glutathione (a free radical scavenger) production [26]. This antioxidant therefore prevented ROS accumulation, telomere shortening, and cell death.

Agents of DNA Damage

As important as it is to understand the forms of DNA damage, it is equally as crucial to comprehend what can cause this damage. There are internal factors, such as spermatozoal maturation processes and oxidative stress, and there are external causes, including lifestyle choices and environmental factors, which can all contribute to sperm DNA damage.

One major causative agent of damage is the inherent nature of spermatozoal maturation, which leaves the sperm enable to protect themselves from stress factors. This maturation eliminates the spermatozoal cytoplasm, without which it is difficult to combat oxidative stress. Furthermore, the human sperm plasma membrane contains an abundance of unsaturated fatty acids, which not only provide membrane fluidity necessary for motility and fusion, but also leaves the sperm predisposed to free radical attach and peroxidation of the plasma membrane lipids [27]. In addition to cytoplasmic reduction, maturation encompasses DNA remodeling. Irregular protamination can result in increased torsional stress, leading to strand breaks [28].

Another main instigator of DNA damage is oxidative stress. The presence of highly reactive oxygen species has been reported in the semen of between 25% and

40% of infertile men, resulting in cascade events which lead to lipid peroxidation and breakdown of macromolecules including nucleotides [10]. Furthermore, leukocytospermia yields an increased presence of pro-inflammatory mediators, such as cytokines, which lead to alterations in the regulation of spermiogenesis and subsequent DNA aberration [30].

Formation of 8-hydroxy-2-deoxyguanosine (8-OHdG) is a biological marker for oxidative stress DNA damage. 8-OHdG is an adduct which represents a modified DNA structure potentially leading to a DNA break [31]. The likelihood of pregnancy occurring with a single menstrual cycle is inversely associated with the levels of 8-OHdG [32]. Additional information concerning the roles of oxidative stress is provided in greater detail in proceeding chapters.

Many external factors are associated with DNA damage, including smoking, and certain medication and treatments. Cigarettes and their associated smoke contain many chemicals which can increase oxidative stress. Saleh et al. found that the percent DNA fragmentation index is significantly higher in infertile men who smoke [33]. The metabolites found in cigarette smoke, including vinyl chloride and benzopyrene, result in DNA adducts and can induce the increased activity of chemical inflammation mediators such as interleukin-6 and interleukin-8 which lead to the subsequent recruitment of leukocytes [24, 34, 35]. Also, there is an association between paternal smoking and an increased risk of childhood cancer in the offspring [34].

Many cancer treatments utilize chemicals which are detrimental to sperm DNA, primarily alkylating agents. Chemotherapy drugs such as fludarabine, cyclophosphamide, and busulfan can cause testicular damage, manifested as reduced volume, oligozoospermia, elevated follicle-stimulating hormone and luteinizing hormone, and decreased testosterone concentrations [36]. The effects of these drugs may persist for several months after cessation of their use [37].

How Can Sperm DNA Damage Be Detected and Prevented?

There are plethora tests available to measure DNA damage in sperm samples. These include TUNEL, Comet, in situ nick translation assay, sperm chromatin structure assay, 3D FISH, and many more. Each can measure and quantify the DNA damage in terms of strand breaks, denaturation of strands, or presence of adducts. Unfortunately, many of these tests lack useful thresholds or a clinically accepted standardization. Also, in order to determine the damage levels, the spermatozoa must first be prepared, which often involves strenuous conditions such as high heat which can lead to additional damage.

There are, however, many test preparation methods with reduced levels of DNA damage. The swim-up method is associated with an increased high post-in vitro fertilization (IVF) rate and better DNA integrity compared to density gradient centrifugation [38, 39]. Furthermore, glass wool preparation significantly decreases the percent DNA fragmentation index when compared with raw semen samples [40].

One must also keep in mind that minute DNA damage can be repaired with appropriate mechanisms available inside the oocyte; however, extensive damage is not reparable. Between the period of sperm entry into the cytoplasm and the beginning of the next S phase, DNA damage can be repaired by the oocyte via pre- and post-replication mechanisms [24]. Both nonhomologous end joining (NHEJ) and homologous recombination are used by the oocyte to rescue the genetic integrity of the paternal genome after fertilization [3]. However, maternal age must be considered as it is found that increased age reflects decreased stores of mRNA for many repair mechanisms, as well as reduced efficient of DNA repair [41].

Clinical Applications

DNA Damage in Relation to Artificial Reproduction Techniques

Today's advances in artificial reproduction techniques (ART) make it easier to transmit defective spermatozoa and still induce pregnancy [25]. Intracytoplasmic sperm injection (ICSI) and IVF allow couples to bypass natural selection processes inherent to the fusion procedure which would normally select out abnormal spermatozoa. These abnormal spermatozoa thereby may hinder implantation, embryo development, and progeny viability.

It has been shown that during the first mitotic cycle, 77.5% of ROSI-generated embryos exhibit abnormal chromosome segregation. This abnormal segregation originates from double-strand breaks of the male-derived genomic DNA [12]. ICSI and ROSI procedures resulted in no embryonic development when chromosome segregation was abnormal during this first mitotic division [42]. Therefore, residual DNA breaks in spermatozoa, those which fall outside the realm of oocyte repair, may lead to impaired zygote development via abnormal chromosome segregation and genetic impairment. This supports the notion that the use of genetically abnormal spermatozoa could lead to unsuccessful reproductive outcomes [43].

Furthermore, Duran et al. found that in intrauterine insemination (IUI), there is a failure of pregnancy in women inseminated with a semen sample with >12% sperm with fragmented DNA and miscarriages in those with moderate degrees of DNA damage (10–12%). One hundred and nineteen couples comprised a total of 154 IUI cycles, both natural and stimulated. From these it was found that an increased rate of miscarriages and pregnancy failure correlated with the level of DNA damage brought upon by defective chromatin organization, ineffective apoptosis, and oxidative stress [44].

Bungum et al. also conducted a similar study, looking at 387 IUI cycles. Their results confirmed those of Duran, with a pregnancy success rate of 19% when the DFI value was <30%, compared to a success rate of only 1.5% when the DFI was >30%. These results indicate that the DFI value can be used a reliable and accurate independent predictor of fertility [45].

Moreover, many studies have found that sperm DNA damage is associated with a significantly higher rate of pregnancy loss after IVF or ICSI (Table 10.1) [46]. Specifically, Zini et al. derived, from a meta-analysis of 2,549 cycles of IVF or ICSI involving 640 pregnancies and 122 failures, that sperm genetic damage was

Table 10.1 Study parameters on sperm DNA damage and pregnancy loss after IVF and ICSI

Study	n	ART	Assay	PL%	Abn test %	Sens	Spec	PPV	NPV
Check, '05	104	ICSI	SCSA	47	24	0.31	0.83	0.63	0.58
Zini, '05	60	ICSI	SCSA	16	19	0.40	0.85	0.33	0.88
Borini, '06	82	IVF	TUNEL	6	11	0.91	0.94	0.50	0.99
Borini, '06	50	ICSI	TUNEL	25	25	0.97	0.99	0.97	0.99
Benchaib, '07	84	IVF	TUNEL	15	15	0.50	0.91	0.50	0.91
Benchaib, '07	218	ICSI	TUNEL	12	15	0.38	0.88	0.30	0.91
Bungum, '07	388	IVF	SCSA	24	14	0.11	0.85	0.19	0.76
Bungum, '07	223	ICSI	SCSA	19	40	0.50	0.63	0.24	0.84
Frydman, '08	117	IVF	TUNEL	19	32	0.64	0.75	0.37	0.90
Lin, '08	137	IVF	SCSA	10	17	0.29	0.84	0.17	0.92
Lin, '08	86	ICSI	SCSA	18	23	0.50	0.83	0.40	0.88

From [46], with permission

ART assisted reproductive technology, *Abn test* proportion of abnormal sperm DNA test among documented pregnancies, *PL* pregnancy loss, *Sens* sensitivity, *Spec* specificity, *PPV* positive predictive value, *NPV* negative predictive value

significantly associated with pregnancy loss ($p < 0.0001$). They also concluded that in populations with abnormal sperm DNA damage, the miscarriage rate increases to 37% compared to an average rate of 18%. In comparison, this rate fell to only 10% when the testing results are negative [46]. This difference may be valuable for patients when making decisions regarding ART procedures.

Also, Virro et al. concluded in their study of 249 couples undergoing IVF/ICSI that men with a DFI <33% has a significantly greater chance of initiating a pregnancy, lower miscarriage rates, and an increase of ongoing pregnancies at week 12 (47% vs. 28%) than those compared with a DFI <33% [47]. These results indicate the importance of DNA integrity in not only pregnancy initiation but also in long-term viability of the embryo.

Lastly, the Y chromosome is particularly susceptible to damage because the haploid genome is unable to retrieve genetic information, leading to gene deletion. In turn, Y chromosome deletions and microdeletions can lead to infertility in the offspring [48].

Unfortunately, when selecting spermatozoa for ART, often, morphology is the main determinant between "normal" and "abnormal" cells. This selection cannot however illustrate the DNA properties, and one cannot avoid selecting spermatozoa undergoing chromatin remodeling, or those with substantial genetic damage.

Antioxidant Use in DNA Repair

An antioxidant regimen to reduce damage is an integral part of applications to repair sperm DNA. tocopherols (TP), vitamin E, and tocotrienol are the main chain breaking antioxidants in biological membranes. TP prevents the dissemination of lipid peroxidation by directly interacting with lipid-free radicals derived from oxidation of polyunsaturated fatty acids. These radicals include the alkoxy radical (LO$^{\bullet}$), lipid peroxyl radical (LOO$^{\bullet}$), and alkyl radicals (L$^{\bullet}$) [49].

TP interacts with these radical in the lipid/water interphase and results in the formation of lipid hydroperoxides (LO–OH) and also the tocopheroxyl radical (TO$^{\bullet}$), which can be reduced by ascorbic acid, or coenzyme Q. The reaction is as follows: TP–OH + L–OO$^{\bullet}$ → L–OOH + TO$^{\bullet}$ [49].

Fraga et al. demonstrated that oral vitamin C intake leads to an increase in semen vitamin C levels. They found decreased dietary ascorbic acid intake (from 250 to 5 mg/day) in a group of 24 men ages 20–50 correlated with decreased seminal ascorbic acid levels by half and increased (91%) levels of 8-OHdG in sperm DNA. The increased intake was associated with a decrease in DNA oxidation and therefore improved sperm DNA integrity [50].

Also, Greco et al. concluded that an antioxidant regimen of vitamin C and E was associated with a significant decrease in the percentage of DNA-fragmented spermatozoa. Oral intake of vitamin C 500 mg and vitamin E 500 mg (twice a day for 2 months) resulted in a significant decrease in sperm DNA fragmentation in a group of 64 men with unexplained infertility (pretreatment 22.1% ± 7.7 vs. posttreatment 9.1% ± 7.2) [51]. The incidence of DNA fragmentation was lower in all men after the antioxidant treatment, showing a generalized benefit of these compounds in preventing damage to sperm DNA.

In addition to vitamin C and vitamin E, there are many other antioxidants which are effective in reducing the free radical load and preventing subsequent damage. Glutathione, selenium, alpha-tocopherol, folic acid, and zinc have all been proven to be effective (Table 10.2) [52] and are generally prescribed to help reduce sperm DNA damage and assist men in their reproductive goals. Many of these oral antioxidants come in compact, multicompound pill form; popular brand names include Fertibiol®, Procrelia®, Condesyl®, and Nurelia® [53].

Recently, Zini et al. demonstrated a reduction in sperm DNA damage when lycopene was added to the semen sample. In this study, sperm samples from 12 fertile men were pretreated with 5 µmol/L lycopene prior to 2-h incubation with hydrogen peroxide. The authors demonstrated a significant decrease in% DFI (treatment 8.0% ± 7.9 vs. control 10.8% ± 39.4; $p < 0.05$), suggesting that pretreatment with lycopene could protect sperm against DNA damage in vitro [54].

The authors recently conducted a survey of three leading male infertility urologists concerning their use of antioxidants in male infertility treatment. These urologists agree that patients should begin an antioxidant regimen upon initial evaluation, along with any other treatments necessary to treat their overlying conditions, such as antibiotics or a varicocelectomy. They recommend their patients to follow an antioxidant regimen for an average of 3–6 months. This typically includes 500 mg of vitamin C, 400 IU of vitamin E, 50 mg of zinc, 100 µg of selenium, and 5 mg of folate. Their patients reported only minor side effects with the antioxidant use, such as mild stomachaches, and were usually very responsive to the suggestion. Overall, patients showed good responsiveness to these antioxidants, and these compounds have become a critical part of the armamentarium used to treat DNA damage-based male infertility.

Table 10.2 Effect of dietary antioxidant supplements on sperm DNA integrity

Study	Patients/test	Treatment(s)	*n*	Results
Infertile men with high sperm DNA fragmentation levels or oxidative stress				
Greco '05	1 failed ICSI	Vits C 1 g, E 1 g	38	Rx (2 months): ↓ DD in 76%, 48% ICSI pregnancy
	TUNEL > 15%			No control group
Greco '05	Infertility	Vits C 1 g, E 1 g	32	Rx (2 months): ↓ DD (22% → 9%)
	TUNEL > 15%		32	Placebo group: no effect on DD (22% → 22%)
Menezo '07	2 failed ICSI DFI > 15%	Vits C, E (400 mg), zinc, Se, β-carotene	57	Rx (90 days):↓ sperm%DFI (32 → 26%: by 19%) but ↑ sperm%HDS (17.5 → 25.5%: by 23%)
	Decond > 15%			No control group
Tremellen '07	Male Infert TUNEL > 25%	Menevit (lycopene, vits C, E, zinc, Se, folate, garlic)	36	Rx (3 months): 39% ICSI pregnancy rate, but no ↑ in embryo quality, no post-Rx DD
			16	Placebo group: 16% ICSI pregnancy rate
Gil Villa '09	Pregn. loss	Vits C, E, zinc, β-carotene	9	Rx (3 months): 6 (of 9) couples got pregnancy
	↑ LPO or DFI			No control group
Unselected infertile men				
Piomboni '08	Asthenosp.	Vits C, E, β-glucan, papaya, lactoferrin	36	Rx (90 days): ↑ motility and morph but not DD
	AO stain		15	Control group: no effect
Kodama '97	Male infert	Vits C, E (200 mg), glutathione (400 mg)	14	Rx (2 months): ↓ in 8-OHdG (1.5 → 1.1/10^5 dG)
	8-OHdG		7	Control group: no change in 8-OHdG levels

From [52], with permission

8-OHdG 8-hydroxy-2-deoxyguanosine, *AO* acridine orange, *DD* DNA damage, *Decond* decondensation, *DFI* DNA fragmentation index, *LPO* lipid peroxidation, *OS* oxidative stress, *Rx* treatment, *ROS* reactive oxygen species, *Se* selenium, *TUNEL* terminal nucleotidyl transferase dUTP nick end labeling, *vit* vitamin

Future Considerations and Conclusions

Artificial reproduction is a growing field, with daily advancements and technological breakthroughs. However, the implications of DNA damage on male fertility and pregnancy outcomes are substantially overlooked. ART procedures allow spermatozoa to bypass natural selection processes and initiate pregnancy; therefore, one must be cautious concerning the quality of the spermatozoa utilized. Multiple studies have shown a strong correlation between DNA damage and pregnancy failure, implying the importance of this parameter on fertility.

Clinical antioxidant use in the repair of DNA damage has increased over the past years. Growing data shows antioxidants protect the DNA from free radicals, thereby increasing the rate of successful pregnancies. Scavenging of these radicals reduces strand breaks, decreases chemical modifications, and halts telomere attrition, thereby increasing the viability of the embryo. Therefore, antioxidant use is strongly recommended in couples facing male factor infertility.

Future studies are needed to further validate the benefits of dietary antioxidants for male fertility. Although the results in the literature suggest that sperm DNA integrity testing may potentially have the greatest clinical utility for predicting pregnancy loss after IVF and ICSI, properly controlled studies are urgently required to confirm these results [55]. Larger studies with longer treatments could help clearly define the correlation between antioxidants and DNA repair. Also, designations of the repair mechanisms are of utmost necessity. Additional in vitro supplementation studies will better define a standard protocol for antioxidant use and will allow for the clinicians, andrologist, and the patients to work together to achieve an increased rate of successful pregnancy. Also, additional studies involving antioxidant benefits on normal, fertile men would serve as guidelines for comparison with the infertile cases.

Expert Commentary

The aim of this chapter is to elucidate the necessity of DNA integrity tests prior to ART techniques and to highlight the benefits of antioxidant use in damage prevention and repair. Current advances in artificial reproduction are making it easier to utilize damaged spermatozoa, yet techniques for detection of this damage are not routinely used. This chapter brings forth clinical evidence which supports the association between sperm DNA damage, male fertility, and pregnancy success, as well as the benefits derived from a prescribed antioxidant regimen. This data will provide information to both clinicians and patients to make choices which will maximize the patients' fertility and pregnancy success. The techniques and methods necessary to detect and improve the DNA damage are already integral parts of semen analysis, and only a standardized protocol for testing and antioxidant use needs to be evolved. Artificial reproduction is a very distinct and specialized field, one that requires further research and standards of practice which may lead to better patient care and improved pregnancy success.

Key Issues

- With the increasing ease of artificial reproduction, factors effecting embryo viability and health of offspring related to the quality of sperm used and associated integrity of DNA must be strictly analyzed.
- Sperm chromatin packaging and DNA organization requires special proteins and unique structural organization to provide accurate folding and unfolding in a time-specific manner.

- Sperm histones and MARs are inherent to the embryo and are needed for proper development.
- DNA damage comes in three main forms: strand breaks, base modifications, and telomere shortening.
- This damage can be attributed to various internal and external factors including spermatozoal maturation, oxidative stress, smoking, and medical treatments.
- Various test procedures are used to elucidate the levels of DNA damage. These include TUNEL, Comet, in situ nick translation, and 3D FISH.
- There have been many studies relating the effects of DNA damage on IVF, ICSI, and IUI. These studies show a strong correlation between increased DNA damage and decreased pregnancy success.
- Antioxidants are clinically prescribed to reduce the levels of DNA damage and repair the genetic integrity. Antioxidants function to reduce the oxidative load and are correlated with an increased pregnancy success rate in ART as shown.

References

1. Dunson DB, Baird DD, Colombo B. Increased infertility with age in men and women. Obstet Gynecol. 2004;103:51–6.
2. World Health Organization, DoRHaR. WHO laboratory manual for the examination and processing of human semen. 5th ed. Geneva: World Health Organization; 2010.
3. Marchetti F, Essers J, Kanaar R, Wyrobek AJ. Disruption of maternal DNA repair increases sperm-derived chromosomal aberrations. Proc Natl Acad Sci USA. 2007;104:17725–9.
4. Aitken RJ, De Iuliis GN, McLachlan RI. Biological and clinical significance of DNA damage in the male germ line. Int J Androl. 2009;32:46–56.
5. Fernandez-Gonzalez R, Moreira PN, Perez-Crespo M, et al. Long-term effects of mouse intracytoplasmic sperm injection with DNA-fragmented sperm on health and behavior of adult offspring. Biol Reprod. 2008;78:761–72.
6. Thomas NS, Durkie M, Van Zyl B, et al. Parental and chromosomal origin of unbalanced de novo structural chromosome abnormalities in man. Hum Genet. 2006;119:444–50.
7. Fuentes-Mascorro G, Serrano H, Rosado A. Sperm chromatin. Arch Androl. 2000;45:215–25.
8. Ward WS. Function of sperm chromatin structural elements in fertilization and development. Mol Hum Reprod. 2010;16:30–6.
9. Sotolongo B, Lino E, Ward WS. Ability of hamster spermatozoa to digest their own DNA. Biol Reprod. 2003;69:2029–35.
10. Mudrak O, Chandra R, Jones E, Godfrey E, Zalensky A. Reorganisation of human sperm nuclear architecture during formation of pronuclei in a model system. Reprod Fertil Dev. 2009;21:665–71.
11. Martins RP, Ostermeier GC, Krawetz SA. Nuclear matrix interactions at the human protamine domain: a working model of potentiation. J Biol Chem. 2004;279:51862–8.
12. Ogura A, Matsuda J, Yanagimachi R. Birth of normal young after electrofusion of mouse oocytes with round spermatids. Proc Natl Acad Sci USA. 1994;91:7460–2.
13. Ajduk A, Yamauchi Y, Ward MA. Sperm chromatin remodeling after intracytoplasmic sperm injection differs from that of in vitro fertilization. Biol Reprod. 2006;75:442–51.
14. Hammoud SS, Nix DA, Zhang H, Purwar J, Carrell DT, Cairns BR. Distinctive chromatin in human sperm packages genes for embryo development. Nature. 2009;460:473–8.
15. Ostermeier GC, Goodrich RJ, Diamond MP, Dix DJ, Krawetz SA. Toward using stable spermatozoal RNAs for prognostic assessment of male factor fertility. Fertil Steril. 2005;83:1687–94.

16. Arpanahi A, Brinkworth M, Iles D, et al. Endonuclease-sensitive regions of human spermatozoal chromatin are highly enriched in promoter and CTCF binding sequences. Genome Res. 2009; 19:1338–49.
17. van der Heijden GW, Ramos L, Baart EB, et al. Sperm-derived histones contribute to zygotic chromatin in humans. BMC Dev Biol. 2008;8:34.
18. Shaman JA, Yamauchi Y, Ward WS. The sperm nuclear matrix is required for paternal DNA replication. J Cell Biochem. 2007;102:680–8.
19. Zalenskaya IA, Bradbury EM, Zalensky AO. Chromatin structure of telomere domain in human sperm. Biochem Biophys Res Commun. 2000;279:213–8.
20. Churikov D, Siino J, Svetlova M, et al. Novel human testis-specific histone H2B encoded by the interrupted gene on the X chromosome. Genomics. 2004;84:745–56.
21. Mudrak O, Tomilin N, Zalensky A. Chromosome architecture in the decondensing human sperm nucleus. J Cell Sci. 2005;118:4541–50.
22. Zalensky A, Zalenskaya I. Organization of chromosomes in spermatozoa: an additional layer of epigenetic information? Biochem Soc Trans. 2007;35:609–11.
23. Spano M, Seli E, Bizzaro D, Manicardi GC, Sakkas D. The significance of sperm nuclear DNA strand breaks on reproductive outcome. Curr Opin Obstet Gynecol. 2005;17:255–60.
24. Menezo Y, Dale B, Cohen M. DNA damage and repair in human oocytes and embryos: a review. Zygote. 2010;18(4):357–65.
25. Erenpreiss J, Spano M, Erenpreisa J, Bungum M, Giwercman A. Sperm chromatin structure and male fertility: biological and clinical aspects. Asian J Androl. 2006;8:11–29.
26. Liu L, Trimarchi JR, Smith PJ, Keefe DL. Mitochondrial dysfunction leads to telomere attrition and genomic instability. Aging Cell. 2002;1:40–6.
27. Twigg J, Fulton N, Gomez E, Irvine DS, Aitken RJ. Analysis of the impact of intracellular reactive oxygen species generation on the structural and functional integrity of human spermatozoa: lipid peroxidation, DNA fragmentation and effectiveness of antioxidants. Hum Reprod. 1998;13:1429–36.
28. Agarwal A, Said TM. Role of sperm chromatin abnormalities and DNA damage in male infertility. Hum Reprod Update. 2003;9:331–45.
29. Padron OF, Sharma RK, Thomas Jr AJ, Agarwal A. Effects of cancer on spermatozoa quality after cryopreservation: a 12-year experience. Fertil Steril. 1997;67:326–31.
30. Kasturi SS, Charles Osterberg E, Tannir J, Brannigan RE. The effect of genital tract infection and inflammation on male infertility. In: Lipshiltz LI, Howards SS, Neiderberger CS, editors. Infertility in the male. 4th ed. Cambridge: Cambridge University Press; 2009. p. 295–330.
31. Aitken RJ, De Iuliis GN. On the possible origins of DNA damage in human spermatozoa. Mol Hum Reprod. 2010;16:3–13.
32. Loft S, Kold-Jensen T, Hjollund NH, et al. Oxidative DNA damage in human sperm influences time to pregnancy. Hum Reprod. 2003;18:1265–72.
33. Saleh RA, Agarwal A, Sharma RK, Nelson DR, Thomas Jr AJ. Effect of cigarette smoking on levels of seminal oxidative stress in infertile men: a prospective study. Fertil Steril. 2002; 78:491–9.
34. Chang JS. Parental smoking and childhood leukemia. Methods Mol Biol. 2009;472:103–37.
35. Sepaniak S, Forges T, Gerard H, Foliguet B, Bene MC, Monnier-Barbarino P. The influence of cigarette smoking on human sperm quality and DNA fragmentation. Toxicology. 2006;223: 54–60.
36. Chatterjee R, Haines GA, Perera DM, Goldstone A, Morris ID. Testicular and sperm DNA damage after treatment with fludarabine for chronic lymphocytic leukaemia. Hum Reprod. 2000;15:762–6.
37. Campbell DI, Bunn JE, Weaver LT, Harding M, Coward WA, Thomas JE. Human milk vacuolating cytotoxin A immunoglobulin A antibodies modify *Helicobacter pylori* infection in Gambian children. Clin Infect Dis. 2006;43:1040–2.
38. Younglai EV, Holt D, Brown P, Jurisicova A, Casper RF. Sperm swim-up techniques and DNA fragmentation. Hum Reprod. 2001;16:1950–3.
39. Zini A, Finelli A, Phang D, Jarvi K. Influence of semen processing technique on human sperm DNA integrity. Urology. 2000;56:1081–4.

40. Larson KL, Brannian JD, Timm BK, Jost LK, Evenson DP. Density gradient centrifugation and glass wool filtration of semen remove spermatozoa with damaged chromatin structure. Hum Reprod. 1999;14:2015–9.
41. Hamatani T, Falco G, Carter MG, et al. Age-associated alteration of gene expression patterns in mouse oocytes. Hum Mol Genet. 2004;13:2263–78.
42. Yamagata K, Suetsugu R, Wakayama T. Assessment of chromosomal integrity using a novel live-cell imaging technique in mouse embryos produced by intracytoplasmic sperm injection. Hum Reprod. 2009;24:2490–9.
43. Kimura Y, Yanagimachi R. Mouse oocytes injected with testicular spermatozoa or round spermatids can develop into normal offspring. Development. 1995;121:2397–405.
44. Duran EH, Morshedi M, Taylor S, Oehninger S. Sperm DNA quality predicts intrauterine insemination outcome: a prospective cohort study. Hum Reprod. 2002;17:3122–8.
45. Bungum M, Humaidan P, Axmon A, et al. Sperm DNA integrity assessment in prediction of assisted reproduction technology outcome. Hum Reprod. 2007;22:174–9.
46. Zini A, Boman JM, Belzile E, Ciampi A. Sperm DNA damage is associated with an increased risk of pregnancy loss after IVF and ICSI: systematic review and meta-analysis. Hum Reprod. 2008;23:2663–8.
47. Virro MR, Larson-Cook KL, Evenson DP. Sperm chromatin structure assay (SCSA) parameters are related to fertilization, blastocyst development, and ongoing pregnancy in in vitro fertilization and intracytoplasmic sperm injection cycles. Fertil Steril. 2004;81:1289–95.
48. Aitken RJ, Krausz C. Oxidative stress, DNA damage and the Y chromosome. Reproduction. 2001;122:497–506.
49. Fagerstedt K, Blokhina O. Oxidative stress and antioxidant defences in plants. In: Singh KK, editor. Oxidative stress, disease and cancer. London: Imperial College Press; 2006. p. 151–99.
50. Fraga CG, Motchnik PA, Shigenaga MK, Helbock HJ, Jacob RA, Ames BN. Ascorbic acid protects against endogenous oxidative DNA damage in human sperm. Proc Natl Acad Sci USA. 1991;88:11003–6.
51. Greco E, Iacobelli M, Rienzi L, Ubaldi F, Ferrero S, Tesarik J. Reduction of the incidence of sperm DNA fragmentation by oral antioxidant treatment. J Androl. 2005;26:349–53.
52. Zini A, San Gabriel M, Baazeem A. Antioxidants and sperm DNA damage: a clinical perspective. J Assist Reprod Genet. 2009;26:427–32.
53. Boxmeer JC, Smit M, Utomo E, et al. Low folate in seminal plasma is associated with increased sperm DNA damage. Fertil Steril. 2009;92:548–56.
54. Zini A, San Gabriel M, Libman J. Lycopene supplementation in vitro can protect human sperm deoxyribonucleic acid from oxidative damage. Fertil Steril. 2010;94:1033–6.
55. Barratt CL, De Jonge CJ. Clinical relevance of sperm DNA assessment: an update. Fertil Steril. 2010;94(6):1958–9.

Chapter 11
Common Male Infertility Disorders: Aging

Fabio Pasqualotto, Edson Borges Jr., and Eleonora Pasqualotto

Approximately 15% of couples of reproductive age experience infertility, and approximately 1/3 to half of infertility cases may be attributed to male factors [1]. It is well known that maternal age is a significant contributor to human infertility [2], due primarily to the precipitous loss of functional oocytes in women by their late 30s [3]. Human spermatogenesis, on the other hand, continues well into advanced ages, allowing men to reproduce during senescence. Although very little is known about the topic, paternal age may also contribute to human infertility.

It is well known that practically no children are born to mothers aged >50 years and it is common to all older fathers that they have younger partners. The discrepancy in the reproductive arena between males and females is astonishing, and reduced fertility and higher reproductive risks associated with advancing maternal age raise the question whether advanced paternal age is also associated with compromised fertility and increasing risks. In addition, it is well documented a progressive decrease of fertility due to both quantitative and qualitative loss of oocytes, eventually ending in menopause, women experience an age-dependent increase of miscarriages, obstetric morbidities, and chromosomal anomalies of the fetus [4].

F. Pasqualotto, MD, PhD (✉)
Department of Anatomy and Urology, Institute of Biotechnology,
University of Caxias do Sul, Caxias do Sul, RS, Brazil

CONCEPTION—Center for Human Reproduction, Caxias do Sul, RS, Brazil
e-mail: fabio@conception-rs.com.br

E. Borges Jr., MD
Department of Fertility, Center for Assisted Fertilization,
Av. Brigadeiro Luis Antomiom 4545, Sao Paulo, 01401-002, Brazil

E. Pasqualotto, MD, PhD
CONCEPTION—Center for Human Reproduction, Caxias do Sul, RS, Brazil

Department of Clinical Medicine, Center of Health Science, University of Caxias do Sul,
R. Pinheiro Machado, 2569, sl 23/24, Caxias do Sul, RS, Brazil

S.J. Parekattil and A. Agarwal (eds.), *Antioxidants in Male Infertility: A Guide
for Clinicians and Researchers*, © Springer Science+Business Media New York 2013

This question should be discussed to younger age groups since increasing numbers of couples postpone parenthood into their fourth or fifth decade of life.

In contrast to the female, male reproductive functions do not cease abruptly, but androgen production and spermatogenesis continue lifelong. However, to evaluate a possible decline in the semen quality is a little bit difficult. Some men are reluctant to provide semen samples unless actively concerned about their fertility. For instance, population-based studies typically recruit at least 20% of young men willing to provide semen samples [5] constituting an inevitable participation bias in such studies [6, 7]. In addition, most of the published studies about sperm output in older men are largely restricted to patients attending infertility clinics, where few are older than 50 years [8]. An uncertain, but probably high proportion of such men have unrecognized defects in sperm production and/or function. Furthermore, access to such specialized medical services may be strongly influenced by nonbiological factors, and the results from infertility clinics may not be reliably extrapolated to the general male population.

Anyway, the effects of paternal age on a couple's fertility are real and may be greater than has previously been thought. Ford et al. stated that, after adjustments for other factors, the probability that a fertile couple will take >12 months to conceive nearly doubles from 8% when the man is <25 years to 15% when he is >35 years; thus, paternal age is a further factor to be taken into account when deciding the prognosis for infertile couples [9].

To explain the age-dependent changes observed in semen quality, two issues should be considered [8–11]. First, cellular or physiological changes due to aging have been described in testicles, seminal vesicles, prostate, and epididymis. Age-related narrowing and sclerosis of the testicular tubular lumen, decreases in spermatogenic activity, increased degeneration of germ cells, and decreased numbers and function of Leydig cells have been found in autopsies of men who died from accidental causes [12]. Smooth muscle atrophy and a decrease in protein and water content, which occur in the prostate with aging, may contribute to decreased semen volume and sperm motility. Also, the epididymis, a hormonally sensitive tissue, may undergo age-related changes. The hormonal or epididymal senescence may lead to decreased motility in older men. Secondly, increasing age implies more frequent exposure to exogenous damage or disease [8]. In addition to age per se, factors such as urogenital infections, vascular diseases, or an accumulation of toxic substances (cigarettes) may be responsible for worsening semen parameters. Indeed, a retrospective cross-sectional study in 3,698 infertile men showed an infection rate of the accessory glands in 6.1% in patients aged <25 years but in 13.6% of patients >40 years, and total sperm counts were significantly lower in patients with an infection of the accessory glands [13]. In addition, an age-dependent increase of polychlorinated biphenyls (PBC) in men has been described, and in men with normal semen parameters, the PBC concentration is inversely correlated with sperm count and progressive motility [14]. The concentration of cadmium also increases with age in the human testis, epididymis, and prostate, although lead and selenium remain constant over the whole age range in reproductive organs [15, 16].

Handelsman and Staraj demonstrated that, after exclusion of men with different diseases associated with diminishing testicular size, the specific effects of age on testicular volume appear only in the eighth decade of life [17]. In healthy men of this age group, the testis volume is 31% lower than in 18–40-year-old men [18]. However, recently a study showed a decline in testicular volume over time, especially after the age of 45 years old [19].

Morphological characteristics of aging testes vary from Sertoli cells accumulating cytoplasmic lipid droplets and are reduced in number [20], as are the Leydig cells [21], which may also be multinucleated [22]. Tubule involution is associated with an enlargement of the tunica propria, leading to progressive sclerosis parallel to a reduction of the seminiferous epithelium with complete tubular sclerosis as an endpoint [23]. Testicular sclerosis is associated with defective vascularization of the testicular parenchyma and with systemic arteriosclerosis of affected men [24]. Arteriographic patterns of the epididymis and the testes support these findings and are correlated with the degree of systemic arteriosclerosis [24]. In addition, age-dependent alterations of the prostate are well known [25] and are detectable histologically in 50% of 50-year-old men, but in 90% of men aged >90 years [26].

Common Male Infertility Disorders: Aging

Semen Analysis

Considering the age-dependent changes in reproductive organs of men, variations in semen parameters over time are not surprising; however, only few studies are controlled for abstinence time and other possible factors that may influence semen quality such as hypertension or smoking habits. Most studies are retrospective and rarely include males with more than 60 or 70 years old. Pasqualotto et al. recently described a decrease in semen volume across the groups evaluated in the study [19]. In fact, reports in the literature have shown a decrease in semen volume with aging [8, 27, 28]. The higher number of days' abstinence in men over 50 years old could explain these results. In the studies where the analyses were adjusted for days' abstinence, a decrease in semen volume of 3–22% was observed [9].

Regarding sperm motility, many studies adjusted for time of abstinence found a significant decrease in sperm motility associated with age and a yearly decrease ranging between 0.17% [29] and 0.7% [30]. However, these studies were performed in sperm donors [29–32] as well as in infertile patients [33, 34]. Pasqualotto et al. are in the same page than others showing that sperm motility tends to decrease as time goes by. Those studies that have been adjusted for duration of abstinence have reported statistically significant effects, such as negative linear relationships and decreases in motility ranging from 0.17 to 0.6% for each year of age [8, 29, 35, 36].

A computer-assisted semen analysis (CASA) has been developed as a specific tool to make the assessment of semen quality more objective and detailed [37].

Several specific motility parameters describing the movements of spermatozoa in a more detailed manner can be obtained with CASA. In addition, the classification into motile and immotile spermatozoa can be based on well-defined velocity thresholds. However, no correlations are detected between specific motion parameters as evaluated with CASA and the aging effect in the study by Pasqualotto et al. [19].

When focusing on sperm concentration, abstinence-adjusted studies do not provide a uniform picture. Even though some studies have reported a decrease in sperm concentration with increased age, several other studies have reported an increase in sperm concentration with age or found little or no association between age and sperm concentration [9, 11, 35, 38]. In fact, there are two different populations that we have to consider before evaluating the results: fertile vs. infertile men. A significant age-dependent decrease [30, 32] as well as constant values over the age range [31] or even a nonsignificant age-dependent increase with age [29] has been detected in healthy men. Regarding the infertile population, sperm concentration increases [33, 34] or remains unaltered [13], as indicated in abstinence-adjusted studies.

One of the good indicators of the germinal epithelium status is the sperm morphology. Degenerative changes in the germinal epithelium because of aging may affect spermatogenesis and thus sperm morphology. Pasqualotto et al., based on a linear regression analysis, stated that normal sperm morphology tends to decrease by 0.039% each year [19]. Auger et al., in a linear regression model, have shown that the normal sperm morphology decreases 0.9% yearly [32]. Thus, as compared to the average 30-year-old man, an average 50-year-old had an 18% decrease in normally shaped sperm [33]. Ng et al. showed that older men had more abnormal sperm morphology with decreasing numbers of normal forms and reduced vitality, as well as increased numbers of cytoplasmic droplets and sperm tail abnormalities (30% vs. 17%) compared to younger men [28]. The aberrant sperm morphology in older men was most evident in defects of tail morphology, possibly reflecting the complex cellular structural assembly process of the axoneme. Such increasing proportion of defects may reflect degenerative changes with aging in the germinal epithelium and/or in the intrinsic program directing spermiogenesis. In fact, the decrease per year varies from 0.2% [36] to 0.9% [32].

All reported changes of histological and seminal parameters develop gradually without a sudden age threshold. The alterations in semen parameters fall within normal ranges. Nevertheless, the age-dependent alterations of testicular histology and semen parameters are accompanied by a significant increase in FSH [19, 39] and a slight but significant decrease in inhibin B [18, 40], which are also found in men with apparently normal semen parameters.

Fertility of Aging Men

Without any type of doubt, male fertility is basically maintained until very late in life, and it has been documented scientifically up to more than 90 years old [41]. Besides female age, further confounders, such as reduced coital frequency, an increasing incidence of erectile dysfunction, and smoking habits, have to be considered in studies analyzing male fertility. All studies focused on a nonclinical population found a significant negative relationship between male age and couples' fertility.

A retrospective study of a large sample of European couples analyzed the risk of difficulties (due to adverse pregnancy outcomes, such as ectopic pregnancy, miscarriage, or stillbirth, or due to delayed conception) and the risk of delay in pregnancy onset [42]. Age-related changes were also found in a prospective study that estimated day-specific probabilities for pregnancy relative to ovulation [43]. Frequency of sexual intercourse was monitored by sexual diaries, and ovulation was based on basal body temperature measurements. According to this study, fertility for men aged >35 years is significantly reduced, and the age effect of men aged 35–40 years is about the same as when intercourse frequency drops from twice per week to once per week [44]. In studies dealing with subfertile couples, a significant decrease in pregnancy rates [33] or increase in TTP [45] was observed with female but not with male age, possibly indicating that male age-dependent alterations are masked by the infertility as such.

With methods of assisted reproduction, prerequisites for natural conception such as motility or fertilizing capacity are circumvented. In fact, the more invasive the treatment, the less important male age appears. Therefore, the success rates of ICSI [46] or IVF [47–49] are not associated with male age. On the other hand, the success rate of intrauterine insemination (IUI), a method requiring much higher quality and capability of sperm, is without question related to male age [50, 51].

Reactive Oxygen Species Generation from Mitochondria

Mitochondria play an important role in cellular energy generation, apoptosis regulation, and calcium homeostasis [52]. Coupled to the tricarboxylic acid cycle, the electron transport chain (ETC), and adenosine triphosphate (ATP) synthase in the mitochondria generate ATP, being the source of most cellular energy [52]. The mitochondrial respiratory chain is also the major intracellular source of reactive oxygen species (ROS) and free radicals under normal physiological and pathological conditions. It has been thought that loss of mitochondrial function and increased mitochondrial ROS production are important causal factors in aging.

In fact, it has been suggested that loss of mitochondrial function and increased mitochondrial ROS production are important causal factors in aging. Superoxide is continually produced as a by-product of normal cellular respiration [53]. As electrons are passed from complexes I to IV in the mitochondrial ETC, continuous leakage of electrons occurs, forming superoxide (1% of total rate of electron transport) [54]. This superoxide is converted to hydrogen peroxide by manganese superoxide dismutase in the mitochondrial matrix under physiological conditions. Superoxide oxidizes iron–sulfur-containing enzymes such as aconitase that produces hydrogen peroxide and ferrous iron [55].

A wide spectrum of alterations in mitochondria and mitochondrial DNA (mtDNA) with aging has been observed in animals and humans. These include (1) decline in mitochondrial respiratory function; (2) increase in mitochondrial production of reactive oxygen species (ROS) and the extent of oxidative damage to DNA, proteins, and lipids; (3) accumulation of point mutations and large-scale deletions of mtDNA; and (4) enhanced apoptosis. Recent studies have provided abundant evidence to substantiate the importance of mitochondrial production of ROS in aging. On the other hand, somatic mtDNA mutations can cause premature aging without increasing ROS production.

The formation of hydrogen peroxide from superoxide and its transformation to hydroxyl radical is apparent, especially when the mitochondrial ETC is abnormal or compromised [53]. Among five mitochondrial ETC complexes, complex I (nicotinamide adenine dinucleotide [NADH]–ubiquinone oxidoreductase) and complex III (ubiquinol–cytochrome c oxidoreductase) are responsible for most of the superoxide production [53]. Numerous studies have used mitochondrial ETC inhibitors such as rotenone and antimycin to disrupt the flow of electrons through complexes I and III, respectively [53, 56, 57]. Mitochondrial superoxide production generally is greater in antimycin-inhibited complex III than in rotenone-inhibited complex I [53, 57]. However, superoxide production by complex III is minimal in the absence of antimycin. Therefore, it can be suggested that in vivo complex I is responsible for much of mitochondrial ROS production through reversed and forward electron transport [57].

Mitochondria are more susceptible to oxidative damage because of the active production of ROS, as mtDNA is not protected by histones [58]. Therefore, mitochondrial ROS production damages the mitochondria themselves [58]. A dysfunctional mitochondrial respiratory chain would lead to more ROS production. Oxidative damage is more prevalent in mtDNA and protein in vivo than in other cell components [59].

Reactive Oxygen Species and Human Spermatozoa

Small amounts of ROS are continuously produced in the spermatozoa and play a crucial role in capacitation, hyperactivation, motility, acrosome reaction, and ultimately, normal fertilization [60]. Located at the midpiece of the spermatozoa, mitochondria function to produce ATP necessary for the physiological functions of the spermatozoa. Electrons leaking out of the mitochondrial respiratory chain contribute to superoxide production in the spermatozoa, such as in somatic cells [56]. Koppers et al. [56] recently were the first to demonstrate that mitochondria in human spermatozoa can produce ROS. They also suggested that rotenone-inhibited complex I, not antimycin, induces peroxidative damage in the midpiece of the spermatozoa. This continuous ROS generation induces oxidative damage to somatic cells as well as the spermatozoa, although spermatozoa are particularly susceptible to ROS damage because of the high content of polyunsaturated fatty acid in the cell membrane. ROS also reduces sperm motility by decreasing axonemal protein phosphorylation, as well as by lipid peroxidation [60].

Effects of Reactive Oxygen Species on Telomere and Telomerase

Telomeres are noncoding, repetitive DNA sequences (TTAGGG) at the ends of eukaryotic chromosomes that function to stabilize and protect chromosome ends. Progressive reduction of telomere length to a critically short size is related to the cessation of cell division and the onset of senescence. The enzyme telomerase adds specific TTAGGG sequence at the chromosome ends and maintains the length of the telomere. Telomerase is found in the male germ line cell, activated lymphocytes, and certain stem cell populations [61, 62]. It has been demonstrated telomerase activity in human testes [63]. Telomerase activity is highly critical in the germ line cells because of its task of preserving the full length chromosome of the cells and to maintain spermatogenesis. Yashima et al. observed variations in the location of telomerase expression in testis between the end of the prepubertal period and adulthood [64]. Before puberty, telomerase is highly expressed in immature Sertoli cells, whereas in advanced age groups, the telomerase expression is highest in the germ cells of the seminiferous tubules [64].

ROS also can affect telomere function indirectly by their interaction with telomerase. Intracellular ROS leads to a loss of activity of telomerase reverse transcriptase (TERT), whereas antioxidants such as *N*-acetylcysteine delay the onset of cell senescence [65]. Zhu et al. [66] suggested that decreased activity of catalytic subunits of telomerase (mTERT) increases neuronal cell susceptibility to oxidative stress. In embryonic mouse neurons, the decrease in the level of mTERT is directly related to the increase in apoptosis induced by oxidative stress. Consequently, the catalytic subunits of telomerase may play a role in protection from oxidative stress.

In fact, ROS-induced telomere shortening may be due to direct injury to guanine repeat telomere DNA by ROS. Using a culture of human WI-38 fibroblasts, it was demonstrated that telomere shortening is significantly increased under mild oxidative stress compared with that observed under normal conditions [67]. Most importantly, the addition of an antioxidant suppresses the rate of telomere shortening in somatic cells. Furumoto et al. [68] showed that the telomere shortening rate slowed after enrichment by ascorbic acid, a very potent antioxidant. Overexpression of the extracellular superoxide dismutase gene in human fibroblasts decreased the peroxide content, decreasing the rate of telomere shortening [67]. The rate of telomere shortening in sheep and humans is directly related to the cellular oxidative stress levels [69].

Deleterious conditions including dysfunctional telomeres, genomic instability, and apoptosis may result from telomere shortening in both somatic and germ line cells. A shortened telomere may limit the potential for replication and could result in genomic instability. This instability may play a role in about 70% of conceptions lost before birth, and also in 50% of spontaneous abortions with detectable chromosomal abnormalities [70]. It is important to notice here that to keep the telomere length may be essential for healthy human spermatozoa.

Antioxidants and Aging

Antioxidants play a crucial role in minimizing oxidative damage in the spermatozoa [71]. Studies have shown that along with an increase in ROS with aging, the antioxidant defense activity decreases with aging [58, 72]. Using Brown Norway rats, the antioxidant enzymatic activities in epididymal spermatozoa from young (4 months old) and old (21 months old) rats were compared [73]. Their study showed that antioxidants such as glutathione peroxidase (Gpx1, Gpx4) and superoxide dismutase had decreased activity in aging spermatozoa. However, ROS production and lipid peroxidation were significantly increased in their study. Examining the activities of copper–zinc superoxide dismutase, manganese superoxide dismutase, and glutathione peroxidase in Leydig cells isolated from 4- and 20-month-old rats, noting related to the age were detected regarding all antioxidant enzymatic activities [74]. The authors concluded that age-related reductions in testosterone levels of Leydig cells may be associated with the impairment of the antioxidant defense system of these cells.

Lipofuscin, also known as *age pigment*, is a marker of cell senescence [75]. It is an intralysosomal polymeric material that cannot be degraded or exocytosed, and continuously accumulates during the lifespan of a cell. It has been suggested that lipofuscin formation is ruled by ROS, mainly hydrogen peroxide, which is a by-product of normal oxygen metabolism that is produced continuously by mitochondria, peroxisomes, and cytosolic oxidases [75]. It is largely eliminated by catalase and glutathione peroxidase. However, it partially diffuses through lysosomal membranes. The Fenton reaction takes place in the presence of iron; the reducing substance (such as cysteine) is converted into a hydroxyl radical that induces peroxidation of various degraded macromolecules in the lysosome. This results in the formation of a cross-linked, nondegradable material called lipofuscin. Thus, ROS are involved in the accumulation of lipofuscin inside lysosomes. An age-related increase in lipofuscin formation is also seen in male reproductive tissue. Significantly large amounts of lipofuscin were found in the Leydig cells of elderly men compared to younger men [76]. Lipofuscin content matches the apoptosis indices of Leydig and epididymal cells. ROS are produced by Leydig cells during steroid genesis (testosterone synthesis), as well as by spermatozoal mitochondria [77]. Therefore, the ROS production might be responsible for Leydig cell aging, considering that inhibition of steroid genesis has been shown to prevent Leydig cell aging [76].

Amyloid (an insoluble protein aggregate) deposition affords additional evidence that ROS play a significant role in the loss of testicular function with aging. An age-dependent increase in oxidative stress and oxidative damage to cellular proteins contribute to amyloid formation [77]. Amyloid formation is associated with age-related increases in the fraction of abnormally folded proteins and decreases in the functions of proteases that degrade newly synthesized proteins [77]. The protein aggregates promote formation of protein aggregates by serving as nucleation sites. Amyloid fibrils with protease resistant structures are not reversible when formed, and promote further formation of protein aggregates. Age-related accumulation of intracellular amyloid fibrils in Sertoli cells of atrophic testes has also been described [78].

Aging and Sperm DNA Damage: Genomic Defects in Offspring

The association between aging and sperm DNA damage has been extensively studied during the last decade. Singh et al. showed higher levels of double-stranded DNA breaks in older men (by comet assay) [79]. Wyrobek et al. found an inverse relationship between DNA fragmentation index and male age by sperm chromatin structure assay [80]. Increasing oxidative stress levels associated with aging might be responsible for this increase in DNA damage with age [81, 82]. Oxidative stress-mediated DNA damage may be an etiology for repeated assisted reproductive technology failures in older men [83]. Increasing male age may have an influence on DNA fragmentation in the form of single-strand breaks [84]. This may not have any effect on fertilization because the oocyte can repair single-strand breaks. However, if the oocyte repair mechanisms are dysfunctional, this may result in poor, if not failed, blastocyst formation. Thus, oxidative stress-induced DNA damage can lead to various genomic defects [85, 86]. Plas et al. [85] showed a positive correlation between structural chromosomal abnormalities and paternal age, with a fourfold increase in abnormalities in the 45 years of age group compared with men aged 20–24 years. They also suggested that children of men in advanced age groups have 20% higher risk of carrying autosomal dominant diseases potentially due to increasing germ cell mitoses and meioses [85].

It is interesting to note that a direct relationship occurs between paternal aging and offspring development [87]. Considerable evidence shows a connection between aging and offspring learning and cognition. One study conducted by Reichenberg et al. [88] examining Israeli births over a consecutive 6-year period concluded that offspring of men 40 years or older were 5.75 times more likely to develop autism spectrum disorder than those of men younger than 30 years. The possible etiologies for that consisted of genetic imprinting alterations and de novo mutations. An older study showed an increased risk of trisomy 21 in offspring of older men, with a profound age effect in men 41 years and older [89]. Because the spontaneous mutation rate closely relates to paternal age, it can be suggested that the progeny of advanced male age groups experience a higher frequency of imprinting disorders such as Beckwith–Wiedemann syndrome, which involves insulin-like growth factor 2, a paternally expressed gene. This syndrome is characterized by abdominal wall defects, macroglossia, and susceptibility to embryonic tumor.

Structural Chromosomal Anomalies

Structural chromosomal anomalies result from chromosomal breakage and the following abnormal rearrangement within the same or within different chromosomes. In 84% of cases, de novo structural aberrations are of paternal origin [90], and they are found in 2% of spontaneous abortions and in 0.6% of live births [91]. Cytogenetic studies on structural chromosomal anomalies in sperm are rare but consistently describe an increase of mutations with age [92].

FISH was used for the structural analysis of individual chromosomes: duplications and deletions for the centromeric and subtelomeric regions of chromosome 9 increase significantly with age [93]. In spite of these age-dependent structural alterations in sperm, no increase of de novo structural chromosomal anomalies has been detected in newborns from older fathers [94].

Autosomal Dominant Diseases

Achondroplasia, the most common form of dwarfism, is the first genetic disorder that was hypothesized to have a paternal age component [95]. Apert's syndrome and achondroplasia have been amenable to direct sperm DNA mutation analysis [96, 97], and both are characterized by an age-dependent increase of mutations in sperm, but there are some peculiarities. For sporadic cases of Crouzon's or Pfeiffer's syndrome, 11 different mutations of the FGFR 2 gene are responsible, indicating that, unlike Apert's syndrome or achondroplasia, these are genetically heterogeneous conditions [98]. These mutations also arise in the male germ line, and advanced paternal age was noted for fathers of those patients.

The relationship between mutation frequency and paternal age is heterogeneous among autosomal dominantly inherited diseases [99]. In contrast to the above-mentioned diseases, osteogenesis imperfecta, neurofibromatosis, or bilateral retinoblastoma shows a weak paternal age effect [100]. Many of the mutations of the neurofibromatosis gene are intragenic deletions. These deletions are not age-dependent because they occur by mechanisms other than the base substitutions and are maternally derived in 16 of 21 cases [101].

Due to this heterogeneity of the paternal age effect in autosomal dominant diseases, the risk estimates proposed by Friedman for paternal age and autosomal dominant mutations may be overestimated [102]. Friedman calculated a risk for autosomal dominant diseases of 0.3–0.5% among offspring of fathers aged >40 years. This risk is comparable with the risk of Down's syndrome for 35–40-year-old women. However, the calculation was based on the assumption that the paternal age effect found in achondroplasia is typical of all autosomal dominant diseases.

There are conflicting data for Alzheimer's disease. Few studies conclude that paternal age is a risk factor [103]. However, the inconsistent results may be due to small sample sizes of the studies or due to the genetic heterogeneity of the disease.

Regarding schizophrenia, there are more conclusive data. In fact, the studies identified an increased risk of schizophrenia with paternal age [104]. Patients without a family history of schizophrenia had significantly older fathers than familial patients, so that de novo mutations were considered responsible [105]. Preeclampsia, which is considered to be a risk factor for schizophrenia, is also associated with paternal age [106].

One very important point we should never forget is that advanced paternal age increases the risk of other cancers in offspring. According to the Swedish Family-Cancer Database, there is an effect of paternal age on the incidence of sporadic breast and sporadic nervous system cancer in offspring [107]. Interestingly, an association between paternal age and the son's risk of prostate cancer was found [108]. The association of paternal age with early-onset prostate cancer (<65 years) was greater than that with late onset.

Expert Commentary

Most studies suggest that reduced fertility begins to become evident in the late 30s in men. Increased male age is associated with an increased risk of miscarriages, and both the risk of infertility and the risk of miscarriage strongly depend on female age. Couples should be aware of these age-dependent alterations in fertility and predisposition to genetic risks. Although at the moment increased paternal age is not an indication for prenatal diagnosis, there may be further developments in the future.

Although abundant experimental data have been gathered in the past decade to support the concept that mitochondrial dysfunction, ROS overproduction, and accumulation of mtDNA mutations in tissue cells are important contributors to human aging, the detailed mechanisms by which these biochemical events cause human aging remain to be established. The functional genomics and proteomics approaches to study aging on a genome-wide basis will provide novel information so we may gain a deeper understanding of the age-related alterations in the structure and function of mitochondria in the aging process. This is critical for the elucidation of the molecular mechanism of aging and for better management of aging and age-related diseases in humans.

Five-Year View

ROS are continually produced in the mitochondria of spermatozoa and play an important role in age-related male reproductive pathophysiology. The increased ROS level in semen observed with aging is associated with a possible decrease in antioxidant enzyme activity. This imbalance between prooxidants and antioxidants induces oxidative damage, resulting in abnormalities in telomeres and telomerase in male germ line cells. This sequence of events may explain the decrease in sperm concentration seen with aging. Oxidative stress in aging male reproductive system may inhibit sperm axonemal phosphorylation and increase lipid peroxidation, which can decrease sperm motility. This oxidative stress can also lead to lipofuscin and amyloid accumulation in the male reproductive tract, potentially the cause of decreased Leydig cell function and a subsequent decrease in blood testosterone levels. A higher rate of lipofuscin accumulation, in turn, may increase the amount of dysfunctional mitochondria in spermatozoa, thus increasing ROS formation.

Along with its negative effect on the fertilizing potential of spermatozoa, ROS also leads to offspring malformation (if fertilization is successful). Oxidative stress-induced mtDNA damage and nuclear DNA damage in aging men may put them at a higher risk for transmitting multiple genetic and chromosomal defects. Thus, this review suggests that ROS might play a central role in decreased male fertility with aging. This hypothesis provides guidance for future study and experiments, focusing on specific biomarkers of aging in men (telomere function, lipofuscin, amyloid) and their comparison with semen parameters and male fertility.

Key Issues

As life expectancy increases and our lives become busiest every day, many couples are waiting longer to establish their families. The recent trend toward delayed parenthood raises concerns because of the adverse effects of aging on fertility. Aging is a biological process that is characterized by the gradual loss of physiological function and increases in the susceptibility to disease of an individual. During the aging process, a wide spectrum of alterations in mitochondria and mitochondrial DNA (mtDNA) has been observed in somatic tissues of humans and animals. This is associated with the decline in mitochondrial respiratory function; excess production of the reactive oxygen species (ROS); increase in the oxidative damage to mtDNA, lipids, and proteins in mitochondria; accumulation of point mutations and large-scale deletions of mtDNA; and altered expression of genes involved in intermediary metabolism.

It has been demonstrated that the ROS may cause oxidative damage and mutations of mtDNA and alterations of the expression of several clusters of genes in aging tissues and senescent cells. The respiratory function decline and increase in the production of the ROS in mitochondria, accumulation of mtDNA mutation and oxidative damage, and altered expression of a few clusters of genes that culminated in the metabolic shift from mitochondrial respiration to glycolysis for major supply of ATP were key contributory factors in the aging process in the human and animals.

Although based on a small number of cases, the data presented for testicular morphology, semen parameters and fertility in aging males are conclusive and reflect a gradual deterioration with age within a broad individual spectrum. Most studies suggest that reduced fertility begins to become evident in the late 30s in men. Increased male age is associated with an increased risk of miscarriages, and both the risk of infertility and the risk of miscarriage strongly depend on female age. Advancing paternal age is associated with an increased risk for trisomy 21 and with diseases of complex etiology such as schizophrenia. Couples should be aware of these age-dependent alterations in fertility and predisposition to genetic risks. Although at the moment increased paternal age is not an indication for prenatal diagnosis, there may be further developments in the future.

References

1. Templeton A. Infertility-epidemiology, aetiology and effective management. Health Bull (Edinb). 1995;53(5):294–8.
2. Joffe M, Li Z. Male and female factors in fertility. Am J Epidemiol. 1995;141(11):1107–8.
3. Lansac J. Delayed parenting. Is delayed childbearing a good thing? Hum Reprod. 1995;10(5):1033–5.
4. Lubna P, Santoro N. Age-related decline in fertility. Endocrinol Metab Clin North Am. 2003; 32:669–88.
5. Jensen TK, Jorgensen N, Punab M, Haugen TB, Suominen J, Zilaitiene B, Horte A, Andersen AG, Carlsen E, Magnus O, et al. Association of in utero exposure to maternal smoking with reduced semen quality and testis size in adulthood: a cross-sectional study of 1 770 young men from the general population in five European countries. Am J Epidemiol. 2004; 159:49–58.
6. Handelsman DJ. Sperm output of healthy men in Australia: magnitude of bias due to self-selected volunteers. Hum Reprod. 1997;12:2701–5.
7. Cohn BA, Overstreet JW, Fogel RJ, Brazil CK, Baird DD, Cirillo PM. Epidemiologic studies of human semen quality: considerations for study design. Am J Epidemiol. 2002;155: 664–71.
8. Kidd SA, Eskenazi B, Wyrobek AJ. Effects of male age on semen quality and fertility: a review of the literature. Fertil Steril. 2001;75:237–48.
9. Ford WCL, North K, Taylor H, Farrow A, Hull MGR, Golding J, The ALSPAC Study Team. Increasing paternal age is associated with delayed conception in a large population of fertile couples: evidence for declining fecundity in older men. Hum Reprod. 2000;15:1703–8.
10. Eskenazi B, Wyrobek AJ, Sloter E, Kidd SA, Moore L, Young S, Moore D. The association of age and semen quality in healthy men. Hum Reprod. 2003;18:447–54.
11. Hassan MAM, Killick SR. Effect of male age on fertility: evidence for the decline in male fertility with increasing age. Fertil Steril. 2003;79:1520–7.
12. Neaves WB, Johnson L, Porter JC, Parker CR, Petty S. Leydig cell numbers, daily sperm production and serum gonadotropin levels in aging men. J Clin Endocrinol Metab. 1984;59:756–63.
13. Rolf C, Kenkel S, Nieschlag E. Age-related disease pattern in infertile men: increasing incidence of infections in older patients. Andrologia. 2002;34:209–17.
14. Dallinga JW, Moonen EJ, Dumoulin JC, Evers JL, Geraedts JP, Kleinjans JC. Decreased human semen quality and organochlorine compounds in blood. Hum Reprod. 2002; 17:1973–99.
15. Oldereid NB, Thomassen Y, Attramadal A, Olaisen B, Purvis K. Concentrations of lead, cadmium and zinc in the tissues of reproductive organs of men. J Reprod Fertil. 1993; 99:421–55.
16. Oldereid NB, Thomassen Y, Purvis K. Selenium in human male reproductive organs. Hum Reprod. 1998;13:2172–6.
17. Handelsman DJ, Staraj S. Testicular size: the effects of aging, malnutrition, and illness. J Androl. 1985;6:144–51.
18. Mahmoud AM, Goemaere S, El-Garem Y, Van Pottelbergh I, Comhaire FH, Kaufman JM. Testicular volume in relation to hormonal indices of gonadal function in community-dwelling elderly men. J Clin Endocrinol Metab. 2003;88:179–84.
19. Pasqualotto FF, Sobreiro BP, Hallak J, Pasqualotto EB, Lucon AM. Sperm concentration and normal sperm morphology decrease and follicle-stimulating hormone level increases with age. BJU Int. 2005;96:1087–91.
20. Harbitz TB. Morphometric studies of the Sertoli cells in elderly men with special reference to the histology of the prostate. Acta Pathol Microbiol Scand Sect A Pathol. 1973;81:703–17.
21. Johnson L. Spermatogenesis and aging in the human. J Androl. 1986;7:331–54.

22. Paniagua R, Amat P, Nistal M, Martin A. Ultrastructure of Leydig cells in human ageing testes. J Anat. 1986;146:173–83.

23. Paniagua R, Nistal M, Amat P, Rodriguez MC, Martin A. Seminiferous tubule involution in elderly men. Biol Reprod. 1987;36:939–47.

24. Regadera J, Nistal M, Paniagua R. Testis, epididymis, and spermatic cord in elderly men. Correlation of angiographic and histologic studies with systemic arteriosclerosis. Arch Pathol Lab Med. 1985;109:663–7.

25. Hermann M, Untergasser G, Rumpold H, Berger P. Aging of the male reproductive system. Exp Gerontol. 2000;35:1267–79.

26. Coffey DS, Berry SJ, Ewing LL. An overview of current concepts in the study of benign prostate hyperplasia. In: Rodgers CH, Coffey DS, Cunha G, Grayhack JT, Hinman F, Horton R, editors. Benign prostatic hyperplasia. Vol II. Washington, DC: US Department of Health and Human Services, NIH publication No. 87-2881; 1987. p. 1–13.

27. Kühnert B, Nieschlag E. Reproductive functions of the ageing male. Hum Reprod Update. 2004;10:327–39.

28. Ng KK, Donat R, Chan L, Lalak A, Di Pierro I, Handelsman DJ. Sperm output of older men. Hum Reprod. 2004;8:1811–5.

29. Fisch H, Goluboff ET, Olson JH, Feldshuh J, Broder SJ, Barad DH. Semen analysis in 1,283 men from the United States over a 25-year period: no decline in quality. Fertil Steril. 1996;65:1009–14.

30. Eskenazi B, Wyrobek AJ, Kidd SA, Lowe X, Moore II D, Weisiger K, Aylstock M. Sperm aneuploidy in fathers of children with paternally and maternally inherited Klinefelter syndrome. Hum Reprod. 2002;17:576–83.

31. Schwartz D, Mayaux MJ, Spira A, Moscato ML, Jouannet P, Czyglik F, David G. Semen characteristics as a function of age in 833 fertile men. Fertil Steril. 1983;39:530–5.

32. Auger J, Kunstmann JM, Czyglik F, Jouannet P. Decline in semen quality among fertile men in Paris during the past 20 years. N Engl J Med. 1995;332:281–5.

33. Rolf C, Behre HM, Nieschlag E. Reproductive parameters of older couples compared to younger men of infertile couples. Int J Androl. 1996;19:135–42.

34. Andolz P, Bielsa MA, Vila J. Evolution of semen quality in North-eastern Spain: a study in 22 759 infertile men over a 36 year period. Hum Reprod. 1999;14:731–5.

35. Berling S, Wolner-Hanssen P. No evidence of deteriorating semen quality among men in infertile relationships during the last decade: a study of males from southern Sweden. Hum Reprod. 1997;12:1002–5.

36. Carlsen E, Giwercman A, Keiding N, Skakkebaek NE. Evidence for decreasing quality of semen during past 50 years. BMJ. 1992;305:609–13.

37. Agarwal A, Ozturk E, Loughlin KR. Comparison of semen analysis between the two Hamilton-Thorn semen analysers. Andrologia. 1992;24:327–9.

38. Hommonai ZT, Fainman N, David MP, Paz GF. Semen quality and sex hormone pattern of 29 middle aged men. Andrologia. 1982;14:164–70.

39. Nieschlag E, Lammers U, Freischem CW, Langer K, Wickings EJ. Reproductive functions in young fathers and grandfathers. J Clin Endocrinol Metab. 1982;55:676–81.

40. Baccarelli A, Morpurgo PS, Corsi A, Vaghi I, Fanelli M, Cremonesi G, Vaninetti S, Beck-Peccoz P, Spada A. Activin A serum levels and aging of the pituitary–gonadal axis: a cross-sectional study in middle-aged and elderly healthy subjects. Exp Gerontol. 2001;36:1403–12.

41. Seymour FI, Duffy C, Koerner A. A case of authenticated fertility in a man, aged 94. J Am Med Assoc. 1935;105:1423–4.

42. de la Rochebrochard E, Thonneau P. Paternal age and maternal age are risk factors for miscarriage; results of a multicentre European study. Hum Reprod. 2002;17:1649–56.

43. Dunson DB, Colombo B, Baird D. Changes with age in the level and duration of fertility in the menstrual cycle. Hum Reprod. 2002;17:1399–403.

44. Dunson DB, Baird DD, Colombo B. Increased infertility with age in men and women. Obstet Gynecol. 2004;103:51–6.

45. Olson J. Subfecundity according to the age of the mother and the father. Dan Med Bull. 1990;37:281–2.
46. Spandorfer SD, Avrech OM, Colombero LT, Palermo GD, Rosenwaks Z. Effect of parental age on fertilization and pregnancy characteristics in couples treated by intracytoplasmic sperm injection. Hum Reprod. 1998;13:334–8.
47. Piette C, de Mouzon J, Bachelot A, Spira A. In-vitro fertilization: influence of women's age on pregnancy rates. Hum Reprod. 1990;5:56–9.
48. Gallardo E, Simón C, Levy M. Effect of age on sperm fertility potential: oocyte donation as a model. Fertil Steril. 1996;66:260–4.
49. Paulson RJ, Milligan RC, Sokol RZ. The lack of influence of age on male fertility. Am J Obstet Gynecol. 2001;184:818–22.
50. Mathieu C, Ecochard R, Bied V, Lornage J, Czyba JC. Cumulative conception rate following intrauterine artificial insemination with husband's spermatozoa: influence of husband's age. Hum Reprod. 1995;10:1090–7.
51. Brzechffa PR, Buyalos RP. Female and male partner age and menotrophin requirements influence pregnancy rates with human menopausal gonadotrophin therapy in combination with intrauterine insemination. Hum Reprod. 1997;12:29–33.
52. McBride HM, Neuspiel M, Wasiak S. Mitochondria: more than just a powerhouse. Curr Biol. 2006;16:R551–60.
53. Raha S, Robinson BH. Mitochondria, oxygen free radicals, disease and ageing. Trends Biochem Sci. 2000;25:502–8.
54. Green K, Brand MD, Murphy MP. Prevention of mitochondrial oxidative damage as a therapeutic strategy in diabetes. Diabetes. 2004;53 suppl 1:S110–8.
55. Vasquez-Vivar J, Kalyanaraman B, Kennedy MC. Mitochondrial aconitase is a source of hydroxyl radical. An electron spin resonance investigation. J Biol Chem. 2000;275:14064–9.
56. Koppers AJ, De Iuliis GN, Finnie JM, et al. Significance of mitochondrial reactive oxygen species in the generation of oxidative stress in spermatozoa. J Clin Endocrinol Metab. 2008;93:3199–207.
57. St-Pierre J, Buckingham JA, Roebuck SJ, et al. Topology of superoxide production from different sites in the mitochondrial electron transport chain. J Biol Chem. 2002;277:44784–90.
58. Wei YH, Ma YS, Lee HC, et al. Mitochondrial theory of aging matures—roles of mtDNA mutation and oxidative stress in human aging. Zhonghua Yi Xue Za Zhi (Taipei). 2001;64:259–70.
59. James AM, Murphy MP. How mitochondrial damage affects cell function. J Biomed Sci. 2002;9:475–87.
60. Agarwal A, Makker K, Sharma R. Clinical relevance of oxidative stress in male factor infertility: an update. Am J Reprod Immunol. 2008;59:2–11.
61. Zalenskaya IA, Zalensky AO. Telomeres in mammalian male germline cells. Int Rev Cytol. 2002;218:37–67.
62. Liu Y, Bohr VA, Lansdorp P. Telomere, telomerase and aging. Mech Ageing Dev. 2008;129:1–2.
63. Fujisawa M, Tanaka H, Tatsumi N, et al. Telomerase activity in the testis of infertile patients with selected causes. Hum Reprod. 1998;13:1476–9.
64. Yashima K, Maitra A, Rogers BB, et al. Expression of the RNA component of telomerase during human development and differentiation. Cell Growth Differ. 1998;9:805–13.
65. Haendeler J, Hoffmann J, Diehl JF, et al. Antioxidants inhibit nuclear export of telomerase reverse transcriptase and delay replicative senescence of endothelial cells. Circ Res. 2004;94:768–75.
66. Zhu H, Fu W, Mattson MP. The catalytic subunit of telomerase protects neurons against amyloid beta-peptide-induced apoptosis. J Neurochem. 2000;75:117–24.
67. Serra V, von Zglinicki T, Lorenz M, et al. Extracellular superoxide dismutase is a major antioxidant in human fibroblasts and slows telomere shortening. J Biol Chem. 2003;278:6824–30.

68. Furumoto K, Inoue E, Nagao N, et al. Age-dependent telomere shortening is slowed down by enrichment of intracellular vitamin C via suppression of oxidative stress. Life Sci. 1998;63:935–48.
69. Richter T, von Zglinicki T. A continuous correlation between oxidative stress and telomere shortening in fibroblasts. Exp Gerontol. 2007;42:1039–42.
70. Baird DM, Britt-Compton B, Rowson J, et al. Telomere instability in the male germline. Hum Mol Genet. 2006;15:45–51.
71. Cocuzza M, Sikka SC, Athayde KS, et al. Clinical relevance of oxidative stress and sperm chromatin damage in male infertility: an evidence based analysis. Int Braz J Urol. 2007;33:603–21.
72. Cao L, Leers-Sucheta S, Azhar S. Aging alters the functional expression of enzymatic and non-enzymatic antioxidant defense systems in testicular rat Leydig's cells. J Steroid Biochem Mol Biol. 2004;88:61–7.
73. Weir CP, Robaire B. Spermatozoa have decreased antioxidant enzymatic capacity and increased reactive oxygen species production during aging in the Brown Norway rat. J Androl. 2007;28:229–40.
74. Luo L, Chen H, Trush MA, et al. Aging and the brown Norway rat Leydig cell antioxidant defense system. J Androl. 2006;27:240–7.
75. Terman A, Gustafsson B, Brunk UT. The lysosomal-mitochondrial axis theory of postmitotic aging and cell death. Chem Biol Interact. 2006;163:29–37.
76. Zirkin BR, Chen H. Regulation of Leydig cell steroidogenic function during aging. Biol Reprod. 2000;63:977–81.
77. Squier TC. Oxidative stress and protein aggregation during biological aging. Exp Gerontol. 2001;36:1539–50.
78. Bohl J, Steinmetz H, Storkel S. Age-related accumulation of congophilic fibrillar inclusions in endocrine cells. Virchows Arch A Pathol Anat Histopathol. 1991;419:51–8.
79. Singh NP, Muller CH, Berger RE. Effects of age on DNA doublestrand breaks and apoptosis in human sperm. Fertil Steril. 2003;80:1420–30.
80. Wyrobek AJ, Eskenazi B, Young S, et al. Advancing age has differential effects on DNA damage, chromatin integrity, gene mutations, and aneuploidies in sperm. Proc Natl Acad Sci USA. 2006;103:9601–6.
81. Desai N, Sabanegu Jr E, Kim T, Agarwal A. Free radical theory of aging: implications in male infertility. Urology. 2010;75:14–9.
82. Angelopoulou R, Lavranos G, Manolakou P. ROS in the aging male: model diseases with ROS-related pathophysiology. Reprod Toxicol. 2009;28:167–71.
83. Shamsi MB, Kumar R, Dada R. Evaluation of nuclear DNA damage in human spermatozoa in men opting for assisted reproduction. Indian J Med Res. 2008;127:115–23.
84. Schmid TE, Eskenazi B, Baumgartner A, et al. The effects of male age on sperm DNA damage in healthy non-smokers. Hum Reprod. 2007;22:180–7.
85. Plas E, Berger P, Hermann M, et al. Effects of aging on male fertility? Exp Gerontol. 2000;35:543–51.
86. Bosco L, Ruvolo G, Morici G, et al. Apoptosis in human unfertilized oocytes after intracytoplasmic sperm injection. Fertil Steril. 2005;84:1417–23.
87. Lawrence LT, Moley KH. Epigenetics and assisted reproductive technologies: human imprinting syndromes. Semin Reprod Med. 2008;26:143–52.
88. Reichenberg A, Gross R, Weiser M, et al. Advancing paternal age and autism. Arch Gen Psychiatry. 2006;63:1026–32.
89. Stene J, Stene E, Stengel-Rutkowski S, et al. Paternal age and Down's syndrome: data from prenatal diagnoses (DFG). Hum Genet. 1981;59:119–24.
90. Olsen SD, Magenis RE. Preferential paternal origin of de novo structural chromosome rearrangements. In: Daniel A, editor. The cytogenetics of mammalian autosomal rearrangements. New York: Alan R. Liss; 1988. p. 583–99.
91. Jacobs PA. The chromosome complement of human gametes. Oxf Rev Reprod Biol. 1992;14:47–72.

92. Sartorelli EM, Mazzucatto LF, de Pina-Neto JM. Effect of paternal age on human sperm chromosomes. Fertil Steril. 2001;76:1119–23.
93. Bosch M, Rajmil O, Martinez-Pasarell O, Egozcue J, Templado C. Linear increase of diploidy in human sperm with age: a four-colour FISH study. Eur J Hum Genet. 2001;9:533–8.
94. Hook EB, Regal RR. A search for a paternal-age effect upon cases of 47, þ 21 in which the extra chromosome is of paternal origin. Am J Hum Genet. 1984;36:413–21.
95. Penrose LS. Parental age and mutation. Lancet. 1955;269:312–3.
96. Glaser RL, Broman KW, Schulman RL, Eskenazi B, Wyrobek AJ, Jabs EW. The paternal-age effect in Apert syndrome is due, in part, to the increased frequency of mutations in sperm. Am J Hum Genet. 2003;73:939–47.
97. Goriely A, McVean GA, Rojmyr M, Ingemarsson B, Wilkie AO. Evidence for selective advantage of pathogenic FGFR2 mutations in the male germ line. Science. 2003;301:643–6.
98. Glaser RL, Jiang W, Boyadjiev SA, Tran AK, Zachary AA, Van Maldergem L, Johnson D, Walsh S, Oldridge M, Wall SA, et al. Paternal origin of FGFR2 mutations in sporadic cases of Crouzon syndrome and Pfeiffer syndrome. Am J Hum Genet. 2000;66:768–77.
99. Risch N, Reich EW, Wishnick MM, McCarthy JG. Spontaneous mutation and parental age in humans. Am J Hum Genet. 1987;41:218–48.
100. Sivakumaran TA, Ghose S, Kumar HAS, Kucheria K. Parental age in Indian patients with sporadic hereditary retinoblastoma. Ophthalmic Epidemiol. 2000;7:285–91.
101. Lazaro C, Gaona A, Ainsworth P, Tenconi R, Vidaud D, Kruyer H, Ars E, Volpini V, Estivill X. Sex differences in the mutation rate and mutational mechanism in the NF gene in neurofibromatosis type 1 patients. Hum Genet. 1996;98:696–9.
102. Friedman JM. Genetic disease in the offspring of older fathers. Obstet Gynecol. 1981;57:745–9.
103. Bertram L, Busch R, Spiegl M, Lautenschlager NT, Müller U, Kurz A. Paternal age is a risk factor for Alzheimer disease in the absence of a major gene. Neurogenetics. 1998;1:277–80.
104. Dalman C, Allebeck P. Paternal age and schizophrenia: further support for an association. Am J Psychiatry. 2002;159:1591–2.
105. Malaspina D, Corcoran C, Fahim C, Berman A, Harkavy-Friedman J, Yale S, Goetz D, Goetz R, Harlap S, Gorman J. Paternal age and sporadic schizophrenia: evidence for de novo mutations. Am J Med Genet. 2002;114:299–303.
106. Harlap S, Paltiel O, Deutsch L, Knaanie A, Masalha S, Tiram E, Caplan LS, Malaspina D, Friedlander Y. Paternal age and preeclampsia. Epidemiology. 2002;13:660–7.
107. Hemminki K, Kyyronen P. Parental age and risk of sporadic and familial cancer in offspring: implications for germ cell mutagenesis. Epidemiology. 1999;10:747–51.
108. Zhang Y, Kreger BE, Dorgan JF, Cupples LA, Myers RH, Splansky GL, Schatzkin A, Ellison RC. Parental age at child's birth and son's risk of prostate cancer. The Framingham Study. Am J Epidemiol. 1999;150:1208–12.

Chapter 12
Apoptosis and Male Infertility

S. Vaithinathan, Shereen Cynthia D'Cruz, and P.P. Mathur

Infertility is a global health issue, affecting approximately 8–10% of couples worldwide. In India, the infertility rate is between 7 and 10% [1]. In the United States, approximately 15% of the couples are infertile, and although infertility is considered to be preliminarily a women's problem, men are responsible in about 20% of infertile cases [2]. In some African countries, one-third of the couples are infertile [3, 4]. Increasing evidence from clinical and epidemiological studies suggests that male infertility could be due to increasing incidence of male reproductive problems. The pathogenesis of male infertility can be reflected by defective spermatogenesis due to pituitary disorders, testicular cancer, germ cell aplasia, varicocele, and environmental factors or due to defective sperm transport resulting from congenital abnormalities, immunological or neurological factors. Recent findings show that male infertility could be increased incidence of genetic disorders and apoptosis [5]. Of these, apoptosis has been identified as a major factor contributing to male fertility and has been studied extensively in recent years.

Apoptosis, also known as programmed cell death (PCD), is required for normal spermatogenesis in mammals and is believed to ensure cellular homeostasis, and an adequate amount of germ cells are eliminated via the process of apoptosis in order to maintain a precise germ cell population in compliance with the supportive capacity of the Sertoli cells. This chapter briefs both physiological and pathological events that can trigger apoptosis and their effects on the male reproductive system.

S. Vaithinathan, PhD • S.C. D'Cruz, MPhil
Department of Biochemistry and Molecular Biology, Pondicherry University,
Kalapet, Pondicherry 605014, India
e-mail: msvnathan@gmail.com; shereencynthia@gmail.com

P.P. Mathur, PhD (✉)
Department of Biochemistry & Molecular Biology and Center for Bioinformatics,
School of Life Sciences, Pondicherry University, Kalapet, Pondicherry 605014, India
e-mail: ppmathur@gmail.com

S.J. Parekattil and A. Agarwal (eds.), *Antioxidants in Male Infertility: A Guide for Clinicians and Researchers*, © Springer Science+Business Media New York 2013

Physiological Role of Apoptosis in Male Reproduction

Testes perform one of the complex events called spermatogenesis, which is necessary for life. Spermatogenesis, a highly dynamic and synchronized process of germ cell maturation from diploid spermatogonia to mature haploid spermatozoa, takes place in the seminiferous epithelium of the testis. This highly intricate cellular development is fostered by the somatic cell type, the Sertoli cells, which envelope the germ cells [6]. During testicular development, the Sertoli cell number increases gradually and thereafter their proliferative capacity declines to produce a stable population of nondividing Sertoli cells [7]. On the other hand, the germ cells continuously proliferate and differentiate to become mature spermatozoa. Overproliferation of germ cells is tempered by selective apoptosis of their progeny in order to maintain a precise germ cell population in compliance with the supportive capacity of the Sertoli cells [7]. Apoptosis also occurs as a defense mechanism such as in immune reactions or when cells are damaged by disease or environmental agents.

Necrosis and apoptosis are the two major mechanisms of cell death. Necrosis occurs in cells that are damaged by external injury, whereas apoptosis occurs in cells that are induced to commit programmed death from internal or external stimuli. Apoptosis consists of highly intricate, sophisticated, and energy-dependent cascade mechanisms and occurs through two main pathways (Fig. 12.1). The first, referred to as the extrinsic or cytoplasmic pathway, is triggered through the Fas death receptor, a member of the tumor necrosis factor (TNF) receptor superfamily [8].

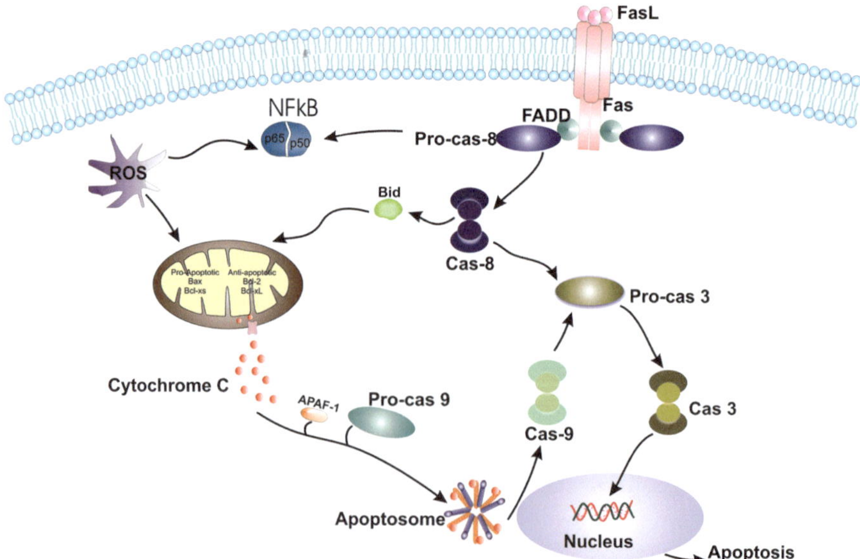

Fig. 12.1 Pathways of apoptosis: Components involved in the mitochondrial and cell death-mediated pathways are shown in the figure

The second pathway is the intrinsic or mitochondrial pathway that when stimulated leads to the release of cytochrome c from the mitochondria and activation of the death signal [9]. Both pathways converge to a final common pathway involving the activation of a cascade of proteases called caspases that cleave regulatory and structural molecules, culminating in the death of the cell. The pathways are linked; thus, the distinction between the two pathways is simplistic. Overexpression of Bcl-2 in the intrinsic pathway may lead to the inhibition of extrinsic mediated apoptosis [10]; conversely, TNFα may increase the expression of NF-κB and stimulates antiapoptotic members of the Bcl-2 family proteins.

Extrinsic Pathway

This pathway comprises several protein members including the death receptors, the membrane-bound Fas ligand, the Fas complexes, the Fas-associated death domain, and caspases 8 and 10, which ultimately activate the rest of the downstream caspases leading to apoptosis. Activation of the extrinsic pathway is initiated with the ligation of cell surface receptors called death receptors (DRs). Fas is a member of the tumor necrosis factor receptor superfamily and is also called Apo-1. Fas signaling play an important role in apoptosis.

The Fas ligand (FasL)–Fas system is mainly recognized for its death-related functions. When a death stimulus triggers the pathway, the membrane-bound FasL interacts with the inactive Fas complexes and forms the death-inducing signaling complex. The Fas death-inducing signaling complex contains the adaptor protein Fas-associated death domain protein and caspases 8 and 10 and leads to activation of caspase 8, which, in turn, can activate the rest of the downstream caspases. Caspase 8 interacts with the intrinsic apoptotic pathway by cleaving Bid (a proapoptotic member of the Bcl-2 family), leading to the subsequent release of cytochrome c [11].

Intrinsic Pathway

One of the most important regulators of this pathway is the Bcl-2 family of proteins. The Bcl-2 family includes proapoptotic members such as Bax, Bak, Bad, Bcl-Xs, Bid, Bik, Bim, and Hrk and antiapoptotic members. Antiapoptotic Bcl-2 members act as repressors of apoptosis by blocking the release of cytochrome c, whereas proapoptotic members act as promoters. Following a death signal, proapoptotic proteins undergo posttranslational modifications that include dephosphorylation and cleavage resulting in their activation and translocation to the mitochondria leading to apoptosis [9]. In response to apoptotic stimuli, the outer mitochondrial membrane becomes permeable, leading to the release of cytochrome c. Once cytochrome c is released into the cytosol, it interacts with Apaf-1, leading to the activation of caspase 9 proenzymes. Active caspase 9 then activates caspase 3, which subsequently activates the rest of the caspase cascade and leads to apoptosis [10].

Fas/FasL

Fas is a type I transmembrane receptor protein that belongs to the TNF/nerve growth factor family [12, 13], and Fas ligand (FasL) has been identified as a tumor necrosis factor-related type II transmembrane protein [14]. Ligation of FasL to Fas induces apoptosis of the Fas-bearing cells by the activation of various caspases. Caspase 8 is involved in the upstream of the apoptosis process [15, 16]. Activation of caspase 8 is followed by activation of caspase 3, which is known as executioner protease in this process [17]. In the rodent testis, apoptosis, induced by FasL, has been suggested to be one of the mechanisms that limit the number of germ cells during normal spermatogenesis or after testicular injuries. Recent studies have also shown that, in the human testis, apoptosis is a conspicuous event during spermatogenesis; Fas–FasL interaction is reportedly involved in the regulation of this event [18, 19].

Caspases Family

Caspases (cysteinyl aspartate-specific proteinases) are aspartic acid-directed cysteine proteases. These proteases are synthesized as precursors that have insignificant catalytic activity. The precursor caspase is converted to the active enzyme by proteolytic processing either by another protease or by autocatalysis and triggered by the binding of cofactors or removal of inhibitors. Caspases share similarities in amino acid sequence, structure, and substrate specificity. They are all expressed as proenzymes (30–50 kDa). It contains three domains and they are: the amino terminal domain, a large subunit ($\sim$20 kDa), and a small subunit ($\sim$10 kDa). During the caspase activation, proteolytic processing occurs between domains, followed by association of the large and small subunits to form a heterodimer [20]. Although the majority of caspases are situated within the cytoplasm, some of the members can be found in the Golgi apparatus (caspase 12) or in association with the mitochondria (caspases 2, 3, and 9) [21, 22]. Caspase 3 is the most important effector caspase. Its activation is important in PCD signaling [23].

Cytochrome c

Different proapoptotic proteins, such as cytochrome c and Smac/Diablo that are normally present in the intermembrane space of mitochondria, are released during the early stages of apoptosis. In the cytosol, cytochrome c participates in the formation of the apoptosome complex together with its adaptor molecule, Apaf-1, resulting in the recruitment, processing, and activation of procaspase 9 in the presence of adenosine triphosphate [24]. Subsequently, caspase 9 cleaves and activates procaspases 3 and 7; these effector caspases are responsible for the cleavage of various proteins leading to the biochemical and morphological features characteristic of apoptosis [25]. The release of cytochrome c is, therefore, considered a key initiative step in the apoptotic process.

Nuclear Factor-κB

The classical NF-κB transcriptional factors are composed of homodimers or heterodimers of Rel protein, of which p65/p50 heterodimer is the predominant complex, in testicular germ cells [26]. In unstimulated cells, NF-κB dimers are sequestered in the cytoplasm by inhibitory kappa B (IκB) protein. Upon exposure to various extracellular signals that leads to phosphorylation and degradation of IκB, free NF-κB dimers rapidly translocate to the nucleus, wherein they activate transcription of target genes [27].

Spermatogenesis

Spermatogenesis is a dynamic and well-regulated process that involves multiplication, maturation, and differentiation of germ cells resulting in the formation of mature spermatozoa. The process is subdivided into spermatogoniogenesis known as mitotic multiplication of spermatogonia, maturation of spermatocytes, spermiogenesis, and spermiation. Germ cells undergo mitosis to produce primary spermatocytes. The primary spermatocytes enter meiosis to form secondary spermatocytes and proceed through meiosis to produce haploid spermatids. These in turn undergo a complex process of morphological and functional differentiation resulting in the production of mature spermatozoa, which is known as spermiogenesis. In mammalian species, to maintain proper germ cell numbers, apoptosis takes place in the testis [16]. Loss of spermatogenic cells is incurred mostly during maturity of spermatogonia and to a lesser extent during maturation of spermatocytes and spermatid in adult rat testis. The sign of spermatogenesis is started when germ cells differentiate into spermatogonia. While some spermatogonia become self-renewing spermatogonial stem cells, most differentiate into spermatocytes and at ~10 days after birth in mice and at puberty in man, initiate meiosis and is accompanied by extensive germ cell apoptosis [16].

Steroidogenesis

Leydig cells are the principal cells involved in the process of steroidogenesis. Leydig cells secrete androgens, particularly testosterone, which is extremely essential for the initiation and maintenance of spermatogenesis [28]. Any factor affecting the Leydig cell viability, in turn, can interrupt the endocrine regulation of spermatogenesis and consequently affect the reproductive performance. Aroclor 1254, a commercial mixture of polychlorinated biphenyls, brought about a state of oxidative stress in cultured Leydig cells characterized by decline in the levels of enzymatic and nonenzymatic antioxidants accompanied by an elevation in the levels of lipid peroxidation and ROS. In addition, the activities of steroidogenic enzymes were inhibited at the level of gene expression causing diminished testosterone production [29]. Exposure of rats to single dose of cadmium (0.20 mg/100 g body weight) inhibited the activities of testicular 3β and 17β-hydroxysteroid dehydrogenase along with reduced expression of StAR protein resulting in lowered serum testosterone levels. The observed effects have been attributed to the excess generation of ROS in the testis resulting from depletion of antioxidant enzymes like SOD and glutathione peroxidase. Exposure of primary cultured Leydig cells to cadmium at the concentrations of 10 mM, caused increased oxidative DNA damage resulting in decreased viability of cells and testosterone secretion [30]. The high levels of corticosterone associated with stress are known to induce apoptosis in Leydig cells. The activation of Fas system, cleavage of procaspase 3, loss of mitochondrial membrane potential, and increased ROS generation are reported to be the possible mechanisms involved in corticosterone-induced Leydig cell death [31]. The decline in testosterone production following toxicant exposure may be in part due to apoptosis of Leydig cells caused by induction of stress by corticosterone.

Effect of Environmental Contaminants

Apoptosis of spermatogenic cells is essential for the maintenance of testicular homeostasis, although increased cell death can result in defective spermatogenesis leading to infertility [32]. In the testis, apoptotic death is a common programmed event that reduces 75% of germ cells [33]. However, excessive or inadequate apoptosis of testicular cells results in abnormal spermatogenesis or testicular tumors [34]. Various testicular toxicants have been reported to induce massive germ cell apoptosis indicating that the seminiferous epithelium responds to most of the adverse stimuli by eliminating germ cells through programmed cell death [35]. Recent studies showed that DDT and its metabolite to induce apoptosis either in vitro or in vivo experiments [36, 37]. Song et al. demonstrated that exposure to p,p'-DDE, a metabolite of DDT, at over 30 μM dose level showed induction of apoptotic cell death in cultured rat Sertoli cells by inducing mitochondria-mediated apoptotic changes including elevation in reactive oxygen species (ROS) generation, decrease in mitochondrial membrane potential, and release of cytochrome c into the cytosol which could be blocked by N-acetyl-L-cysteine, an antioxidant with an elevated ratios of Bax/Bcl-w and Bak/Bcl-w, and cleavages of procaspases 3 and 9 were induced by p,p'-DDE [38]. Metabolite of DDT (p,p'-DDE) at a dose of 30 μM for 24 h exposure could induce apoptosis of Sertoli cells through a FasL-dependent pathway including nuclear translocation of NF-κB, increase of the FasL mRNA, and protein expression, which could be blocked by an antioxidant agent N-acetyl-L-CYSTEINE. In addition, caspases 3 and 8 were activated by p,p'-DDE treatment in these cells [39]. Ichimura et al. demonstrated the expression and localization of FasL, Fas, and caspase 3 proteins in mouse testis 12 h after the exposure to 4–0.004 mg/g of di(2-ethylhexyl) phthalate (DEHP) and correlated the expression of these proteins with TUNEL labeling of the DNA-fragmented nucleus [40]. Immunocytochemical examination of the DEHP-exposed (4 mg/g) mouse revealed a distribution of FasL in Sertoli cell and Fas in nearby spermatocyte and Fas and caspase 3 in the same spermatocyte. Exposure to mono(2-ethylhexyl) phthalate (MEHP), a Sertoli cell-specific toxicant, induced massive germ cell apoptosis associated with increased expression of both the Fas and FasL genes in rat testis. Mono(2-ethylhexyl) phthalate (MEHP), a well-known Sertoli cell toxicant, could decrease the levels of procaspase 8 and increase the levels of procaspase 8 cleavage products in mice testis [41]. β-Benzene hexachloride (β-BHC), a major metabolite of benzene hexachloride induced apoptosis by activation of JNKs, translocation of NF-κB, expression of FasL, and further activation of caspase cascade [42].

Spontaneous germ cell apoptosis has been observed in several species of mammalian testis. Vaithinathan et al. demonstrated a significant increase in the levels of cytosolic cytochrome c and procaspase 9 as early as 6 h following exposure to a single dose of methoxychlor at 50 mg/kg body weight. Time-dependent elevations in the levels of Fas, FasL, and pro- and cleaved caspase 3 demonstrate induction of testicular apoptosis in adult rats following a single dose of methoxychlor [43]. Recent findings reveal that methoxychlor exposure to pregnant female rats from embryonic day 8–15 at the dosage of 100 and 200 mg/kg/day showed an increase in spermatogenic cell apoptosis and decreased sperm number and motility in adult animals of F1 and F2 generation [44, 45]. In another study, oral administration of bisphenol A 480 and 960 mg/kg/day induces apoptosis of Leydig and germ cells in the mouse testis through the Fas-signaling pathway [46].

Lindane, a well-known endocrine disruptor could induce apoptosis of testicular cells by stimulating the mitochondrion-dependent pathway by elevating the levels of cytochrome c with a parallel increase in procaspase 9. A time-dependent elevation of Fas, FasL, and caspase 3 in peritubular germ cells illustrates induction of testicular apoptosis in adult rats following exposure to a single dose of lindane [47].

Oxidative Stress

Control of apoptosis may involve various pathways such as the mitochondria-mediated, Bcl-2 family, Fas/FasL system that can be engaged by oxidative stress. Reactive oxygen species (ROS) is considered a potential signal for apoptosis. Elevated levels of ROS can cause oxidation of the mitochondrial pores thereby disrupting the mitochondrial membrane potential and releasing cytochrome c thereby activating the mitochondrial mediated pathway of apoptosis. In addition, ROS have been shown to induce the expression of Fas receptor and ligand stimulating the Fas/FasL-mediated apoptotic signal transduction pathway. Several environmental disruptors are known to inappropriately activate apoptosis in testicular locale by increasing the levels of ROS [47, 48].

During the transit from undifferentiated germ cells to mature spermatozoa, the sperms are vulnerable to multitudinous threats which are counteracted by the powerful antioxidant defense system of the testis [49]. Many toxicants have been shown to damage this protective shield, thus increasing the susceptibility of this organ to oxidative stress [50, 51]. Experimental studies have demonstrated that exposure to hexachlorocyclohexane (i.p., 20 mg/kg/day) during the critical stages of testicular development induces elevation in the levels of lipid peroxidation and hydrogen peroxide (H_2O_2) along with reduction in the levels of superoxide dismutase (SOD), catalase, and ascorbic acid [52]. Doreswamy et al. have demonstrated the induction of oxidative stress, DNA damage, and apoptosis in testis following exposure to multiple doses of nickel chloride [53]. Our earlier studies on various toxicants in rodent models have exemplified the role of oxidative stress in mediating its effects on testis. Oral exposure to lindane (5 mg/kg body weight/day) for 30 days resulted in elevated levels of hydrogen peroxide and lipid peroxidation with concomitant decline in the activities of antioxidant and steroidogenic enzymes in testis [54]. Similar impairment of antioxidant system and mitochondria-dependent apoptosis of rat testis have been observed with lindane following single dose of lindane [47, 55]. Methoxychlor, at dose levels of 50 mg/kg body weight, caused significant diminution in testicular antioxidant enzymes along with Fas–FasL and mitochondria-mediated apoptosis in a time-dependent manner [43]. Compilation of these studies indicates the generation of free radicals and associated oxidative stress as the pathological mechanism underpinning the adverse effects of testicular toxicants. Innumerable studies have disclosed the involvement of oxidative stress in carrying out the malicious role of apoptosis in testis.

Most of the toxicants have been reported to perturb the testicular locale either directly or indirectly targeting pivotal constituents of testis—the germ cells, Sertoli cells, and Leydig cells. A study on the exposure of testis to a single dose (2 g/kg body weight) of di(2-ethylhexyl) phthalate revealed an augmented generation of ROS with simultaneous decrement in the concentrations of glutathione and ascorbic acid leading to selective apoptosis of spermatocytes [56]. Further exploration revealed the accrual of mono(2-ethylhexyl) phthalate, a toxic metabolite of DEHP, in testis causing mitochondrial respiratory damage and release of cytochrome c inciting apoptosis [56]. Exposure of spermatogenic cells to synthetic organic chemical, methyl *tert*-butyl ether (MTBE), enervated cell viability and induced generation of ROS and enhanced lipid peroxidation [57]. Similar damaging effects of oxidative stress followed by apoptosis in maturing germ cells have been observed with multifarious array of toxicants including metals.

The uninterrupted close association of germ cells with Sertoli cells is yet another obligatory factor in spermatogenesis. Apart from its fostering role, Sertoli cells play a highly remarkable phagocytic role in eliminating spermatogenic cells undergoing apoptosis in response to chemical insult [58]. Consequently, any agent that confronts Sertoli cells may have a profound effect on spermatogenesis.

In vitro exposure to β-BHC can enhance ROS and oxidative stress and then induce activation of JNKs and NF-κB, expression of FasL in rat Sertoli cells. Upon ligation of FasL to Fas, an FasL-mediated apoptotic death is stimulated in a target cell leading to the activation of caspase 8. Finally, apoptosis of Sertoli cells is mediated by executioner caspase 3, thereby disturbing the spermatogenic process [42]. Sertoli cells on exposure to an environmental contaminant, nonylphenol (10–40 μM), caused accumulation of ROS within 2 h of exposure which subsequently resulted in the loss of mitochondrial membrane potential and enhanced lipid peroxidation at 12 h posttreatment [59]. In vitro studies on the effects of 4-*tert*-octylphenol, a degradation product of alkylphenol polyethoxylate, at a concentration of 30–60 μM for 6–24 h decreased the viability of Sertoli cells and increased apoptosis via caspase 3 pathway in a concentration- and time-dependent manner [60]. Diverse studies have cumulated over time which accentuates the feasible role of oxidative stress in Sertoli cell apoptosis in response to toxicants.

Mechanisms Involved in Inducing Apoptosis

The possible mechanisms involved in the action of various factors in mediating testicular apoptosis are summed up. Most of the studies involving toxicants illustrate the undoubted role of ROS in executing its detrimental effects [29, 54, 59, 61]. These elevated levels of ROS can cause oxidation of the mitochondrial pores thereby disrupting the mitochondrial membrane potential and releasing cytochrome c [56, 62]. Once free of the mitochondrial membrane, cytochrome c rapidly assembles a multiprotein complex involving Apaf-1 and procaspase 9 leading to the activation of the caspase 9, which subsequently triggers the effector caspase 3, 6, and/or 7 [24, 25]. These caspases, in turn, activate endonucleases and proteases resulting in DNA fragmentation and degradation of nuclear and cytoskeletal proteins [63, 64]. Apart from ROS, Bax, a member of proapoptotic Bcl-2 family, can directly influence the release of cytochrome c from mitochondria [65]. It is interesting to note that the Bcl-2 protein family is itself regulated by ROS [66]; however, whether this regulation has any role in toxicant-mediated apoptosis is not known.

ROS have been shown to induce the expression of Fas receptor and ligand stimulating the Fas/FasL-mediated apoptotic signal transduction pathway [67]. Interaction of Fas with FasL leads to a cascade of events which begins with the proteolytic cleavage of procaspase 8 to its active form, which consequently activates downstream effector caspase 3, 6, or 7 [68–70]. These caspases execute the cells by degrading the constituent proteins [71]. Elimination of apoptotic action of Fas by antioxidants further emphasizes the role of ROS in Fas-mediated death process [72, 73]. Therefore, deprivation of antioxidants and/or generation of free radicals by toxicants is capable of reducing the Fas pathway. In addition, they impair steroidogenesis and may deprive germ cell of the essential growth factor, testosterone, and increase their susceptibility to ROS attack [74].

Key Issues

The purpose of this chapter was to evaluate the role of various factors influencing apoptosis in male infertility. Mounting evidence suggests that apoptosis occurs as the predominant cell death mechanism in testis in response to several diseases and toxic injuries. Research implies that reactive oxygen species and other secondary free radicals such as nitric oxide and hydroperoxides could be inducers or mediators of apoptosis in testis through downregulation of antioxidant defense system or increased expression of apoptosis-related proteins. However, the exact mechanism of action of apoptosis in inducing male infertility remains a mystery. Further studies are warranted to evaluate the adverse effects of apoptosis on testis.

Acknowledgments P.P. Mathur acknowledges the receipt of financial support from the Department of Science and Technology, Government of India, under the projects (1) SP/SO/B-65/99, (2) DST-FIST-2009, and (3) Indian Council of Medical Research, New Delhi. Shereen Cynthia D'Cruz acknowledges the Indian Council of Medical Research, New Delhi, India, for Senior Research Fellowship. The authors also thank the staff of Bioinformatics Center, Pondicherry University, Pondicherry, for providing various facilities.

References

1. Nene UA, Coyaji K, Apte H. Infertility: a label of choice in the case of sexually dysfunctional couples. Patient Educ Couns. 2005;59(3):234–8.
2. Sharlip ID, Jarow JP, Belker AM, et al. Best practice policies for male infertility. Fertil Steril. 2002;77(5):873–82.
3. Larsen U. Sterility in sub-Saharan Africa. Popul Stud. 1994;48:459–74.
4. Larsen U. Infertility in Central Africa. Trop Med Int Health. 2003;8:354–67.
5. Iammarrone E, Balet R, Lower AM, Gillott C, Grudzinskas JG. Male infertility. Best Pract Res Clin Obstet Gynaecol. 2003;17(2):211–29.
6. Saez JM, Avallet O, Lejeune H, Chatelain PG. Cell-cell communication in the testis. Horm Res. 1991;36(3–4):104–15.
7. McLachlan RI, Wreford NG, Meachem SJ, De Kretser DM, Robertson DM. Effects of testosterone on spermatogenic cell populations in the adult rat. Biol Reprod. 1994;51(5):945–55.
8. Zapata JM, Pawlowski K, Haas E, et al. A diverse family of proteins containing tumor necrosis factor receptor-associated factor domains. J Biol Chem. 2001;276(26):24242–52.
9. Scorrano L, Korsmeyer SJ. Mechanisms of cytochrome c release by proapoptotic BCL-2 family members. Biochem Biophys Res Commun. 2003;304(3):437–44.
10. Reed JC. Bcl-2 family proteins: regulators of apoptosis and chemoresistance in hematologic malignancies. Semin Hematol. 1997;34(4 Suppl 5):9–19.
11. Wajant H. The Fas signaling pathway: more than a paradigm. Science. 2002;296(5573):1635–6.
12. Watanabe-Fukunaga R, Brannan CI, Copeland NG, Jenkins NA, Nagata S. Lymphoproliferation disorder in mice explained by defects in Fas antigen that mediates apoptosis. Nature. 1992;356(6367):314–7.
13. Nagata S, Golstein P. The Fas death factor. Science. 1995;267(5203):1449–56.
14. Suda T, Takahashi T, Golstein P, Nagata S. Molecular cloning and expression of the Fas ligand, a novel member of the tumor necrosis factor family. Cell. 1993;75(6):1169–78.

15. Tanaka M, Itai T, Adachi M, Nagata S. Downregulation of Fas ligand by shedding. Nat Med. 1998;4(1):31–6.
16. Sinha Hikim AP, Lue Y, Diaz-Romero M, et al. Deciphering the pathways of germ cell apoptosis in the testis. J Steroid Biochem Mol Biol. 2003;85(2-5):175–82.
17. Philchenkov AA. Caspases as regulators of apoptosis and other cell functions. Biochemistry (Mosc). 2003;68(4):365–76.
18. Pentikainen V, Erkkila K, Dunkel L. Fas regulates germ cell apoptosis in the human testis in vitro. Am J Physiol. 1999;276(2 Pt 1):E310–6.
19. Francavilla S, D'Abrizio P, Rucci N, et al. Fas and Fas ligand expression in fetal and adult human testis with normal or deranged spermatogenesis. J Clin Endocrinol Metab. 2000; 85(8):2692–700.
20. Thornberry NA, Lazebnik Y. Caspases: enemies within. Science. 1998;281(5381):1312–6.
21. Nicholson DW. Caspase structure, proteolytic substrates, and function during apoptotic cell death. Cell Death Differ. 1999;6(11):1028–42.
22. Cohen GM. Caspases: the executioners of apoptosis. Biochem J. 1997;326(Pt 1):1–16.
23. Earnshaw WC, Martins LM, Kaufmann SH. Mammalian caspases: structure, activation, substrates, and functions during apoptosis. Annu Rev Biochem. 1999;68:383–424.
24. Hengartner MO. The biochemistry of apoptosis. Nature. 2000;407(6805):770–6.
25. Budihardjo I, Oliver H, Lutter M, Luo X, Wang X. Biochemical pathways of caspase activation during apoptosis. Annu Rev Cell Dev Biol. 1999;15:269–90.
26. Delfino F, Walker WH. Stage-specific nuclear expression of NF-kappaB in mammalian testis. Mol Endocrinol. 1998;12(11):1696–707.
27. Karin M. How NF-kappaB is activated: the role of the IkappaB kinase (IKK) complex. Oncogene. 1999;18(49):6867–74.
28. Huleihel M, Lunenfeld E. Regulation of spermatogenesis by paracrine/autocrine testicular factors. Asian J Androl. 2004;6(3):259–68.
29. Murugesan P, Balaganesh M, Balasubramanian K, Arunakaran J. Effects of polychlorinated biphenyl (Aroclor 1254) on steroidogenesis and antioxidant system in cultured adult rat Leydig cells. J Endocrinol. 2007;192(2):325.
30. Yang JM, Arnush M, Chen QY, et al. Cadmium-induced damage to primary cultures of rat Leydig cells. Reprod Toxicol. 2003;17(5):553–60.
31. Gao HB, Tong MH, Hu YQ, et al. Mechanisms of glucocorticoid-induced Leydig cell apoptosis. Mol Cell Endocrinol. 2003;199(1–2):153–63.
32. Print CG, Loveland KL. Germ cell suicide: new insights into apoptosis during spermatogenesis. Bioessays. 2000;22(5):423.
33. Allan DJ, Harmon BV, Roberts SA. Spermatogonial apoptosis has three morphologically recognizable phases and shows no circadian rhythm during normal spermatogenesis in the rat. Cell Prolif. 1992;25(3):241–50.
34. Lin WW, Lamb DJ, Wheeler TM, Lipshultz LI, Kim ED. In situ end-labeling of human testicular tissue demonstrates increased apoptosis in conditions of abnormal spermatogenesis. Fertil Steril. 1997;68(6):1065–9.
35. Blanchard TL, Johnson L. Increased germ cell degeneration and reduced germ cell:Sertoli cell ratio in stallions with low sperm production. Theriogenology. 1997;47(3):665–77.
36. Tebourbi O, Rhouma KB, Sakly M. DDT induces apoptosis in rat thymocytes. Bull Environ Contam Toxicol. 1998;61(2):216–23.
37. Perez-Maldonado IN, Diaz-Barriga F, de la Fuente H, et al. DDT induces apoptosis in human mononuclear cells in vitro and is associated with increased apoptosis in exposed children. Environ Res. 2004;94(1):38–46.
38. Song Y, Liang X, Hu Y, et al. p, p'-DDE induces mitochondria-mediated apoptosis of cultured rat Sertoli cells. Toxicology. 2008;253(1–3):53–61.
39. Shi Y, Song Y, Wang Y, et al. p, p'-DDE induces apoptosis of rat Sertoli cells via a FasL-dependent pathway. J Biomed Biotechnol. 2009;2009:181282.

40. Ichimura T, Kawamura M, Mitani A. Co-localized expression of FasL, Fas, Caspase-3 and apoptotic DNA fragmentation in mouse testis after oral exposure to di(2-ethylhexyl)phthalate. Toxicology. 2003;194(1–2):35–42.
41. Giammona CJ, Sawhney P, Chandrasekaran Y, Richburg JH. Death receptor response in rodent testis after mono-(2-ethylhexyl) phthalate exposure. Toxicol Appl Pharmacol. 2002;185(2):119–27.
42. Shi Y, Song Y, Wang Y, et al. Beta-benzene hexachloride induces apoptosis of rat sertoli cells through generation of reactive oxygen species and activation of JNKs and FasL. Environ Toxicol. 2011;26(2):124–35. doi:10.1002/tox.20536.
43. Vaithinathan S, Saradha B, Mathur PP. Methoxychlor induces apoptosis via mitochondria- and FasL-mediated pathways in adult rat testis. Chem Biol Interact. 2010;185(2):110–8.
44. Anway MD, Cupp AS, Uzumcu M, Skinner MK. Epigenetic transgenerational actions of endocrine disruptors and male fertility. Science. 2005;308(5727):1466–9.
45. Cupp AS, Uzumcu M, Suzuki H, et al. Effect of transient embryonic in vivo exposure to the endocrine disruptor methoxychlor on embryonic and postnatal testis development. J Androl. 2003;24(5):736–45.
46. Li YJ, Song TB, Cai YY, et al. Bisphenol A exposure induces apoptosis and upregulation of Fas/FasL and caspase-3 expression in the testes of mice. Toxicol Sci. 2009;108(2):427–36.
47. Saradha B, Vaithinathan S, Mathur PP. Lindane induces testicular apoptosis in adult Wistar rats through the involvement of Fas-FasL and mitochondria-dependent pathways. Toxicology. 2009;255(3):131–9.
48. Lee J, Richburg JH, Shipp EB, Meistrich ML, Boekelheide K. The Fas system, a regulator of testicular germ cell apoptosis, is differentially up-regulated in Sertoli cell versus germ cell injury of the testis. Endocrinology. 1999;140(2):852–8.
49. Peltola V, Huhtaniemi I, Ahotupa M. Antioxidant enzyme activity in the maturing rat testis. J Androl. 1992;13(5):450–5.
50. Abdollahi M, Ranjbar A, Shadnia S, Nikfar S, Rezaie A. Pesticides and oxidative stress: a review. Med Sci Monit. 2004;10(6):RA141–7.
51. Saradha B, Mathur PP. Effect of environmental contaminants on male reproduction. Environ Toxicol Pharmacol. 2006;21(1):34.
52. Samanta L, Roy A, Chainy GB. Changes in rat testicular antioxidant defence profile as a function of age and its impairment by hexachlorocyclohexane during critical stages of maturation. Andrologia. 1999;31(2):83–90.
53. Doreswamy K, Shrilatha B, Rajeshkumar T, Muralidhara. Nickel-induced oxidative stress in testis of mice: evidence of DNA damage and genotoxic effects. J Androl. 2004;25(6):996–1003.
54. Sujatha R, Chitra KC, Latchoumycandane C, Mathur PP. Effect of lindane on testicular antioxidant system and steroidogenic enzymes in adult rats. Asian J Androl. 2001;3(2):135–8.
55. Saradha B, Vaithinathan S, Mathur PP. Lindane alters the levels of HSP70 and clusterin in adult rat testis. Toxicology. 2008;243(1–2):116–23.
56. Kasahara E, Sato EF, Miyoshi M, et al. Role of oxidative stress in germ cell apoptosis induced by di(2-ethylhexyl)phthalate. Biochem J. 2002;365(Pt 3):849–56.
57. Li D, Yin D, Han X. Methyl tert-butyl ether (MTBE)-induced cytotoxicity and oxidative stress in isolated rat spermatogenic cells. J Appl Toxicol. 2007;27(1):10–7.
58. Tay TW, Andriana BB, Ishii M, et al. Phagocytosis plays an important role in clearing dead cells caused by mono(2-ethylhexyl) phthalate administration. Tissue Cell. 2007;39(4):241–6.
59. Gong Y, Han XD. Nonylphenol-induced oxidative stress and cytotoxicity in testicular Sertoli cells. Reprod Toxicol. 2006;22(4):623–30.
60. Qian J, Bian Q, Cui L, et al. Octylphenol induces apoptosis in cultured rat Sertoli cells. Toxicol Lett. 2006;166(2):178–86.
61. Sen Gupta R, Sen Gupta E, Dhakal BK, Thakur AR, Ahnn J. Vitamin C and vitamin E protect the rat testes from cadmium-induced reactive oxygen species. Mol Cells. 2004;17(1):132–9.

62. Zamzami N, Marchetti P, Castedo M, et al. Sequential reduction of mitochondrial transmembrane potential and generation of reactive oxygen species in early programmed cell death. J Exp Med. 1995;182(2):367–77.
63. Bortner CD, Oldenburg NB, Cidlowski JA. The role of DNA fragmentation in apoptosis. Trends Cell Biol. 1995;5(1):21–6.
64. Kohler C, Hakansson A, Svanborg C, Orrenius S, Zhivotovsky B. Protease activation in apoptosis induced by MAL. Exp Cell Res. 1999;249(2):260–8.
65. Green DR, Reed JC. Mitochondria and apoptosis. Science. 1998;281(5381):1309–12.
66. Tripathi P, Hildeman D. Sensitization of T cells to apoptosis—a role for ROS? Apoptosis. 2004;9(5):515–23.
67. Krammer PH. CD95(APO-1/Fas)-mediated apoptosis: live and let die. Adv Immunol. 1999;71:163–210.
68. Scaffidi C, Fulda S, Srinivasan A, et al. Two CD95 (APO-1/Fas) signaling pathways. EMBO J. 1998;17(6):1675–87.
69. Sanchez-Gomez MV, Alberdi E, Ibarretxe G, Torre I, Matute C. Caspase-dependent and caspase-independent oligodendrocyte death mediated by AMPA and kainate receptors. J Neurosci. 2003;23(29):9519–28.
70. Henkler F, Behrle E, Dennehy KM, et al. The extracellular domains of FasL and Fas are sufficient for the formation of supramolecular FasL-Fas clusters of high stability. J Cell Biol. 2005;168(7):1087–98.
71. Riedl SJ, Shi Y. Molecular mechanisms of caspase regulation during apoptosis. Nat Rev Mol Cell Biol. 2004;5(11):897–907.
72. Um HD, Orenstein JM, Wahl SM. Fas mediates apoptosis in human monocytes by a reactive oxygen intermediate dependent pathway. J Immunol. 1996;156(9):3469.
73. Chiba T, Takahashi S, Sato N, Ishii S, Kikuchi K. Fas-mediated apoptosis is modulated by intracellular glutathione in human T cells. Eur J Immunol. 1996;26(5):1164.
74. Chainy GB, Samantaray S, Samanta L. Testosterone-induced changes in testicular antioxidant system. Andrologia. 1997;29(6):343–9.

Chapter 13
Impact of Spinal Cord Injury

Viacheslav Iremashvili, Nancy L. Brackett, and Charles M. Lynne

Although medical advances have greatly improved the prognosis for people who sustain spinal cord injury, it remains a major social and health-care problem. There are estimated 10,000–12,000 spinal cord injuries every year in the USA alone. More than a quarter of a million Americans are currently living with spinal cord injury [1], with many millions more worldwide. The cost of managing the care of patients with spinal cord injury is approximately \$4 billion per year. Car accidents are the most common cause of spinal cord injury followed by violent encounters, sporting and work-related accidents, and falls [1].

The majority of spinal cord injury victims are young adults. Of them, more than 80% are men. As a result, young males constitute the largest part of this patient population. Reproductive function is essential for men with spinal cord injury, but unfortunately, less than 10% of them can father children without medical assistance [2]. Infertility in male patients with spinal cord injury results from a combination of erectile dysfunction, ejaculatory dysfunction, and poor semen quality [3]. As a result of advancements in assisted ejaculation techniques including electroejaculation and high-amplitude penile vibratory stimulation, semen can be safely obtained from nearly all men with spinal cord injury without resorting to surgical procedures [4]; however, semen quality is poor in the majority of cases [5].

V. Iremashvili, MD, PhD
Department of Urology, University of Miami Miller School of Medicine,
016960 (M-14), Miami, Florida 33101, USA
e-mail: iremashvili@hotmail.com

N.L. Brackett, PhD, HCLD (✉)
The Miami Project to Cure Paralysis, University of Miami Miller School of Medicine,
Lois Pope Life Center, Room 2-17, 1095 NW 14th Terrace, Miami, Florida 33136, USA
e-mail: nbrackett@miami.edu

C.M. Lynne, MD
Department of Urology, University of Miami Miller School of Medicine, Miami, FL, USA
e-mail: clynne@miami.edu

S.J. Parckattil and A. Agarwal (eds.), *Antioxidants in Male Infertility: A Guide for Clinicians and Researchers*, © Springer Science+Business Media New York 2013

Semen Abnormalities in Men with Spinal Cord Injury

The origin and/or cause of low sperm quality in men with spinal cord injury has not been clearly defined. Several possible etiologies have been postulated, including hormonal dysfunction [6], elevated scrotal temperature [7], methods of bladder management [8], and alterations in sperm transport and storage due to reproductive tract stasis [9, 10], but none of these causes has been conclusively proven.

Role of Hormonal Alterations

Alterations in the hypothalamic-pituitary-gonadal axis may result in the disruption of spermatogenesis. The endocrine status of men with spinal cord injury has been examined in several studies that provided contradictory results (Table 13.1). Some studies in humans [6, 11–14] and animals [15, 16] have reported different hormone abnormalities associated with spinal cord injury, but no consistent correlation with the semen quality was shown. It was also not clear if these abnormalities were primary or secondary. We studied this problem in a group of 66 men with spinal cord injury and found no association between semen quality and serum levels of luteinizing hormone, follicle-stimulating hormone, testosterone, or prolactin [17].

Table 13.1 Principal results of the studies of endocrine status of men with spinal cord injuries

	Luteinizing hormone	Follicle-stimulating hormone	Testosterone	Prolactin
No difference from control	Huang et al. [19] Tsitouras et al. [20]	Naftchi et al. [21] Tsitouras et al. [20] Huang et al. [22]	Huang et al. [19] Naftchi et al. [21] Brackett et al. [17]	Huang et al. [19] Brackett et al. [17] Naderi et al. [14]
Lower than control	Naftchi et al. [21] Brackett et al. [17] Safarinejad et al. [23] Naderi et al. [14] Kostovski et al. [12]	Brackett et al. [17] Safarinejad et al. [23] Naderi et al. [14] Kostovski et al. [12]	Tsitouras et al. [20] Safarinejad et al. [23] Naderi et al. [14] Kostovski et al. [12]	
Higher than control		Huang et al. [19]		
Outside reference range		Huang et al.—high, 18.7% [19]	Tsitouras et al. low, 45% [20]	Huang et al.—high, 25% [19]

Endocrine profiles of spinal cord injury men were not shown to follow any specific pattern and/or to be significantly related to impairments in semen quality

The only exception was in a subgroup of subjects who had elevated levels of follicle-stimulating hormone. In each case, the patient was azoospermic, even patients with only small elevations of follicle-stimulating hormone. Hormonal alterations are unlikely to be a major contributor to poor semen quality in men with spinal cord injury [18–22].

Role of Scrotal Temperature

Elevated scrotal/testicular temperature was one of the first hypotheses to explain the origin of semen abnormalities in men with spinal cord injury. It is common knowledge that spermatogenesis is temperature-sensitive and proceeds optimally at 35°C. Higher scrotal temperatures could have detrimental effects on sperm production [23]. It was assumed that men with spinal cord injury could have scrotal hyperthermia as a result of generalized scrotal thermoregulatory dysfunction or because of sitting in a wheelchair for prolonged periods [24]. Some studies showed that men with spinal cord injury sitting in wheelchairs had higher scrotal temperatures compared to able-bodied men, sitting in armchairs [7, 25]. Brindley reported an inverse correlation between scrotal temperatures and motile sperm counts in men with spinal cord injury [25]. However, we did not find any difference between control subjects and spinal cord-injured subjects in oral temperature, scrotal temperature, or the difference between these two parameters [26]. Furthermore, men with spinal cord injury who were ambulatory (i.e., not in wheelchairs) still had impaired semen quality [26], indicating that some aspect of spinal cord injury, other than the simple act of sitting in a wheelchair, contributes to abnormal semen quality in these men. Supporting this idea is the fact that no study has found improvement in semen quality by cooling the scrotum of men with spinal cord injury.

Studies of scrotal temperature in noninjured men have suggested that short-term versus long-term exposure to elevated temperature causes reversible versus irreversible changes in the seminiferous tubules [27, 28]. In men with spinal cord injury, however, both cross-sectional [29] and longitudinal [30] studies have shown that semen parameters were not significantly related to the duration of the postinjury period, suggesting a stable (and null) pattern for the measures across time. In light of these facts, it appears that no strong evidence exists to support the role of elevated scrotal temperature as a leading etiologic factor of the semen abnormalities in men with spinal cord injury.

Role of Bladder Management

No bladder management regime has been associated with normal semen quality in men with spinal cord injury. However, some studies have shown that the use of intermittent catheterization is associated with better sperm motility than the use of indwelling urethral catheters, suprapubic catheters, or spontaneous voiding [31, 32]. Although semen quality is improved with intermittent catheterization versus the other methods mentioned, it does not become normalized. Bladder management, then, does not seem to be a significant cause of impaired semen quality in men with spinal cord injury.

Role of Ejaculation Frequency

The majority of men with spinal cord injury cannot ejaculate without medical assistance. It has been hypothesized that long periods between ejaculations may result in reproductive tract stasis which can negatively affect sperm. However, most studies investigating the effect of repeated ejaculation on semen quality in men with spinal cord injury found no improvement in semen parameters [9, 33–37]. Only one group reported a moderate increase in sperm motility and sperm morphology after 3 months of weekly ejaculations with penile vibratory stimulation [38]. These findings indicate that frequency of ejaculation is not the sole factor causing abnormal semen quality in men with spinal cord injury.

Interesting data were presented by Ohl et al., suggesting that spinal cord injury could result in fundamental changes in sperm transport and storage [10]. In eight patients with spinal cord injury, bilateral seminal vesicle aspiration was performed immediately before electroejaculation or penile vibratory stimulation. The seminal vesicle aspirates contained large numbers of poor quality sperm. It should be noted that normal men do not have large numbers of sperm in seminal vesicles. Duration of abstinence did not correlate with the number of seminal vesicle sperm. Furthermore, the semen parameters in samples obtained immediately after seminal vesicle aspiration were significantly better compared to historical ejaculated parameters [10]. The authors concluded that altered transport with stagnation of sperm in the seminal vesicles could be a primary source of semen with poor quality in men with spinal cord injury. It was also shown that factors within the seminal plasma contribute to poor semen abnormalities in men with spinal cord injury [39]. This issue will be discussed in more detail later in this chapter.

Studies of Oxidative Stress in Men with Spinal Cord Injury

In addition to the aforementioned putative causes that have been investigated, there is increasing evidence that oxidative stress is an important mechanism contributing to sperm damage in this group of patients. The generation of reactive oxygen species and their relation to semen quality in men with spinal cord injury has been investigated in several studies.

Electric Current and Reactive Oxygen Species

The first study to demonstrate elevated reactive oxygen activity in the semen of men with spinal cord injury was published by Rajasekaran et al. [40]. At the time of this study, electroejaculation was the most common method of obtaining semen from men with spinal cord injury. Electroejaculation is performed by passing electricity into the pelvic region via a probe inserted into the rectum. The authors hypothesized that this electric current induced sperm damage in men with spinal cord injury. The study consisted of two experiments. During the first experiment, sperm from healthy men was incubated with a normal and an electrolyzed medium. Reactive oxygen species levels and sperm motility were measured in each group of samples. The second experiment included measurements of reactive oxygen species generation in semen from men with spinal cord injury and normal controls. In subjects with spinal cord injury, semen samples were obtained by electroejaculation.

The results of this study showed that when sperm from control subjects were incubated with electrolyzed physiologic medium, a significant and time-dependent decrease occurred in sperm motility and sperm viability, and these decreases were associated with an increased generation of reactive oxygen species. The second experiment demonstrated a significant increase in reactive oxygen species generation in semen from subjects with spinal cord injury compared to semen from control subjects. In the latter group, ejaculates were collected by masturbation. These findings led authors to conclude that, in patients with spinal cord injury, the electric current was a likely cause of poor quality of semen obtained by electroejaculation, and this effect was mediated by increased the production of reactive oxygen species [40].

Reactive Oxygen Species in Whole Semen Versus Washed Sperm

The purpose of a study performed by de Lamirande et al. was to determine whether whole semen samples versus washed spermatozoa obtained from men with spinal cord injury produced excessive amounts of reactive oxygen species [41]. This study included three groups of men: healthy volunteers ($n = 20$), infertile able-bodied men ($n = 166$), and subjects with spinal cord injury ($n = 21$). In the latter group, semen was obtained by masturbation after butylbromide and physostigmine injections in 19 patients and by electroejaculation in the remaining two men. Formation of reactive oxygen species was measured in neat semen and in Percoll-washed spermatozoa of all subjects.

The presence of reactive oxygen species in whole semen was detected in 97% of subjects with spinal cord injury compared to 40% and 15% in infertile able-bodied men and volunteers, respectively. Compared to a threshold value of 10 mV/s/10^9, reactive oxygen species production was elevated in 81% of patients with spinal cord injury, 25% of infertile able-bodied men, and 10% of healthy controls. In healthy controls and in infertile able-bodied subjects, the levels of reactive oxygen species measured in semen were, respectively, 40 and 14 times lower than those detected in semen from subjects with spinal cord injury. No correlation was found between reactive oxygen species production and level or duration of injury.

After centrifugation on Percoll gradients, sperm from men with spinal cord injury continued to generate large amounts of reactive oxygen species. High reactive oxygen species production by Percoll-washed spermatozoa was found in 75% of men with spinal cord injury, 20% of infertile men, and 5% of healthy controls. The mean reactive oxygen species levels in washed spermatozoa from men with spinal cord injury were sixfold higher than that of infertile patients, and 140-fold higher than that of normal volunteers. There was a significant inverse relationship between levels of reactive oxygen species and percentage of motile sperm in Percoll-washed specimens from patients with spinal cord injury.

Results of this study showed that semen samples and Percoll-washed sperm samples from subjects with spinal cord injury produced reactive oxygen species at a higher frequency and at higher levels than equivalent samples from normal men or infertile men. In men with spinal cord injury, levels of reactive oxygen species correlated negatively with sperm motility [41]. These data suggest that the role of reactive oxygen species as a mechanism of sperm damage leading to infertility could be more important in men with spinal cord injury compared to the general population or to the infertile population.

Reactive Oxygen Species and Sperm Characteristics

The generation of reactive oxygen species and its relation to semen characteristics in men with spinal cord injury was investigated by our group [42]. This study included 24 men with spinal cord injury and 19 able-bodied controls. In the spinal cord-injured patients, semen was obtained by penile vibratory stimulation ($n = 15$), electroejaculation ($n = 8$), and masturbation ($n = 1$). Measurements of reactive oxygen species formation were performed before and after stimulation with N-formyl-methionyl-leucyl-phenylalanine and 12-myristate 13-acetate phorbol ester. These two substances trigger the generation of reactive oxygen species by leukocytes and spermatozoa, respectively.

The study showed that mean levels of reactive oxygen species in unstimulated and stimulated specimens were significantly higher in spinal cord-injured men compared to controls. The actual values reflecting the reactive oxygen species activity in the spinal cord-injured group were from 250 to 2,000 times higher than that of the control group. The incidence of samples positive for reactive oxygen species specimens in unstimulated controls and men with spinal cord injury was 47.3% versus 100%, respectively. It was also found that the levels of reactive oxygen species in semen from men with spinal cord injury correlated negatively with sperm motility and positively with white blood cell concentrations. Interestingly, the levels of reactive oxygen species did not differ between antegrade and retrograde samples or between different methods of ejaculation (penile vibratory stimulation and electroejaculation). Therefore, the high levels of reactive oxygen species in semen specimens obtained by electroejaculation and vibratory stimulation may not be due exclusively to the effects of electrical current, as was suggested by Rajasekaran et al. [40].

As can be seen from the above studies, reactive oxygen species production is elevated in semen from patients with spinal cord injury, and increased oxidative stress may be an important mechanism of impaired sperm quality in this group of men. The next section of this chapter will discuss the potential sources of reactive oxygen species in semen from patients with spinal cord injury, the consequences of this oxidative stress elevation, and the possible applications of this information in the treatment of infertility in these patients.

Sources of Reactive Oxygen Radicals in Semen from Men with Spinal Cord Injury

Human ejaculate consists of several types of cells including mature and immature spermatozoa, germ cells from different stages of the spermatogenic process, epithelial cells, and leukocytes. Of these different cell types, leukocytes and spermatozoa have been shown to be the two principal sources of production of free radicals [43].

Effect of Leukocytes

Ejaculates from men with spinal cord injury are known to have increased leukocyte counts (Fig. 13.1) [44, 45]. The main sources of leukocytes in human ejaculate are the prostate gland, seminal vesicles, and epididymis [46]. Our studies

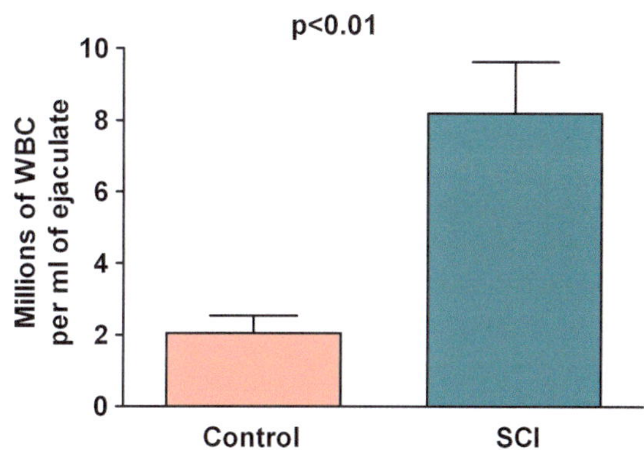

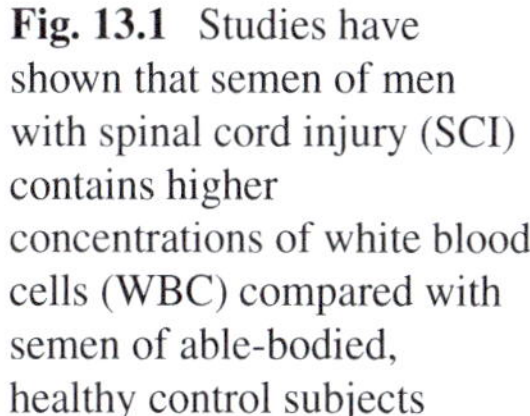

Fig. 13.1 Studies have shown that semen of men with spinal cord injury (SCI) contains higher concentrations of white blood cells (WBC) compared with semen of able-bodied, healthy control subjects

showed no evidence of chronic or acute prostate gland inflammation in leukocyto-spermic patients with spinal cord injury [47], and we did not find any white blood cells in the vasal aspirates from these subjects [48]. These data indicate that the seminal vesicles are the most likely origin of leukocytospermia in men with spinal cord injury.

Leukocytes can produce large amounts of reactive oxygen species. A positive correlation has been reported between seminal leukocyte counts and reactive oxy-gen species production [49, 50]. Of different leukocyte subtypes, peroxidase-positive cells, namely, neutrophils and macrophages, are predominant sources of reactive oxygen species production [51]. In ejaculates obtained by electroejacula-tion, these two leukocyte subpopulations, as identified by immunohistochemical staining, were the predominant contributors to leukocytospermia in men with spinal cord injury [52]. Lymphocytes were also found to be significant contributors to leukocytospermia in men with spinal cord injury. Immunophenotypic analysis by flow cytometry showed that the greater fraction were T cells, many of which coex-pressed the human leukocyte antigen HLA-DR and CD25, suggesting they were in an activated state. No significant B-cell population was evident [44].

The activation state of leukocytes plays a crucial role in determining reactive oxygen species output because activated white blood cells can produce up to 100-fold increases in reactive oxygen species compared with nonactivated cells [53]. This effect is mediated by an increase in reduced nicotinamide adenine dinucleo-tide phosphate production via the hexose monophosphate shunt [54]. The myelo-peroxidase system of neutrophils and macrophages is also activated, resulting in a respiratory burst and production of large amounts of superoxide and other reactive oxygen species.

Effect of Cytokines

Elevated concentrations of the proinflammatory cytokines interleukin 1 beta, inter-leukin 6, and tumor necrosis factor α have been detected in the semen of men with spinal cord injury [55], reflecting activation of T-lymphocytes [44] (Fig. 13.2). Inactivation of these cytokines, by adding monoclonal antibodies or receptor block-ers to semen from men with spinal cord injury, improves sperm motility [56, 57]. Interleukins are important mediators of free radical generation in many tissues, and the role of cytokines as mediators of oxidative stress is well known. Supporting this notion is the observation of a positive correlation between seminal reactive oxygen species production and seminal plasma concentrations of cytokines such as interleu-kin 6 [58, 59], interleukin 1, and tumor necrosis factor α [60, 61] in infertile able-bodied men. Interleukin 1 and tumor necrosis factor α were also shown to stimulate reactive oxygen species production in fertile donor semen [62]. Thus, activated seminal leukocytes have the potential to cause oxidative stress elevation in men with spinal cord injury.

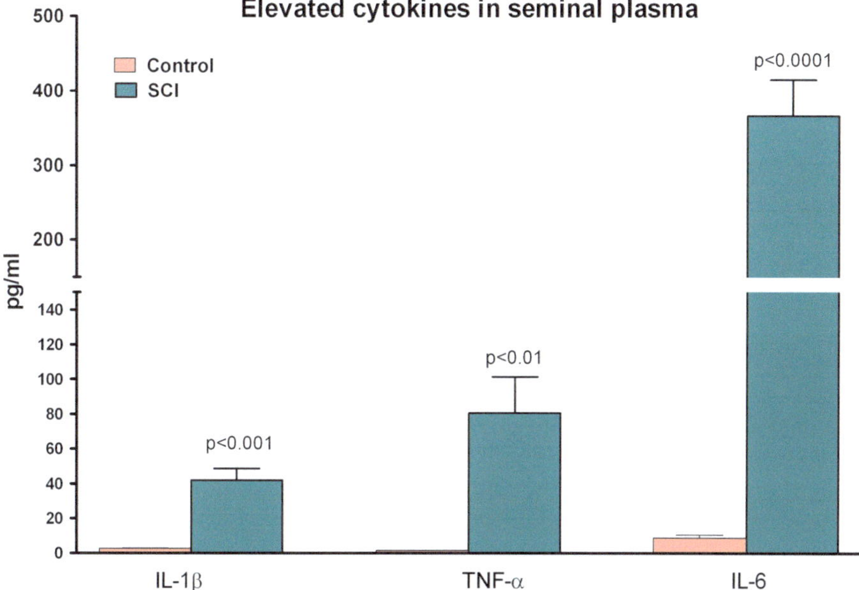

Fig. 13.2 Cytokines can be detrimental to sperm cells. Concentrations of the proinflammatory cytokines, interleukin 1β (1IL-1β), tumor necrosis factor α (TNF-α), and interleukin 6 (IL-6) were significantly elevated in semen of men with spinal cord injury (SCI) compared with semen of control subjects. pg/ml = picograms per milliliter

Effect of Immature Sperm

Even after complete separation of sperm from leukocytes by density gradient and magnetic beads coated with leukocyte-specific CD45 antibodies, reactive oxygen species production can still be recorded, indicating the ability of spermatozoa to generate reactive oxygen species [63]. This ability inversely correlates with the sperm maturation state. During the process of spermiogenesis, surplus cytoplasm is normally extruded, and the sperm cell takes on a condensed, elongated form. If this process is defective, residual cytoplasm forms a cytoplasmic droplet in the sperm mid-region. These spermatozoa are immature and functionally and morphologically abnormal. The residual cytoplasm contains high concentration of cytosolic enzyme glucose-6-phosphate dehydrogenase, which controls the rate of glucose flux and intracellular production of b-nicotinamide adenine dinucleotide phosphate through the hexose monophosphate shunt [64]. Nicotinamide adenine dinucleotide phosphate contributes to the reactive oxygen species production by nicotinamide adenine dinucleotide phosphate oxidase located within the sperm membrane and nicotinamide adenine dinucleotide phosphate-dependent oxidoreductase in the mitochondria [65, 66]. As a consequence, immature sperm with retained cytoplasm produce increased amounts of reactive oxygen species as compared to mature, morphologically normal sperm.

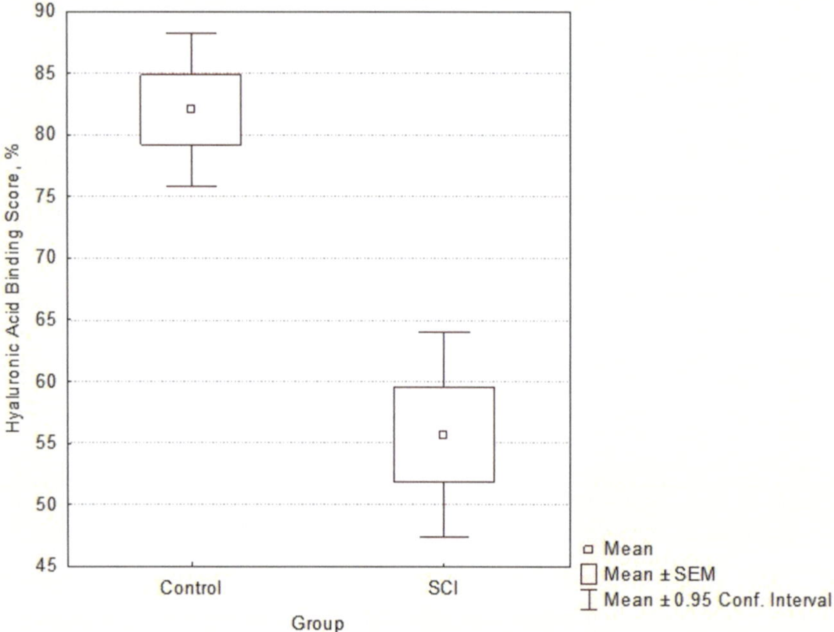

Fig. 13.3 The hyaluronic acid binding score was significantly lower in sperm from men with spinal cord injury (SCI) compared with that of healthy, noninjured control subjects. This deficit may be related to the presence of increased reactive oxygen species and immature sperm in the semen. *SEM* standard error of the mean, *Conf. Interval* confidence interval

The maturation stage of sperm development, along with cytoplasmic extrusion, involves other changes, including the sperm plasma membrane remodeling. This remodeling step facilitates the formation of the sites for zona pellucida and hyaluronic acid binding [67]. Immature sperm with cytoplasmic retention are characterized by low densities of zona pellucida binding sites and also of hyaluronic acid receptors [68]. Sperm hyaluronic acid binding capacity can be tested by evaluating the percentage binding of sperm to hyaluronic acid-coated slides. After application of semen to the slide, it can be seen that mature sperm with a high density of hyaluronic acid receptors exhibits permanent binding, while the immature sperm does not bind and swims freely. We have recently investigated hyaluronic acid binding in sperm from men with spinal cord injury and compared it to that of healthy noninjured control subjects [69]. This study included 13 spinal cord-injured subjects and 13 control subjects. Hyaluronic acid binding was significantly lower in spinal cord-injured subjects compared to the control group (55.7 ± 3.8 versus 82.0 ± 2.8, $p < 0.001$) (Fig. 13.3). A hyaluronic acid binding score of 65% is considered a threshold value, as evidenced by clinical outcomes [70]. Only 3 of the 13 spinal cord-injured subjects had a hyaluronic acid binding score higher than 65%, while in the control group, 12 of 13 had a hyaluronic acid binding score higher than 65%.

These results seem to be consistent with an earlier finding showing increased incidences of sperm with cytoplasmic droplets compared to ejaculates of healthy control subjects [42]. It should be noted that the effects of reactive oxygen species produced by immature sperm (intrinsic) and leukocytes (extrinsic) may differ. For example, it has been shown that while both intrinsic and extrinsic reactive oxygen species negatively affect the integrity of deoxyribonucleic acid (DNA) (explained below), the correlation is much stronger for the intrinsic reactive oxygen species production [71]. These data suggest that reactive oxygen species produced by immature sperm cells may have a greater capacity to damage fertility potential.

Consequences of Oxidative Stress in Semen of Men with Spinal Cord Injury

While leukocytospermia and increased numbers of immature sperm are potential sources of reactive oxygen species in semen of men with spinal cord injury, several other abnormalities, which are characteristic of this group of patients, could be the result of sperm oxidative stress.

Seminal reactive oxygen species, when present in excess, damage different molecules, including lipids, proteins, nucleic acids, and sugars [72]. These toxic effects can result in decreased sperm motility, decreased sperm viability, DNA damage, impaired sperm function, and hyperviscosity of the semen [73]. All of these defects are highly prevalent in semen of men with spinal cord injury [24].

Spermatozoa are vulnerable to the damage induced by excessive reactive oxygen species because their plasma membranes contain large quantities of polyunsaturated fatty acids. Peroxidation of these molecules could decrease membrane flexibility and therefore tail motion. This mechanism of how reactive oxygen species exert their effects on sperm motility was introduced in 1979 [74]. The levels of lipid peroxidation in spermatozoa have been shown to be directly correlated with the loss of motility [75]. Later, several other hypotheses explaining the link between increased reactive oxygen species levels and impaired sperm motility were proposed, including inhibition of enzymes important for intracellular energy production by H_2O_2 and axonemal protein phosphorylation [76, 77]. High levels of seminal reactive oxygen species can also disrupt the inner and outer mitochondrial membranes in spermatozoa [78, 79]. They cause the release of the cytochrome-C protein and activate caspases and apoptosis, resulting in necrospermia [80].

Decreased sperm motility and decreased sperm viability are characteristic features of semen from men with spinal cord injury [24]. In contrast to able-bodied men, most immotile spermatozoa in the semen from men with spinal cord injury are dead. It was shown that the dead-to-live immotile sperm ratio in spinal cord-injured subjects was more than double that in able-bodied subjects (7:3 versus 3:7) [81]. Apoptosis may play an important role in these changes. Experimental data shows that spinal cord injury in rats is associated with decreased sperm mitochondrial transmembrane potential and decreased sperm viability, suggesting excessive apoptosis [16, 82].

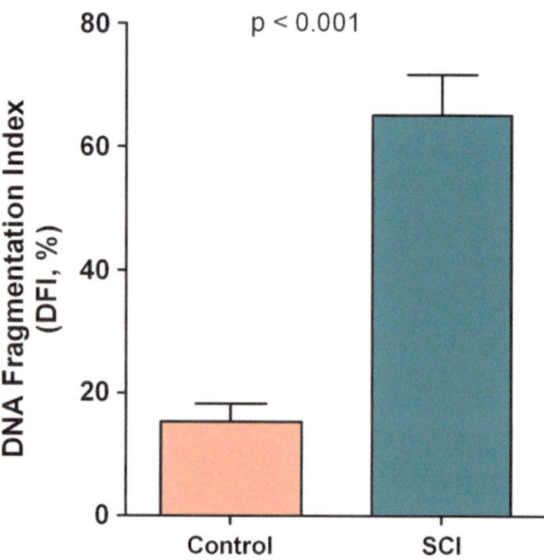

Fig. 13.4 A higher percentage of sperm cells from men with spinal cord injury (SCI) contain DNA damage compared with sperm cells of noninjured control subjects

Increased levels of reactive oxygen species can also negatively affect the integrity of DNA in the sperm nucleus. Several forms of sperm DNA damage could be caused by reactive oxygen species, including chromatin cross-linking, chromosome deletion, DNA single- and double-stranded breaks, and base oxidation [83, 84]. With the use of flow cytometry, it has been shown that sperm from men with spinal cord injury have a high degree of abnormal chromatin condensation and reduced binding [85].

DNA fragmentation in sperm from men with spinal cord injury was also investigated by our group [86]. The study consisted of three experiments. In experiment 1, we compared the DNA fragmentation index in sperm from men with spinal cord injury to that of able-bodied controls. This experiment showed that the mean DNA fragmentation index was fourfold higher in the spinal cord injury group compared with the control group, and there was no overlap in the DNA fragmentation index between these two groups (Fig. 13.4). As was discussed earlier, chronic anejaculation is considered to be one of the possible explanations of semen abnormalities seen in men with spinal cord injury. To examine this possibility, we performed experiment 2 in which we compared the sperm DNA fragmentation index in two semen specimens obtained 3 days apart from the same spinal cord-injured subjects. No significant difference was found in the sperm DNA fragmentation between the two specimens. The purpose of experiment 3 was to determine if necrospermia, leukocytospermia, or semen processing in men with spinal cord injury contribute to their sperm DNA fragmentation index. In this experiment, the DNA fragmentation index in unprocessed semen samples was compared with that of semen samples processed on a gradient (i.e., free of dead sperm and leukocytes). The results of experiment 3 found no significant difference between mean DNA fragmentation index in aliquots of neat versus processed semen in spinal cord-injured subjects. Although removal of leukocytes did not result in a change in the DNA fragmentation index, it is possible that their negative effects on sperm were exerted prior to sperm processing. Thus, it appears that men with spinal cord injury have significantly greater sperm DNA damage, which may be related to high levels of oxidative stress in semen.

Complex relationships exist between apoptosis and DNA damage. Induction of apoptosis by reactive oxygen species results in a high frequency of single- and double-stranded DNA strand breaks in a process referred to karyorrhexis. Severe DNA damage can initiate the apoptosis pathway. Agarwal and Said have suggested that in the context of male infertility, there may be an interaction between seminal reactive oxygen species, sperm DNA damage, and apoptosis, and this interaction may constitute a unified pathogenic molecular mechanism [87].

Semen from men with spinal cord injury is typically highly viscous. Hyperviscous seminal plasma has been reported to be associated with elevated levels of malondi-aldehyde, an unsaturated carbonyl product of oxidative stress indicating excessive lipid peroxidation [88]. Hyperviscosity has also been shown to be linked to reduced seminal plasma antioxidant capacity [89]. The mechanism of change in seminal viscosity due to oxidative stress could be related to altered interactions between oxidized proteins in the seminal plasma [90].

Increased levels of reactive oxygen species can impair sperm function. This phenomenon could be attributed to changes in membrane fluidity and acrosome integrity, resulting in decreased capacity for sperm-oocyte fusion [91]. Sperm from men with spinal cord injury may have functional impairments that could diminish the capacity of their sperm to bind to the oocyte. A study by Denil et al. [92] showed decreased bovine cervical mucus penetration and decreased hamster egg penetration in sperm from spinal cord-injured subjects versus controls. Sperm from men with spinal cord injury was also reported to have a high degree of acrosomal abnormalities [85].

Acrosin (EC 3.4.21.10) is a sperm acrosomal proteinase with trypsin-like substrate specificity, located in the acrosomal matrix as an enzymatically inactive zymogen. Evidence suggests that its active form, acrosin, is necessary for normal fertilization in humans. If acrosin is reduced, absent, or inhibited, sperm binding to, and penetration of, the zona pellucida is severely impaired [93]. We have recently shown that sperm from men with spinal cord injury is characterized by lower acrosin activity compared to healthy men [69]. These findings indicate that sperm from men with spinal cord injury could have functional defects in sperm-oocyte fusion, resulting from oxidative damage.

Oxidative stress results from an imbalance between the production of reactive oxygen species and their efficient removal by available antioxidant systems. Seminal plasma contains different reactive oxygen species scavengers which take part in the protection of spermatozoa from oxidative stress [94]. Exhaustion of seminal plasma antioxidant capacity facilitates sperm damage by free radicals.

It is known that seminal plasma is a major contributor to semen abnormalities in men with spinal cord injury (Fig. 13.5). For example, seminal plasma of spinal cord-injured men rapidly inhibits motility of sperm from normal men. Similarly, seminal plasma from normal men improves the motility of sperm from spinal cord-injured men [39]. Further evidence that an abnormal seminal plasma environment impairs sperm of men with spinal cord injury comes from a study measuring sperm

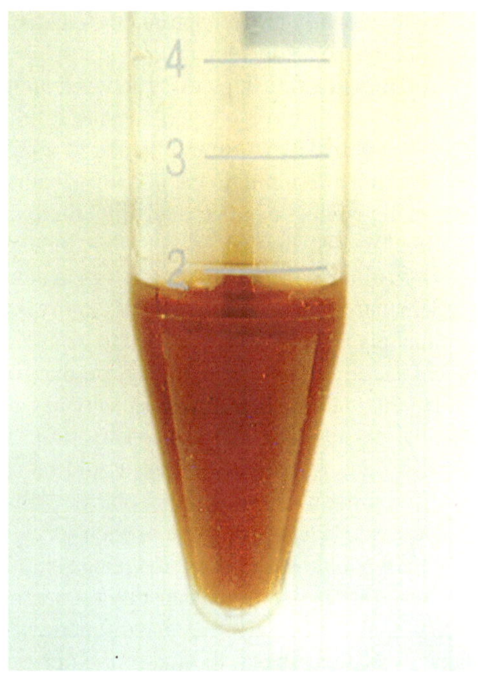

Fig. 13.5 Twenty-seven percent of men with spinal cord injury have *brown-colored semen*. The cause of the *brown color* is unknown and may be related the presence of abnormal constituents in the seminal plasma. Evidence suggests that an abnormal seminal plasma environment contributes to sperm impairments in men with spinal cord injury

motility and sperm viability in ejaculates versus vas deferens aspirates of the same group of spinal cord-injured subjects [48]. Because sperm from the vas deferens has not yet been subjected to the effects of the seminal plasma, a direct comparison of these sperm sources provided information about the effects of seminal plasma on sperm function in men with spinal cord injury. The results of this study showed that in patients with spinal cord injury, but not in able-bodied controls, sperm motility and sperm viability were significantly lower in ejaculated specimens (Fig. 13.6). These data provided evidence that, in men with spinal cord injury, seminal plasma is toxic to the sperm.

Interestingly, sperm obtained from men with spinal cord injury not only lose motility more rapidly than sperm from normal men but this deterioration is also exacerbated when semen is stored at body temperature compared to room temperature. In normal men, this correlation was not found [95]. The possible explanation of this discrepancy is higher reactive oxygen species production by activated leukocytes at body temperature in the semen from men with spinal cord injury. Based on the information presented above, it is reasonable to suggest that elevated levels of reactive oxygen species and/or decreased antioxidant capacity of seminal plasma could be, at least in part, responsible for its detrimental effects on sperm motility and viability. Table 13.2 summarizes characteristics of the semen in men with spinal cord injury, suggesting the presence of increased oxidative stress.

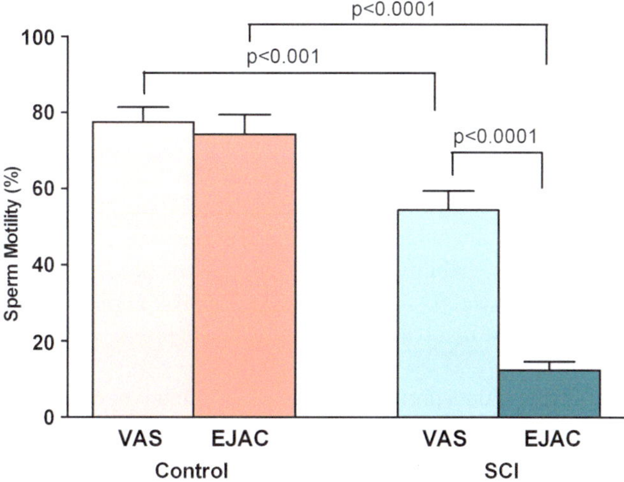

Fig. 13.6 In men with spinal cord injury (SCI), sperm motility was significantly higher when obtained from the vas deferens (VAS) than from the ejaculate (EJAC). In contrast, in control subjects, there was little difference in sperm motility between the two sites. This study provided definitive evidence that seminal plasma was a major contributor to low sperm motility in men with spinal cord injury

Table 13.2 Characteristics of semen from men with spinal cord injury suggesting increased oxidative stress	
	Leukocytospermia
	Teratozoospermia, increased numbers of immature sperm
	Low sperm motility
	Necrospermia
	Increased DNA fragmentation
	Semen hyperviscosity

Treating Oxidative Stress to Improve Semen Quality in Men with Spinal Cord Injury

Understanding the role of increased levels of reactive oxygen species in the pathogenesis of semen quality deterioration after spinal cord injury indicates that correction of oxidative stress could be used in the treatment of these abnormalities. Some studies have shown that treatment with antioxidants, including vitamin E, was associated with improvement of semen parameters in infertile men [96]. The effects of vitamin E on semen quality were studied by Wang et al. in an experimental rat model of spinal cord injury [97]. In this study, rats were given oral vitamin E in two different schedules starting immediately after the injury (maintenance) or 8–10 weeks postinjury (restoration) for 8 weeks. Various sperm parameters were studied including motility, viability, mitochondrial potential, and head decondensation. Weight of accessory glands was also measured.

Feeding with vitamin E was associated with improvement in sperm motility only during the chronic phase of injury, while viability and mitochondrial potential were partially preserved as a result of vitamin E treatment in both restoration and maintenance groups. Sperm head decondensation was significantly less pronounced in rats receiving vitamin E feeding compared to a sham control group. Vitamin E feeding during the chronic phase of injury also resulted in a significant increase in the weight of prostate and seminal vesicles. The results of this study indicate that the antioxidant, vitamin E, attenuated some of the damaging effects of spinal cord injury on sperm motility, viability, and morphology. The partial restoration of prostate and seminal vesicle weight during the chronic phase implies that reactive oxygen species could also be involved in the damaging effects of the spinal cord injury on these glands [97].

Taken together, these data provide evidence that oxidative stress may account for decreased semen quality after spinal cord injury. It is hoped that further laboratory and clinical studies will help to define the role of vitamin E and other antioxidants in the management of male infertility resulting from spinal cord injury.

Expert Commentary

A number of reasons for poor sperm quality in men with spinal cord injury have been postulated; however, we believe that no single factor has been convincingly shown to be the root cause, and it is likely that the etiology of this problem is multifactorial. Among these factors, elevated oxidative stress is clearly an important pathogenic mechanism leading to sperm damage and subsequent infertility resulting from spinal cord injury. Several studies have established a relationship between poor semen quality and the generation of reactive oxygen species in men with spinal cord injury. Semen from these men is characterized by higher concentrations of leukocytes and immature spermatozoa, both of which are important sources of reactive oxygen species production. Furthermore, other seminal abnormalities found in men with spinal cord injury may result from increased oxidative stress.

Five-Year View and Key Issues

While much evidence indicates a role for oxidative stress in the development of infertility in men with spinal cord injury, many unanswered questions still remain. Future research should take several directions:

- Measurements of the changes in antioxidant capacity of seminal plasma in men with spinal cord injury.
- Analysis of the correlation between antioxidant capacity of the seminal plasma and its toxic effects on sperm.

- Studies of the effects of antioxidants as an in vitro and possibly in vivo treatment of semen abnormalities in men with spinal cord injury.
- Investigation of the role of apoptosis in the development of semen abnormalities in men with spinal cord injury and the correlation between apoptosis and seminal plasma antioxidant capacity/seminal reactive oxygen species production.

Results of these studies will enhance our understanding of the underlying pathophysiology of infertility in men with spinal cord injury. These data may also help introduce new methods of treatment of semen abnormalities in this group of patients.

References

1. Spinal cord injury—facts and figures at a glance. 2009. http://www.spinalcord.uab.edu/. Accessed 10 Sept 2009.
2. Elliott S. Sexual dysfunction and infertility in men with spinal cord disorders. In: Lin V, editor. Spinal cord medicine: principles and practice. New York: Demos Medical Publishing; 2003. p. 349–65.
3. Brackett NL, Lynne CM, Ibrahim E, Ohl DA, Sonksen J. Treatment of infertility in men with spinal cord injury. Nat Rev Urol. 2010;7:162–72.
4. Brackett NL, Ibrahim E, Iremashvili V, Aballa TC, Lynne CM. Treatment of ejaculatory dysfunction in men with spinal cord injury: a single-center experience of more than 18 years. J Urol. 2010;183:2304–8.
5. Kafetsoulis A, Brackett NL, Ibrahim E, Attia GR, Lynne CM. Current trends in the treatment of infertility in men with spinal cord injury. Fertil Steril. 2006;86:781–9.
6. Wang YH, Huang TS, Lien IN. Hormone changes in men with spinal cord injuries. Am J Phys Med Rehabil. 1992;71:328–32.
7. Wang YH, Huang TS, Lin MC, Yeh CS, Lien IN. Scrotal temperature in spinal cord injury. Am J Phys Med Rehabil. 1993;72:6–9.
8. Ohl DA, Denil J, Fitzgerald-Shelton K, et al. Fertility of spinal cord injured males: effect of genitourinary infection and bladder management on results of electroejaculation. J Am Paraplegia Soc. 1992;15:53–9.
9. Beretta G, Chelo E, Zanollo A. Reproductive aspects in spinal cord injured males. Paraplegia. 1989;27:113–8.
10. Ohl DA, Menge AC, Jarow JP. Seminal vesicle aspiration in spinal cord injured men: insight into poor sperm quality. J Urol. 1999;162:2048–51.
11. Kostovski E, Iversen PO, Birkeland K, Torjesen PA, Hjeltnes N. Decreased levels of testosterone and gonadotrophins in men with long-standing tetraplegia. Spinal Cord. 2008;46: 559–64.
12. Bors E, Engle ET, Rosenquist RC, Holliger VH. Fertility in paraplegic males; a preliminary report of endocrine studies. J Clin Endocrinol Metab. 1950;10:381–98.
13. Shim HB, Kim YD, Jung TY, Lee JK, Ku JH. Prostate-specific antigen and prostate volume in Korean men with spinal cord injury: a case-control study. Spinal Cord. 2008;46:11–5.
14. Naderi AR, Safarinejad MR. Endocrine profiles and semen quality in spinal cord injured men. Clin Endocrinol (Oxf). 2003;58:177–84.
15. Huang HF, Li MT, Giglio W, Anesetti R, Ottenweller JE, Pogach LM. The detrimental effects of spinal cord injury on spermatogenesis in the rat is partially reversed by testosterone, but enhanced by follicle-stimulating hormone. Endocrinology. 1999;140:1349–55.

16. Huang HF, Li MT, Wang S, Barton B, Anesetti R, Jetko JA. Effects of exogenous testosterone on testicular function during the chronic phase of spinal cord injury: dose effects on spermatogenesis and Sertoli cell and sperm function. J Spinal Cord Med. 2004;27:55–62.
17. Brackett NL, Lynne CM, Weizman MS, Bloch WE, Abae M. Endocrine profiles and semen quality of spinal cord injured men. J Urol. 1994;151:114–9.
18. Huang HF, Linsenmeyer TA, Li MT, et al. Acute effects of spinal cord injury on the pituitary-testicular hormone axis and Sertoli cell functions: a time course study. J Androl. 1995;16: 148–57.
19. Tsitouras PD, Zhong YG, Spungen AM, Bauman WA. Serum testosterone and growth hormone/insulin-like growth factor-I in adults with spinal cord injury. Horm Metab Res. 1995;27:287–92.
20. Naftchi NE, Viau AT, Sell GH, Lowman EW. Pituitary-testicular axis dysfunction in spinal cord injury. Arch Phys Med Rehabil. 1980;61:402–5.
21. Huang HF, Linsenmeyer TA, Anesetti R, Giglio W, Ottenweller JE, Pogach L. Suppression and recovery of spermatogenesis following spinal cord injury in the rat. J Androl. 1998;19: 72–80.
22. Safarinejad MR. Level of injury and hormone profiles in spinal cord-injured men. Urology. 2001;58:671–6.
23. Zorgniotti A, Reiss H, Toth A, Sealfon A. Effect of clothing on scrotal temperature in normal men and patients with poor semen. Urology. 1982;19:176–8.
24. Brackett NL, Nash MS, Lynne CM. Male fertility following spinal cord injury: facts and fiction. Phys Ther. 1996;76:1221–31.
25. Brindley GS. Deep scrotal temperature and the effect on it of clothing, air temperature, activity, posture and paraplegia. Br J Urol. 1982;54:49–55.
26. Brackett NL, Lynne CM, Weizman MS, Bloch WE, Padron OF. Scrotal and oral temperatures are not related to semen quality of serum gonadotropin levels in spinal cord-injured men. J Androl. 1994;15:614–9.
27. Dada R, Gupta NP, Kucheria K. Spermatogenic arrest in men with testicular hyperthermia. Teratog Carcinog Mutagen. 2003;(Suppl 1):235–43.
28. Morgentaler A, Stahl BC, Yin Y. Testis and temperature: an historical, clinical, and research perspective. J Androl. 1999;20:189–95.
29. Brackett NL, Ferrell SM, Aballa TC, Amador MJ, Lynne CM. Semen quality in spinal cord injured men: does it progressively decline postinjury? Arch Phys Med Rehabil. 1998; 79:625–8.
30. Iremashvili V, Brackett NL, Ibrahim E, et al. Semen quality remains stable during the chronic phase of spinal cord injury: a longitudinal study. J Urol. 2010;184(5):2073–7.
31. Rutkowski SB, Middleton JW, Truman G, Hagen DL, Ryan JP. The influence of bladder management on fertility in spinal cord injured males. Paraplegia. 1995;33:263–6.
32. Ohl DA, Bennett CJ, McCabe M, Menge AC, McGuire EJ. Predictors of success in electroejaculation of spinal cord injured men. J Urol. 1989;142:1483–6.
33. Momen MN, Fahmy I, Amer M, Arafa M, Zohdy W, Naser TA. Semen parameters in men with spinal cord injury: changes and aetiology. Asian J Androl. 2007;9:684–9.
34. Das S, Dodd S, Soni BM, Sharma SD, Gazvani R, Lewis-Jones DI. Does repeated electroejaculation improve sperm quality in spinal cord injured men? Spinal Cord. 2006;44:753–6.
35. Siosteen A, Forssman L, Steen Y, Sullivan L, Wickstrom I. Quality of semen after repeated ejaculation treatment in spinal cord injury men. Paraplegia. 1990;28:96–104.
36. Heruti RJ, Katz H, Menashe Y, et al. Treatment of male infertility due to spinal cord injury using rectal probe electroejaculation: the Israeli experience. Spinal Cord. 2001;39:168–75.
37. Sonksen J, Ohl DA, Giwercman A, Biering-Sorensen F, Skakkebaek NE, Kristensen JK. Effect of repeated ejaculation on semen quality in spinal cord injured men. J Urol. 1999;161: 1163–5.
38. Hamid R, Patki P, Bywater H, Shah PJ, Craggs MD. Effects of repeated ejaculations on semen characteristics following spinal cord injury. Spinal Cord. 2006;44:369–73.

39. Brackett NL, Davi RC, Padron OF, Lynne CM. Seminal plasma of spinal cord injured men inhibits sperm motility of normal men. J Urol. 1996;155:1632–5.
40. Rajasekaran M, Hellstrom WJ, Sparks RL, Sikka SC. Sperm-damaging effects of electric current: possible role of free radicals. Reprod Toxicol. 1994;8:427–32.
41. de Lamirande E, Leduc BE, Iwasaki A, Hassouna M, Gagnon C. Increased reactive oxygen species formation in semen of patients with spinal cord injury. Fertil Steril. 1995;63:637–42.
42. Padron OF, Brackett NL, Sharma RK, Lynne CM, Thomas Jr AJ, Agarwal A. Seminal reactive oxygen species and sperm motility and morphology in men with spinal cord injury. Fertil Steril. 1997;67:1115–20.
43. Aitken RJ, Buckingham DW, Brindle J, Gomez E, Baker HW, Irvine DS. Analysis of sperm movement in relation to the oxidative stress created by leukocytes in washed sperm preparations and seminal plasma. Hum Reprod. 1995;10:2061–71.
44. Basu S, Lynne CM, Ruiz P, Aballa TC, Ferrell SM, Brackett NL. Cytofluorographic identification of activated T-cell subpopulations in the semen of men with spinal cord injuries. J Androl. 2002;23:551–6.
45. Aird IA, Vince GS, Bates MD, Johnson PM, Lewis-Jones ID. Leukocytes in semen from men with spinal cord injuries. Fertil Steril. 1999;72:97–103.
46. Pentyala S, Lee J, Annam S, et al. Current perspectives on pyospermia: a review. Asian J Androl. 2007;9:593–600.
47. Randall JM, Evans DH, Bird VG, Aballa TC, Lynne CM, Brackett NL. Leukocytospermia in spinal cord injured patients is not related to histological inflammatory changes in the prostate. J Urol. 2003;170:897–900.
48. Brackett NL, Lynne CM, Aballa TC, Ferrell SM. Sperm motility from the vas deferens of spinal cord injured men is higher than from the ejaculate. J Urol. 2000;164:712–5.
49. Whittington K, Harrison SC, Williams KM, et al. Reactive oxygen species (ROS) production and the outcome of diagnostic tests of sperm function. Int J Androl. 1999;22:236–42.
50. Sharma RK, Pasqualotto AE, Nelson DR, Thomas Jr AJ, Agarwal A. Relationship between seminal white blood cell counts and oxidative stress in men treated at an infertility clinic. J Androl. 2001;22:575–83.
51. Agarwal A, Makker K, Sharma R. Clinical relevance of oxidative stress in male factor infertility: an update. Am J Reprod Immunol. 2008;59:2–11.
52. Trabulsi EJ, Shupp-Byrne D, Sedor J, Hirsch IH. Leukocyte subtypes in electroejaculates of spinal cord injured men. Arch Phys Med Rehabil. 2002;83:31–4.
53. Plante M, de Lamirande E, Gagnon C. Reactive oxygen species released by activated neutrophils, but not by deficient spermatozoa, are sufficient to affect normal sperm motility. Fertil Steril. 1994;62:387–93.
54. Said TM, Agarwal A, Sharma RK, Thomas Jr AJ, Sikka SC. Impact of sperm morphology on DNA damage caused by oxidative stress induced by beta-nicotinamide adenine dinucleotide phosphate. Fertil Steril. 2005;83:95–103.
55. Basu S, Aballa TC, Ferrell SM, Lynne CM, Brackett NL. Inflammatory cytokine concentrations are elevated in seminal plasma of men with spinal cord injuries. J Androl. 2004; 25:250–4.
56. Brackett NL, Cohen DR, Ibrahim E, Aballa TC, Lynne CM. Neutralization of cytokine activity at the receptor level improves sperm motility in men with spinal cord injuries. J Androl. 2007;28:717–21.
57. Cohen DR, Basu S, Randall JM, Aballa TC, Lynne CM, Brackett NL. Sperm motility in men with spinal cord injuries is enhanced by inactivating cytokines in the seminal plasma. J Androl. 2004;25:922–5.
58. Nandipati KC, Pasqualotto FF, Thomas Jr AJ, Agarwal A. Relationship of interleukin-6 with semen characteristics and oxidative stress in vasectomy reversal patients. Andrologia. 2005; 37:131–4.
59. Camejo MI, Segnini A, Proverbio F. Interleukin-6 (IL-6) in seminal plasma of infertile men, and lipid peroxidation of their sperm. Arch Androl. 2001;47:97–101.

60. Martinez P, Proverbio F, Camejo MI. Sperm lipid peroxidation and pro-inflammatory cytokines. Asian J Androl. 2007;9:102–7.
61. Sanocka D, Jedrzejczak P, Szumala-Kaekol A, Fraczek M, Kurpisz M. Male genital tract inflammation: the role of selected interleukins in regulation of pro-oxidant and antioxidant enzymatic substances in seminal plasma. J Androl. 2003;24:448–55.
62. Buch JP, Kolon TF, Maulik N, Kreutzer DL, Das DK. Cytokines stimulate lipid membrane peroxidation of human sperm. Fertil Steril. 1994;62:186–8.
63. Aitken RJ, Buckingham DW, West K, Brindle J. On the use of paramagnetic beads and ferrofluids to assess and eliminate the leukocytic contribution to oxygen radical generation by human sperm suspensions. Am J Reprod Immunol. 1996;35:541–51.
64. Fisher HM, Aitken RJ. Comparative analysis of the ability of precursor germ cells and epididymal spermatozoa to generate reactive oxygen metabolites. J Exp Zool. 1997;277:390–400.
65. Aitken RJ, Buckingham DW, West KM. Reactive oxygen species and human spermatozoa: analysis of the cellular mechanisms involved in luminol- and lucigenin-dependent chemiluminescence. J Cell Physiol. 1992;151:466–77.
66. Gavella M, Lipovac V. NADH-dependent oxidoreductase (diaphorase) activity and isozyme pattern of sperm in infertile men. Arch Androl. 1992;28:135–41.
67. Huszar G, Sbracia M, Vigue L, Miller DJ, Shur BD. Sperm plasma membrane remodeling during spermiogenetic maturation in men: relationship among plasma membrane beta 1,4-galactosyltransferase, cytoplasmic creatine phosphokinase, and creatine phosphokinase isoform ratios. Biol Reprod. 1997;56:1020–4.
68. Huszar G, Ozenci CC, Cayli S, Zavaczki Z, Hansch E, Vigue L. Hyaluronic acid binding by human sperm indicates cellular maturity, viability, and unreacted acrosomal status. Fertil Steril. 2003;79 Suppl 3:1616–24.
69. Iremashvili V, Brackett NL, Ibrahim E, Aballa TC, Bruck D, Lynne CM. Hyaluronic acid binding and acrosin activity are decreased in sperm from men with spinal cord injury. Fertil Steril. 2010;94(5):1925–7.
70. Huszar G, Ozkavukcu S, Jakab A, Celik-Ozenci C, Sati GL, Cayli S. Hyaluronic acid binding ability of human sperm reflects cellular maturity and fertilizing potential: selection of sperm for intracytoplasmic sperm injection. Curr Opin Obstet Gynecol. 2006;18:260–7.
71. Henkel R, Kierspel E, Stalf T, et al. Effect of reactive oxygen species produced by spermatozoa and leukocytes on sperm functions in non-leukocytospermic patients. Fertil Steril. 2005;83:635–42.
72. Pryor WA, Houk KN, Foote CS, et al. Free radical biology and medicine: it's a gas, man! Am J Physiol Regul Integr Comp Physiol. 2006;291:R491–511.
73. Tremellen K. Oxidative stress and male infertility–a clinical perspective. Hum Reprod Update. 2008;14:243–58.
74. Jones R, Mann T, Sherins R. Peroxidative breakdown of phospholipids in human spermatozoa, spermicidal properties of fatty acid peroxides, and protective action of seminal plasma. Fertil Steril. 1979;31:531–7.
75. Gomez E, Irvine DS, Aitken RJ. Evaluation of a spectrophotometric assay for the measurement of malondialdehyde and 4-hydroxyalkenals in human spermatozoa: relationships with semen quality and sperm function. Int J Androl. 1998;21:81–94.
76. Aitken RJ, Fisher HM, Fulton N, et al. Reactive oxygen species generation by human spermatozoa is induced by exogenous NADPH and inhibited by the flavoprotein inhibitors diphenylene iodonium and quinacrine. Mol Reprod Dev. 1997;47:468–82.
77. de Lamirande E, Gagnon C. Reactive oxygen species and human spermatozoa. I. Effects on the motility of intact spermatozoa and on sperm axonemes. J Androl. 1992;13:368–78.
78. de Lamirande E, Gagnon C. Reactive oxygen species and human spermatozoa. II. Depletion of adenosine triphosphate plays an important role in the inhibition of sperm motility. J Androl. 1992;13:379–86.
79. de Lamirande E, Jiang H, Zini A, Kodama H, Gagnon C. Reactive oxygen species and sperm physiology. Rev Reprod. 1997;2:48–54.

80. Wang X, Sharma RK, Sikka SC, Thomas Jr AJ, Falcone T, Agarwal A. Oxidative stress is associated with increased apoptosis leading to spermatozoa DNA damage in patients with male factor infertility. Fertil Steril. 2003;80:531–5.
81. Brackett NL, Bloch WE, Lynne CM. Predictors of necrospermia in men with spinal cord injury. J Urol. 1998;159:844–7.
82. Nunez R, Murphy TF, Huang HF, Barton BE. Use of SYBR14, 7-amino-actinomycin D, and JC-1 in assessing sperm damage from rats with spinal cord injury. Cytometry A. 2004;61: 56–61.
83. Aitken RJ, Krausz C. Oxidative stress, DNA damage and the Y chromosome. Reproduction. 2001;122:497–506.
84. Kemal Duru N, Morshedi M, Oehninger S. Effects of hydrogen peroxide on DNA and plasma membrane integrity of human spermatozoa. Fertil Steril. 2000;74:1200–7.
85. Engh E, Clausen OP, Purvis K, Stien R. Sperm quality assessed by flow cytometry and accessory sex gland function in spinal cord injured men after repeated vibration- induced ejaculation. Paraplegia. 1993;31:3–12.
86. Brackett NL, Ibrahim E, Grotas JA, Aballa TC, Lynne CM. Higher sperm DNA damage in semen from men with spinal cord injuries compared with controls. J Androl. 2008;29:93–9. discussion 100–101.
87. Agarwal A, Said TM. Oxidative stress, DNA damage and apoptosis in male infertility: a clinical approach. BJU Int. 2005;95:503–7.
88. Aydemir B, Onaran I, Kiziler AR, Alici B, Akyolcu MC. The influence of oxidative damage on viscosity of seminal fluid in infertile men. J Androl. 2008;29:41–6.
89. Siciliano L, Tarantino P, Longobardi F, Rago V, De Stefano C, Carpino A. Impaired seminal antioxidant capacity in human semen with hyperviscosity or oligoasthenozoospermia. J Androl. 2001;22:798–803.
90. Traverso N, Menini S, Maineri EP, et al. Malondialdehyde, a lipoperoxidation-derived aldehyde, can bring about secondary oxidative damage to proteins. J Gerontol A Biol Sci Med Sci. 2004;59:B890–5.
91. Agarwal A, Saleh RA. Role of oxidants in male infertility: rationale, significance, and treatment. Urol Clin North Am. 2002;29:817–27.
92. Denil J, Ohl DA, Menge AC, Keller LM, McCabe M. Functional characteristics of sperm obtained by electroejaculation. J Urol. 1992;147:69–72.
93. Liu DY, Baker HW. Inhibition of acrosin activity with a trypsin inhibitor blocks human sperm penetration of the zona pellucida. Biol Reprod. 1993;48:340–8.
94. Balercia G, Armeni T, Mantero F, Principato G, Regoli F. Total oxyradical scavenging capacity toward different reactive oxygen species in seminal plasma and sperm cells. Clin Chem Lab Med. 2003;41:13–9.
95. Brackett NL, Santa-Cruz C, Lynne CM. Sperm from spinal cord injured men lose motility faster than sperm from normal men: the effect is exacerbated at body compared to room temperature. J Urol. 1997;157:2150–3.
96. Kessopoulou E, Powers HJ, Sharma KK, et al. A double-blind randomized placebo cross-over controlled trial using the antioxidant vitamin E to treat reactive oxygen species associated male infertility. Fertil Steril. 1995;64:825–31.
97. Wang S, Wang G, Barton BE, Murphy TF, Huang HF. Beneficial effects of vitamin E in sperm functions in the rat after spinal cord injury. J Androl. 2007;28:334–41.

Chapter 14
Obesity and Male Fertility

Stephanie Cabler, Ashok Agarwal, and Stefan S. du Plessis

In the past 5–10 years, obesity has become a worldwide epidemic that has brought attention to learning more about the various causes, effects, and treatments. A combination of an increasingly acceptable sedentary lifestyle and unhealthy diet in the Western world has resulted in an increasing number of overweight and obese children and adults. According to the WHO, approximately 1.6 billion adults were classified as being overweight and 400 million adults were obese in 2005 [1]. It is predicted that globally, in the next 5 years, more than 700 million adults will suffer from obesity [1]. Once considered a problem only in high-income countries, overweight and obesity are now dramatically on the rise in all countries. Evidence of this is the five unit increase in body mass index (BMI) for the period 1997–2006 in the 95th percentile BMI level among children aged 6–9 years in China. These children in the 95th percentile have a BMI of 24.8, which is surprisingly higher than that of the USA (22.2), Australia (20.1), and the UK (20.1) [2].

Parallel to the global increase in obesity is the reported world decrease in male fertility and fecundity [3]. Interestingly, men with increased BMI were significantly more likely to be infertile than normal-weight men, according to research conducted at the National Institute of Environmental Health Sciences (NIEHS) [4]. According to Carlson et al., the quality of semen has substantially declined, which has subsequently lead to decreased male fertility [5]. This could likely contribute to overall reduced male reproductive potential. Some studies estimate that male sperm counts continue to decrease at a rate of approximately 1.5% per year in the USA and

S. Cabler, BSc (✉) • A. Agarwal, PhD
Center for Reproductive Medicine, Glickman Urological and Kidney Institute, Cleveland Clinic Foundation, 9500 Euclid Avenue, Desk A19, Cleveland, OH 44195, USA
e-mail: agarwaa@ccf.org

S.S. du Plessis, PhD, MBA
Department of Medical Physiology, Faculty of Health Sciences, Stellenbosch University, 19063, Tygerberg, Western Cape 7505, South Africa
e-mail: ssdp@sun.ac.za

S.J. Parekattil and A. Agarwal (eds.), *Antioxidants in Male Infertility: A Guide for Clinicians and Researchers*, © Springer Science+Business Media New York 2013

similar findings have been found in other Western countries as well [3]. In addition, there is also a significant increase in the incidence of obesity in patients with male factor infertility, and couples with obese male partners are more likely to experience subfecundity, a correlation that seems necessary to address [6]. Due to the fact that this decline has occurred in close parallel with increasing rates of obesity, it is necessary to focus on the possibility of obesity as an etiology of male infertility and reduced fecundity. The "obesity pandemic" seen in many countries is a serious threat to public health, and a reduced capacity to reproduce is a potential but less well-known health hazard that can often be attributed to obesity.

It is therefore necessary to explore the links between obesity and male infertility, as well as to explain how it disrupts the male reproductive system at a mechanistical level. Treatment and prevention of obesity and associated fertility disorders will also be discussed in a clinical context.

What Is Obesity?

Obesity is a medical condition in which excess body fat, or white adipose tissue, accumulates in the body to the extent that the excess fat adversely affects health, often reducing life expectancy. The fundamental cause of obesity and overweight is an energy imbalance, where the energy consumed exceeds the energy expended. Global increases in overweight and obesity are attributable to a number of factors, including a shift in diet toward increased intake of energy-dense foods that are high in fat and sugars, and a trend toward decreased physical activity, resulting from increasingly sedentary nature of work, changing modes of transportation, and increasing urbanization.

Currently, overweight and obesity are defined more broadly as abnormal or excessive fat accumulation that may impair health. However, there are other specific requirements that qualify an individual as obese. The most accurate measures are to weigh a person underwater or to use an X-ray test called dual energy X-ray absorptiometry. These methods are not practical for the average individual and are conducted only in research centers with special equipment. There are simpler methods to estimate body fat such as BMI, skin fold measurements, waist-to-hip ratio (WHR), waist circumference, and also methods such as bioelectrical impedance analysis, risk factors and comorbidities [7]. The two tools that are most commonly used to identify obese patients are BMI, a waist-to-height ratio, and waist circumference. An individual is normally defined as being overweight if their BMI is between 25 and 30 kg/m^2 and obese if it exceeds 30 kg/m^2.[8] A problem with this method is that individuals with a high BMI may be mesomorphic and have a high amount of muscle mass. Therefore, BMI may not be the most accurate marker for total body fat percentage and is an even less suitable tool to assess body fat distribution.

Waist circumference is a slightly less common method used to predict obesity in an individual, but may be more accurate in predicting obesity-related health issues.

For females, a waist circumference of 88 cm or greater is considered unhealthy. For men, a waist circumference of 102 cm or greater is considered unhealthy. If waist circumference is used as the criterion, then according to a study conducted in 2006, the prevalence of being overweight among Australian adults, and probably other Caucasian populations, may be significantly greater than indicated by surveys relying on self-reported height and weight. The development of valid self-reported measures of waist circumference for use in population surveys may allow more accurate monitoring of overweight and obesity and should be considered instead of BMI [9]. A WHR can also be used to predict unhealthy consequences as a result of increased body fat (normal WHR: males = <0.9; females <0.85), especially related to the risk of coronary heart disease as it relates to obesity [10]. WHR may be the most useful measure of obesity and the best simple anthropometric index in predicting a wide range of risk factors and related health conditions [11].

How Does Obesity Affect Male Fertility?

The relationship between male infertility and obesity has more concrete evidence than solely studies showing reduced fecundity among couples, one of whom is an obese male. Although spermatogenesis and fertility are not impaired in a majority of obese men, a disproportionate number of men seeking infertility treatment are obese. There have been a number of studies analyzing the relationship between semen quality and obesity, with a common finding that there is an inverse correlation between BMI and quality of semen parameters.

Abnormal Semen Parameters

Altered semen parameters attributed to obesity include decreased sperm concentration, abnormal morphology, compromised chromatin integrity, and abnormal motility. Although there is a convincing amount of evidence to demonstrate the adverse affect of excess body fat on spermatogenesis, not all studies have come to the same conclusions. Individual studies are conflicting in evidence, but a recent meta-analysis by MacDonald et al. [12] combined 31 studies containing data and information relating to obesity and male infertility. Reproductive hormones studied included testosterone, free testosterone, estradiol, FSH, LH, inhibin B, and sex hormone-binding globulin (SHBG). This meta-analysis was conducted to investigate sperm concentration and total sperm count but found no evidence for a relationship between BMI and sperm concentration or total sperm count. Examination of further studies may present more insight in the relationship between obesity and semen quality.

Decreased Sperm Count and Concentration

Obese men are three times more likely than healthy men of normal weight to have a sperm count of fewer than 20 million/ml, an indicator of oligospermia [13]. In one of the largest studies on male fertility and obesity, done on Danish men, Jensen et al. measured BMI in relation to semen quality and reproductive hormones and found significant relationships between sperm concentration and BMI. A lower sperm concentration was observed in not only obese and overweight males, but also in males who were significantly underweight. This could serve as an indication that there may be an ideal range of BMI for normal spermatogenesis. Subjects whose BMI was within the normal range showed a higher sperm concentration, as well as a higher total sperm count, and a lower percentage of abnormal spermatozoa [14]. According to a study by Chavarro et al., men with a BMI greater than 25 kg/m^2 had a lower total sperm count than men of normal weight, and the measured volume of ejaculate decreased steadily with an increasing BMI [15]. These findings have been corroborated by other studies as well [16, 17]. Although several reports exist indicating a considerable negative effect of BMI on sperm count and concentration, some discrepancies have been noted. In these studies, a correlation between sperm count and concentration in obese men compared to controls was demonstrated but was not deemed significant [18–20].

Sperm Motility

Some consensus on the effects of obesity on sperm motility has been established, but there is no overall agreement. Hofny et al. [16] found that the BMI correlated negatively with sperm motility, and Hammoud et al. [21] concluded that the incidence of low progressively motile sperm count increased with increasing BMI. Fejes et al. [22] found that the waist to hip circumference of men correlated negatively with the total motile sperm count as well as the rapid progressively motile sperm count. Another study by Martini et al. found that there was a negative association between BMI and motility and rapid motility [23]. Despite this evidence, not all studies have come to the same conclusions, and a majority of studies measuring semen parameters neglect to include motility in their measurements [14, 19].

DNA Fragmentation

Kort et al. found that an increase in the DNA fragmentation index (DFI) accompanied an increase in BMI, demonstrating that obesity might compromise the integrity of sperm chromatin, their only genetic material [24].

DFI is the percent of sperm in a semen sample that have increased levels of single or double strand breaks in their nuclear DNA. A young and healthy man has about 3–5% of sperm with fragmented DNA while a level of 25–30% DFI places a man attempting natural conception at a statistical risk for infertility [25]. An increase in the BMI above 25 kg/m^2 causes an increase in sperm DFI and a decrease in the number of normal chromatin-intact sperm cells per ejaculate, relative to the degree of obesity [24]. Men with type 2 diabetes also present with a significantly higher number of severe structural defects in sperm compared with sperm from controls ($p < 0.05$) [47]. Typically, males presenting with a high DFI will have reduced fertility, and their partners will display an increased incidence of miscarriage as a consequence [26].

A new breakthrough in gel electrophoresis has been used to identify obesity-associated changes of the sperm proteome. Semen samples from obese males differed from those of normal-weight men with 12 spots seen after running their "difference gel electrophoresis" (DIGE) of fluorescently labeled human sperm proteins. Tryptic digestion of the 12 spot proteins and mass spectrometric analysis of the corresponding peptides identified nine sperm proteins associated with obesity. This can now be considered a noninvasive experimental tool in the diagnosis of male infertility and monitoring device for fertility-restoring therapy in obese males [27]. This finding clearly demonstrates the differences or changes in the protein composition of spermatozoa in obese men.

Sperm Morphology

Measuring differences in the morphology of sperm between obese and normal-weight men can be difficult owing to differences in what is classified as "normal" morphology and high individual variability within individual patient samples. However, most studies have shown no correlation between obesity and abnormal sperm morphology [14, 15, 19, 21]. In the large retrospective study of Danish military recruits, no association between obesity and poor sperm motility or morphology was reported [14]. Identifying the specific hormones, proteins, and mechanisms involved in regulating sperm morphology might help to explain how and why obesity affects normal spermatogenesis.

What Are the Proposed Mechanisms?

Although environmental and lifestyle factors might help to explain the growing numbers of obese adults and children, there is less evidence explaining how obesity causes male infertility. The mechanisms responsible for effects on male infertility are mostly ambiguous and undefined. Several mechanisms have been proposed,

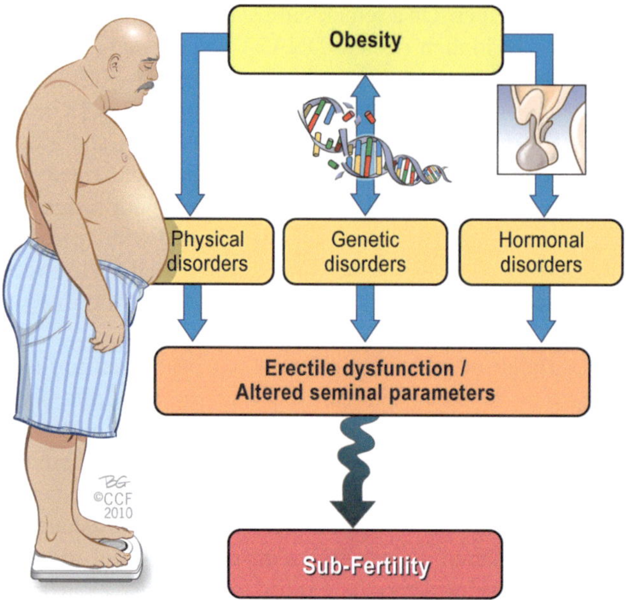

Fig. 14.1 The effects of obesity on male fertility and mechanisms involved

all of which are described below (Fig. 14.1). Most of these mechanisms contribute to the dysregulation of the hypothalamic–pituitary–gonadal (HPG) axis, one of the most important functions of which is to regulate aspects of reproduction.

Genetic Link

Despite there being a known effect of obesity on infertility, many obese males are fertile and have normal reproductive function and fecundity. However, because obesity can result from an unfavorable genotype and because obesity can cause infertility, a genetic link between these two factors might explain this discrepancy. Patients with Klinefelter, Prader–Willi, or Laurence–Moon–Bardet–Biedel syndromes all display, to varying degrees, both obesity and infertility. In addition, men who are both infertile and obese show significantly lower testosterone levels than obese fertile men [28]. Although the specific genes involved and mechanism(s) explaining these syndromes are quite well understood, it is possible that other, less severe genetic mutations exist. These small mutations might explain the discrepancies between obese fertile and infertile men and shed light upon a possible genetic link between obesity and infertility.

Also, mutations in the human ALMS1 gene are responsible for Alström syndrome, a disorder in which key metabolic and endocrinological features include childhood-onset obesity, metabolic syndrome, and diabetes, as well as infertility [29]. Scientists still need to accurately establish which particular genes are involved in these different syndromes, but the linkage of obesity and infertility in extreme genetic cases points to some degree of genetic linkage. Hammoud et al. [30] recently discovered that an aromatase polymorphism modulates the relationship between weight and estradiol levels in obese men. This could explain why only certain obese men experience this rise in estradiol and subsequent fertility problems, while others experience no fertility issues. It seems possible that there are other less severe genetic markers than chromosome 15 abnormalities and ALMS1 mutations that may clarify the discrepancies between obese fertile and infertile men and give explanation to a possible genetic link between obesity and infertility.

Hormonal Mechanisms

Abdominal or visceral fat is more likely to lead to changes in hormone levels and to cause inflammation than fat stored in other parts of the body. This is predominantly due to the fact that white adipose tissue, found in high levels in obese men, exhibits elevated aromatase activity and secretes adipose-derived hormones, as well as adipokines.

Reproductive Hormones

The reproductive hormonal profiles of most obese men deviate from what is considered the norm. Obese men tend to present with elevated estrogen and low testosterone and FSH levels. Androgen deficiency or hypogonadism found in males who are obese or have metabolic syndrome can account for problems with erectile dysfunction and spermatogenesis. However, many other hormones associated with obesity may alter the male reproductive potential. In morbidly obese individuals, reduced spermatogenesis associated with severe hypotestosteronemia may contribute to infertility [31, 32]. This estrogen excess is explained by overactivity of the aromatase cytochrome P450 enzyme, which is expressed at high levels in white adipose tissue and is responsible for a key step in the biosynthesis of estrogens. High levels of estrogens in obese males result from the increased conversion of androgens into estrogens, owing to the high bioavailability of these aromatase enzymes [33]. Visceral obesity can serve as a major endocrine disrupter and can also influence the endocrine interactions by reducing the levels of luteinizing hormone (LH) and testosterone, resulting in hypogonadotropic hypogonadism, a condition which contributes to male infertility. Although abnormal levels of reproductive hormones could be the source of fertility problems in obese males, Qin et al. [34] established that the associations between BMI and semen quality were found statistically significant even after an adjustment for reproductive hormones, thereby demonstrating that reproductive hormones cannot fully explain the association between BMI and semen quality [35]. Perhaps, altered hormone levels themselves do not explain poor semen quality but instead a deregulation of the normal HPG axis. Regardless, studies indicate that the association between BMI and semen quality is clearly more complex than what can be accounted for simply by reproductive hormones. Instead, it may be a result of other factors such as one's lifestyle and increased adipokine release.

White Adipose Tissue as an Endocrine Organ

White adipose tissue is a major secretory and endocrine organ that secretes approximately 30 biologically active peptides and proteins that can be grouped as either adipose-derived hormones (e.g., leptin, adiponectin, resistin) or adipokines (immunomodulating agents). Adipose-derived hormones play a central role in body homeostasis including the regulation of food intake and energy balance, insulin action, lipid and glucose metabolism, angiogenesis and vascular remodeling, coagulation, and the regulation of blood pressure [35]. Due to an excess of white adipose tissue in obese men, levels of adipose-derived hormones are often elevated, and their action is thought to modify many obesity-related diseases, including reproductive functioning.

Leptin

One such adipose-derived hormone is leptin, which is best known as a regulator of food intake and energy expenditure via hypothalamic-mediated effects [36, 37]. Although normal levels of leptin are required for overall reproductive health, excess leptin may be an important contributor to the development of reduced androgens in male obesity [38]. In addition to a higher prevalence of infertility, obese individuals are reported to have higher circulating levels of leptin than non-obese individuals [39, 40]. An increasing body of data suggests that leptin is also involved in glucose metabolism as well as in normal sexual maturation and reproduction [16]. Leptin receptors are not only present in testicular tissue but also on the plasma membrane of sperm suggesting that leptin may directly affect sperm via the endocrine system, independent of changes in the HPG axis [38, 41]. Diet-induced obesity in mice caused a significant reduction in male fertility and resulted in a fivefold increase in leptin levels compared to control mice. Sperm from these obese males exhibited decreased motility and reduced hyperactivated progression compared to the lean mice.

Oxidative Stress and Reactive Oxygen Species

As mentioned previously, adipocytes secrete various adipokines (e.g., tumor necrosis factor α (TNF-α), interleukin 6 (IL-6), plasminogen activator inhibitor-1 (PAI-1), and tissue factor) [37]. A number of these adipokines have been connected to infertility and testicular cancer. Bialas et al. [42] found that changes in the activity of intratesticular cytokines may promote various distinct pathologies such as testicular cancer or infertility. Also, increased release of adipokines from excess white adipose tissue, resulting in inflammation, can have a toxic effect on spermatozoa through the release of excess reactive oxygen species (ROS) and reactive nitrogen species (RNS) [43]. ROS and RNS are free radicals, highly reactive and unstable molecules that arise as a consequence of oxidative stress or inflammation that can induce significant cellular damage throughout the body. Two adipocyte-released adipokines, TNF-α and IL-6, significantly reduced human sperm progressive motility in a dose- and time-dependent manner by promoting the elevation of nitric oxide production to pathological levels [44]. Numerous authors have noted that obesity and several of its causative agents, namely insulin resistance and dyslipidemia, are associated with increased oxidative stress [45, 46]. This association is most likely the result of the elevated metabolic rates that are required to maintain normal biological processes and increased levels of stress in the local testicular environment, both of which naturally produce ROS. The local influences of biologically active substances (cytokines) released by activated leukocytes in the course of the inflammatory response to obesity may damage sperm and inhibit spermatogenesis. Agarwal et al. [47] found that abnormal patterns of increased ROS were associated with male factor infertility and are responsible for abnormal sperm concentration, motility, and morphology found in obese males.

Inhibin B

In a study by Winters et al. [48], the levels of inhibin B, another hormone involved in the HPG axis, declined with increasing obesity in young adult men, and values were 26% lower in men who were obese compared to normal-weight men. As it was shown that inhibin B is positively correlated with the number of Sertoli cells in normal adult rhesus monkeys, the reduced levels of inhibin B in the Winters study may indicate that obese men have fewer Sertoli cells than men of normal weight [49]. Since each Sertoli cell is thought to support a finite number of germ cells, fewer Sertoli cells as a result of obesity may result in a lower sperm count [48].

Resistin Secretion and Insulin Resistance

Resistin is another adipose-tissue-specific factor, which is reported to induce insulin resistance. Almost 80% of men with type 2 diabetes are also obese, and an increase in resistin secretion owing to a higher number of adipocytes links obesity to type 2 diabetes [37, 50]. As a consequence of insulin resistance in patients with type 2 diabetes, increased renin secretion was associated with increased oxidative stress [45, 46]. This association is most likely the result of the higher-than-usual metabolic rates required to maintain normal biological processes and an increased level of stress in the local testicular environment. Hyperinsulinemia, which often occurs in obese men, has an inhibitory effect on normal spermatogenesis and can be linked to decreased male fertility. In a group of diabetic men, semen parameters (concentration, motility, and morphology) did not differ from the control group, but the amount of nuclear and mitochondrial DNA damage in the sperm was significantly higher [51]. This sperm DNA damage can impair male fertility and reproductive health. In addition to inducing sperm DNA damage, high insulin levels also have been shown to influence the levels of sex hormone binding globulin (SHBG), a glycoprotein that binds to sex hormones, specifically testosterone and estradiol, thereby inhibiting their biologic activity as a carrier.

High circulating insulin levels inhibit SHBG synthesis in the liver, whereas weight loss has been shown to increase SHBG levels [52]. In obese males, the decrease in SHBG means that less estrogen will be bound, resulting in more biologically active, free estrogen. In addition to the conversion of testosterone to estrogen in obese patients, the decreased ability of SHBG to sustain homeostatic levels of free testosterone also contributes to abnormal testosterone levels [14]. This failure to maintain homeostatic levels might magnify the negative feedback effect of elevated total estrogen levels. Even when the presence of SHBG is accounted for, an independent relationship between insulin resistance and testosterone production can still be demonstrated [32]. Therefore, the levels of SHBG might be important only as a marker of altered hormone profiles in obese infertile men.

Environmental Toxins

Most environmental toxins are fat soluble and therefore accumulate in fatty tissue. Their accumulation not only around the scrotum and testes, but also elsewhere in the body may disrupt the normal hormone profile because they are proven endocrine disruptors in male fertility [21]. Since morbidly obese males present with excess scrotal fat, environmental toxins accumulating in white adipose tissue surrounding the scrotum may also have a direct localized effect on spermatogenesis in the testes. Lipophilic contaminants such as organochlorines, organic compounds containing at least one covalently bonded chlorine atom whose uses are controversial because of the often toxic effects of these compounds on the environment, are associated with decreased sperm production and thus decreased male reproductive potential, even if fat is not localized in the scrotal area [34]. Other toxic species that may induce abnormal spermatogenesis are ROS discussed in the previous section. Despite reports that certain toxins can negatively affect fertility, Magnusdottir et al. [6] found that poor semen quality was found to be associated with sedentary work and obesity, but not with increased plasma levels of persistent organochlorines.

Dysregulation of HPG Axis

Excess body weight can impair the feedback regulation of the HPG axis, and all of the factors above might contribute to or be a result of this dysregulation, contributing to apparent semen quality abnormalities. Sex steroids and glucocorticoids control the interaction between the hypothalamic–pituitary–adrenal (HPA) and the HPG axes, and any amount of disturbance might, in turn, affect spermatogenesis and male reproductive function. Men of normal weight with low levels of testosterone regularly present with elevated levels of LH and FSH, in contrast with obese men, who usually present with low LH and FSH levels [53]. Inhibin B, a growth-like factor, is produced by Sertoli cells in the testis and normally acts to inhibit both FSH production and stimulation of testosterone production by Leydig cells in the testis. Surprisingly, the expected compensatory increase in FSH levels in response to low levels of inhibin B is not observed in obese men. A low level of inhibin B might result from the suppressive effects of elevated estrogen levels. A study by Globerman et al. [54] also found that there was no increase in FSH levels in obese men whose inhibin B levels remained low after weight loss. Obese, infertile men exhibit endocrine changes that are not observed in men with either obesity or infertility alone. This defective response to hormonal changes might be explained by partial or complete dysregulation of the HPG axis.

Physical Mechanisms

Many obese men face physical problems that could be related to their decreased fecundity and fertility, including erectile dysfunction, scrotal lipomatosis leading to increased scrotal temperatures, and sleep apnea that can cause disruptions in the nightly testosterone rise.

Sleep Apnea

Sleep apnea is a disorder affecting 4% of middle-aged men. The disorder is characterized by repetitive collapse of the pharyngeal airway during sleep resulting in hypoxia and hypercapnia. About two-thirds of middle-aged men with obstructive sleep apnea suffer from obesity, particularly central obesity [55]. Sleep apnea is characterized by a fragmented sleep course owing to repeated episodes of upper airway obstructions and hypoxia and is often diagnosed in obese and diabetic males. Patients with sleep apnea have a disrupted nightly rise in testosterone levels and, therefore, lower mean levels of testosterone and LH compared with controls. In a study analyzing sleep apnea in obese, control, and lean patients, Luboshitzky et al. [56] concluded that the condition is associated with decreased pituitary–gonadal function and that the accompanying decline in testosterone concentrations is the result of obesity and, to a lesser degree, sleep fragmentation and hypoxia. This disruption has been associated with abnormal spermatogenesis and male reproductive potential.

Erectile Dysfunction

Whereas the effects of sleep apnea on reproduction are confounding owing to obesity itself being a cause of infertility, erectile dysfunction is significantly associated with obesity. Patients who are overweight or obese make up of 76% of men who report erectile dysfunction and a decrease in libido [19]. Many studies have found an association between an increased incidence of erectile dysfunction and an increase in BMI; hormonal dysfunction is central to the connection between obesity and erectile dysfunction [57]. Erectile dysfunction is highly prevalent in men with both type 2 diabetes and obesity and might act as a forerunner to cardiovascular disease in this high-risk population. Conversely, improved diabetes control and weight loss have been found to improve erectile function [58].

Elevated Scrotal Temperature

An elevated BMI can impair or arrest spermatogenesis by causing an increase in scrotal temperature. Increased fat distribution in the upper thighs, suprapubic area, and scrotum in conjunction with the sedentary lifestyle often associated with obesity can result in increased testicular temperature [21, 28]. Studies of cyclists, truck drivers, and individuals that almost constantly experience elevated scrotal temperatures, like those with undescended testes demonstrate a negative influence of genital heat stress on spermatogenesis. Many studies have focused on genital heat stress as a potential cause of impaired semen quality in cases of sedentary occupations, the occurrence of frequent fever, and varicocele [59]. Hjollund et al. [60] concluded that even a moderate physiological elevation in scrotal skin temperature is associated with substantially reduced sperm concentrations. Additionally Magnusdottir et al. [6] found that the duration of sedentary posture correlated positively with increased scrotal temperatures, leading to a decrease in sperm density.

Are There Solutions?

From the preceding literature, it is evident that obesity is an influencing factor in male infertility. Many experts believe that overweight and obesity, as well as their related chronic diseases, are largely preventable and measures can be taken to reverse both the unhealthy consequences associated with obesity and the negative

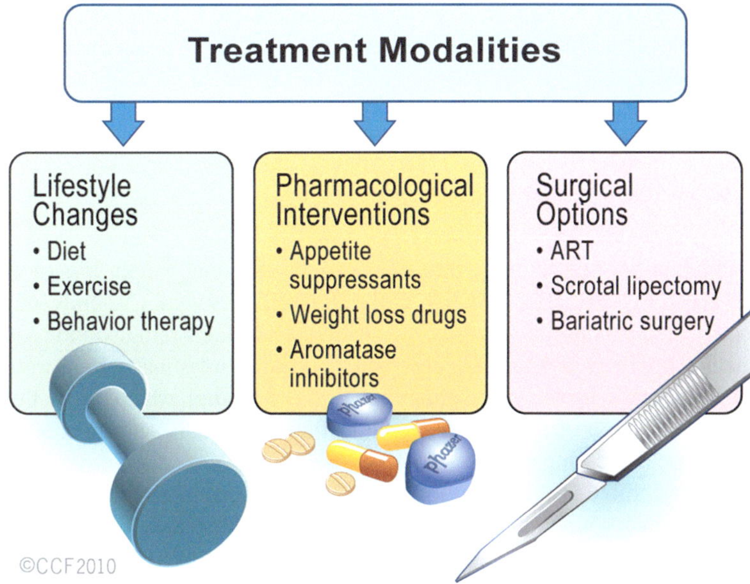

Fig. 14.2 Approaches to treatment of obesity-related male infertility

impacts on male fertility. Therefore, the treatment approach will predominantly focus on the management of obesity (Fig. 14.2). The rapid rise in the incidence of obesity has prompted researchers to not only look at natural treatment methods but also for new treatments in order to manage the pandemic and its subsequent comorbidities.

Lifestyle Changes

Lifestyle changes that can lead to weight loss can include diet modifications (eating smaller meals, cutting down on certain types of food) as well as making a conscious effort to exercise more in order to achieve a normal energy balance. Several studies showed that natural weight loss through diet and/or exercise resulted in an increase in androgen, inhibin B, and SHBG levels and decreased serum concentrations of insulin and leptin, thereby improving semen parameters in obese men [15, 28, 38, 61, 62]. In addition, reducing adipose tissue mass through weight loss in association with exercise or a low-energy and low-fat diet decreases levels of TNF-α, IL-6, and other inflammatory cytokines associated with infertility [63, 64].

Gradual weight loss is best achieved through a sensible eating plan that can be maintained over long periods of time. The likelihood of maintaining weight loss is increased when the diet is combined with regular exercise, cognitive behavior therapy, and connecting with a supportive group environment [65]. Therefore, adoption of these principles in a primary health-care setting can aid in the treatment of infertility related to obesity.

Pharmacological Interventions

Medication can be used to either treat obesity by addressing weight loss or dealing with the obesity-related effects on the male reproductive system. Currently, only two anti-obesity medications are approved by the Food and Drug Administration for long-term use [66]. One is orlistat (Xenical), which reduces intestinal fat absorption by inhibiting pancreatic lipase; the other is sibutramine (Meridia), which acts in the brain to inhibit deactivation of the neurotransmitters norepinephrine, serotonin, and dopamine, therefore decreasing appetite. However, weight loss with these drugs is modest.

Aromatase inhibitors are an option for obese males facing infertility problems, especially if they have elevated estrogen and lowered testosterone levels. Aromatase inhibitors prevent the excess aromatase enzymes from converting testosterone to estrogen. They interfere with the aromatase p450 enzyme that is highly expressed in white adipose tissue. Currently available aromatase inhibitors include anastrozole, testolactone, and letrozole. Numerous case studies have found this to be an effective treatment in not only restoring normal hormone levels, but also fertility. Raman and Schlegel tested the effects of anastrozole on nonobstructive azoospermic patients who presented with normal or decreased levels of testosterone and elevated levels of estradiol. Anastrozole treatment normalized the testosterone-to-estrogen ratio and total testosterone levels and improved semen parameters [67]. Zumoff et al. [68] found that by inhibiting estrogen biosynthesis (through administration of the aromatase inhibitor testolactone), there was an alleviation of possible infertility as a result of hypogonadotropic hypogonadism in obese male subjects. In another case study, a patient diagnosed with infertility secondary to morbid obesity was treated with the aromatase inhibitor, anastrozole. This led to normalization of the patient's testosterone, LH, and FSH hormone levels, as well as suppression of the serum estradiol levels and the normalization of spermatogenesis and fertility [33]. In a study including normal, overweight, and obese men, treatment with anastrozole led to an increase in testosterone-to-estradiol ratio that occurred in association with increased semen parameters. Anastrozole and testolactone have similar effects on hormonal profiles and semen analysis, but anastrozole appears to be at least as effective as testolactone for treating men with abnormal testosterone-to-estradiol ratio [67].

New directions in pharmacological treatment might include testosterone replacement therapy and maintenance and regulation of adipose-derived hormones, particularly leptin, which is produced by fat cells in the body and known to affect appetite and the body's energy balance, and also reproductive function. Testosterone replacement therapy has been shown to suppress the levels of circulating leptin, although no information regarding the effect of the treatment on semen parameters was reported [16, 38]. Quennell et al. [69] discovered that leptin indirectly regulates gonadotropin-releasing hormone neuronal function, affecting forebrain neurons that induce infertility. By decreasing elevated leptin levels in obese patients, it might be possible to reverse some of the potential suppressive effects of excess leptin on the HPG axis and restore normal spermatogenesis and sperm function. Ghrelin, a hormone which is secreted by cells in the lining of the stomach, also affects appetite and the body's energy balance. Further studies of these hormones may lead to the development of new medications to control appetite and provide an option for treating obesity-related health problems and infertility.

Surgical Options

In vitro fertilization may be an option for obese patients facing problems such as erectile dysfunction or other purely physical fertility problems. Although morbid obesity is associated with unfavorable IVF/ICSI cycle outcome as evidenced by lower pregnancy rates in females, there is no evidence for a contributing male factor when assisted reproductive methods are used [70]. It is recommended that morbidly obese patients undergo appropriate counseling before the initiation of this expensive and invasive therapy. Fortunately, studies show that obesity in men may not adversely affect the results of their partners who are undergoing in vitro fertilization or embryo transfer [71].

Scrotal lipectomy is a treatment option available for infertility in obese men whose excess fat accumulation may be contributing to their infertility, either through increased scrotal temperature or excess toxin accumulation. One-fifth of patients who were previously considered infertile and underwent scrotal lipectomy to remove excess fat were able to achieve a successful pregnancy [28]. For individuals who are severely obese, dietary changes and behavior modification may be accompanied by surgery to reduce or bypass portions of the stomach or small intestine. The risks of obesity surgery have declined in recent years, but it is still only performed on patients for whom other strategies have failed and whose obesity seriously threatens their health.

Bariatric surgery ("weight loss surgery") is the use of surgical intervention in the treatment of obesity by reducing or bypassing portions of the stomach or small intestine. As it is a rather extreme intervention, it is only recommended for severely obese people (BMI > 40) who have failed to lose sufficient weight following dietary modification and pharmacological treatment [72]. Gastric bypass and banding surgeries are very effective in the treatment of morbid obesity and its comorbid conditions. One study reported that a significant decrease in estrogen, increase in testosterone, and normalization of other hormone and adipokine levels were experienced by patients who underwent vertical banded gastroplasty [73]. However, others speculate that the drastic weight loss that accompanies this procedure might induce secondary infertility, even though natural weight loss has shown promising results in terms of restoring fertility [74]. Bariatric surgery should therefore not be recommended as a treatment for obesity-linked infertility until extensive, long-term studies have been performed to determine the definite effects on male fertility.

Conclusion

Obesity is a modern-day pandemic with serious comorbidities, both physical and psychological. Studies clearly show that obese men have an increased chance of subfertility and subfecundity due to various mechanisms (physical, genetic, hormonal, adipokine, cytokine) that ultimately lead to ED and abnormal semen parameters. The central factor behind these mechanisms is the abnormal regulation of the HPG axis. An abnormal hormonal profile, and more specifically increased adipose-derived hormones and adipokine levels, may explain the association between BMI, altered semen parameters, and infertility more accurately as it is clearly more complex than can be accounted for simply by abnormal levels of reproductive hormones.

New studies point to many causes for abnormal semen parameters, including genetic markers, excess adipose-derived hormone and adipokine release, as well as oxidative stress. The consistent decrease in inhibin B levels and increase in leptin levels, and specific proteomic sperm changes observed in obese infertile males, all may have negative impacts on spermatogenesis. Increased cytokines, such as IL-6, are connected with oxidative stress and impaired reproduction and could also contribute to abnormal semen parameters observed in obese men facing fertility issues. These markers point toward a true suppression of normal spermatogenesis and sperm quality despite some inconsistency in the results of studies performed to measure the effects of obesity on semen parameters.

In treating obesity-linked sperm disorders and male infertility, few controlled studies have been performed, and effective therapeutic treatments, advice for lifestyle changes, and surgical options should be explored further. In addition, determining the most accurate measure for qualifying patients as obese could more accurately clarify the cause of their infertility and other health issues that might accompany their state of obesity. Neither the reversibility of obesity-associated male infertility in response to weight loss nor effective therapeutic treatments or interventions have been extensively studied. The increasing prevalence of obesity worldwide in conjunction with a perceived declining male sperm count in modern man calls for more research and attention to obesity as an etiology of male infertility. Clinicians should consider obesity when a male patient with idiopathic infertility is confronted.

Expert Commentary

The purpose of this chapter was to discuss obesity as a newly discovered etiology of male infertility. The growing incidence of obesity and apparent decrease in male fertility makes this topic especially relevant when dealing with the infertile male. Although data on abnormal semen parameters and evidence of obesity as it affects male fertility is abundant, the specific mechanisms are not definite. Discovery and proof of significant mechanisms that contribute to this issue are important when treating infertility as it relates to obesity. The recognition of adipose tissue as an endocrine organ and discovery of adipokines have contributed greatly in explaining the mechanisms behind this problem, but it appears many other factors are involved. Further understanding of adipose tissue as an endocrine organ and obesity as a constant inflammatory state will allow in-depth studies of specific adipokines and cytokines involved.

In addition, controlled studies demonstrating all effects of aromatase inhibitors, weight loss, bariatric surgery, and other new therapeutic measures are needed to definitely recommend specific treatments. Lifestyle changes leading to weight loss appear to be of the greatest benefit, not only for male fertility issues but overall health. The pressing issue of obesity in not only the USA, but the whole world, has lasting effects that now appear to include male infertility. It is important, especially as the obesity epidemic grows, for clinicians to consider obesity as explanation to a male with idiopathic infertility or subfertility.

Key Issues

- Obesity is a medical condition in which excess body fat, or white adipose tissue, accumulates in the body to the extent that the excess fat often adversely affects health, often reducing life expectancy.
- The obesity epidemic is growing to concerning proportions, affecting an estimated 700 million people in the next 5 years.
- Altered semen parameters ascribed to obesity include decreased sperm concentration, abnormal morphology, compromised chromatin integrity, and abnormal sperm motility.
- The discovery of adipose tissue as an active endocrine organ secreting adipokines and adipose-derived hormones is an important mechanistic link explaining infertility in many obese men.
- Mechanisms that may explain abnormal semen parameters in obese men include genetic, hormonal, and physical mechanisms that may all contribute to the deregulation of the HPG axis that controls normal spermatogenesis.
- Physical problems that may contribute to decreased fertility include ED; scrotal lipomatosis, which leads to increased scrotal temperatures; and sleep apnea that can cause disruptions in the essential nightly testosterone rise.
- There are solutions that often lead to restoration of fertility that include lifestyle changes, pharmacological interventions, and surgical procedures.
- The rapid rise in the incidence of obesity has prompted researchers to not only look at natural or lifestyle changes as treatment methods but also for new therapies in order to manage the pandemic and its subsequent comorbidities.
- Clinicians should consider obesity when a male patient with idiopathic infertility is confronted.

References

1. World Health Organization. http://www.who.int/nmh/publications/fact_sheet_diet_en.pdf (2009). Accessed 15 July 2009.
2. Popkin BM. Recent dynamics suggest selected countries catching up to US obesity. Am J Clin Nutr. 2010;91(1):284S–8.
3. Swan SH, Elkin EP, Fenster L. The question of declining sperm density revisited: an analysis of 101 studies published 1934–1996. Environ Health Perspect. 2000;108(10):961–6.
4. Sallmen M, Sandler DP, Hoppin JA, Blair A, Baird DD. Reduced fertility among overweight and obese men. Epidemiology. 2006;17(5):520–3.
5. Carlsen E, Giwercman A, Keiding N, Skakkebaek NE. Evidence for decreasing quality of semen during past 50 years. BMJ. 1992;305(6854):609–13.
6. Magnusdottir EV, Thorsteinsson T, Thorsteinsdottir S, Heimisdottir M, Olafsdottir K. Persistent organochlorines, sedentary occupation, obesity and human male subfertility. Hum Reprod. 2005;20(1):208–15.
7. Kyle UG, Bosaeus I, De Lorenzo AD, et al. Bioelectrical impedance analysis—part I: review of principles and methods. Clin Nutr. 2004;23(5):1226–43.
8. World Health Organization. Diet, nutrition and the prevention of chronic diseases. World Health Organ Tech Rep Ser. 2003;916:i–viii. 1–149, backcover.
9. Booth ML, Hunter C, Gore CJ, Bauman A, Owen N. The relationship between body mass index and waist circumference: implications for estimates of the population prevalence of overweight. Int J Obes Relat Metab Disord. 2000;24(8):1058–61.
10. Huxley R, Mendis S, Zheleznyakov E, Reddy S, Chan J. Body mass index, waist circumference and waist: hip ratio as predictors of cardiovascular risk–a review of the literature. Eur J Clin Nutr. 2010;64(1):16–22.
11. Akpinar E, Bashan I, Bozdemir N, Saatci E. Which is the best anthropometric technique to identify obesity: body mass index, waist circumference or waist-hip ratio? Coll Antropol. 2007;31(2):387–93.
12. Macdonald AA, Herbison GP, Showell M, Farquhar CM. The impact of body mass index on semen parameters and reproductive hormones in human males: a systematic review with meta-analysis. Hum Reprod Update. 2010;16(3):293–311.
13. Hammoud AO, Gibson M, Peterson CM, Hamilton BD, Carrell DT. Obesity and male reproductive potential. J Androl. 2006;27(5):619–26.
14. Jensen TK, Andersson AM, Jorgensen N, et al. Body mass index in relation to semen quality and reproductive hormones among 1,558 Danish men. Fertil Steril. 2004;82(4):863–70.
15. Chavarro JE, Toth TL, Wright DL, Meeker JD, Hauser R. Body mass index in relation to semen quality, sperm DNA integrity, and serum reproductive hormone levels among men attending an infertility clinic. Fertil Steril. 2010;93(7):2222–31.
16. Hofny ER, Ali ME, Abdel-Hafez HZ, et al. Semen parameters and hormonal profile in obese fertile and infertile males. Fertil Steril. 2010;94(2):581–4.
17. Fejes I, Koloszar S, Szollosi J, Zavaczki Z, Pal A. Is semen quality affected by male body fat distribution? Andrologia. 2005;37(5):155–9.
18. Aggerholm AS, Thulstrup AM, Toft G, Ramlau-Hansen CH, Bonde JP. Is overweight a risk factor for reduced semen quality and altered serum sex hormone profile? Fertil Steril. 2008;90(3):619–26.
19. Pauli EM, Legro RS, Demers LM, Kunselman AR, Dodson WC, Lee PA. Diminished paternity and gonadal function with increasing obesity in men. Fertil Steril. 2008;90(2):346–51.
20. Nicopoulou SC, Alexiou M, Michalakis K, et al. Body mass index vis-a-vis total sperm count in attendees of a single andrology clinic. Fertil Steril. 2009;92(3):1016–7.
21. Hammoud AO, Wilde N, Gibson M, Parks A, Carrell DT, Meikle AW. Male obesity and alteration in sperm parameters. Fertil Steril. 2008;90(6):2222–5.
22. Fejes I, Koloszar S, Zavaczki Z, Daru J, Szollosi J, Pal A. Effect of body weight on testosterone/estradiol ratio in oligozoospermic patients. Arch Androl. 2006;52(2):97–102.

23. Martini AC, Tissera A, Estofan D, et al. Overweight and seminal quality: a study of 794 patients. Fertil Steril. 2010;94(5):1739–43.
24. Kort HI, Massey JB, Elsner CW, et al. Impact of body mass index values on sperm quantity and quality. J Androl. 2006;27(3):450–2.
25. Evenson D, Wixon R. Meta-analysis of sperm DNA fragmentation using the sperm chromatin structure assay. Reprod Biomed Online. 2006;12(4):466–72.
26. Gopalkrishnan K, Padwal V, Meherji PK, Gokral JS, Shah R, Juneja HS. Poor quality of sperm as it affects repeated early pregnancy loss. Arch Androl. 2000;45(2):111–7.
27. Kriegel TM, Heidenreich F, Kettner K, et al. Identification of diabetes- and obesity-associated proteomic changes in human spermatozoa by difference gel electrophoresis. Reprod Biomed Online. 2009;19(5):660–70.
28. Kasturi SS, Tannir J, Brannigan RE. The metabolic syndrome and male infertility. J Androl. 2008;29(3):251–9.
29. Arsov T, Silva DG, O'Bryan MK, et al. Fat aussie–a new Alstrom syndrome mouse showing a critical role for ALMS1 in obesity, diabetes, and spermatogenesis. Mol Endocrinol. 2006; 20(7):1610–22.
30. Hammoud A, Carrell DT, Meikle AW, et al. An aromatase polymorphism modulates the relationship between weight and estradiol levels in obese men. Fertil Steril. 2010;94(5):1734–8.
31. Strain GW, Zumoff B, Kream J, et al. Mild hypogonadotropic hypogonadism in obese men. Metabolism. 1982;31(9):871–5.
32. Tsai EC, Matsumoto AM, Fujimoto WY, Boyko EJ. Association of bioavailable, free, and total testosterone with insulin resistance: influence of sex hormone-binding globulin and body fat. Diabetes Care. 2004;27(4):861–8.
33. Roth MY, Amory JK, Page ST. Treatment of male infertility secondary to morbid obesity. Nat Clin Pract Endocrinol Metab. 2008;4(7):415–9.
34. Qin DD, Yuan W, Zhou WJ, Cui YQ, Wu JQ, Gao ES. Do reproductive hormones explain the association between body mass index and semen quality? Asian J Androl. 2007;9(6):827–34.
35. Athyros VG, Tziomalos K, Karagiannis A, Anagnostis P, Mikhailidis DP. Should adipokines be considered in the choice of the treatment of obesity-related health problems? Curr Drug Targets. 2010;11(1):122–35.
36. Bhat GK, Sea TL, Olatinwo MO, et al. Influence of a leptin deficiency on testicular morphology, germ cell apoptosis, and expression levels of apoptosis-related genes in the mouse. J Androl. 2006;27(2):302–10.
37. Trayhurn P, Beattie JH. Physiological role of adipose tissue: white adipose tissue as an endocrine and secretory organ. Proc Nutr Soc. 2001;60(3):329–39.
38. Isidori AM, Caprio M, Strollo F, et al. Leptin and androgens in male obesity: evidence for leptin contribution to reduced androgen levels. J Clin Endocrinol Metab. 1999; 84(10):3673–80.
39. Wang P, Mariman E, Renes J, Keijer J. The secretory function of adipocytes in the physiology of white adipose tissue. J Cell Physiol. 2008;216(1):3–13.
40. Wozniak SE, Gee LL, Wachtel MS, Frezza EE. Adipose tissue: the new endocrine organ? A review article. Dig Dis Sci. 2009;54(9):1847–56.
41. Jope T, Lammert A, Kratzsch J, Paasch U, Glander HJ. Leptin and leptin receptor in human seminal plasma and in human spermatozoa. Int J Androl. 2003;26(6):335–41.
42. Bialas M, Fiszer D, Rozwadowska N, Kosicki W, Jedrzejczak P, Kurpisz M. The role of IL-6, IL-10, TNF-alpha and its receptors TNFR1 and TNFR2 in the local regulatory system of normal and impaired human spermatogenesis. Am J Reprod Immunol. 2009;62(1):51–9.
43. Fraczek M, Kurpisz M. Inflammatory mediators exert toxic effects of oxidative stress on human spermatozoa. J Androl. 2007;28(2):325–33.
44. Lampiao F, du Plessis SS. TNF-alpha and IL-6 affect human sperm function by elevating nitric oxide production. Reprod Biomed Online. 2008;17(5):628–31.
45. Dandona P, Aljada A, Chaudhuri A, Mohanty P, Garg R. Metabolic syndrome: a comprehensive perspective based on interactions between obesity, diabetes, and inflammation. Circulation. 2005;111(11):1448–54.

46. Davi G, Falco A. Oxidant stress, inflammation and atherogenesis. Lupus. 2005;14(9):760–4.
47. Agarwal A, Sharma RK, Nallella KP, Thomas Jr AJ, Alvarez JG, Sikka SC. Reactive oxygen species as an independent marker of male factor infertility. Fertil Steril. 2006;86(4):878–85.
48. Winters SJ, Wang C, Abdelrahaman E, Hadeed V, Dyky MA, Brufsky A. Inhibin-B levels in healthy young adult men and prepubertal boys: is obesity the cause for the contemporary decline in sperm count because of fewer Sertoli cells? J Androl. 2006;27(4):560–4.
49. Ramaswamy S, Marshall GR, McNeilly AS, Plant TM. Evidence that in a physiological setting Sertoli cell number is the major determinant of circulating concentrations of inhibin B in the adult male rhesus monkey (Macaca mulatta). J Androl. 1999;20(3):430–4.
50. Bener A, Al-Ansari AA, Zirie M, Al-Hamaq AO. Is male fertility associated with type 2 diabetes mellitus? Int Urol Nephrol. 2009;41(4):777–84.
51. Agbaje IM, Rogers DA, McVicar CM, et al. Insulin dependant diabetes mellitus: implications for male reproductive function. Hum Reprod. 2007;22(7):1871–7.
52. Lima N, Cavaliere H, Knobel M, Halpern A, Medeiros-Neto G. Decreased androgen levels in massively obese men may be associated with impaired function of the gonadostat. Int J Obes Relat Metab Disord. 2000;24(11):1433–7.
53. Jarow JP, Kirkland J, Koritnik DR, Cefalu WT. Effect of obesity and fertility status on sex steroid levels in men. Urology. 1993;42(2):171–4.
54. Globerman H, Shen-Orr Z, Karnieli E, Aloni Y, Charuzi I. Inhibin B in men with severe obesity and after weight reduction following gastroplasty. Endocr Res. 2005;31(1):17–26.
55. Vgontzas AN, Papanicolaou DA, Bixler EO, et al. Sleep apnea and daytime sleepiness and fatigue: relation to visceral obesity, insulin resistance, and hypercytokinemia. J Clin Endocrinol Metab. 2000;85(3):1151–8.
56. Luboshitzky R, Lavie L, Shen-Orr Z, Herer P. Altered luteinizing hormone and testosterone secretion in middle-aged obese men with obstructive sleep apnea. Obes Res. 2005; 13(4):780–6.
57. Cheng JY, Ng EM. Body mass index, physical activity and erectile dysfunction: an U-shaped relationship from population-based study. Int J Obes (Lond). 2007;31(10):1571–8.
58. Tamler R. Diabetes, obesity, and erectile dysfunction. Gend Med. 2009;6 Suppl 1:4–16.
59. Jung A, Schuppe HC. Influence of genital heat stress on semen quality in humans. Andrologia. 2007;39(6):203–15.
60. Hjollund NH, Bonde JP, Jensen TK, Olsen J. Diurnal scrotal skin temperature and semen quality. The Danish First Pregnancy Planner Study Team. Int J Androl. 2000;23(5):309–18.
61. Kaukua J, Pekkarinen T, Sane T, Mustajoki P. Sex hormones and sexual function in obese men losing weight. Obes Res. 2003;11(6):689–94.
62. Niskanen L, Laaksonen DE, Punnonen K, Mustajoki P, Kaukua J, Rissanen A. Changes in sex hormone-binding globulin and testosterone during weight loss and weight maintenance in abdominally obese men with the metabolic syndrome. Diabetes Obes Metab. 2004;6(3): 208–15.
63. Sharman MJ, Volek JS. Weight loss leads to reductions in inflammatory biomarkers after a very-low-carbohydrate diet and a low-fat diet in overweight men. Clin Sci (Lond). 2004;107(4): 365–9.
64. Ziccardi P, Nappo F, Giugliano G, et al. Reduction of inflammatory cytokine concentrations and improvement of endothelial functions in obese women after weight loss over one year. Circulation. 2002;105(7):804–9.
65. Lau DC, Douketis JD, Morrison KM, et al. 2006 Canadian clinical practice guidelines on the management and prevention of obesity in adults and children [summary]. CMAJ. 2007;176(8):S1–13.
66. National Institute of Diabetes and Digestive and Kidney Diseases. Prescription medications for the treatment of obesity. http://win.niddk.nih.gov/publications/prescription.htm#fdameds. Accessed 20 July 2009.
67. Raman JD, Schlegel PN. Aromatase inhibitors for male infertility. J Urol. 2002;167(2 Pt 1): 624–9.

68. Zumoff B, Miller LK, Strain GW. Reversal of the hypogonadotropic hypogonadism of obese men by administration of the aromatase inhibitor testolactone. Metabolism. 2003;52(9): 1126–8.
69. Quennell JH, Mulligan AC, Tups A, et al. Leptin indirectly regulates gonadotropin-releasing hormone neuronal function. Endocrinology. 2009;150(6):2805–12.
70. Awartani KA, Nahas S, Al Hassan SH, Al Deery MA, Coskun S. Infertility treatment outcome in sub groups of obese population. Reprod Biol Endocrinol. 2009;7:52.
71. Dechaud H, Anahory T, Reyftmann L, Loup V, Hamamah S, Hedon B. Obesity does not adversely affect results in patients who are undergoing in vitro fertilization and embryo transfer. Eur J Obstet Gynecol Reprod Biol. 2006;127(1):88–93.
72. Encinosa WE, Bernard DM, Chen CC, Steiner CA. Healthcare utilization and outcomes after bariatric surgery. Med Care. 2006;44(8):706–12.
73. Bastounis EA, Karayiannakis AJ, Syrigos K, Zbar A, Makri GG, Alexiou D. Sex hormone changes in morbidly obese patients after vertical banded gastroplasty. Eur Surg Res. 1998; 30(1):43–7.
74. di Frega AS, Dale B, Di Matteo L, Wilding M. Secondary male factor infertility after Roux-en-Y gastric bypass for morbid obesity: case report. Hum Reprod. 2005;20(4):997–8.

Chapter 15
Environmental Factors

Claudio Telöken, Samuel Juncal, and Túlio M. Graziottin

Approximately 50% of the human infertility issues involve male factors. A number of different components may result in reduction of sperm count or motility and affect sperm morphology. The etiology of male infertility is difficult to understand, due to its etiological heterogeneity, complexity, and incomplete knowledge of the underlying causes. In addition, World Health Organization (WHO) recently suggested changes in semen analysis lower limit parameters. In this way, it is not easy, based on the sperm count, to compare male infertility of earlier with the current ones. Most likely, some subfertile and/or infertile individuals under these new numbers would not be screened as such 5 years ago [1]. Moreover, conventional reference values for seminal parameters have little diagnostic value because of their marked biological individuality variations, although seminal parameters may be useful for assessing differences in an individual's serial results, in particular of progressive motility, morphology, and vitality [2–4].

Not long, we have seen significant refinement regarding male full evaluation combined with new sophisticated diagnostic techniques. Even then, most of the infertile men are described as idiopathic. Therefore, reproductive toxicity has been a topic of increasing interest and concern, as human exposure to a considerable number of potential toxicants is unavoidable due to contamination of air, water, ground, food, beverages, and household [5]. Several lifestyle-related factors such as obesity, smoking, sedentary exposure to traffic exhaust fumes, dioxins, combustion products, cell phone electromagnetic radiations, chronic noise stress, anabolic steroids, illicit drugs, heat, notebook use, dietary habits, oxidative stress, etc., appear to exhibit some involvement in human reproduction. Apart from this, public

C. Telöken, MD, PhD (✉) • T.M. Graziottin, MD, PhD
Andrology Section of Fertilitat – Human Reproduction Center, Department of Urology,
Santa Casa Hospital and Federal University of Health Sciences, Porto Alegre, RS, Brazil
e-mail: urologyteloken@yahoo.com

S. Juncal, MS, MD
Andrology Section of Fertilitat – Human Reproduction Center,
Federal University of Health Sciences, Porto Alegre, RS, Brazil

S.J. Parekattil and A. Agarwal (eds.), *Antioxidants in Male Infertility: A Guide for Clinicians and Researchers*, © Springer Science+Business Media New York 2013

concern about adverse effects of environmental chemicals, pesticides, food additives, and persistent pollutants on spermatogenesis in adult men is sometimes not supported by the available data for humans [6–10].

About 80,000 new chemical compounds have been introduced to human civilization in the last 100 years, and only 145 have been rigorously assessed for their reproductive health effects [11]. It has been suggested that sperm counts have decreased and population fecundity has been declining during the second half of the last century in Western societies, in human as well as in animals, possibly due to environmental pollutants. However, studies are diverse, complex, and complicated to interpret. Whether environmental contaminants are really involved can neither be confirmed nor rejected. Under these circumstances, it should be a matter of great concern triggering studies into its causes and possibilities for prevention [12–16].

Take into account that in the field of reproductive environmental health, there remain many unanswered questions that suggest the need to include studies that target populations with high exposure to chemicals and to identify susceptibility factors and critical exposure windows (life stages) that may increase a man's risk of infertility. We need methods to better study mixtures of chemicals and develop methods to assess clinical reproductive outcomes of human exposure to the ever-growing list of chemicals [17]. Study designs need to incorporate markers of susceptibility into these chemicals and metals. Susceptibility may be increased by the timing or life stage exposure occurrences, such as neonatal or peripubertal periods. In addition, genetic susceptibility may result from differences incurred because of genetic polymorphisms in enzymes metabolizing or activating these compounds. With the current revolution in genomics and molecular biology, these techniques must be incorporated into the next generation of epidemiologic studies on male reproductive health [18], in such a way to possibly decrease the idiopathic male infertility rate.

The main scope of this chapter is to review some of the most frequent environmental or occupational pollutants in sex hormone levels, birth rates, and human reproduction in view of the fact that male infertility may be a surrogate marker of serious additional underlying medical problems.

Environmental Factors

The numerous external causes of infertility include exposure to work-related substances, contact with toxic substances like pesticides, or exposure to extremely hot areas such as blast furnace operations. Many substances such as metals, volatile organic compounds, physical factors (heat, vibration, and radiation), and pesticides including pyrethroids, organophosphates, phenoxyacetic acids, carbamates, and organochlorines have been investigated since studies reported an association between human exposure and semen quality, DNA damage, hormonal change, numerical chromosome aberrations, and possible human reproduction impairment. Studies varied widely in methods, exposures, and outcomes. Although suggestive of semen parameters, the epidemiologic evidence accumulated thus far remains equivocal as to the spermatotoxic and aneugenic potential of pesticides given the small number of published studies. This question warrants more investigation and suggestions for future studies [18, 19].

The hormone-disrupting properties of some factors have raised interest in how contemporary pollutants, which primarily take the form of low-level environmental or occupational exposures, impact human reproduction. Many studies in humans and animals support the role of environmental contaminants as potential endocrine disruptor. Endocrine-disrupting chemicals are among the most complex environmental health threat known today. By mimicking natural hormones such as estrogen and testosterone, these chemicals can interact with the body's endocrine system and exert toxic effects.

The rise in male infertility and the decline in human sperm counts could be linked with chemicals in the environment known as antiandrogens. These antiandrogens, for instance, have been linked with the feminization of fish in British rivers and could be affecting the development of male reproductive organs in humans. A link has been established between antiandrogens released into rivers from sewage outflows. There are several chemicals in widely used pharmaceuticals and pesticides that are known to have antiandrogenic activity, coming from domestic sources. One possibility is that drugs excreted from the body may end up in rivers. Antiandrogens may also be seeping into rivers as runoff from agricultural land. Sex change was first detected in fish more than 20 years ago. During the same period, human sperm counts have been falling in several countries over a period of 30 years or more. This has been matched by a corresponding rise in other male reproductive problems, such as the congenital condition testicular dysgenesis, which can affect fertility [20].

Other studies demonstrate the interaction of environmental toxicants with steroid receptors in the testis and thereby interference with proliferation and differentiation of spermatogenic cells. Acceleration of sperm transition through epididymis has been reported with several environmental contaminants such as methoxychlor, vinclozolin, etc. These and other observations support the endocrine-mediated toxic effects of environmental contaminants on reproductive and development abnormalities.

Apart from endocrine disruption, another mechanism that has emerged in the last two decades is the discovery of reactive oxygen species (ROS) and the role of associated oxidative stress in the etiology of defective sperm function and male infertility. Oxidative effects on spermatozoa may result in lower sperm motility and increased damage to sperm DNA [21]. Many contaminants have been reported to disturb the pro-oxidant/antioxidant balance, leading to excessive generation of ROS (oxidative stress). In higher concentrations, ROS may cause sperm cell damage through lipid peroxidation of the plasma membrane, single- and double-stranded DNA breaks [22], as well as the induction of germ cell apoptosis [23]. A greater proportion of infertile men demonstrate elevated levels of seminal ROS as compared with populations of fertile men. Nevertheless, other works have obtained contradictory results, indicating that these changes have not taken place homogeneously in the world. Geographical differences in semen quality also support the fact that semen quality may have declined only in some areas [24–28].

Volatile organic compounds, certain halogenated compounds, several heavy metals, xenoestrogens, organochlorine compounds, and phthalate esters may compromise reproductive male function, in vivo and in vitro. [15, 29, 30]. More studies are required for experimental confirmation of this link, which could give answer to several adverse effects of the contaminants whose mechanisms are yet to be established. Maternal beef consumption, and possibly xenobiotics (anabolic steroids) in beef, may alter a male fetus' testicular development in utero and adversely affect his reproductive capacity. In sons of "high beef consumer mothers," sperm concentration was 24.3% lower than that in the men whose mothers ate less beef [27, 31]. Ultrastructural analyses revealed damage to sperm head membranes in relation to the metal used: acrosome breakage with formation of various sized microvesicles, a large round hole and numerous folds in the acrosome membrane. Metal compounds may reduce sperm kinetic characteristics and probably fertilizing capacity by triggering specific morphological damages to the head and/or by inhibiting motility. It is worth mentioning that only specific chemical forms of a metal can pass through the blood–testis barrier and are more likely to target organs of the reproductive track and concentrate in the semen. In the testis, Leydig cells along with germ cells have been identified as the main targets of metal cytotoxicity, leading to a reduced steroidogenesis and, thereby, disruption of spermatogenesis. Inter-Sertoli tight junctions may also be affected by metals with consequent exfoliation of immature cells into the lumen of seminiferous tubules and reduction of viable sperm count in the epididymis. The underlying mechanisms of these effects are uncertain. Oxidative stress, inflammation, induced apoptosis, and ionic and molecular mimicry could be the basis of metal toxic activity. Some metals seem to experience a direct effect on sperm cells, reducing their motility and/or affecting their morphology. These adverse effects have been reported either by epidemiological studies of occupationally exposed individuals, highlighting a positive correlation, in most of the cases, with high concentrations of metals in semen [31].

Vanadium

Vanadium (V) is a rare element found combined in certain minerals and used mainly to produce certain alloys. Most of the vanadium produced is used as ferrovanadium or as a steel additive. Vanadium mixed with aluminum in titanium alloys is used in jet engines, high-speed airframes, and nuclear reactors. Vanadium oxide (V_2O_5) is used as a catalyst in manufacturing sulfuric acid and maleic anhydride and in making ceramics. Glass coated with vanadium dioxide (VO_2) can block infrared radiation at some specific temperature. Vanadium compounds are not regarded as a serious hazard; however, workers exposed to vanadium peroxide dust were found to suffer with severe eye, nose, and throat irritation. The uptake of vanadium by humans mainly takes place through foodstuffs, such as buckwheat, soya beans, olive oil, sunflower oil, apples, and eggs. Vanadium can have a number of effects on human health, when the uptake is too high.

Vanadium can be found in the environment in algae, plants, invertebrates, fishes, and many other species. In mussels and crabs, vanadium strongly bioaccumulates, which can lead to greater concentrations than those found in seawater. Vanadium causes the inhibition of certain enzymes with animals, which has several neurological effects. Laboratory tests with test animals have shown that vanadium can cause harm to the reproductive system of male animals and that it accumulates in the female placenta. In male mice, it can result in DNA damage, decrease in fertility rate, implantations, live fetuses, and fetal weight. It is concluded that vanadium pentoxide is a reprotoxic and genotoxic agent in mice [32]. Vanadium pentoxide inhalation in the human workplace enters the body through lungs, disrupts mitochondria function and the permeability of the epithelium, and promotes access of inflammatory mediators to the underlying neuronal tissue causing injury and neuronal death. Exposure results in necrosis of spermatogonium, spermatocytes, and Sertoli cells contributing to male infertility [33].

Manganese

Manganese (Mn) is a metal found as a free element in nature or often in combination with iron. It is important in the industry particularly in stainless steels. The fertility of male workers exposed to manganese dust was assessed by using a questionnaire. The manganese-exposed workers exhibited a statistically significant deficit in the number of children during their period of exposure to the metal [34]. High manganese level was associated with increased risk of low sperm motility and low sperm concentration. Ambient exposure to manganese levels is associated with a reduction in sperm motility and concentration [35].

Boron

Boron (B), the fifth element in the periodic table, is a metalloid, which occurs abundantly in the evaporite ores borax and ulexite and has widespread commercial uses. Boron is used as a dopant in the semiconductor industry, while boron compounds play specialized roles as structural and refractory materials and reagents for the synthesis of organic compounds, including pharmaceuticals.

Male reproductive toxicity has been demonstrated in experimental animals exposed to, and there is considerable interest in possible human reproductive effects. Although there appears to be considerable human exposure to boron compounds, epidemiological studies have not been sufficient for an evaluation of reproductive risk. Boron treatment of rats, mice, and dogs has been associated with testicular toxicity, characterized by inhibited spermiation at lower dose levels and a reduction in epididymal sperm count at higher dose levels. Earlier studies in human workers and populations have not identified adverse effects of boron exposure on fertility, but outcome measures in these studies were relatively insensitive, based mainly on family size and did not include an evaluation of semen end points. Reproductive outcomes in the wives of boron workers were not significantly different from those in the wives of background control men after adjustment for potential confounders. There were no statistically significant differences in semen characteristics between exposure groups, except that sperm Y:X ratio was reduced in boron workers. While boron has been shown to adversely affect male reproduction in laboratory animals, there is no clear evidence of male reproductive effects attributable to boron in studies of highly exposed workers.

In the USA, boron mine workers were not adversely affected. Overall, boron workers fathered 52.7% female offspring, compared to the US national average of 48.8%. However, the data did not indicate effects attributable to boron. Workers in the two lowest exposure categories had the highest percentage female offspring, while workers in the highest exposure category had virtually the same percentage (49.2%) as the national average. Thus, the fertility rate was not adversely affected when workers were most exposed to boron. The ratio of boys to girls was not reduced. Lack of strict epidemiological study design and the use of fertility rate to measure fecundity detracted from the utility of these papers for an evaluation of human reproductive toxicity [36] and since then, two studies that examined fertility and secondary sex ratios in response to long-term exposure to boron among the population in two geographical regions in Turkey have found no negative effects on fertility [37]. An influence of boron intake on certain human key enzymes, however, cannot be excluded [38]. There are no significant differences in sex ratio, with more females than males in the boron-rich region than in the boron-poor [38]. The only significant differences were that average pregnancies and live births among production workers exceeded those of office workers. The reported infertility rates are very low compared to usual general population infertility rates of 15%, and the reliability is questioned [39].

Cadmium

Cadmium (Cd) is one of the metallic components in the Earth's crust and oceans, and present everywhere in our environment. With the exception of its use in nickel–cadmium batteries and cadmium telluride solar panels, the use of cadmium is generally decreasing in its other applications, due to competing technologies and toxicity in certain forms and concentration. Cadmium is extremely toxic even in low concentrations and bioaccumulates in organisms and ecosystems. In the 1950s and 1960s, industrial exposure to cadmium was high, but as the toxic effects became apparent, industrial limits have been reduced in most industrialized nations. Buildup of cadmium levels in the water, air, and soil has been occurring particularly in industrial areas. Some sources of phosphate in fertilizers contain cadmium. Environmental exposure to cadmium has been particularly problematic in Japan where many people have consumed rice that was grown in cadmium-contaminated irrigation water, known under the name *itai-itai* disease [40]. Food and cigarettes are also a significant source of cadmium exposure. The general population and people living near hazardous waste sites may be exposed to cadmium in contaminated food, dust, or water from unregulated releases or accidental releases. Acute exposure to cadmium fumes may cause flu-like symptoms; kidney damage, and create hypophosphatemia causing muscle weakness. As a consequence of its unpredictability in children, in the future, it can have fertility impact. Cadmium was detected in the paint used on promotional drinking glasses for the movie *Shrek Forever After*, sold by McDonald's Restaurants, requiring the glasses to be recalled.

Chromium

Chromium (Cr) is a hard metal and was regarded with great interest because of its high corrosion resistance and hardness. A major development was the discovery that steel could be made highly resistant to corrosion and discoloration by adding chromium to form stainless steel. It is toxic in larger amounts. Cr(VI) treatment disrupted spermatogenesis, leading to accumulation of prematurely released spermatocytes, spermatids, and uni- and multinucleate giant cells in the lumen of seminiferous tubules in animals [41]. Two recent reports also correlated chronic occupational exposure to Cr(VI) to abnormal semen quality in men [42, 43], though the amount and type of Cr(VI) used were questioned [44]. The accumulation of uni- and multinucleate germ cells in the epididymal lumen of the monkeys treated with Cr(VI) causing ductal obstruction probably attributed to the disruption of spermatogenesis and testicular histoarchitecture [45]. Testes, seminal vesicle, and preputial gland weights were significantly reduced in chromium chloride- and potassium dichromate-exposed males [46].

Lead

Lead (Pb) is counted as one of the heavy metals. Lead is widely used in the production of batteries, metal products (solder and pipes), ammunition, and devices to shield X-rays, leading to its exposure to the people working in these industries. Use of lead in gasoline, paints and ceramic products, caulking, and pipe solder has been dramatically reduced in recent years because of health concerns. Ingestion of contaminated food and drinking water is the most common source of lead exposure in humans. Exposure can also occur via inadvertent ingestion of contaminated soil/dust or lead-based paints. Lead has long been known to be toxic to male fertility associated with the impairment of spermatogenesis and reduced concentrations of androgens. Male reproductive toxicity studies in humans have addressed effects on sex hormone levels, birth rates, time taken to conceive in couples not using contraception, and semen characteristics. Although findings across studies and end points are not entirely consistent, the main body of evidence points to current blood lead concentrations of about 40–50 µg/dl as a most likely no adverse effect threshold. This applies to semen characteristics such as sperm count, motility, abnormal sperm forms, as well as to fertility rate and time taken to conceive, whereas primary effects on the hormonal regulation of the male reproductive system at these exposure levels are questionable [47]. This view on male reproductive toxicity of lead is challenged by the findings on decreased fecundity among male lead workers [48, 49]. They observed an astonishing clear exposure response relation between current blood lead level and time taken to conceive among male battery workers in Taiwan. The fecundability ratio, in exposed compared to nonexposed, declined steadily from 0.9 in men with blood lead levels below 20 µg/dl to 0.4 among men with a blood level above 40 µg/dl. The fact that a large European study failed to show effects of lead on time to pregnancy in any of the three independent study populations is not reassuring if the consistency of findings across countries reflects repetition of errors inherent in the study design. The divergent findings in Europe and Taiwan could of course also be due to differences in susceptibility to the toxic effects of lead. During recent years, it has been shown that lead may interfere with the reorganization and tight packaging of sperm DNA during spermatogenesis by competition with zinc on protamine-binding sites. This results in reduced stability of the chromatin, and abnormal chromatin structure is strongly related to reduced fertility in humans. And there is indeed limited evidence that chromatin structure abnormalities are related to lead exposures in the lower range of blood lead values in men with high concentrations of lead within spermatozoa. Other mechanisms might be of significance as well. Thus, it was recently found that lead at environmental levels strongly interferes with the sperm acrosome reaction, which is essential for fertilization and negatively affects outcomes of artificial insemination [50]. There is definitely a need to keep open this line of research [48]. However, unlike many other metals such as zinc, chromium, manganese, copper, and iron, lead has no known essential effects for living organisms, and current exposure levels are still high compared to preindustrial populations.

Mercury

Mercury (Hg) is a heavy metal, proven to be toxic, has a very long half-life in the body, and is found in air, water, and soil. Mercury is in many products: metallic mercury is used in thermometers, dental fillings, and batteries. Mercury salts may be used in skin creams and ointments. It is also used in many industries. Mercury in the air settles into water and can pass through the food chain and build up in fish, shellfish, and animals that eat fish. The nervous system is sensitive to all forms of mercury. Exposure to high levels can damage the brain and kidneys.

Pregnant women can pass the mercury in their bodies to their babies. Research on mercury increased after the accident in Japan in 1968, when more was learned about exposure to this metal in rats and humans. Mercury can concentrate in the kidneys, cerebellum, testes, and epididymis, leading to neurological disorders, kidney failure, and infertility, particularly on susceptible individuals and on susceptible groups such as fetuses and young children [51]. Young syndrome can be associated with obstructive lesion of the upper epididymis [52]. Some authors reviewed that existing scientific evidence does not demonstrate that mercury from dental amalgam poses a public health hazard, although there exists some controversy on this issue [51, 53, 54].

Copper

Copper (Cu) levels in serum and seminal plasma in the subfertile male group were significantly higher than those in the fertile male group [55]. Copper can act on FSH receptors, interfering in spermatogenesis. In animals, the main endocrine alterations are in testosterone, LH, and FSH secretion. Significant correlations between copper concentrations in semen and sperm concentration ($P < 0.001$), percentage progressive motility ($P < 0.005$), and normal morphology ($P < 0.005$) were observed. However, semen copper concentrations of infertile men and fertile men did not differ significantly [56].

Dioxins

Dioxins are the result of various industrial processes and are considered the most toxic anthropogenic agents. Exposure to dioxins decreases spermatogenesis and testicular weight, reduces fertility, and can affect libido, causing changes in the sexual behavior of male fish, birds, and mammals, and also reptiles when in uterus. Sperm counts have dropped, and alterations in the male reproductive tract have increased since the 1950s.

2,3,7,8-Tetrachlorodibenzo-*p*-dioxin (TCDD) is a polychlorinated dibenzodioxin, the most toxic dioxin. The half-life in rodents is usually 2–4 weeks, but in humans has been estimated to be 7–11 years although with wide individual variation. It became known as a contaminant in Agent Orange, a herbicide used in the Vietnam War. It is a colorless solid with no distinguishable odor formed as an unintentional by-product of incomplete combustion of fossil fuels and wood, and during incineration processes of municipal and industrial wastes. Human studies have shown an association between TCDD and soft-tissue sarcomas, lymphomas, and stomach carcinomas. TCDD may be formed during the chlorine bleaching process used by pulp and paper mills and as a by-product from the manufacture of certain chlorinated organic chemicals, such as chlorinated phenols. Very low levels of

TCDD are found throughout the environment, but most of the exposure of the general population is from food, mainly meat, dairy products, and fish. Chloracne is also the major effect seen from long-term exposure to TCDD in humans. Animal studies have reported hair loss, loss of body weight, and a weakened immune system from oral exposure to TCDD. The results of available reproductive and developmental studies in humans are inconclusive. Reproductive effects, including altered levels of sex hormones, reduced production of sperm, and increased rates of miscarriages, have been seen in animals exposed to TCDD.

Ethylene Oxide

Ethylene oxide (EtO) is produced in large volumes and is both flammable and highly reactive. Primarily used as an intermediate in the production of several industrial chemicals, the most notable of which is ethylene glycol. It is also used as a fumigant in certain agricultural products and as a sterilant for medical equipment and supplies and possesses several physical and health hazards that merit special attention. Acute exposures to EtO gas may result in respiratory irritation and lung injury, headache, nausea, vomiting, diarrhea, shortness of breath, and cyanosis. Chronic exposure has been associated with the occurrence of cancer, sperm damaging, reduces fertility, mutagenic changes, neurotoxicity, and sensitization [57].

Arsenic

Arsenic (As), a chemical element, is found in the uncombined condition in various localities but more generally in combination with other metals and sulfur. Arsenic is a constituent of the minerals arsenical iron, arsenical pyrites or mispickel, tin-white cobalt or smaltite, arsenical nickel, realgar, orpiment, pharmacolite, and cobalt bloom. The ordinary commercial arsenic is either the naturally occurring form, which is, however, more or less contaminated with other metals, or is the product obtained by heating arsenical pyrites, out of contact with air, in earthenware retorts which are fitted with a roll of sheet iron at the mouth and an earthenware receiver. A very high exposure to inorganic arsenic can cause infertility and miscarriages with women, and it can cause skin disturbances, declined resistance to infections, heart disruptions, and brain damage. Finally, inorganic arsenic can damage DNA, peripheral neuritis, sensory disturbances, tingling, numbness, formication, and occasionally cutaneous anesthesia. Later, the affected muscles become tender, and then atrophy, while the knee jerk or an other reflex is lost. Arsenic and most of its soluble compounds are very poisonous. Despite their toxic effect, inorganic arsenic bonds occur on earth naturally in small amounts. Humans may be exposed through food, water, and air. Exposure may also occur through skin contact with soil or water that contains arsenic. Levels of arsenic in food are fairly low, but levels in fish and seafood may be high because fish absorb arsenic from the water they live in. Luckily, this is mainly the fairly harmless organic form, but fish that contain significant amounts of inorganic arsenic may be a danger to human health [57]. Human data are limited to a few studies of populations exposed to arsenic from drinking water or from working at or living near smelters. Associations with spontaneous abortion and stillbirth have been reported in more than one of these studies. Interpretation of most of these studies is complicated because study populations were exposed to multiple chemicals.

Methoxychlor

Methoxychlor is a synthetic organochlorine used as an insecticide to protect crops, ornamentals, livestock, and pets against fleas, mosquitoes, and other insects and has been used to some degree as a replacement for dichlorodiphenyltrichloroethane (DDT) as it is metabolized faster and does not lead to bioaccumulation. The amount of methoxychlor in the environment changes seasonally due to its use in farming and foresting. It does not dissolve readily in water, so it is mixed with a petroleum-based fluid and sprayed, or used as a dust. Sprayed methoxychlor settles on the ground or in aquatic ecosystems, where it can be found in sediments. Its degradation may take many months. Methoxychlor is ingested and absorbed by living organisms, but is readily released and does not accumulate in the food chain. Some metabolites may have unwanted side effects. The use of methoxychlor as a pesticide was banned in the USA in 2003 and in Europe in 2002.

Human exposure to methoxychlor occurs via air, soil, and water [58], primarily in people who work with the substance or who are exposed to air, soil, or water that has been contaminated. Some of the agent's metabolites have an estrogenic effect as shown in adult and developing animals before and after birth [58]. One metabolite is 2,2-bis(p-hydroxyphenyl)-1,1,1-trichloroethane (HPTE) which is considered to have reproductive toxicity in the animal model by reducing testosterone biosynthesis. Such effects adversely affect both the male and female reproductive systems. It is expected that this "could occur in humans" but has not been proven.

Little information is available regarding effects on human pregnancy and children, but it is assumed from animal studies that methoxychlor crosses the placenta, and it has been detected in human milk. Exposure to children may be different from that in adults because they tend to play on the ground; further, their reproductive system may be more sensitive to the effects of methoxychlor as an endocrine disruptor. Food contamination may occur at low levels. Some of the breakdown products of methoxychlor cause effects similar to those produced by estrogen. Exposure in animals to methoxychlor adversely affects prostate and fertility in adults and in developing animals exposed prenatally or shortly after birth. Likewise, it is expected that reproductive effects seen in animals could occur in humans exposed to methoxychlor but yet has not been clearly reported [59, 60].

Glycol Ether

"Glycol ethers" is a name for a large group of chemicals. Most glycol ether compounds are clear, colorless liquids. Some have mild, pleasant odors, or no smell at all; others (mainly the acetates) have strong odors. The common belief that glycol ethers never evaporate fast enough to create harmful levels in the air is false. Some evaporate quickly and can easily reach hazardous levels in the air; others evaporate very slowly and therefore are less hazardous by inhalation. The glycol ethers are widely used industrial solvents. Each of them may be used alone or as an ingredient in products such as coatings (paints, varnishes, dyes, stains, inks, and semiconductor chip coatings), cleaners (for degreasing, dry cleaning, film cleaning, and circuit board manufacture), jet fuel deicing additives, brake fluids, and perfumes and cosmetics. Certain glycol ethers have been found to cause birth defects and damage to the testicles in laboratory animals [61]. Glico exposure is related to low motile sperm count in men attending fertility clinics. This suggests that it continues to be a hazard to male fertility [62]. Controversially, another study suggests that most glycol ethers currently used do not have an impact on human semen characteristics. Those that were more prevalent from the 1960s until recently may have long-lasting negative effects on human semen quality [63].

Polychlorinated Biphenyls

Polychlorinated biphenyls (PCBs) are a class of synthetic, persistent, lipophilic, halogenated aromatic compounds that were widely used in industrial and consumer products for decades before their production was banned in the USA in the late 1970s. PCBs were used in cutting oils, lubricants, and as electrical insulators. As a result of their extensive use and persistence, PCBs remain ubiquitous environmental contaminants. They are distributed worldwide and have been measured in air, water, aquatic and marine sediments, fish, and wildlife. Furthermore, they are biologically concentrated and stored in human adipose tissue. The general population is exposed primarily through the ingestion of contaminated foods (fish, meat, and dairy products), as PCBs bioaccumulate up the food chain. As a result of their persistence and ubiquity, measurable levels of serum PCBs are found in the majority of the US general population. Epidemiologic data support an inverse association of PCBs with reduced semen quality, specifically reduced sperm motility. The associations found were generally consistent across studies despite a range of PCB levels [64].

Bisphenol

Bisphenol (BPA) is an organic compound with two phenol functional groups and is a dysfunctional building block of several important plastic additives. BPA is an industrial chemical used to make a hard, clear plastic known as polycarbonate, which has been used in many consumer products, including reusable water bottles and baby bottles and is also found in epoxy resins, which act as a protective lining on the inside of metal-based food and beverage cans. These uses of BPA are subject to premarket approval by FDA as indirect food additives or food contact substances. The original approvals were issued under FDA's food additive regulations and date from the 1960s. Suspected of being hazardous to humans since the 1930s, concerns about the use of bisphenol A in consumer products were regularly reported in the news media in 2008 after several governments issued reports questioning its safety, thus prompting some retailers to remove products containing it from their shelves. A 2010 report by the United States Food and Drug Administration (FDA) raised further concerns regarding exposure of fetuses, infants, and young children [65–67].

Tobacco

The data on the effect of cigarette smoking on semen parameters and fertility is conflicting as well as uncertain [68]. However, increasing evidence suggests detrimental effects on human reproduction. DNA-binding carcinogens from cigarette smoke have been found in spermatozoa of smokers as well as in the embryos formed during IVF cycles using the sperm from these men. The heavy metal cadmium and the toxic alkaloid nicotine are present in increased amounts in the semen of smokers [69–71]. Studies have correlated smoking with adverse effects on parameters such as seminal volume, sperm count, motility, morphology, and increased numbers of white blood cells (WBCs) in the semen [72]. Other studies, however, have found no influence of cigarette smoking on semen parameters [73]. Smoking has been found to have an adverse effect on female fecundity, whereas the effects on male fecundity are conflicting [73, 74]. There is a delay in conception when the male smoked and evidence of a delay in conception when the nonsmoking female was passively exposed to cigarette smoke. In addition, a decreased success of IVF was reported when the male was a smoker [75]. We believe the evidence is strong enough that smoking should be considered a risk factor for infertility, and patients should be strongly encouraged to discontinue this habit [68]. However, smoking may serve as a cofactor for patients with other causes of male infertility. Effects of tobacco on fertility include higher levels of seminal oxidative stress than infertile nonsmokers, increasing DNA damage, higher sperm aneuploidy, testicular atrophy, and poorer sperm quality such as abnormal semen volume, concentration, motility, morphology, and elevated prolactin and estrogen. That is why some IVF programs restrict smoking for 3 months prior to semen collection. It is well established that smoking has a detrimental effect on male reproductive system. Cigarette smoking leads to an increase in ROS level. The high level of leukocytospermia in smokers suggests that oxidative stress is due to ROS generation by activated leukocytes. Various compounds of cigarette smoke (polycyclic aromatic hydrocarbons) and smoking metabolites may act as chemotactic stimuli and thereby induce an inflammatory response, recruitment of leukocyte, and subsequent generation of ROS. Motility is one of the first sperm parameters affected, and asthenozoospermia may be an early indicator of reduced semen quality in light smokers. There is a significantly high teratozoospermia in heavy smokers compared to nonsmokers. Studies have shown that maternal smoking affects reproductive parameters of their offspring (male) during adolescence [74, 76]. Remains unclear possible impact on nonsmokers industrial cigarette workers.

Radiation

Exposure to radiation, even small amounts of ionizing, particularly that used for medical therapy, may destroy sperm-forming cells. Spermatogonia are particularly radiosensitive and may further impair testicular function [77]. Spermatogenesis may take up to 4–5 years to return after radiation therapy or chemotherapy [78].

Radiation induces chromosomal changes, which lead to congenital abnormalities. Radiation exposure of pregnant mothers and the developing male fetus can cause adverse reproductive effects. A study among more than 100 prisoners, who volunteered themselves for testicle X-irradiation, showed that a dose of 0.11 Gy could cause substantial suppression of sperm counts and a dose of 3–5 Gy could lead to permanent sterility.

Phthalates

Phthalates are chemical substances widespread in general population exposure. High molecular weight phthalates, for example, di-[2-ethylhexylphthalate (DEHP)], are primarily used as plasticizers in the manufacture of flexible vinyl plastic, which in turn is used in consumer products, flooring and wall coverings, food contact applications, manufacturing of automobiles plastics, beverage containers, coating of metal cans, etc., and medical devices. Manufacturers use low molecular weight phthalates (e.g., diethyl phthalate [DEP] and dibutyl phthalate [DBP]) in personal care products (perfumes, lotions, and cosmetics), as solvents and plasticizers for cellulose acetate, and in making lacquers, varnishes, and coatings, including those used to provide timed releases in some pharmaceuticals [55, 57, 58]. Parenteral exposure from medical devices containing phthalates is an important source of high exposure to phthalates, primarily DEHP [79]. As a result of the ubiquitous use of phthalates in personal forms of exposure are food, inhalation, dermal contact, medical materials and by occupational contact. Phthalates can alter reproductive development regardless of binding to androgen or estrogen receptors. Some phthalate esters inhibit steroidogenesis in Leydig cells. Through exposure by food, they can cause testicular atrophy and reduced fertility. Data have demonstrated that perinatal exposure to a variety of phthalate esters alters the development of the male reproductive tract in an antiandrogenic way, causing underdevelopment and agenesis of the epididymis at relatively low doses [80]. Compared with the laboratory animal data on the reproductive toxicity of phthalates, the human data is limited. In spite of that, the concentration of the sum of several phthalate diesters in seminal plasma was inversely correlated with sperm morphology in infertile males, an inverse relationship with sperm concentration [81]. DBP concentrations have been found in the cellular fractions of ejaculates [80, 82]. In contrast, according to a singular study, there were no relationships of MBP or MBzP with any of the semen parameters. However, this particular study should not be compared with others due to many epidemiologic differences, such as median age, type of recruitment, etc. Phthalates can alter reproductive development regardless of binding to androgen or estrogen receptors.

Xenoestrogens

Xenoestrogens are industrially made compounds that have estrogenic effects and differ chemically from naturally occurring estrogenic substances produced by living organisms. In the environment, xenoestrogens can be divided into natural compounds (plants or fungi) and synthetically derived agents including pesticides and industrial by-products. They have been a ubiquitous part of the environment even before the existence of the human race [83]. Xenoestrogens have also been identified as endocrine disruptors that might not only cause the "testicular dysgenesis syndrome" (TDS) but also disturb meiosis in developmental germinal cells. The male reproductive system is most vulnerable to estrogenic agents during the critical period of cell differentiation and organ development in fetal and neonatal life [84]. In this period, the testes are structurally organized, establishing Sertoli cell and spermatogonia numbers to support spermatogenesis that will be initiated at puberty. The maintenance of tightly regulated estrogen levels is essential for its completion. Analysis of maternal and fetal biological fluids has shown that xeno- and phytoestrogens cross the placenta barrier into fetal circulation and that they can bioaccumulate in fetal organs. An analysis on amniotic fluid samples undergoing routine amniocentesis shows that overall, one in three amniotic fluid samples tested positive for at least one environmental contaminant. It has also been described that these compounds cross a blood–tissue barrier similar to that of the testis, suggesting that intratubular germ cells might be exposed [21]. Soy isoflavone has estrogenic activity and is widely consumed. The association of soy foods and soy isoflavones suggested that higher intake of these foods was associated with lower sperm concentration. A further recent change in diet is the increased use of soy-based infant formula milk (SFM) for the increasing numbers of babies that are lactose intolerant. Infants on SFM have a phytoestrogen (a kind of xenoestrogen) intake per kg body weight 6–11 times higher than that seen in adults consuming a high phytoestrogen diet. Plasma levels of phytoestrogen are 1,000-fold greater than those of endogenous estradiol raising concerns about the effects of prolonged neonatal exposure to such high concentrations of estrogens and its potential disruption of male reproductive tract. Consequently, it is being speculated that male reproductive anomalies (hypospadias and cryptorchidism) and the global fall in sperm counts have both a causal link in the marked increase of phytoestrogens in our diet, causing a disruption of the male reproductive system. Endogenous hormones have a vital role in fetal life and ensure future fertility. Exposure to the wrong hormones (female fetus exposed to male hormones) or inadequate amounts of these could affect the reproductive system, and genitalia may not develop correctly, resulting in fertility problems in adulthood. Children are extremely sensitive to estradiol and may respond with increased growth and/or breast development even at serum levels below the current detection limits and that those changes in hormone levels during fetal and prepubertal development may have severe effects in adult life [85]. A cautionary approach should be taken in order to avoid unnecessary exposure of fetuses and children to exogenous sex steroids and endocrine disruptors, even at very low levels. That caution includes food intake, as possible adverse effects on human health may be expected by consumption of meat from hormone-treated animals [86]. Maternal beef consumption, and possibly xenobiotics (anabolic steroids) in beef, may alter testicular development in uterus and adversely affect reproductive capacity. Sperm concentration was inversely related to mother's weekly beef intake. In sons of "high consumers" (>7 beef meals/week), sperm concentration was 24.3% lower than that of men whose mothers ate less beef [87]. General population is exposed to many potential endocrine disruptors concurrently. Studies have shown that the action of estrogenic compounds is additive, but little is known about the possible synergistic or additive effects of these compounds in humans [88]. There is a human association between maternal exposure to pesticides and cryptorchidism among male children. Pesticide levels in breast milk were significantly higher in boys with cryptorchidism [89].

Vinclozolin

Vinclozolin [3-(3-5-dichlorophenyl)-5-methyl-oxazolidine-2,4-dione] is a common dicarboximide fungicide used to control various diseases on raspberries, chicory grown, lettuce, kiwi, canola, snap beans, dry bulb onions, ornamentals, and turf. Vinclozolin is formulated as a dry flowable and extruded granule which may be applied with aerial, chemigation, or ground equipment (broadcast, band, or soil drench); as a dip treatment on ornamental bulbs and corms, cut flowers, rose budwood, or nursery stock; and with thermal fogger in greenhouses. It has been registered since 1981 in the USA for use as fungicide [90]. Vinclozolin is a known environmental endocrine disrupter. Endocrine disruptors are hormonally active environmental compounds that have been shown to influence both male and female reproductive development and function [91]. Endocrine disruptors affect normal reproductive physiological development and functions by acting as antiandrogenic compounds. Vinclozolin binds with high affinity to the androgen receptor and blocks the action of gonadal hormones on male reproductive organs [92].

An alternative mechanism of the action of vinclozolin involves transgenerational effects on the male reproductive tract, which has defined as the transfer of heritable material from parents to offspring continuing through multiple subsequent generations. To transfer an induced phenotype from parents to offspring, the germ line genetic material must be altered via an epigenetic (DNA methylation) or stable genetic alteration (mutation, change in the DNA sequence) mechanism [93]. Vinclozolin exposure results in a transgenerational effect on spermatogenic capacity and testis function. The embryonic exposure to vinclozolin resulted in a reduced spermatogenetic capacity in the male offspring, and this phenotype was transmitted to the subsequent generations. This is a stage where spermatogenesis has advanced germ cell maturation and early spermatocyte development [94, 95].

Heat

There is human and animal experimental evidence that heat exposure may be detrimental to spermatogenesis [96]. The relationship between fertility and occupations in which heat exposure occurs reported a detrimental effect on sperm morphology and time to conception [97]. Occupations that have been reported to be associated with heat exposure and infertility include bakers, drivers (industrial machinery, taxis, and trucks), ceramic oven operators, welders, and workers in submarines [98]. In addition, a dysfunction of testicular thermoregulation has been suggested to occur in paraplegic men in wheelchairs [99].

Expert Commentary

Environmental factors that affect male fertility are complex and not well known. Our modern society produces several new chemical components each day, and the impact of these products in male fertility is not enough studied. This plethora of new components can affect the environmental delicate equilibrium, and the results for humans, flora, and fauna are a public issue. The twenty-first century is still facing many controversial issues, although there is a growing body of literature relating to the deleterious effect of substances on semen quality, fertility, offspring anomalies, etc. There is no question that it is a matter of interest for any country in spite of its economic, social, and cultural background. However, there is a tremendous heterogeneous situation among countries: some carrying out outstanding control as well as studies, some working as slaves and do not have "the right" to learn what they are working with, no personal exposure protection, and the family living just behind the industry plant, without any water, soil, and dust control. It is well known that the protection against exposure may prevent diseases with high morbidity and mortality, such as tumors, endocrine disruption, immune and endocrine system, behavior, human reproduction, etc.

In spite of all the growing progress, we need to learn more about food additives, toxicants, contaminants, outdoor and indoor air pollutants, pesticides, xenoestrogens, and hazardous substances in the workplace and particularly the possible synergism among many substances.

We are already aware that sperm DNA fragmentation, ROS (oxidative stress), apoptosis, and some Y microdeletions are happening, and the scientific world is running far behind.

Five-Year View

For the next 5 years, strong education development program worldwide for lay population is crucial since some pollutant hazards can be prevented. The scientific community should be committed to share the data, information, not just among the sophisticated academic world but to make it happen across the target general population.

Many current study designs present bias and need to be reviewed in such a way that we can compare data and come across with definite conclusions. Certainly, they need to incorporate markers of susceptibility for several chemicals, metals, etc. Thus, it will be possible temporally be sure when and what hazards chemicals are being deleterious to human being as well as determined in what life stage (fetus, neonatal, peripubertal, etc.) will be risky.

Regarding preventive attitudes, it depends upon the country policy. Most of the situations are just government investment and decisions because pollutants are spread all over (air, water, soil, food, etc.).

Key Issues

- Male infertility and pollutants.
- Environmental hazards can cause infertility as well as many serious diseases.
- The decreasing male fertility can be a consequence of external toxic ubiquitous substances.

References

1. World Health Organization, Department of Reproductive Health and Research. WHO laboratory manual for the examination and processing of human semen. 5th ed. Geneva: World Health Organization; 2010. p. 1–271. ISBN 978 92 4 154778 9 (NLM classification: QY 190).
2. Lampiao F. Variation of semen parameters in healthy medical students due to exam stress. Malawi Med J. 2009;21(4):166–7.
3. Castilla JA, Álvarez C, Aguilar J, et al. Influence of analytical and biological variation on the clinical interpretationol seminal parameters. Hum Reprod. 2006;21(4):847–51.

4. Oshio S, Ashizawa Y, Yotsukura M, et al. Individual variation in semen parameters of healthy young volunteers. Arch Androl. 2004;50:417–25.
5. Public Health Statement about Methoxychlor. Agency for toxic substances and disease registry (ATSDR). 2002. http://www.atsdr.cdc.gov/toxprofiles/tp47-c1-b.pdf. Accessed 22 Aug 2010.
6. Agarwal A, Desai NR, Ruffoli N, et al. Lifestyle and testicular dysfunction: a brief update. Biomed Pharmacother. 2008;62:550–3.
7. Ausmees K, Zarkovski M, Timberg G, et al. Associations between semen quality, body mass index and metabolic syndrome parameters in young male. Eur Urol Suppl. 2010;9:I–XX.
8. Phillips KP, Tanphaichitr N. Mechanisms of obesity-induced male infertility. Expert Rev Endocrinol Metabol. 2010;5(2):229–51.
9. Sharpe RM. Environmental/lifestyle effects on spermatogenesis. Philos Trans R Soc Lond B Biol Sci. 2010;365(1546):1697–712.
10. Sheynkin Y, Jung M, Yoo P, et al. Increase in scrotal temperature in laptop computer users. Hum Reprod. 2004. http://humrep.oxfordjournals.org/cgi/content/abstract/deh616v1. Accessed 1 June 2011.
11. Turek PJ. Does the male infertility clinical evaluation adequately assess toxicologic exposures? Fertil Steril. 2008;89:69.
12. Velde E, Burdorf A, Nieschlag E, et al. Is human fecundity declining in Western countries? Hum Reprod. 2010;25(6):1348–53.
13. Sinclair S. Male infertility nutritional and environmental considerations. Altern Med Rev. 2000;5(1):28–38.
14. Rhind SM, Evans NP, Bellingham M. Effects of environmental pollutants on the reproduction and welfare of ruminants. Animal. 2010;4(7):1227–39.
15. Toppari J, Larsen JC, Christiansen P, et al. Male reproductive health and environmental xenoestrogens. Environ Health Perspect. 1996;104(4):741–803.
16. Carlsen E, Giwercman A, Keiding N, et al. Evidence for decreasing quality of semen during past 50 years. BMJ. 1992;305:609–13.
17. Hauser R, Sokol R. Science linking environmental contaminant exposures with fertility and reproductive health impacts in the adult male. Fertil Steril. 2008;89:59–65.
18. Saradha B, Mathur PP. Effect of environmental contaminants on male reproduction. Environ Toxicol Pharmacol. 2006;21:34–41.
19. Perry MJ. Effects of environmental and occupational pesticide exposure on human sperm: a systematic review. Hum Reprod Update. 2008;14(3):233–42.
20. Jobling S, Burn RW, Thorpe R, et al. Statistical modelling suggests that anti-androgens in wastewater treatment works effluents are contributing causes of widespread sexual disruption in fish living in English rivers. Environ Health Perspect. 2009. doi: 10.1289/ehp.0800197. http://dx.doi.org/. Accessed 7 Jan 2009.
21. Sharpe RM, Skakkebaek NE. Are oestrogens involved in falling sperm counts and disorders of the male reproductive tract? Lancet. 1993;341:1392–5.
22. Aitken RJ, Baker MA. Reactive oxygen species generation by human spermatozoa: a continuing. Int J Androl. 2002;25(4):191–4.
23. Agarwal A, Said TM. Role of sperm chromatin abnormalities and DNA damage in male infertility. Hum Reprod Update. 2003;9:331–45.
24. Rao AVSK, Shaha C. Role of glutathione S-transferases in oxidative stress–induced male germ cell apoptosis. Free Radic Biol Med. 2000;29(10):1015–27.
25. Iwasaki A, Gagnon C. Formation of reactive oxygen species in spermatozoa of infertile patients. Fertil Steril. 1992;57(2):409–16.
26. Chen SS, Chang LS, Wei YH. Oxidative damage to proteins and decrease of antioxidant capacity in patients with varicocele. Free Radic Biol Med. 2001;30:1328–34.
27. Agarwal A, Saleh RA, Bedaiwy MA. Role of recreative oxygen species in the pathophysiology of human reproduction. Fertil Steril. 2003;79:829–43.
28. Mendiola J, Torres-Cantero AM, Moreno-Grau JM, et al. Food intake and its relationship with semen quality: a case-control study. Fertil Steril. 2009;91:812–8.

29. Agarwal A. New insights in molecular mechanisms of male infertility. Urology News. 2003;22(8):22.
30. Akingbemi BT, Ge RS, Klinefelter GR, et al. A metabolite of methoxychlor, 2,2-bis (p-hydroxyphenyl)-1,1,1-trichloroethane, reduces testosterone biosynthesis in rat Leydig cells through suppression of steady-state messenger ribonucleic acid levels of the cholesterol side-chain cleavage enzyme. Biol Reprod. 2000;62:571–8.
31. Cummings AW. Methoxychlor as a model for environmental estrogens. Crit Rev Toxicol. 1997;27:367–79.
32. Castellini C, Mourvakia E, Sartini B, et al. In vitro toxic effects of metal compounds on kinetic traits and ultrastructure of rabbit spermatozoa. Reprod Toxicol. 2009;27:46–54.
33. Altamirano-Lozano M, Alvarez-Barrera L, Basurto-Alcántara F, et al. Reprotoxic and genotoxic studies of vanadium pentoxide in male mice. Teratog Carcinog Mutagen. 1996;16:7–17.
34. Cooper RG. Vanadium pentoxide inhalation. Indian J Occup Environ Med. 2007;11:97–102.
35. Lauwerys R, Roels H, Genet P, et al. Fertility of male workers exposed to mercury vapor or to manganese dust: a questionnaire study. Am J Ind Med. 1985;7(2):171–6.
36. Wirth JJ, Rossano MG, Daly DC, et al. Ambient manganese exposure is negatively associated with human sperm motility and concentration. Epidemiology. 2007;18:270–3.
37. Şayli BS. Assessment of fertility and infertility in boron-exposed turkish subpopulations. Evaluation of fertility among sibs and in "borate families". Biol Trace Elem Res. 2001; 81(3):255–67.
38. Şayli BS. Low frequency of infertility among workers in a borate processing facility. Biol Trace Elem Res. 2003;93:19–29.
39. Tüccar EAH, Yavuz Y, et al. Comparison of infertility rates in communities from boron-rich and boron-poor territories. Biol Trace Elem Res. 1998;66:401–7.
40. Scialli AR, Bondeb JP, Bruske-Hohlfeldc I, et al. An overview of male reproductive studies of boron with an emphasis on studies of highly exposed Chinese workers. Reprod Toxicol. 2010;29:10–24.
41. Jarup L. Health effects of cadmium exposure—a review of the literature and a risk estimate. Scand J Work Environ Health. 1998;24:11–51.
42. Aruldhas MM, Subramanian S, Sekar P, et al. Chronic chromium exposure-induced changes in testicular histoarchitecture are associated with oxidative stress: study in a non-human primate (Macaca radiata Geoffroy). Hum Reprod. 2005;20(10):2801–13.
43. Danadevi K, Roya R, Reddy PP, et al. Semen quality of Indian welders occupationally exposed to nickel and chromium. Reprod Toxicol. 2003;17(4):451–6.
44. Li H, Chen Q, Li S, et al. Effect of Cr(VI) exposure on sperm quality: human and animal studies. Ann Occup Hyg. 2001;45:505–11.
45. Duffus JH. Effect of Cr(VI) exposure on sperm quality. Ann Occup Hyg. 2002;46(2):269–70.
46. Aruldhas MM, Subramanian S, Sekar P, et al. Microcanalization in the epididymis to overcome ductal obstruction caused by chronic exposure to chromium—a study in the mature bonnet monkey (Macaca radiata Geoffroy). Reproduction. 2004;128:127–37.
47. Bataineh H, Al-Hamood MH, Elbetieha A. Effect of long-term ingestion of chromium compounds on aggression, sex behavior and fertility in adult male rat. Drug Chem Toxicol. 1997;20(3):133–49.
48. Sheiner EK, Sheiner E, Hammel RD, et al. Effect of occupational exposures on male fertility. Ind Health. 2003;41:55–62.
49. Shiau CY, Wang JD, Chen PC. Decreased fecundity among male lead workers. Occup Environ Med. 2004;61:915–23.
50. Benoff S, Centola GM, Millan C, et al. Increased seminal plasma lead levels adversely affect the fertility potential of sperm in IVF. Hum Reprod. 2003;18(2):374–83.
51. Bonde JP, Apostoli P. Any need to revisit the male reproductive toxicity of lead? Occup Environ Med. 2005;62:2–3.
52. Podzimek S, Prochazkova J, Bultasova L, et al. Sensitization to inorganic mercury could be a risk factor for infertility. Neuroendocrinology. 2005;4(26):277–82.

53. Hendry WF, A'Hern RP, Cole PJ. Was Young's syndrome caused by exposure to mercury in childhood? BMJ. 1993;307(6919):1579–82.
54. Mutter J, Naumann J, Sadaghiani C, et al. Amalgam studies: disregarding basic principles of mercury toxicity. Int J Hyg Environ Health. 2004;207(4):391–7.
55. Choy CM, Lam CW, Cheung LT, et al. Infertility, blood mercury concentrations and dietary seafood consumption. BJOG. 2002;109(10):1121–5.
56. Aydemir B, Kiziler AR, Onaran I, et al. Impact of Cu and Fe concentrations on oxidative damage in male infertility. Biol Trace Elem Res. 2006;112(3):193–203.
57. Jockenhövel F, Bals-Pratsch M, Bertram HP, et al. Seminal lead and copper in fertile and infertile men. Andrologia. 1990;22(6):503–11.
58. Water treatment solutions—Lenntech. http://www.lenntech.com/periodic/elements/as.htm. Accessed 22 Aug 2010.
59. Public Health Statement about Methoxychlor. Atlanta, GA: ATSDR. http://www.atsdr.cdc.gov/toxprofiles/tp47-c1-b.pdf. Accessed 1 June 2011.
60. EU Pesticides Database. European Union—DG SANCO. http://ec.europa.eu/sanco_pesticides/public/index.cfm?event=activesubstance.selection&a=1. Accessed 2 Oct 2009.
61. Consumer Factsheet on: METHOXYCHLOR. United States Environmental Protection Agency. http://www.epa.gov/safewater/contaminants/dw_contamfs/methoxyc.html. Accessed 26 Nov 2006.
62. Hazard Evaluation System and Information Service. http://www.dhs.ca.gov/ohb/HESIS/glycols.htm. Accessed 5 Jun 2008.
63. Cherry N, Moore H, McNamee R, et al. Occupation and male infertility: glycol ethers and other exposures. Occup Environ Med. 2008;65:708–14.
64. Multigner L, Brik EB, Arnaud I, et al. Glycol ethers and semen quality: a cross-sectional study among male workers in the Paris municipality. Occup Environ Med. 2007;64:467–73.
65. Hauser R. The environment and male fertility: recent research on emerging chemicals and semen quality. Semin Reprod Med. 2006;24(3):156–67.
66. Update on bisphenol A for use in food contact applications. U.S. Food and Drug Administration—FDA. 2010. http://www.fda.gov/NewsEvents/PublicHealthFocus/ucm197739.htm. Accessed 1 June 2011.
67. European Food Safety Authority. Toxicokinetics of bisphenol A, scientific opinion of the panel on food additives, flavourings, processing aids and materials in contact with food. EFSA J. 2008. http://www.efsa.europa.eu/cs/BlobServer/Scientific_Opinion/afc_ej759_bpa_%20toxicokinetics_op_en.pdf?ssbinary=true. Accessed 9 Jul 2008.
68. Vom Saal VS, Akingbemi BT, Belcher SM, et al. Bisphenol A expert panel consensus statement: integration of mechanisms, effects in animals and potential to impact human health at current levels of exposure. Reprod Toxicol. 2007;24:131–8.
69. Sigman M, Jarow JP. Male infertility. In: Wein AJ, Kavoussi LR, Novick AC, Partin AW, Peters CA, editors. Campbell-Walsh urology, vol. 9. Philadelphia: Elsevier Inc; 2007. p. 609–50.
70. Sepaniak S, Forges T, Gerard H, et al. The influence of cigarette smoking on human sperm quality and DNA fragmentation. Toxicology. 2006;223:54–60.
71. Zenzes MT. Smoking and reproduction: gene damage to human gametes and embryos. Hum Reprod Update. 2000;6:122–31.
72. Zenzes MT, Bielecki R, Reed TE. Detection of benzo(a)pyrene diol epoxide-DNA adducts in sperm of men exposed to cigarette smoke. Fertil Steril. 1999;72:330–5.
73. Vine MF, Tse CK, Hu P, et al. Cigarette smoking and semen quality. Fertil Steril. 1996;65:835–42.
74. Goverde HJM, Dekker HS, Janssen HJ, et al. Semen quality and frequency of smoking and alcohol consumption—an explorative study. Int J Fertil. 1995;40(3):135–8.
75. Bolumar F, Olsen J, Boldsen J. Smoking reduces fecundity: a European multicenter study on infertility and subfecundity. The European Study Group on Infertility and Subfecundity. Am J Epidemiol. 1996;143:578–87.

76. Zitzmann M, Rolf C, Nordhoff V, et al. Male smokers have a decreased success rate for in vitro fertilization and intracytoplasmic sperm injection. Fertil Steril. 2003;79(3):1550–4.
77. Bonde JP, Kold JT, Brixen LS, et al. Year of birth and sperm count in 10 Danish occupational studies. Scand J Work Environ Health. 1998;24:407–13.
78. Turek PJ. Evaluation and treatment of male factor infertility. In: Shoskes DA, Morey AF, editors. The American Urological Association Educational review manual in urology. 2nd ed. New York: Castle Connolly Graduate Medical Publishing; 2009. p. 825–52.
79. Costabile RA. The effects of cancer and cancer therapy on male reproductive function. J Urol. 1993;149:1327–30.
80. Hauser R, Meeker JD, Duty S, et al. Altered semen quality in relation to urinary concentrations of phthalate monoester and oxidative metabolites. Epidemiology. 2006;17:682–91.
81. Queiroz EKR, Waissmann W. Occupational exposure and effects on the male reproductive system. Cad Saúde Pública. 2006;22(3):485–93.
82. Murature DA, Tang SY, Steinhardt G, Dougherty RC. Phthalate esters and semen quality parameters. Biomed Environ Mass Spectrom. 1987;14:473–7.
83. Singleton DW, Sohaib AK. Xenosestrogen exposure and mechanisms of endocrine disruption. Front Biosci. 2003;8:110–8.
84. Skakkebæk NE, Rajpert-De Meyts E, Main KM. Testicular dysgenesis syndrome: an increasingly common developmental disorder with environmental aspects. Hum Reprod. 2001;16:972–8.
85. Aksglaede L, Juul A, Leffers H, et al. The sensitivity of the child to sex steroids: possible impact of exogenous estrogens. Hum Reprod. 2006;12:341–9.
86. Andersson AM, Skakkebæk NE. Exposure to exogenous estrogens in food: possible impact on human development and health. Eur J Endocrinol. 1999;140:477–85.
87. Swan SH, Liu F, Overstreet JW, et al. Semen quality of fertile US males in relation to their mothers beef consumption during pregnancy. Hum Reprod. 2007;22:1497–502.
88. Toppari J, Skakkebæk NE. Sexual differentiation and environmental endocrine disrupters. Baillieres Clin Endocrinol Metab. 1998;12:143–56.
89. Damgaard IN, Skakkebæk NE, Toppari J, et al. Persistent pesticides in human breast milk and cryptorchidism. Environ Health Perspect. 2006;114:1133–8.
90. Kelce WR, Monosson E, Gamcsik MP, Laws SC, et al. Environmental hormone disruptors: evidence that vinclozolin developmental toxicity is mediated by antiandrogenic metabolites. Toxicol Appl Pharmacol. 1994;126:276–85.
91. Bayley M, Junge M, Baatrup E. Exposure of juvenile guppies to three antiandrogens causes demasculinization and a reduced sperm count in adult males. Aquat Toxicol. 2002;56(4):227–39.
92. Blake LS, et al. Reproductive toxicity of vinclozolin in the fathead minnow: confirming an anti-androgenic mode of action. Environ Toxicol Chem. 2008;27(2):478–88.
93. Anway MD, Cupp AS, Uzumcu M, et al. Epigenetic transgenerational actions of endocrine disruptors and male fertility. Science. 2005;308:1466–9.
94. Uzumcu M, Suzuki H, Skinner MK. Effect of the anti-androgenic endocrine disruptor vinclozolin on embryonic testis cord formation and postnatal testis development and function. Reprod Toxicol. 2004;18(6):765–74.
95. Anway MD, Memon AM, Uzumcu M, et al. Transgenerational effect of the endocrine disruptor vinclozolin on male spermatogenesis. J Androl. 2006;27(6):868–79.
96. MacLeod J, Hotchkiss RS. The effect of hyperpyrexia upon spermatozoa counts in men. Endocrinology. 1941;28:780–4.
97. Thonneau P, Bujan L, Multigner L, et al. Occupational heat exposure and male fertility: a review. Hum Reprod. 1998;13(8):2122–5.
98. de la Calle JF Velez, Rachou E, le Martelot MT, et al. Male infertility risk factors in a French military population. Hum Reprod. 2001;16(3):481–6.
99. Brindley GS. Deep scrotal temperature and the effect on it of clothing, air temperature, activity, posture and paraplegia. Br J Urol. 1982;54(1):49–55.

Part IV

Antioxidants in Male Reproductive Health

Chapter 16
Nutritional Pathways to Protect Male Reproductive Health

Tung-Chin Hsieh and Paul Shin

Nutrition is an essential component of one's overall health. Many common disease processes can be alleviated or prevented by a healthy diet. First reports of antioxidant deficiency and decreased male fertility can be traced back to over 50 years ago [1]. With the understanding of oxidative damage to spermatogenesis, most of the nutritional research has focused on the role of antioxidants in improving male fertility. However, there are not any randomized controlled trials studying whole food diet in infertile male patients. Patients are often counseled based on data extrapolated from antioxidant supplement studies. This chapter is intended to give an overview of contemporary research on nutrient and male reproductive health with guidance to natural food source that contain high levels of antioxidants.

Nutrients and Male Reproductive Health

Arginine

Arginine is a semi-essential amino acid because it can be synthesize by the human body from glutamine, glutamate, and praline. It plays an important role in cell division, wound healing, immune function, hormone production, and ammonia metabolism. Arginine has significant effects on endothelial function since it is a precursor for nitric oxide synthesis. Not surprisingly, it is involved in the pathophysiology of many vascular disorders including vasogenic erectile dysfunction [2].

T.-C. Hsieh, MD (✉)
Department of Urology, Baylor College of Medicine,
One Baylor Plaza, Houston, TX 77030, USA

P. Shin, MD
Urologic Surgeons of Washington, 2021 K St. NW, Suite 408, Washington, DC 20006, USA
e-mail: pshin@dcurology.net

S.J. Parckattil and A. Agarwal (eds.), *Antioxidants in Male Infertility: A Guide for Clinicians and Researchers*, © Springer Science+Business Media New York 2013

Arginine is required for normal spermatogenesis. Researchers found that adult men on an arginine-deficient diet had decreased sperm counts and increased percentage of nonmotile sperm [1]. Oral administration of arginine (500 mg/day) to infertile men for 6–8 weeks has shown improvement in sperm counts, motility, and conception rates [3–6]. However, similar benefits were not observed in patients with baseline sperm counts less than 10 million/mL [7].

De novo biosynthesis, however, does not produce sufficient arginine; dietary intake remains the primary determinant of plasma arginine levels. It is considered an essential nutrient for human children but not adults by US Department of Agriculture (USDA) [8]. Currently, there is not a consensus on the daily recommended intake of arginine; studied doses range from 1 to 15 g/day. Although no significant adverse effects have been observed in studied doses, patients with impaired renal or hepatic dysfunction might be unable to metabolize arginine properly. The effect of arginine on the airway is also unclear, therefore precaution should be taken in asthmatic patients. Animal sources of arginine include dairy products, turkey, pork, and beef. Vegetable sources include seeds, soybeans, and nuts.

Zinc

Zinc is an essential micromineral. There are 2–4 g of zinc throughout the human body with the highest concentrations in the prostate and parts of the eye [9]. It is a metalloprotein cofactor for DNA binding. Copper/zinc superoxide dismutase is involved in the repair of damaged DNA. It has an important role in testes development and sperm physiologic functions. Zinc deficiency is associated with hypogonadism, testicular/seminiferous tubular atrophy, and inadequate development of secondary sexual characteristics [10].

Semen analysis of fertile and infertile men showed a positive correlation between low zinc levels and poor sperm quality [11]. Treating asthenozoospermia men with zinc (200 mg twice per day) for 3 months showed an improvement in sperm parameters: an increase in the seminal antioxidant capacity and a reduction of oxidative status. Researchers postulated that poor zinc nutrition can impair antioxidant defenses, be a risk factor in oxidant release, and compromise the mechanism of DNA repair, making the sperm cells highly susceptible to oxidative damage [11, 12]. Currently, there is limited data available in humans to establish a dietary dosage to achieve adequate concentration in seminal plasma.

The daily recommended dietary allowance of zinc is 8 mg/day for women and 11 mg/day for men [8]. Excess zinc absorption (>15 mg/day) can interfere with copper and iron absorption, cholesterol metabolism, and cause anosmia. Animal sources of zinc include red meat, oysters, and liver. Vegetable sources include seeds, nuts, and whole grains.

Selenium

Similar to zinc, selenium is also an essential micronutrient. It functions as a cofactor for reduction of antioxidant enzymes, such as glutathione peroxidase. Although rare in healthy, well-nourished adult human, selenium deficiency is associated with reduced or impaired reproduction throughout the animal kingdom [13]. A sperm-specific selenoprotein has been identified and suspected to play a key role in selenium deficiency-induced subfertility [14].

Population studies on the effect of selenium in subfertile men have yielded conflicting data [15, 16]. In a randomized, double-blinded study, treating subfertile men with selenium (100 µg) once a day showed no influence on sperm count but an improvement on sperm motility with 56% response rate when compared with placebo [17].

The recommended daily allowance for selenium is 70 µg/day for men. Selenosis can occur when intake reaches the level greater than 400 µg resulting in cirrhosis, pulmonary edema, and death. In Europe, there is a documented decline in the mean intake from 60 µg/day in the 1970s to 30 µg/day in the 1990s due to a change in the source of cereals for bread making [18]. Animal sources of selenium include meat, fish, and eggs. Vegetable sources include Brazil nuts, wheat/cereals, and soy products.

Vitamin C

Ascorbic acid is an essential nutrient for humans and other animal species. It has been associated with fertility for many years, since it is a key compound in gonadal physiology. However, the precise mechanism of action has not been elucidated. Most consider the effect of vitamin C on fertility is related to its three principal functions: promotion of collagen synthesis, role in hormone production, and protection or prevention against oxidation.

Early reports on the effects of vitamin C on male fertility were based on animal studies. Ascorbate deficiency was associated with poor breeding performance and degeneration of the testicular germinal epithelium [19, 20]. The gonadal growth-enhancing effects of gonadotropins were enhanced by simultaneous treatment with ascorbic acid [21]. In human studies, low ascorbate level has been associated with low sperm counts, increased number of abnormal sperm, reduced motility, and agglutination [22]. Dietary treatment with vitamin C has yielded mixed data on improvement of sperm parameters [23]. No current randomized controlled trials show an improvement in the semen parameters or pregnancy rates of healthy infertile men who take oral supplementation of vitamin C.

The recommended daily allowance of vitamin C is 90 mg/day for adult male and 75 mg/day for adult female [8]. Dietary intake should not exceed 2,300 mg/day since intoxication can lead to gastrointestinal disturbances, iron poisoning, and hemolytic anemia in patients with glucose-6-phosphate dehydrogenase deficiency. A well-balanced diet without supplementation is generally accepted to be sufficient to meet the daily requirement for vitamin C, except those who are pregnant or smoke tobacco. The highest natural sources are fruit and vegetables: black currant, red pepper, and guava.

Vitamin E

Vitamin E is a lipid-soluble antioxidant. It protects cell membranes from oxidation by reacting with free radicals generated during lipid peroxidation. Various forms of vitamin E had been identified, and the exact role and importance of the isoforms is still unclear. The motility of the spermatozoa depends on the integrity of the mitochondrial sheath which is composed of phospholipids and can be damaged by lipid peroxidation [24]. Therefore, vitamin E has been hypothesized to be an important factor in maintaining overall health of sperm.

In asthenozoospermic male, an increased concentration of the peroxidation by-product (malondialdehyde, MDA) was observed in the semen plasma. Treating these patients with vitamin E (100 mg/day) in a randomized, double-blinded fashion showed improvement in sperm motility and decreased MDA concentration, resulting in 11/52 successful pregnancies [25]. Although more well-designed studies were available, randomized controlled trials showed conflicting results regarding improvement in semen parameters [26, 27]. Since vitamin C has been shown to work synergistically with vitamin E, many studies examining the effect of combination therapy in infertile men were conducted and failed to show any improvement in semen parameters [28, 29].

The recommended daily intake of vitamin E is 15 mg (30 international unit, IU) per day for adults [8]. At dose of greater than 1,000 mg (1,500 IU) per day, there is an increased risk of hemorrhage and death. The best sources of vitamin E are nuts, seeds, and vegetable oil along with green leafy vegetable and fortified cereals.

L-Carnitine

Carnitine is a semi-essential nutrient that can be biosynthesized from lysine and methionine by the liver and kidneys. Two stereoisoforms exist with L-carnitine as the bioactive form. It is involved in the metabolism of long-chain fatty acids and serves as an antioxidant by removing acetyl-CoA that is responsible for mitochondrial lipid peroxidation [30]. The highest concentration of carnitine occurs in the epididymis with epididymal concentrations 2,000-fold higher than in plasma [31].

A multicenter, uncontrolled trial showed that oral administration of L-carnitine (3 g/day) for 4 months in asthenozoospermia patients resulted in an improvement in sperm motility, linearity index, rapid linear progression, and mean velocity

[32]. In a randomized, double-blinded, placebo-controlled trial, L-carnitine therapy (2 g/day) for 4 months in infertile men showed improvements in sperm concentration and motility [33]. Despite the observed success in improvement of sperm motility with carnitine supplementation, other randomized controlled studies have not been able to replicate similar results [34].

Seventy-five percent of carnitine that is present in human is derived from diet [35]. Currently, there is not a recommended daily allowance of carnitine intake or any detrimental reports of carnitine overdose. Oral intake greater than 1 g/day did not show any advantage since absorption studies indicate saturation at this level. The highest concentration of carnitine is found in red meat and dairy products. Vegetable sources include nuts, seeds, and asparagus.

Factors Contributing to Subfertility

Obesity

Multiple population-based studies suggest an increased risk of subfertility among obese couples [36]. In women, there are extensive researches performed on the effects of extremes of body composition on fertility by altered menstrual function [37]. Epidemiologic studies have observed a higher incidence of male factor infertility in obese male [38, 39]. Obese men often exhibit an altered reproductive hormonal profile: decreased androgen, sex hormone-binding globulin (SHBG), and inhibin B levels along with elevated estrogen levels [40, 41]. Other contributing factors of male obesity to increase risk for infertility are altered lifestyle and increased risks for sexual dysfunction.

Currently, there is limited data on the reversibility of obesity-associated male infertility with weight loss. A small randomized controlled trial showed increases in SHBG and testosterone (free and total) after weight loss from 10 weeks of a very low-energy diet and behavior modification program [42]. Other studies on the effect of weight loss, both surgical and diet/lifestyle modification programs showed mixed improvement in hormonal profile and sperm parameters [36].

Alcohol

Alcohol abuse has been shown to cause impaired testosterone production and testicular atrophy resulting in impotence, infertility, and reduced secondary sexual characteristics [43]. It has been shown to have a deleterious effect on all levels of male reproductive system: altered hypothalamic–pituitary–gonadal axis, Leydig and Sertoli cell dysfunction, and altered spermatogenesis leading to spermatogenic arrest and Sertoli cell-only syndrome in advanced cases [44, 45].

In an uncontrolled study, semen analysis of alcohol users showed altered sperm count, morphology, and motility. The association is most significant when alcohol consumption is greater than 40 g/day [43]. There are reports of potential beneficial effects of alcohol consumption on fertility since red wine has been shown to exert protection against oxidative damage [46]. Currently, the dose-dependent effects of alcohol on male factor infertility are not well understood.

Five-Year View and Key Issues

Diet modification and nutritional supplements are popular areas of concern for the infertile patient. Altering one's nutritional habits is usually easily done, for little to no cost, and empowers the patient to feel as though they are actively tackling their condition. From our survey of the literature, it should be apparent that no consensus exists regarding the best pathway or outcome to maximize fertility. Basic science research does not always translate into clinical success especially in the arena of infertility. Avoidance of toxicants, proper nutrition, and stress reduction are general guidelines that all infertile men should follow.

References

1. Holt L, Albanese A. Observations on amino acid deficiencies in man. Trans Assoc Am Physicians. 1944;58:143–56.
2. Appleton J. Arginine: clinical potential of a semi-essential amino acid. Altern Med Rev. 2002;7(6):512–22.
3. Tanimura J. Studies on arginine in human semen. Part II. The effects of medication with L-arginine-HCl on male infertility. Bull Osaka Med School. 1967;13:84–9.
4. De Aloysio D, Mantuano R, Mauloni M, et al. The clinical use of arginine aspartate in male infertility. Acta Eur Fertil. 1982;13:133–67.
5. Scibona M, Meschini P, Capparelli S, et al. L-Arginine and male infertility. Minerva Urol Nefrol. 1994;46:251–3.
6. Schacter A, Goldman JA, Zukerman Z, et al. Treatment of oligospermia with amino acid arginine. J Urol. 1973;110:311–3.
7. Pryor J, Blandy J, Evans P, et al. Controlled clinical trail of arginine for infertile men with oligozoospermia. Br J Urol. 1978;50:47–50.
8. National Academy of Sciences. Institute of Medicine. Food and Nutrition Board. Dietary guidance: DRI tables. US Department of Agriculture, National Agricultural Library and National Academy of Sciences, Institute of Medicine, Food and Nutrition Board. 2009.
9. Wapnir R. Protein nutrition and mineral absorption. Boca Raton: CRC; 1990.
10. Bedwal R, Bahuguna A. Zinc, copper and selenium in reproduction. Experientia. 1994; 50:626–40.
11. Colagar A, Marzony E, Chaichi M. Zinc levels in seminal plasma are associated with sperm quality in fertile and infertile men. Nutr Res. 2009;29:82–8.
12. Omu A, Al-Azemi M, Kehinde E, et al. Indications of the mechanism involved in improved sperm parameters by zinc therapy. Med Princ Pract. 2008;17:108–16.
13. Underwood EJ. Trace elements in human and animal nutrition. New York: Academic; 1977. p. 321.

14. Behne D, Weiss-Nowak C, Kalcklosch M, et al. Studies on new mammalian seleno proteins. Proceedings of the eighth international symposium on trace elements in man and animals. 1993. pp. 516–23.
15. Abou-Shakra R, Ward N, Everard D. The role of trace elements in male infertility. Fertil Steril. 1989;52:502–10.
16. Xu B, Chia SE, Tsakok M, et al. Trace elements in blood and seminal plasma and the relationship to sperm quality. Reprod Toxicol. 1993;7:613–8.
17. Scott R, Macpherson A, Yates R, et al. The effect of oral selenium supplementation on human sperm motility. Br J Urol. 1998;82:76–80.
18. Macpherson A, Barclay M, Dixon J, et al. Decline in dietary selenium intake in Scotland and effects on plasma concentrations. In: Anke M, Meissner D, Mills CF, editors. Trace elements in man and animals—TEMA 8. Gersdorf Germany: Verlag Media Tourisik; 1993. p. 269–70.
19. Counsell J, Hornig D. Vitamin C ascorbic acid. Essex: Applied Science; 1981.
20. Phillips P, Lardy H, Jeizer E, et al. Sperm stimulation in the bull through the subcutaneous administration of ascorbic acid. J Dairy Sci. 1040;23:873–8.
21. Dr Cio A, Schteingart M. The influence of ascorbic acid on the activity of gonadotrophic hormones. Endocrinology. 1942;30:263–4.
22. Wilson I. Sperm agglutinations in human serum and blood. Proc Soc Exp Biol Med. 1954;85:652–5.
23. Luck M, Jeyaseelan I, Scholes R. Ascorbic acid and fertility. Biol Reprod. 1995;52:262–6.
24. Palamanda J, Kehrer J. Involvement of vitamin E and protein thiols in the inhibition of microsomal lipid peroxidation by glutathione. Lipids. 1993;28:427–31.
25. Suleiman S, Ali M, Zaki Z, et al. Lipid peroxidation and human sperm motility: protective role of vitamin E. J Androl. 1996;17(5):530–7.
26. Geva E, Bartoov B, Zabuludovsky N, et al. The effect of antioxidant treatment on juman spermatozoa and fertilization rate in and in vitro fertilization program. Fertil Steril. 1996;66:430–4.
27. Kessopoulou E, Powers H, Sharma K, et al. A double-blind randomized placebo cross-over controlled trail using the antioxidant vitamin E to treat reactive oxygen species associated male infertility. Fertil Steril. 1996;64:825–31.
28. Greco E, Iacobelli M, Rienzi I, et al. Reduction of the incidence of sperm DNA fragmentation by oral antioxidant treatment. J Androl. 2005;26:349–53.
29. Rolf C, Cooper T, Yeung C, et al. Antioxidant treatment of patients with asthenozoospermia or moderate oligoasthenozoospermia with high-dose vitamin C and vitamin E: a randomized, placebo-controlled, double-blind study. Hum Repod. 1999;14:1028–33.
30. Agarwal A, Said T. Carnitines and male infertility. Reprod Biomed Online. 2004;8:376–84.
31. Hinton B, Snoswell A, Setchell B. The concentration of carnitine in the luminal fluid of the testis and epididymis of the rate and some other mammals. J Reprod Fertil. 1979;56:105–11.
32. Costa M, Canale D, Filicori M, et al. L-Carnitine in idiopathic asthenozoospermia: a multicenter study Italian study group on carnitine and male infertility. Andrologia. 1994; 26:155–9.
33. Lenzi A, Lombardo F, Sgro P, et al. Use of carnitine therapy in selected cases of male factor infertility: a double-blind crossover trail. Fertil Steril. 2003;79(2):292–300.
34. Patel S, Sigman M. Antioxidant therapy in male infertility. Urol Clin North Am. 2008; 35:319–30.
35. Peluso G, Nicolai R, Reda E, et al. Cancer and anticancer therapy-induced modifications on metabolism mediated by carnitine system. J Cell Physiol. 2000;182:339–50.
36. Hammoud A, Gibson M, Peterson M, et al. Impact of male obesity on infertility: a critical review of the current literature. Fertil Steril. 2008;90(4):897–904.
37. Pasquali R, Pelusi C, Genghini S, et al. Obesity and reproductive disorders in women. Hum Reprod Update. 2003;9:359–72.
38. Alavanja M, Sandler D, McMaster S, et al. The agricultural health study. Environ Health Perspect. 1996;104:362–9.
39. Magnusdottir E, Thorsteinsson T, Thorsteinsdottir S, et al. Persistent organochlorines, sedentary occupation, obesity and human male subfertility. Hum Reprod. 2005;20:208–15.

40. Stellato R, Feldman H, Hamdy O, et al. Testosterone, sex hormone-binding globulin and the development of type 2 diabetes in middle-age men: prospective results from the massachussetts male aging study. Diabetes Care. 2000;23:490–4.
41. Globerman H, Shen-Orr Z, Karnieli E, et al. Inhibin B in men with severe obesity and after weight reduction following gastroplasty. Endocr Res. 2005;31:17–26.
42. Kaukua J, Pekkarinen T, Sane T, et al. Sex hormones and sexual function in obese men losing weight. Obes Res. 2003;11:689–94.
43. Gaur D, Talekar M, Pathak V. Alcohol intake and cigarette smoking: impact of 2 major lifestyle factors on male infertility. Indian J Pathol Microbiol. 2010;53(1):35–40.
44. Emanuele M, Emanuele N. Alcohol's effects on male reproduction. Alcohol Health Res World. 1998;22:195–218.
45. Zhu Q, Van Thiel D, Gavaler J. Effect of ethanol on rate sertoli cell function: studies in vitro and in vivo. Alcohol Clin Exp Res. 1997;21:1409–17.
46. Perez D, Strobel P, Foncea R, et al. Wine, diet, antioxidant defenses and oxidative damage. Ann N Y Acad Sci. 2002;957:136–45.

Chapter 17
Natural Antioxidants

Giancarlo Balercia, Antonio Mancini, and Gian Paolo Littarru

An excess of reactive oxygen species (ROS) and other oxidant radicals has been associated with male infertility [1–8]. The total oxyradical scavenging capacity (TOSC) is a recently developed assay measuring the overall capability of biological fluids or cellular antioxidants to neutralize the toxicity of various oxyradicals [9, 10]. The TOSC assay can discriminate between different forms of ROS, allowing to identify the role of specific antioxidants, or their pathway of formation in the onset of toxicological or pathological processes. The previous application of TOSC assay in andrology led us to show a reduced antioxidant efficiency in seminal fluid of infertile men with a significant correlation between the scavenging capacity towards hydroxyl radicals and parameters of sperm cell motility [11].

Despite the fact that oxidative stress is well recognized as a cause of male infertility, the use of antioxidants as a treatment is still debated, and it is considered as a "supplementation" therapy, rather than an etiological or physiopathological therapy, since no clear correlation has been investigated between a real deficiency of a

G. Balercia, MD (✉)
Andrology Unit, Endocrinology, Department of Internal Medicine and Applied
Biotechnologies, Umberto I Hospital, School of Medicine, Marche Polytechnic University,
Ancona 60100, Italy

Department of Clinical and Molecular Sciences, Marche Polytechnic University,
Umberto I Hospital, Ancona 60100, Italy
e-mail: g.balercia@univpm.it

A. Mancini, MD
Department of Internal Medicine, Division of Endocrinology, The Catholic University
of Sacred Heart, Rome, Italy
e-mail: amancini@rm.unicatt.it

G.P. Littarru, MD
Dipartimento di Scienze Cliniche Specialistiche ed Odontostomatologiche,
Universita Politecnica delle Marche, Vai Ranieri 65, Ancona 60131, Italy
e-mail: g.littarru@univpm.it

S.J. Parckattil and A. Agarwal (eds.), *Antioxidants in Male Infertility: A Guide
for Clinicians and Researchers*, © Springer Science+Business Media New York 2013

specific antioxidant and the effect of oral supplementation. Various models have been introduced to explore the protective role of different antioxidants in vitro, and some differences can be discovered regarding the protective effects exerted by specific enzymatic or non-enzymatic molecules [12]. We focus our attention on two main natural antioxidants, the efficacy of which has been supported by clinical trials: coenzyme Q_{10} and carnitine.

Coenzyme Q_{10}

Among natural antioxidant, a special role is covered by coenzyme Q_{10} (CoQ_{10}), also called ubiquinone for its wide distribution in different plants, animals and tissues. Coenzyme Q_{10} is a crucial component of the mitochondrial oxidative phosphorylation process because of its role in redox link between flavoproteins and cytochromes in the inner mitochondrial membrane; it has also many other functions, first of all the antioxidant activity, and new roles in different cellular functions were recently highlighted: this molecule can participate in redox reactions also in not mitochondrial cellular reactions, as in lysosomes, in Golgi apparatus and in plasma membranes [13], also contributing to membrane fluidity. Moreover, coenzyme Q_{10} can participate in many aspects of the redox control of the cellular signalling origin and transmission; in fact, the auto-oxidation of semiquinone, formed in various membranes during electron transport, can be a primary source for H_2O_2 generation, which activates some transcription factors, such as NF-kB, to induce gene expression [14]. It is also possible that ROS generation could suppress other genes. There are also some indications regarding the involvement of CoQ_{10} in cellular proliferation at least two aspects of the stimulation of cellular proliferation concerning CoQ_{10} [15, 16]. Cellular growth stimulation could be based on the activation of an oxidase in the plasma membrane, which should need CoQ_{10} to transfer electrons through the membrane, in which is also present [17]. On the other hand, the exposition of cells to serum can induce the apoptosis, while coenzyme Q_{10} allows a normal cellular division. Further studies are necessary to better understand these issues.

Clinically, the significance of antioxidant action of ubiquinone has been clarified by many studies concerning lipoproteins both in vitro and in vivo. In fact, LDLs are molecules particularly susceptible to the oxidative damage with cytotoxic products generation, associated with vascular contractile response alterations and atherosclerosis [18]. It has been demonstrated that reduced CoQ_{10} present in LDL is oxidized before vitamin E and the appearance of fatty acid hydroperoxides occurs only after the oxidation of ubiquinol [19]. Moreover, treatment per os with CoQ_{10} in normal subjects induces an increase of ubiquinol in plasma and lipoproteins and an augmented resistance to LDL peroxidation [20]. Based on the above-mentioned biochemical features, different trials have highlighted the potential therapeutic usefulness of CoQ_{10} in the treatment of various diseases (cardiovascular, neurologic, muscular, immunologic, diabetic endotheliopathy).

There is a relationship between low concentrations of CoQ_{10} and coronary pathologies, even if this correlation is not so strong to be considered a casual relation [21]. The ubiquinol/ubiquinone ratio is considered an oxidative stress marker in coronary pathologies, and the LDL/CoQ_{10} ratio is an index of coronary risk [22].

Both the bioenergetic and the antioxidant roles of CoQ_{10} suggested a possible involvement in male fertility: it is known that a large amount of mitochondria are present in spermatozoa, in which motility requires a high energy expenditure [23]; moreover, as shown in the previous paragraph, the protection of membrane from oxidative stress could play a role in preserving sperm integrity; finally, the biosynthetic machinery for CoQ_{10} is present at remarkably high levels in rat testis [24].

Original studies on CoQ_{10} administration in unselected population of infertile patients showed an amelioration of the results in membrane integrity tests (swelling test) [25] and an improvement in seminal parameters in men with sperm pathology [26]; however, these studies did not report the endogenous CoQ_{10} levels in such patients.

The first analytical data on CoQ_{10} levels in seminal fluid were produced by our group [27], in a sample including 60 subjects (21 patients with normozoospermia, 15 patients with azoospermia or oligozoospermia, 2 patients with germ-free genital tract inflammation and 22 subjects with varicocele, 7 of whom presented oligoazoospermia). We showed that CoQ_{10} was assayable in total seminal fluid and in seminal plasma; its levels showed a good correlation with sperm count ($R = 0.504$, $p < 0.0005$) and motility ($R = 0.261$, $p < 0.05$), except in the population of varicocele patients, in whom the correlation with sperm count was maintained ($R = 0.666$, $p < 0.0005$) but that with sperm motility was completely lacking ($R = 0.008$, N.S.). Moreover, in the varicocele patients, a significantly higher proportion of total CoQ_{10} was present in seminal plasma when compared with normal subjects or other infertile patients without varicocele (the ratio plasma/seminal fluid Q_{10} was $69 \pm 7.1\%$ vs $41.2 \pm 5.6\%$, $p < 0.01$, respectively).

These data were also confirmed in larger series of patients [12, 28, 29].

Since CoQ_{10} in seminal plasma did not correlate with LDH levels, we concluded that the amounts of CoQ_{10} in plasma were not due to spermatozoa damage and to a consequent release of ubiquinone from the cells. We hypothesized that seminal plasma CoQ_{10} levels reflect an interchange between cellular and extracellular compartments, with a pathophysiological meaning similar to serum ubiquinone values [30, 31]; a relative deficiency or utilization of CoQ in sperm cell was therefore supposed to be present in varicocele condition [32]. We also hypothesized that the significantly higher percent of CoQ_{10} in plasma found in VAR patients could reflect an altered compartment distribution: the intracellular, bioenergetic use of CoQ_{10} could be defective in these patients, and its shift towards the plasma compartment could be considered of relevance regarding a possible antioxidant role in that environment.

Finally, we studied VAR patients, after surgical repair; only a partial reversion was observed, since the ratio plasma-to-total CoQ_{10} decreased, but the correlation between total CoQ_{10} and motility was not restored; on the contrary, the peculiar correlation between cellular CoQ_{10} and motility was no more detectable in post-operative VAR patients [33]. Vitamin E has also been demonstrated to be positively affected by surgical VAR repair [34].

In order to explore physiological hormone control of seminal CoQ_{10}, since FSH seemed to be involved in regulation of total antioxidant capacity of seminal plasma [35], another trial was conducted in 13 oligoasthenozoospermic subjects, studied before and after 3 months of rh-FSH (225 UI/week) [36]. Following FSH treatment, CoQ_{10} showed an increase, although not significant, in seminal plasma levels (0.035 ± 0.010 µg/ml vs 0.028 ± 0.005). A possible role of systemic thyroid hormones has been also hypothesized, since seminal TAC inversely correlated with free T3 in infertile patients [37].

All these referred studies consider total CoQ_{10} levels, irrespective of its redox status. The first report on the assay of reduced and oxidized forms of ubiquinone was performed in our laboratory [38]. We showed a significant correlation between the reduced form (ubiquinol) and sperm count in seminal plasma, an inverse correlation between ubiquinol and hydroperoxide levels both in seminal plasma and seminal fluid, a strong correlation—using multiple regression analysis—between sperm count, motility and ubiquinol-10 content in seminal fluid, and, finally, an inverse correlation between ubiquinol/ubiquinone ratio and the percentage of abnormal forms. These results indicate an important role of ubiquinol-10 in inhibiting hydroperoxide formation. We also found a lower ubiquinol/ubiquinone ratio in sperm cells from idiopathic asthenozoospermic (IDA) patients and in seminal plasma from IDA and varicocele-associated asthenozoospermic (VARA) patients compared to controls [39]. The important conclusion was that the QH_2/Q_{OX} ratio may be an index of oxidative stress and its reduction a risk factor for semen quality. Sperm cells characterized by low motility and abnormal morphology, equipped with low CoQ_{10} content, could be less capable in counteracting oxidative stress, which could lead to a reduced QH_2/Q_{OX} ratio.

Concerning the therapeutic role of CoQ_{10}, it should be mentioned that CoQ_{10} was first introduced as an ethical drug for heart failure patients but its use has grown since its recognition as a food supplement aimed at improving cellular bioenergetics, counteracting oxidative stress and slowing down some age-related pathologies. Numerous clinical studies have shown its efficacy as an adjunctive therapy in cardiovascular and neurodegenerative diseases and in mitochondrial myopathies [40]. The above-mentioned studies constitute a rationale that eventually led us to treat infertile subjects with exogenous CoQ_{10}.

Lewin and Lavon [41] originally reported the effect of CoQ_{10} on sperm motility in vitro: a significant increase in motility was observed in sperm obtained from asthenozoospermic men, incubated with exogenous CoQ_{10}, while no significant variation was reported in the motility of sperm cells from normal subjects. The same study also reports the effect of exogenous CoQ_{10} in vivo, in a group of patients with low fertilization rates, after in vitro fertilization with intracytoplasmatic sperm injection for male factor infertility: no significant changes were reported in most sperm parameters, but a significant improvement was noticed in fertilization rates after a treatment with 60 mg/day for a mean of 103 days.

CoQ$_{10}$ is one of the compounds contributing to the total antioxidant buffer capacity of semen, and its decrease could lead to an impairment of the system in counteracting oxidative stress [11]; exogenous administration of CoQ$_{10}$ could increase its content in semen and improve sperm cell function. In different clinical models, such as hypogonadism and hypoadrenalism, a significant correlation has been discovered between CoQ$_{10}$ and total antioxidant capacity, measured as latency phase in the formation of radicals using the system H_2O_2-metmyoglobin/ABTS system [42, 43].

To investigate a potential therapeutic role, we administered CoQ$_{10}$ to a group of 22 idiopathic asthenozoospermic infertile patients [44], classified according to the WHO 1999 criteria [45] as having <50% forward motile forms at two distinct sperm analyses and normal sperm morphology >30%.

Patients were given CoQ$_{10}$ (Pharma Nord, Denmark), 200 mg/day divided into two doses, for 6 months. Semen analysis, including computer-assisted sperm analysis and motility (C.A.S.A.), CoQ$_{10}$ and phosphatidylcholine assays, was performed at baseline and after 6 months of therapy. A semen analysis was further performed after 6 months from interruption of therapy (washout). CoQ$_{10}$ levels were assayed in sperm cells and seminal plasma using a Beckman Gold HPLC System HPLC (Beckman Instruments, San Ramon, CA, USA) equipped with an electrochemical detector (EC, ESA 5100, Bedford, MA, USA) [39]. PC was essentially determined according to Frei et al. [46].

An increase of CoQ$_{10}$ was found in seminal plasma after treatment, the mean value rising significantly from 42.0±5.1 at baseline to 127.1±1.9 ng/ml after 6 months of exogenous CoQ$_{10}$ administration ($p < 0.005$). A significant increase of CoQ$_{10}$ content was also detected in sperm cells (from 3.1±0.4 to 6.5±0.3 ng/10^6 cells; $p < 0.05$). Similarly, PC levels increased significantly both in seminal plasma and sperm cells after treatment (from 1.49±0.50 to 5.84±1.15 µM, $p < 0.05$; and from 6.83±0.98 to 9.67±1.23 nmoles/10^6 cells, $p < 0.05$, respectively).

Regarding semen, a significant difference was found in forward (class a + b) motility of sperm cells after 6 months of CoQ$_{10}$ dietary implementation (from 9.13 ± 2.50 to 16.34 ± 3.43%, $p < 0.05$). The improvement of motility was also confirmed by means of computer-assisted determination of kinetic parameters. A significant increase of VCL (from 26.31 ± 1.50 to 46.43 ± 2.28 µm/s, $p < 0.05$) and VSL (from 15.20 ± 1.30 to 20.40 ± 2.17 µm/s, $p < 0.05$) was found after treatment. No significant differences were found in sperm cell concentration and morphology.

Although a direct correlation was not found (data not shown), a positive dependence (using the Cramer's index of association) was evident among the relative variations, baseline and after treatment, of seminal plasma or intracellular CoQ$_{10}$ content and of C.A.S.A. (VCL and VSL) kinetic parameters (Cramer's $V = 0.4637$; 0.3818; 0.3467; 0.5148, respectively) [44].

A significant reduction in sperm forward motility was reported after 6 months of washout (from 16.34 ± 3.43 to 9.50 ± 2.28%, $p < 0.001$), while no significant differences were found in sperm cell concentration and morphology.

In order to find out whether different responses were age related, the relative variations (before and after treatment) of CoQ$_{10}$ and PC content in seminal plasma and sperm cells, as well as forward motility, were analysed, but no correlation was found (data not shown).

Wives of 3 out of 22 patients (13.6%) achieved spontaneous pregnancy within 3 months from the discontinuation of therapy (2.4% pregnancy rate per cycle).

This study indicates a significant improvement of kinetic features of sperm cells after 6 months of administration of CoQ_{10}, both on the basis of manual and computer-assisted evaluation. Moreover, these results constitute the first demonstration that exogenous administration of CoQ_{10} increases its levels in seminal plasma and in spermatozoa.

The increment was important, especially in seminal plasma where post-treatment levels were three times higher than basal ones. Similar increases of CoQ_{10} concentration (two–three times higher than baseline value) are commonly found in blood plasma after chronic administration of the quinone [47]. As CoQ_{10} is a highly lipophilic molecule, we could reasonably hypothesize its diffusion through the phospholipid bilayer of cellular membranes, but we presently do not know whether transport from blood plasma to testicular and accessory male genital glands is passive or involves an active mechanism.

Statistical analysis did not reveal any significant functional relationship among the therapy-induced variations of CoQ_{10} and kinetic parameters of spermatozoa, probably due to the low number of samples. Nevertheless, the good degree of association among these variables, according to Cramer's V index of association, supports the hypothesis of a pathogenetic role of CoQ_{10} in asthenozoospermia, according to previously reported data [39]. Improvement of the spontaneous pregnancy rate also suggests that this therapeutic approach is beneficial.

These results were confirmed by a double-blind, placebo-controlled clinical trial, also from our group [48]. The selected patients underwent a double-blind therapy with CoQ_{10} (Q-absorb soft gels, Jarrow Formulas LA, USA), containing 100 mg of CoQ_{10}, lecithin and medium-chain glycerides Placebo had the same composition but the soft gels did not contain any CoQ_{10}. All patients were given a total of two soft capsules in two separate daily administrations, with meals. The CoQ_{10} dose was similar to that used in our previous open trial on male infertility.

The study design was 1-month run-in, 6 months of therapy (30 patients) or placebo (30 patients), and further 3 months' follow-up (controls at months T−1, T0, T + 3, T + 6, T + 9).

CoQ_{10} levels increased in seminal plasma after treatment, the mean value rising significantly from 61.29 ± 20.24 at baseline to 99.39 ± 31.51 ng/ml after 6 months of exogenous CoQ_{10} administration ($p < 0.0001$). A significant increase of CoQ_{10} content was also detected in sperm cells (from 2.44 ± 0.97 to 4.57 ± 2.46 ng/10^6 cells, $p < 0.0001$). Similarly, QH_2 levels increased significantly both in seminal plasma and sperm cells after treatment (from 31.54 ± 10.05 to 51.93 ± 16.44 ng/ml, $p < 0.0001$; and from 0.95 ± 0.46 to 1.84 ± 1.03 ng/10^6 cells, $p < 0.0001$, respectively). No statistically significant modifications were found in the placebo group.

A significant improvement of sperm cell total motility (from 33.14 ± 7.12 to $39.41 \pm 6.80\%$, $p < 0.0001$) and forward motility (from 10.43 ± 3.52 to

15.11 ± 7.34%, $p = 0.0003$) was observed in the treated group after 6 months (T + 6) of CoQ_{10} administration. The improvement of sperm cell kinetic parameters was also confirmed after computer-assisted analysis, with an increase both in VCL (from 27.99 ± 5.32 to 33.18 ± 4.22 µm/s, $p < 0.0001$) and VSL (from 10.76 ± 2.63 to 13.13 ± 2.86 µm/s $p < 0.0001$) after treatment. No statistically significant modifications in kinetic parameters were found in placebo group.

A significant inverse correlation between baseline (T0) and T + 6 relative variations of seminal plasma or intracellular CoQ_{10} or QII_2 content and kinetic parame ters was also found in treated group. In fact, patients with lower baseline value of motility and levels of CoQ_{10} had a statistically significant higher probability to be responders to the treatment.

After washout (T + 9), sperm cell kinetic features (total and forward motility, VSL) resulted significantly reduced in treatment groups when compared with month T + 6.

Nine spontaneous pregnancies were achieved during the observation period. After opening the randomization list, it was found that six of the patients who had impregnated their female partner had undergone CoQ_{10} therapy (three of them after 4 months, one after 5 months and one after 6 months of treatment). Three out of the nine pregnancies occurred in partners of patients undergoing placebo treatment, respectively, one after 2 months of therapy and the other two after 3 months of washout. Recently, a positive effect of CoQ_{10} treatment on sperm motility was also confirmed in a study by Safarinejad et al. [49].

Carnitine

L-Carnitine (LC) plays a central role in cellular energetic metabolism, being the shuttle of the activated long-chain fatty acids (acyl-CoA) into the mitochondria, where the beta-oxidation takes place [50–52]. An important role in sperm cell metabolism is strongly suggested by the high levels found in epididymal fluid due to an active secretory mechanism [53], and there are evidences that the initiation of the sperm motility is related to an increase of L-carnitine in the epididymal lumen and L-acetyl-carnitine (LAC) in sperm cells [54–56].

We have performed a 6-month double-blind randomized placebo-controlled trial using LC or LAC or combined LC and LAC treatment in infertile males affected by idiopathic asthenozoospermia [57]. The evaluation of the effectiveness of these treatments in improving semen kinetic parameters and the variation of TOSC in semen after treatment were the end points of the study. Sixty patients (mean age, 30 years; range, 24–38 years) affected by idiopathic asthenozoospermia have been enrolled in the study. The patients were selected at the Andrology Unit of Endocrinology, Umberto I Hospital, Polytechnic University of Marche, Ancona (Italy). All subjects underwent medical screening, including history and clinical examination, and presented a clinical history of primary infertility >2 years. Testicular volume was evaluated in each patient using Prader's orchidometer.

To accomplish a complete diagnosis, the following investigations were also performed: semen analysis; Mar-test (SperMar test, CGA, Florence, Italy) for anti-spermatozoa antibodies (Ab); sperm culture and urethral specimens collection for *Chlamydia* and *Mycoplasma ureoliticum* detection; FSH, LH, testosterone (T), estradiol (E2) and prolactin (PRL) assays, using commercial radioimmunoassay kits; testicular, prostatic and seminal vesicle ultrasonography and echo-colour Doppler of venous spermatic plexus, for anatomical abnormalities and varicocele detection. No female-related factor was apparently involved in sterility, since all partners (mean age, 26 years; range, 21–32 years) were ovulating regularly, as formally proven by biphasic basal body temperature and luteal phase progesterone levels; no anatomical abnormalities were detected after ultrasound ovary and uterus evaluation; no abnormal Fallopian tube anatomy was detected after hysterosalpingography.

The selected patients were submitted to a double-blind therapy of LC (10 ml phials containing 3 g/day orally of Carnitene—Sigma Tau, Italy, n. 15 patients), LAC (tablets containing 3 g/day orally of Zibren—Sigma Tau, n. 15 patients), a combination of LC (10 ml phials containing 2 g/day orally of Carnitene) and LAC (tablets containing 1 g/day orally of Zibren) (n. 15 patients) or a seemingly identical placebo (each 10 ml placebo phial contains malic acid, sodium benzoate, sodium saccharinate dihydrate, anhydrous sodium citrate, pineapple flavouring, demineralised water; each placebo tablet contains a core with 1-hydro lactose, magnesium stearate, polyvinylpyrrolidone, cornstarch and a coating with cellulose acetophtalate, dimethicone, ethyl phthalate, Sigma Tau, Pomezia, Rome, Italy). All patients assumed a total of one phial and two tablets three times a day. The study design was 1-month run-in, 6 months of therapy (45 patients) or placebo (15 patients), and further 3 months' follow-up (controls at months T−1, T0, T + 3, T + 6, T + 9). Monthly evaluation of two semen samples before the beginning of treatment (T−1, T0) was carried out to test semen parameter stability in each patient, as recommended by the WHO [45]. At various time points, the following analyses were carried out: semen analysis at months T−1, T0, T + 3, T + 6, T + 9, including computer-assisted sperm analysis (C.A.S.A.) at months T0, T + 3, T + 6, T + 9 to evaluate modifications in semen parameters and TOSC of the seminal fluid towards different ROS at months T0 and T + 6 to evaluate any variations during therapy [9, 10].

Table 17.1 reports mean and standard deviation of sperm variables at each time; the percentage variations with respect to baseline are reported in Table 17.2. The percentage variations of total and forward sperm motility in all groups at each time are shown in Figs. 17.1 and 17.2. The univariate analysis of variance performed on variables (percentage variations with respect to T−1 or T0) for the homogeneity at baseline (T0 or T + 3) showed that there were no significant differences between groups regarding motility (total and forward), sperm concentration, atypical sperm cells, semen volume and VCL. On the contrary, the percentage variation of VSL between T0 and T + 3 was significantly higher in the subgroup C (LC–LAC combined) than in the placebo group (44.86 ± 76.24 vs -4.59 ± 37.05; $F = 3.077$; $p = 0.035$)[1]; in other words, patients treated with the combination of the two molecules improved significantly during the first 3-month period of the administration.

Table 17.1 Descriptive statistics of sperm variables at each time: mean ± standard deviation

Treatment	Month T−1	Month T0	Month T + 3	Month T + 6	Month T + 9
Sperm total motility					
Placebo	43.73 ± 10.06	43.93 ± 10.26	44.60 ± 7.68	43.40 ± 9.85	42.73 ± 10.02
LC	54.33 ± 8.59	51.67 ± 11.08	59.93 ± 8.04	64.53 ± 8.41	54.27 ± 8.96
LAC	45.07 ± 12.01	43.87 ± 11.36	56.47 ± 11.56	60.43 ± 10.46	50.57 ± 5.71
LC and LAC	46.73 ± 10.10	44.53 ± 11.84	55.13 ± 10.15	61.07 ± 9.07	49.00 ± 7.80
Sperm forward motility					
Placebo	24.33 ± 7.93	24.13 ± 7.74	22.33 ± 7.76	24.00 ± 8.50	23.20 ± 8.96
LC	33.47 ± 6.55	31.20 ± 7.43	38.93 ± 7.09	43.80 ± 7.12	34.00 ± 7.02
LAC	27.00 ± 10.87	25.53 ± 10.43	34.93 ± 9.24	37.50 ± 9.20	30.21 ± 7.84
LC and LAC	25.47 ± 8.90	24.60 ± 9.40	33.87 ± 8.37	38.13 ± 8.23	28.47 ± 8.27
Sperm concentration					
Placebo	35.27 ± 21.98	29.53 ± 10.07	31.40 ± 12.85	33.73 ± 14.36	30.13 ± 9.30
LC	35.47 ± 9.21	39.00 ± 10.39	41.00 ± 17.34	45.53 ± 21.42	39.40 ± 13.93
LAC	27.07 ± 6.47	30.40 ± 10.80	39.33 ± 18.05	39.57 ± 19.99	31.21 ± 8.60
LC and LAC	29.93 ± 10.57	29.40 ± 9.39	36.93 ± 19.71	37.40 ± 16.42	33.27 ± 13.62
Atypical sperm cells					
Placebo	66.40 ± 6.50	68.20 ± 5.86	67.40 ± 6.42	67.27 ± 6.71	67.53 ± 7.42
LC	63.13 ± 5.04	62.87 ± 4.69	58.47 ± 6.20	54.87 ± 7.27	58.07 ± 11.82
LAC	65.93 ± 8.19	67.13 ± 7.06	61.73 ± 6.82	58.93 ± 5.62	60.93 ± 10.12
LC and LAC	65.40 ± 6.22	67.13 ± 6.01	61.73 ± 5.86	59.60 ± 5.82	61.53 ± 8.84
Semen volume					
Placebo	2.97 ± 1.36	3.01 ± 0.83	3.08 ± 0.85	2.75 ± 0.68	2.82 ± 0.45
LC	2.96 ± 0.74	3.12 ± 1.04	3.10 ± 0.68	3.18 ± 0.93	3.03 ± 0.83
LAC	2.89 ± 0.85	2.59 ± 0.63	2.71 ± 0.62	3.03 ± 0.66	2.76 ± 0.51
LC and LAC	3.05 ± 0.94	2.87 ± 0.88	2.75 ± 0.80	2.69 ± 0.78	2.50 ± 0.41
Curvilinear velocity					
Placebo		41.67 ± 14.14	39.67 ± 14.07	42.87 ± 6.83	46.33 ± 11.96
LC		41.73 ± 13.47	47.73 ± 13.43	57.13 ± 13.95	41.67 ± 6.28
LAC		39.73 ± 12.57	45.87 ± 11.33	51.79 ± 6.17	44.79 ± 8.19
LC and LAC		43.00 ± 12.02	44.93 ± 15.72	51.40 ± 13.71	42.53 ± 7.78
Straight progressive velocity					
Placebo		24.47 ± 15.19	21.80 ± 12.23	15.87 ± 2.47	17.67 ± 2.58
LC		20.00 ± 7.87	21.13 ± 6.92	21.47 ± 3.52	16.80 ± 2.11
LAC		23.27 ± 16.28	18.60 ± 5.78	20.36 ± 3.41	16.36 ± 2.41
LC and LAC		18.60 ± 6.93	25.67 ± 12.75	22.53 ± 10.26	16.73 ± 2.89

A significant improvement in total sperm motility was found in patients to whom LAC was administered, either alone or combined with LC (from −3.3 ± 17.4 at T0 to 37.7 ± 27.8 at T + 6; $F = 11.19$; $p = 0.001$)[2] (Fig. 17.3). The analysis of forward sperm cell motility showed the same results (from −2.9 ± 26 at T0 to 63 ± 66.8 at T + 6; $F = 12.68$; $p = 0.001$)[2] (Fig. 17.4). An improvement of forward motility was found when combined LC–LAC was compared with LC or LAC therapy alone, although the variations of kinetics sperm parameters were not significantly (see Fig. 17.2). No significant modifications were found in placebo group. In all carnitine

Table 17.2 Percentage variations with respect to baseline for sperm variables at each time: mean ± standard deviation

Treatment	Month T0	Month T + 3	Month T + 6	Month T + 9
Sperm total motility[a]				
Placebo	1.30 ± 13.52	4.15 ± 16.26	0.52 ± 17.43	−1.22 ± 17.46
LC	−5.32 ± 9.91	11.01 ± 8.46	19.90 ± 12.74	0.31 ± 9.65
LAC	−1.31 ± 23.07	30.83 ± 33.99	41.25 ± 29.98	19.78 ± 28.51
LC and LAC	−5.16 ± 10.18	19.59 ± 16.63	34.46 ± 26.20	6.75 ± 14.77
Sperm forward motility[a]				
Placebo	−0.30 ± 9.81	−8.31 ± 13.73	−0.96 ± 18.99	−4.38 ± 21.71
LC	−5.92 ± 16.21	18.01 ± 15.73	33.08 ± 17.29	2.67 ± 14.40
LAC	−4.09 ± 27.85	41.85 ± 42.43	56.84 ± 54.23	22.32 ± 29.03
LC and LAC	−1.86 ± 25.16	43.58 ± 46.86	68.70 ± 78.18	17.73 ± 28.61
Sperm concentration[a]				
Placebo	−4.31 ± 27.75	−3.17 ± 20.06	6.98 ± 36.97	−1.51 ± 32.69
LC	11.14 ± 19.58	17.18 ± 45.99	24.50 ± 35.55	12.06 ± 30.16
LAC	6.95 ± 22.06	46.55 ± 55.80	42.88 ± 50.80	15.90 ± 32.10
LC and LAC	1.26 ± 19.66	24.34 ± 41.83	29.78 ± 41.53	15.18 ± 42.83
LC and LAC	1.26 ± 19.66	24.34 ± 41.83	29.78 ± 41.53	15.18 ± 42.83
Atypical sperm cells[a]				
Placebo	2.92 ± 4.68	1.70 ± 5.97	1.49 ± 6.50	1.86 ± 7.46
LC	−0.28 ± 4.86	−7.42 ± 6.23	−13.24 ± 7.66	−7.51 ± 19.46
LAC	2.20 ± 5.48	−6.00 ± 6.90	−10.24 ± 5.56	−6.32 ± 18.07
LC and LAC	2.90 ± 6.66	−5.27 ± 8.13	−8.35 ± 10.41	−5.36 ± 14.29
Semen volume[a]				
Placebo	11.76 ± 31.35	19.75 ± 62.98	4.85 ± 40.95	12.03 ± 51.56
LC	3.63 ± 12.23	6.58 ± 16.51	11.26 ± 34.40	4.91 ± 25.76
LAC	−5.20 ± 22.97	0.00 ± 27.80	11.63 ± 39.62	2.09 ± 32.97
LC and LAC	−4.94 ± 17.07	−8.27 ± 16.62	−5.38 ± 38.63	−13.74 ± 19.09
Curvilinear velocity[b]				
Placebo		2.20 ± 54.71	20.16 ± 67.30	31.24 ± 79.69
LC		26.00 ± 67.68	64.99 ± 104.59	20.06 ± 74.02
LAC		30.95 ± 66.09	53.31 ± 71.53	31.23 ± 62.97
LC and LAC		8.27 ± 33.87	29.05 ± 51.98	8.44 ± 44.17
Straight progressive velocity[b]				
Placebo		−4.59 ± 37.05	−22.08 ± 27.78	−15.04 ± 25.40
LC		11.08 ± 22.75	17.07 ± 32.81	−6.45 ± 29.37
LAC		2.05 ± 43.11	15.57 ± 46.31	−6.78 ± 38.88
LC and LAC		44.86 ± 76.24	33.26 ± 70.62	−3.15 ± 26.25

[a]Percentage variations with respect to month T−1
[b]Percentage variations with respect to month T0

therapy groups, a significant dependence of the total and forward motility variations on the baseline values was found, and patients with lower baseline values of motility had a significantly higher probability to be responders to the treatment (Table 17.3). After washout (T + 9), sperm cell kinetic features (total and forward motility, VSL) resulted significantly reduced in treatment groups when compared with month T + 6. In the group to whom LAC was administered (alone or combined),

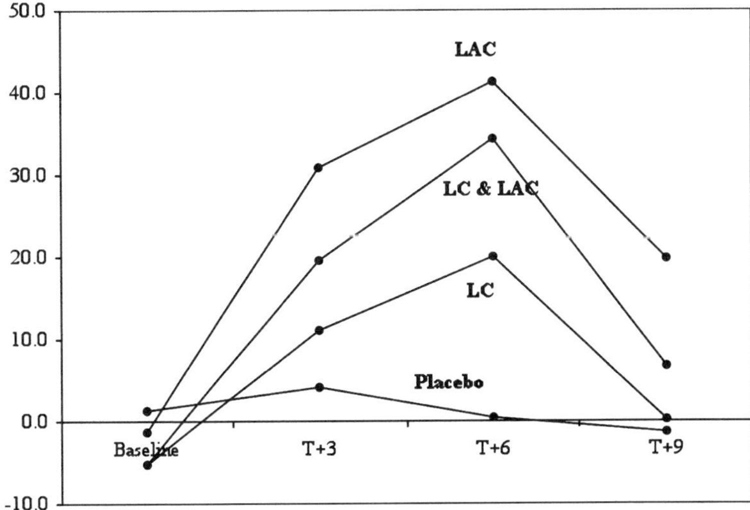

Fig. 17.1 Total sperm motility at each time in the four treatment groups: percentage variations with respect to T−1

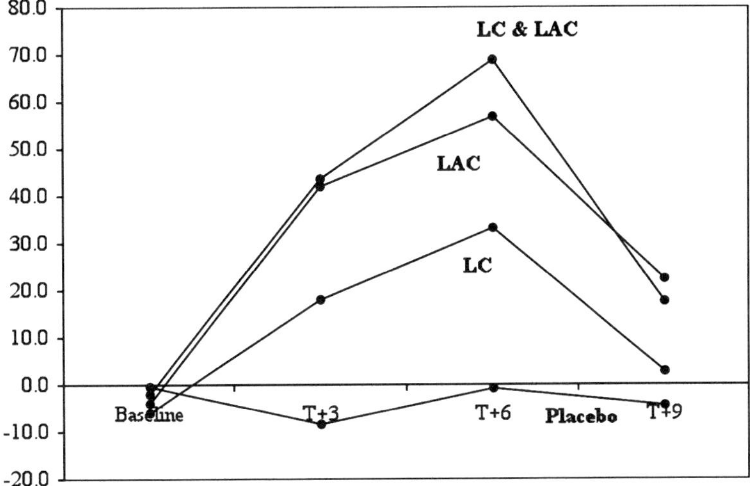

Fig. 17.2 Forward sperm motility at each time in the four treatment groups: percentage variations with respect to T−1

the sperm concentration varied significantly during the treatment period (from 6.95 ± 22.06 at T0 to 42.88 ± 50.80 at T + 6; $F = 3.611$; $p = 0.015$)[2]. A significant reduction of atypical sperm cells was also evident between T0 and T + 6; in particular, the improvement was significantly different in the LC. No significantly different variations in semen volume and in VCL were detected in the studied patients.

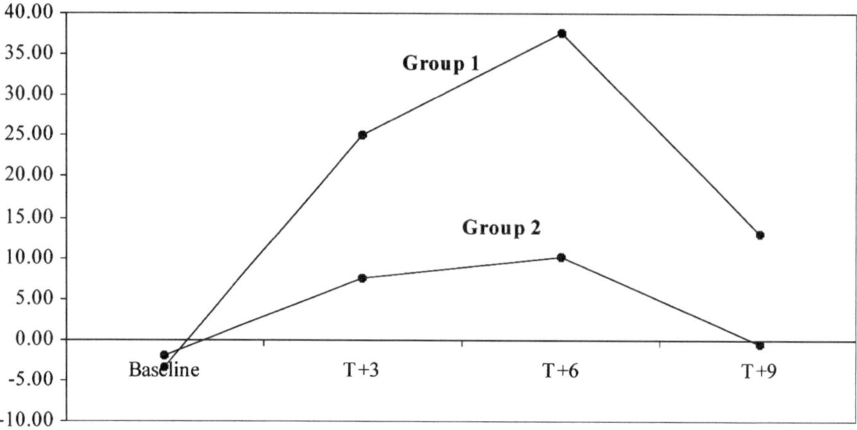

Fig. 17.3 Total sperm motility at each time: percentage variations with respect to T–1 (Time: $p < 0.001$; LACTX: $p = 0.001$). Group 1: patients treated with LAC, alone or combined. Group 2: patients treated with LC or placebo

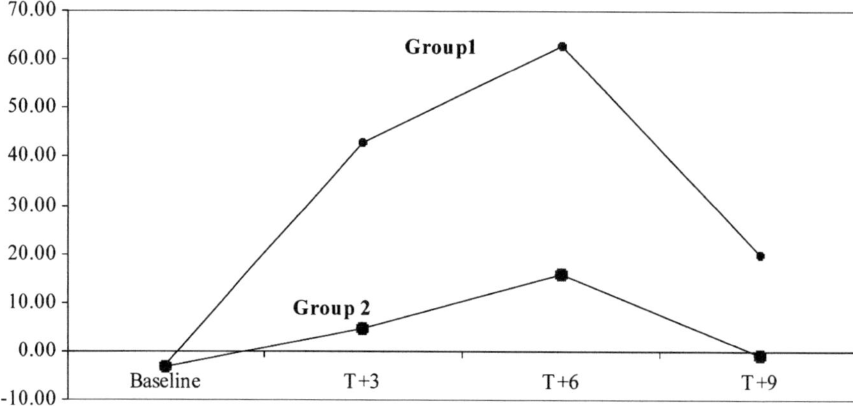

Fig. 17.4 Forward sperm motility at each time: percentage variations with respect to T–1 (Time: $p < 0.001$; LACTX: $p = 0.001$). Group 1: patients treated with LAC, alone or combined. Group 2: patients treated with LC or placebo

Table 17.4 reports mean and standard deviation of TOSC values at each time and the percentage variations with respect to baseline.

TOSC assay of the seminal fluid towards different ROS showed a significant improvement for both hydroxyl and peroxyl radicals in the treatment groups (Table 17.4), while no significant modifications were found in placebo group. The increase in TOSC values, between T0 and T + 6, was positively correlated with the improvement of kinetic features, i.e. with total motility, forward motility for both the radicals, and with VCL or VSL respectively for hydroxyl radicals and peroxyl radicals (Tables 17.5 and 17.6). Moreover, forward motility variation was found depending on the baseline values of TOSC (hydroxyl radicals) (see Table 17.3) [11].

Table 17.3 Analysis of responders: logistic models

	Estimate	Pr(>|z|)	Exp(Estimate)
Dependent variable: variation of total motility during treatment period			
Sperm total motility (T0)	−0.434	0.016	0.648
Dependent variable: variation of forward motility during treatment period			
Sperm forward motility (T0)	−0.235	0.039	0.790
TOSC hydroxyl (T0)	0.0002	0.030	1.0002

Table 17.4 Descriptive statistics of TOSC variables at each time; absolute and percentage variations: mean ± standard deviation

Treatment	Month T0	Month T + 6	Absolute variations	Percentage variations
TOSC (hydroxyl)				
PLAC	31,276.67 ± 5,467.22	28,931 ± 5,351.48	−2,345.53 ± 3,516.51	−7.12 ± 10.43
LC	26,301 ± 6,127.76	30,636.20 ± 5,646.47	4,334.67 ± 3,454.27	18.52 ± 15.49
LAC	27,566 ± 6,139.02	31,645.79 ± 4,680.91	4,382.64 ± 3,883.61	20.67 ± 27.19
LC*LAC	27,207 ± 6,061.33	31,712.67 ± 5,933.07	4,505.07 ± 2,730.59	18.38 ± 12.72
TOSC (peroxyl)				
PLAC	24,879.20 ± 4,865.76	24,358.20 ± 5,466.47	−521.00 ± 1,548.79	−2.43 ± 6.79
LC	26,035.60 ± 4,098.60	31,003.00 ± 5,841.52	4,967.40 ± 3,900.30	19.48 ± 15.86
LAC	22,775.73 ± 5,675.95	24,924.07 ± 6,344.44	2,474.00 ± 3,487.15	12.32 ± 21.72
LC*LAC	25,899.00 ± 5,147.45	29,889.13 ± 5,345.76	3,990.13 ± 2,533.32	16.53 ± 12.64

Table 17.5 Correlations between the increase of TOSC values (hydroxyl radicals) and the variation of sperm variables

		Total motility
TOSC	Pearson correlation	0.391
	Sig. (two-tailed)	0.002
		Forward motility
TOSC	Pearson correlation	0.455
	Sig. (two-tailed)	< 0.001
		Curvilinear velocity (VCL)
TOSC	Pearson correlation	0.357
	Sig. (two-tailed)	0.006

Table 17.6 Correlations between the increase of TOSC values (peroxyl radicals) and the variation of sperm variables

		Total motility
TOSC	Pearson correlation	0.410
	Sig. (two-tailed)	0.001
		Forward motility
TOSC	Pearson correlation	0.439
	Sig. (two-tailed)	0.001
		Straight progressive velocity (VSL)
TOSC	Pearson correlation	0.316
	Sig. (two-tailed)	0.015

Several controlled and uncontrolled studies support at present a potential positive effect of therapy with LC and its acyl derivatives in selected forms of oligo-astheno-teratozoospermia [58–61]. In particular, a very recent controlled study reports the efficacy of LC and LAC combined treatment in improving sperm motility, especially in patients with lower baseline levels [62]. The main rationale is based on the central role of carnitine in energetic metabolism and its accumulation in epididymal fluid and spermatozoa, both as free and acetylated LC [53]. Although some evidences suggest a secondary role of carnitine as antioxidant [63], its effective role and the mechanism of action still remain an interesting open question.

Key Issues

Endogenous CoQ_{10} is significantly related to sperm count and motility, as one could expect considering its important cellular compartmentalization; furthermore, it appears to be one of the most important antioxidants in seminal plasma. Its presence in this compartment does not depend on sperm lysis, as it does not correlate with LDH [27]; moreover, its distribution between intra- and extracellular compartments seems to be an active process, which is profoundly disturbed in VAR patients [28]. CoQ_{10} levels in seminal plasma do correlate with sperm motility. It can be hypothesized that, in certain circumstances, the increased oxidative stress in sperm cells can somehow over-consume CoQ_{10} to the detriment of its bioenergetic role.

Improved sperm motility upon exogenous CoQ_{10} administration could be explained on the basis of the well-known involvement of CoQ_{10} in mitochondrial bioenergetics and of its widely recognized antioxidant properties. Regarding the first point, it is well known that mitochondrial concentration of CoQ_{10} in mammals is close to its K_M, as far as NADH oxidation is concerned, and therefore is not kinetically saturated [64]. In these conditions, one might reasonably hypothesize that a small increase in mitochondrial CoQ_{10} leads to a relevant rise in respiratory velocity. The resulting improvement of oxidative phosphorylation might well affect sperm cells. Since low PC levels in semen were found to be related to a reduction of the phospholipid pool and to low antioxidant capacity [65], the increased PC content in semen after treatment might reasonably involve the restoration of scavenger equilibrium. Another possible reason for this finding is that increased levels of CoQ_{10} also need an appropriate, highly concentration of a lipid carrier.

Thus, the administration of CoQ_{10} may play a positive role in the treatment of asthenozoospermia, probably related not only to its function in mitochondrial respiratory chain but also to its antioxidant properties. The increased concentration of CoQ_{10} in seminal plasma and sperm cells, the improvement of semen kinetic features after treatment, and the evidence of a direct correlation between CoQ_{10} concentrations and sperm motility strongly support a cause/effect relationship.

As far as carnitine is concerned, taken together, the data available in literature seem to suggest that long-term carnitine therapy is effective in improving sperm function and fertilization capacity. Following the end points of our study, we can conclude that (1) LC and LAC administration is effective in increasing sperm motility in patients affected by idiopathic asthenozoospermia, especially in the ones with lower baseline values and lower baseline TOSC; combined LC–LAC therapy improves sperm cell forward motility (not significantly) and VSL (significantly) when compared with LC or LAC therapy alone and (2) the administration of both LAC and LC improves the total scavenging capacity of the seminal fluid in the same population.

A deeper insight into these molecular mechanisms could lead to a greater knowledge of the so-called unexplained infertility.

References

1. Alvarez JG, Storey B. Spontaneous lipid peroxidation in rabbit epididymal spermatozoa: its effect on sperm motility. Biol Reprod. 1982;27:1102–8.
2. Aitken RJ, Clarkson JS. Cellular basis of defective sperm function and its association with the genesis of reactive oxygen species by human spermatozoa. J Reprod Fertil. 1987;81:459–69.
3. Aitken RJ, Clarkson JS, Fishel S. Generation of reactive oxygen species, lipid peroxidation and human sperm function. Biol Reprod. 1989;40:183–97.
4. Rao B, Soufir JC, Martin M, David G. Lipid peroxidation in human spermatozoa as related to midpiece abnormalities and motility. Gamete Res. 1989;24:127–34.
5. Suleiman SA, Ali ME, Zaki ZM, El-Malik EM, Nasr MA. Lipid peroxidation and human sperm motility: protective role of vitamin E. J Androl. 1996;17:530–7.
6. Aitken RJ, Krausz C. Oxidative stress, DNA damage and the Y chromosome. Reproduction. 2001;122:497–506.
7. Aitken RJ, Baker MA. Reactive oxygen species generation by human spermatozoa: a continuing enigma. Int J Androl. 2002;25:191–4.
8. Balercia G, Moretti S, Vignini A, Magagnini M, Mantero F, Boscaro M, et al. Role of nitric oxide concentration on human sperm motility. J Androl. 2004;25:245–9.
9. Winston GW, Regoli F, Dugas Jr AJ, Fong JH, Blanchard KA. A rapid chromatographic assay for determining oxyradical scavenging capacity of antioxidants and biological fluids. Free Radic Biol Med. 1998;24:480–93.
10. Regoli F, Winston GW. Quantification of total antioxidant scavenging capacity (TOSC) of antioxidants for peroxynitrite, peroxyl radicals and hydroxyl radicals. Toxicol Appl Pharmacol. 1999;156:96–105.
11. Balercia G, Mantero F, Armeni T, Principato G, Regoli F. Oxyradical scavenging capacity toward different reactive species in seminal plasma and sperm cells. A possible influence on kinetic parameters. Clin Chem Lab Med. 2003;41:13–9.
12. Mancini A, Meucci E, Bianchi A, Milardi D, De Marinis L, Littarru GP. Antioxidant systems in human seminal plasma: physiopathological meaning and new perspectives. In: Panglossi HV, editor. New perspective in antioxidant research. New York: Nova Science; 2006. p. 131–47.
13. Crane FL. Biochemical functions of coenzyme Q10. J Am Coll Nutr. 2001;20(6):591–8.
14. Kaltschmidt B, Sparna T, Kaltschmidt C. Activation of NF-kB by reactive oxygen intermediates in the nervous system. Antioxid Redox Signal. 1999;1:129–44.
15. Crane FL, Navas P. The diversity of coenzyme Q function. Mol Aspects Med. 1997;18:S1–6.
16. Sun IL, Sun EE, Crane FL. Comparison of growth stimulation of HeLa cells, HL-60 cells and mouse fibroblasts by coenzyme Q. Protoplasma. 1995;184:214–9.
17. Sun IL, Sun EE, Crane FL, Morrè DJ, Lindgren A, Low H. A requirement for coenzyme Q in plasma membrane electron transport. Proc Natl Acad Sci USA. 1990;89:11126–30.

18. Thomas SR, Witting PK, Stocker R. A role for reduced coenzyme Q in atherosclerosis? Biofactors. 1999;9:207–24.

19. Stocker R, Bowry VW, Frei B. Ubiquinol-10 protects human low density lipoprotein more efficiently against lipid peroxidation than does alpha-tocopherol. Proc Natl Acad Sci USA. 1991;88(5):1646–50.

20. Mohr D, Bowry VW, Stocker R. Dietary supplementation with coenzyme Q10 results in increased levels of ubiquinol-10 within circulating lipoproteins and increased resistance of human low-density lipoprotein to the initiation of lipid peroxidation. Biochim Biophys Acta. 1992;1126(3):247–54.

21. Yalcin A, Kilinc E, Sagcan A, Kultursay H. Coenzyme Q10 concentrations in coronary artery disease. Clin Biochem. 2004;37:706–9.

22. Hughes K, Lee BL, Feng X, Lee J, Ong CN. Coenzyme Q10 and differences in coronary heart disease risk in Asian Indians and Chinese. Free Radic Biol Med. 2002;32(2):132–8.

23. Fawcett DW. The mammalian spermatozoon. Dev Biol. 1975;44:394–436.

24. Kalen A, Appelkvist EL, Chojnacki T, Dallner G. Nonaprenyl-4-hydroxybenzoate transferase, an enzyme involved in ubiquinone biosynthesis in endoplasmic reticulum-Golgi system of rat liver. J Biol Chem. 1990;265:1158–64.

25. Mazzilli F, Cerasaro M, Bisanti A, Rossi T, Dondero F. Seminal parameters and the swelling test in patients with sperm before and after treatment with ubiquinone (CoQ10). 2nd International Symposium on Reproductive Medicine, Fiuggi, vol. 71. Rome: Acta Medica, Edizioni e Congressi; 1988.

26. Mazzilli F, Bisanti A, Rossi T, DeSantis L, Dondero F. Seminal and biological parameters in dysspermic patients with sperm hypomotility before and after treatment with ubiquinone (CoQ10). J Endocrinol Invest. 1990;13S(1):88.

27. Mancini A, De Marinis L, Oradei A, Hallgass ME, Conte G, Pozza D, Littarru GP. Coenzyme Q10 concentrations in normal and pathological human seminal fluid. J Androl. 1994;15:591–4.

28. Mancini A, Milardi D, Conte G, Bianchi A, Balercia G, De Marinis L, Littarru GP. Coenzyme Q10: another biochemical alteration linked to infertility in varicocele patients? Metabolism. 2003;52:402–6.

29. Angelitti AG, Colacicco L, Callà C, Arizzi M, Lippa S. Coenzyme Q: potentially useful index of bioenergetic and oxidative status of spermatozoa. Clin Chem. 1995;41:217–9.

30. Mancini A, Conte G, De Marinis L, Hallgass ME, Pozza D, Oradei A, Littarru GP. Coenzyme Q10 levels in human seminal fluid: diagnostic and clinical implications. Mol Aspects Med. 1994;15:s249–55.

31. Littarru GP, Lippa S, Oradei A, Fiorini RM, Mazzanti L. Metabolic and diagnostic implications of human blood CoQ10 levels. In: Folkers K, Littarru GP, Yamagami T, editors. Biomedical and clinical aspects of coenzyme Q, vol. 6. Amsterdam: Elsevier; 1991. p. 167–78.

32. Mancini A, Conte G, Milardi D, De Marinis L, Littarru GP. Relationship between sperm cell ubiquinone and seminal parameters in subjects with and without varicocele. Andrologia. 1998;30:1–4.

33. Mancini A, Milardi D, Conte G, Festa R, De Marinis L, Littarru GP. Seminal antioxidants in humans: preoperative and postoperative evaluation of coenzyme Q10 in varicocele patients. Horm Metab Res. 2005;37:428–32.

34. Mostafa T, Anis TH, El-Nashar A, Imam H, Othman IA. Varicocelectomy reduces reactive oxygen species levels and increases antioxidant attività of seminal plasma from infertile men with varicocele. Int J Androl. 2001;24:261–5.

35. Meucci E, Milardi D, Mordente A, Martorana GE, Giacchi E, De Marinis L, Mancini A. Total antioxidant capacity in patients with varicocele. Fertil Steril. 2003;79:1577–83.

36. Mancini A, Milardi D, Festa R, Balercia G, De Marinis L, Pontecorvi A, Principi F, Littarru GP. Seminal CoQ10 and male infertility: effects of medical or surgical treatment on endogenous seminal plasma concentrations. Abstracts of the 4th International Coenzyme Q10 association. Los Angeles, 14–17 Apr 2005. p. 64–65.

37. Mancini A, Festa R, Silvestrini A, Nicolotti N, Di Donna V, La Torre G, Pontecorvi A, Meucci E. Hormonal regulation of total antioxidant capacity in seminal plasma. J Androl. 2009; 30(5):534–40. e-pub 19 Feb 2009.
38. Alleva R, Scaramucci A, Mantero F, Bompadre S, Leoni L, Littarru GP. The protective role of ubiquinol-10 against formation of lipid hydroperoxides in human seminal fluid. Mol Aspects Med. 1997;18:s221–8.
39. Balercia G, Arnaldi G, Fazioli F, Serresi M, Alleva R, Mancini A, Mosca F, Lamonica GR, Mantero F, Littarru GP. Coenzyme Q10 levels in idiopathic and varicocele-associated asthenozoospermia. Andrologia. 2002;34:107–11.
40. Littarru GP, Tiano L. Clinical aspects of coenzyme Q_{10}: an update. Curr Opin Clin Nutr Metab Care. 2005;8:641–6.
41. Lewin A, Lavon H. The effect of coenzyme Q_{10} on sperm motility and function. Mol Aspects Med. 1997;18:s213–9.
42. Mancini A, Leone E, Festa R, Grande G, Silvestrini A, De Marinis L, Pontecorvi A, Maira G, Littarru GP, Meucci E. Effects of testosterone on antioxidant systems in male secondary hypogonadism. J Androl. 2008;29(6):622–9.
43. Mancini A, Leone E, Silvestrini A, Festa R, Di Donna V, De Marinis L, Pontecorvi A, Littarry GP, Meucci E. Evaluation of antioxidant systems in pituitary-adrenal axis diseases. Pituitary. Heidelberg: Springer; 2010;13:138–45.
44. Balercia G, Mosca F, Mantero F, Boscaro M, Mancini A, Ricciardo-Lamonica G, Littarru GP. Coenzyme Q(10) supplementation in infertile men with idiopathic asthenozoospermia: an open, uncontrolled pilot study. Fertil Steril. 2004;81:93–8.
45. World Health Organization (WHO). Laboratory manual for the examination of human semen and semen-cervical mucus interaction. 4th ed. Cambridge: Cambridge University; 1999.
46. Frei B, Kim MC, Ames BN. Ubiquinol-10 is an effective lipid-soluble antioxidant at physiological concentrations. Proc Natl Acad Sci USA. 1990;87(12):4879–83.
47. Langsjoen P, Langsjoen A, Willis R, Folkers K. Treatment of hypertrophic cardiomyopathy with coenzyme Q_{10}. Mol Aspects Med. 1997;8:145–151s.
48. Balercia G, Buldreghini E, Vignini A, Tiano L, Paggi F, Amoroso S, Ricciardo-Lamonica G, Boscaro M, Lenzi A, Littarru GP. Coenzyme Q_{10} treatment in infertile men with idiopathic asthenozoospermia: a placebo-controlled, double-blind randomized trial. Fertil Steril. 2009;91:1785–92.
49. Safarinejad MR. Efficacy of coenzyme Q_{10} on semen parameters, sperm function and reproductive hormones in infertile men. J Urol. 2009;182:237–48.
50. Bremer J. Carnitine-metabolism and functions. Physiol Rev. 1983;63:1420–80.
51. Jeulin C, Dacheux JL, Soufir JC. Uptake and release of free L-carnitine by boar epididymal spermatozoa in vitro and subsequent acetylation rate. J Reprod Fertil. 1994;100:263–71.
52. DiLisa F, Barbato R, Manebo R, Siliprandi N. Carnitine and carnitine esters in mitochondrial metabolism and function. In: DeJong JW, Ferrari R, editors. The carnitine system. A new therapeutical approach to cardiovascular diseases. Dordrecht: Kluwer Academic; 1995. p. 21–38.
53. Enomoto A, Wempe MF, Tsuchida H, Shin HJ, Cha SH, Anzai N, et al. Molecular identification of a novel carnitine transporter specific to human testis. J Biol Chem. 2002;39: 36262–71.
54. Bohmer T, Johansen L. Carnitine-binding related suppressed oxygen uptake by spermatozoa. Arch Androl. 1978;1:321–4.
55. Jeulin C, Lewin LM. Role of free L-carnitine and acetyl-L-carnitine in post-gonadal maturation of mammalian spermatozoa. Hum Reprod Update. 1996;2:87–102.
56. Radigue C, Es-Slami S, Soufir JC. Relationship of carnitine transport across the epididymis to blood carnitine and androgens in rats. Arch Androl. 1996;37:27–31.
57. Balercia G, Regoli F, Armeni T, Koverech A, Mantero F, Boscaro M. Placebo-controlled double-blind randomized trial on the use of L-carnitine, L-acetylcarnitine, or combined

L-CARNITINE and L-acetylcarnitine in men with idiopathic asthenozoospermia. Fertil Steril. 2005;84:662–71.

58. Costa M, Canale D, Filicori M, D'Iddio S, Lenzi A. L-Carnitine in idiopathic asthenozoospermia: a multicenter study. Andrologia. 1994;26:155–9.

59. Vicari E, Calogero AE. Effects of treatment with carnitines in infertile patients with prostato-vesiculo-epididymitis. Hum Reprod. 2001;16:2338–42.

60. Vicari E, La Vignera S, Calogero AE. Antioxidant treatment with carnitine is effective in infertile patients with prostato-vesiculo-epididymitis and elevated seminal leukocyte concentration after treatment with nonsteroidal anti-inflammatory compounds. Fertil Steril. 2002;78: 1203–8.

61. Lenzi A, Lombardo F, Sgro P, Salacone P, Caponecchia L, Dondero F, et al. Use of carnitine therapy in selected cases of male factor infertility: a double blind cross-over trial. Fertil Steril. 2003;79:292–300.

62. Lenzi A, Sgrò P, Salacone P, Paoli D, Gilio B, Lombardo F, et al. Placebo controlled double blind randomised trial on the use of L-carnitine and L-acetyl-carnitine combined treatment in asthenozoospermia. Fertil Steril. 2004;81:1578–84.

63. Kobayashi A, Fujisawa S. Effect of L-carnitine on mitochondrial acyl-carnitine, acyl-coenzyme A and high energy phosphate in ischemic dog heart. J Mol Cell Cardiol. 1994;26:499–508.

64. Fato R, Cavazzoni M, Castelluccio C, Parenti Castelli G, Lenaz G. Steady-state kinetics of ubiquinol-cytochrome c reductase in bovine heart submitochondrial particles: diffusional effects. Biochem J. 1993;290:225–36.

65. Kelso KA, Redpath A, Noble RC, Speake BK. Lipid and antioxidant changes in spermatozoa and seminal plasma throughout the reproductive period of bulls. J Reprod Fertil. 1997; 109:1–6.

Chapter 18
Synthetic Antioxidants

Edmund Y. Ko, John C. Kefer, Ashok Agarwal, and Edmund Sabanegh

Infertility is a major clinical concern, affecting 15% of all reproductive-aged couples, and male factors, including decreased semen quality, are responsible for 25% of these cases [1, 2]. Many men with male factor infertility have suboptimal semen quality, the etiology of which is poorly understood. Many environmental, genetic, and physiological factors, including oxidative stress induced by reactive oxygen species (ROS), have been implicated [3–5]. Oxidative stress induces significant damage to sperm, including decreased motility [6–8], increased DNA damage [9–11], lipid peroxidation [12–14], and decreased oocyte–sperm fusion [15]. Interestingly, while excessive levels of ROS can negatively impact sperm quality, lower levels of ROS have been shown to be required for sperm capacitation, hyperactivation, sperm–oocyte fusion, and other critical cellular processes [16, 17].

E.Y. Ko, MD (✉) • E. Sabanegh, MD
Section of Male Fertility, Department of Urology, Center for Reproductive Medicine,
Glickman Urological and Kidney Institute, Cleveland Clinic, 9500 Euclid Avenue/Q10-1,
Cleveland, OH 44195, USA
e-mail: edko05@gmail.com; sabanee@ccf.org

J.C. Kefer, MD, PhD
Alpine Urology, 1155 Alpine Ave, Suite 180, Boulder, CO 80304, USA
e-mail: johnckefer@gmail.com

A. Agarwal, PhD
Center for Reproductive Medicine, Glickman Urological and Kidney Institute, Cleveland
Clinic Foundation, 9500 Euclid Avenue, Desk A19, Cleveland, OH 44195, USA
e-mail: agarwaa@ccf.org

S.J. Parekattil and A. Agarwal (eds.), *Antioxidants in Male Infertility: A Guide
for Clinicians and Researchers*, © Springer Science+Business Media New York 2013

Reactive Oxygen Species and Antioxidants

The majority of aerobic metabolism utilizes oxidative phosphorylation within mitochondria. During the enzymatic reduction of oxygen by cells to produce energy, free radicals are a constant by-product [18]. Free radicals are defined as oxygen molecules containing one or more unpaired electrons. Free radicals induce cellular damage when they pass this unpaired electron onto nearby structures, resulting in the oxidation of cell membrane lipids, amino acids in proteins, or within nucleic acids [19]. Oxygen is especially susceptible to free radical formation, as it normally has two unpaired electrons. For example, the addition of one electron to molecular oxygen (O_2) forms a superoxide anion radical ($O_2^{\cdot-}$), the primary form of ROS. Superoxide is then directly or indirectly converted to secondary ROS, including hydroxyl radical ($^{\cdot}OH$), peroxyl radical ($ROO^{\cdot}$) or hydrogen peroxide (H_2O_2) [20].

ROS are also formed during the normal enzymatic reactions of inter- and intracellular signaling [21]. ROS generation by leukocytes as a cytotoxic mechanism of host defense, hypoxic states, and a wide array of drugs with oxidizing effects all generate oxidative stress. Significant cellular damage by oxidative stress is prevented through enzymatic and nonenzymatic antioxidant pathways which scavenge excess ROS. This oxidant–antioxidant system allows a critically important balance to be achieved, allowing beneficial oxidant generation for proper cell function, while preventing damaging oxidative stress.

Under normal conditions, antioxidants maintain an overall low level of oxidative stress in the semen, allowing for normal cell signaling processes and normal spermatic function while avoiding oxidant-induced cell damage. In contrast, the pathological effects of oxidative stress arise under conditions where levels of unscavenged ROS increase, thus perturbing the delicate oxidant/antioxidant balance, significantly impacting both sperm quality and function [15, 19, 21]. ROS-induced sperm damage may be a significant contributing factor in 30–80% of all cases of male infertility [19, 21].

Free radicals are scavenged most commonly by one tripeptide, glutathione, and three enzymes important for cellular metabolism. Glutathione, which contains a sulfhydryl group that directly scavenges free radicals, is the most important intracellular defense against ROS. Once oxidized, glutathione is then regenerated/reduced by glutathione reductase and NADPH to complete the cycle [15]. Of the three antioxidant enzymes, superoxide dismutase (SOD) is a metal-containing enzyme that catalyzes two superoxides into oxygen and hydrogen peroxide, which is less toxic than superoxide [18]. Catalase, an enzyme found in peroxisomes, then degrades hydrogen peroxide to water and oxygen, thereby completing the reaction started by SOD. Glutathione peroxidase, as well as other enzymes such as glutathione transferase, ceruloplasmin, or heme oxygenase, also acts to degrade hydrogen peroxide.

Vitamins E and C also play critical roles as nonenzymatic antioxidants [15]. Vitamin E protects cell membranes from oxidative damage by scavenging free radicals within the cellular membrane. Vitamin C is a water-soluble antioxidant that reduces a variety of free radicals and also recycles oxidized vitamin E.

Oxidative Damage to Sperm Cells

Unfortunately, spermatozoa are particularly sensitive to oxidative stress. The majority of the antioxidant enzymatic buffering capacity (i.e., SOD, glutathione peroxidase and catalase, vitamins E and C) is contained in the seminal fluid [15]. Conversely, levels of these antioxidants in the sperm cytoplasm are minimal due to the extremely low volume of spermatic cytoplasm. The polyunsaturated fatty acids found in sperm cell membranes are exquisitely sensitive to peroxidation, making sperm more susceptible to lipid membrane damage than other nongerm cells [12, 13]. Maintaining a healthy antioxidant level is further exacerbated by the ROS production by spermatozoa during its lifespan.

Two principal sources of free radicals are found in the semen: leukocytes and spermatozoa. Most semen specimens contain variable numbers of leukocytes, with neutrophils noted as the predominant type [22–24]. Neutrophils function by generating and releasing high concentrations of ROS to form cytotoxic reactions against nearby cells and pathogens. Over the last 10 years, many studies have investigated the correlation between leukocytospermia and oxidative stress injury to sperm [20, 22, 25–33]. Nonetheless, the relationship between leukocytes in the semen and male infertility remains incompletely defined.

Leukocytospermia has long been associated with decreased sperm concentration, motility, and morphology, as well as decreased hyperactivation and defective fertilization. In a thorough review of the literature, Wolff et al. delineated several studies describing the association between the presence of white blood cells (WBC) in semen and overall sperm quality [34]. The majority of these epidemiologic, clinical, and experimental studies all described a significant negative association between the number of WBCs and overall sperm function. Moskovtsev et al. recently analyzed the relationship between leukocytospermia and sperm DNA damage in 1,230 unselected nonazoospermic infertility patients [35]. While the authors found no significant relationship between leukocytospermia and DNA integrity, a significant negative effect was again noted between the presence of leukocytospermia and corresponding sperm concentration, motility, and morphology. Nonetheless, this relationship is not definitive, as several other studies have found no evidence of a correlation between leukocytospermia and abnormal sperm parameters [25–27]. In a review of these studies, Aitken et al. emphasized that seminal leukocytes may not necessarily affect the fertilizing potential of spermatozoa, as not all men with leukocytospermia demonstrate abnormal sperm parameters [25]. The authors also postulate that the role of leukocytes on male fertility might instead be related to the etiology of the leukocytospermia or the degree of inflammation in the seminal fluid, as well as the leukocyte subtypes present. This relationship therefore remains controversial. While the significance of leukocytospermia on the fertility potential of the individual patient remains difficult to quantify, it can nonetheless be considered a marker of urological or systemic inflammation and possible sperm dysfunction.

Synthetic Antioxidants

Due to the cost and difficulty of chemically extracting and isolating vitamins and other dietary antioxidants from their food source, a broad number of antioxidants are chemically synthesized and packaged in a pill form as an isolate compound. Several studies have suggested that these synthetic antioxidants offer suboptimal antioxidant properties due to their chemical composition and the fact that they are isolated from other synergistic compounds present in normal food sources [36, 37]. Several large clinical studies have been performed investigating the efficacy of these antioxidant isolates, used alone or in combination with one other antioxidant supplement. Bjelakovic et al. postulated that antioxidant supplements have not been proven to have a distinct benefit and may be overall harmful [38, 39]. They investigated the role of synthetic vitamin A, vitamin E, and beta-carotene supplements on overall morbidity and mortality in patients with gastrointestinal cancers. The authors concluded that antioxidant supplements, with the potential exception of selenium, were without significant effects on gastrointestinal cancers and, most concerning, were noted to increase all-cause mortality.

This same group went further and performed a meta-analysis of 68 randomized trials with 232,606 participants to assess the effect of antioxidant supplements on all-cause mortality in randomized primary and secondary prevention trials [40]. All included trials used beta-carotene, vitamin A, vitamin C (ascorbic acid), vitamin E, and selenium, either alone or in combination, and compared these groups to placebo or no intervention. In 47 trials with 180,938 participants, the antioxidant supplements were overall shown to significantly increase mortality (RR, 1.05; 95% CI, 1.02–1.08). After exclusion of the trials involving selenium, patients taking synthetic beta-carotene, vitamin A, and vitamin E, either singly or combined, had significantly increased overall mortality, whereas patients taking synthetic Vitamin C and selenium had no significant effect on mortality.

These authors and others have postulated that natural antioxidants obtained from food sources contribute multiple antioxidants and other co-factors that have been shown to act in synergy with each other, potentially increasing the overall antioxidant capabilities of these agents.

It has been suggested that antioxidant supplements may show interdependency and may have effects only if given in combination [41]. A single antioxidant in high doses will donate a single electron to scavenge free radicals. However, if these "spent" or oxidized antioxidants are present in higher concentrations than the enzymes and cofactors that "recycle" or reduce the antioxidants through reduction–oxidation pathways, these high-dose synthetic antioxidants may actually increase the oxidative stress environment within the relevant physiological system. These theories offer a possible explanation for the broad number of antioxidant trials noting no improvement in a disease process or showing a detrimental effect [42].

Based on numerous clinical studies reviewed in detail by subsequent authors, our center has derived an empiric regimen of synthetic vitamin C, vitamin E,

L-carnitine, and coenzyme-Q10 for men demonstrating elevated oxidative stress levels in their semen profile. Here, we review the mechanism of action of these vitamins and further delineate the potential toxicities and side effects of these vitamins and dietary supplements. Overall, it should be noted that most of these dietary supplements can have a detrimental effect on patient health, and our center counsels all patients regarding the potential for toxicity with misuse of these supplements.

Mechanisms of Action

Vitamin E

Synthetic vitamin E is a general term used to describe a group of tocopherols, of which α-tocopherol has the highest biological activity. It is interesting to note that vitamin E has been recognized as an essential nutrient for reproduction since its discovery in 1922 [43]. The cellular and antioxidant functions of vitamin E have yet to be fully described, and it is unlikely they are solely limited to antioxidant functions [44]. Of importance, synthetic vitamin E is mainly comprised of α-tocopherol. The other three tocopherols (β, γ, δ) found in vitamin E-containing foods having antioxidant properties may be present at much lower concentrations in synthesized nutritional supplements [45]. Vitamin E is a chain-breaking antioxidant that prevents oxidant-induced lipid peroxidation, thereby preventing damage to cellular membranes and related structures [46]. It should be noted, however, that like all other oxidative–reductive compounds, vitamin E can act as an oxidant as well. Prooxidative functions of α-tocopherol have been noted in healthy volunteers [47].

A potential role for γ-tocopherol has also been postulated. Unlike α-tocopherol, γ-tocopherol is a powerful nucleophile that traps electrophilic mutagens in lipophilic compartments [48]. Thus, protection of cellular lipids, DNA, and proteins from oxidant damage may occur from several isomers of vitamin E.

In regard to maintaining proper male fertility, optimal function of vitamin E has been linked to optimal levels of selenium. It has been shown that vitamin E scavenges free radicals generated from lipid peroxidation and that the by-products of these scavenged radicals, hydrogen peroxide molecules, are in turn reduced by glutathione peroxidase, a selenium-dependent enzyme [44].

Synthetic vitamin E may therefore indeed play an injurious role in cellular function. Since the optimal role of vitamin E has been linked to the presence of optimal concentrations of other micronutrients, and vitamin E has been shown to have prooxidant properties, supplementing with high levels of synthetic vitamin E may in fact lead to a prooxidant state due to a buildup of hydrogen peroxides or oxidized tocopherols. These data should be considered when prescribing vitamin E and when discussing dietary supplements with patients.

Vitamin A

Vitamin A is a fat-soluble vitamin that is required for proper vision. Vitamin A also functions as a hormone-like growth factor and has been postulated to have antioxidant properties; however, the mechanism by which vitamin A may act as an antioxidant is currently unknown [49]. In clinical trials, vitamin A was shown to improve semen parameters, most significantly by improving the oxidant stress levels of the semen [49–51]. One caveat in these trials is that vitamin A was given in conjunction with other antioxidants, which could have induced the changes in parameters.

Vitamin C

Vitamin C, or ascorbic acid, is considered a vitamin because humans cannot synthesize it enzymatically and must instead obtain it through dietary intake. Vitamin C is a monosaccharide catalyst of oxidation–reduction (redox) reactions in human physiology. Vitamin C is also required for the conversion of procollagen to collagen through the oxidation of proline residues to hydroxyproline, where vitamin C deficiency leads to scurvy [52].

Vitamin C has a unique function as an antioxidant. When vitamin C loses one electron (oxidation), it remains very stable, allowing it to gain an electron from a more aggressive free radical while also not damaging critical cellular structures. When vitamin C is oxidized, it is recycled back to an antioxidant form via the NADPH pathway, as well as by the glutathione pathways [52]. It is therefore not surprising then that synthetic vitamin C in very high doses has been shown to have a detrimental clinical effect. Regular intake of high doses of synthetic vitamin C as a single dietary supplement may overwhelm the recycling pathways, leading to excessive levels of oxidized vitamin C, which would then act as an oxidant on the cellular system.

Safety, Dosing, and Side Effects of Toxicity

Adverse events due to vitamin toxicity are almost exclusively seen due to overconsumption of synthetic vitamin supplements [53]. Adverse events associated with vitamin use can be of similar magnitude as conventional pharmaceuticals, and significant toxicity can occur with high intake of most vitamins [53]. For some vitamins, such as the B vitamins, vitamin C, and vitamin K, adverse reactions are minor and usually reversible. Other vitamins, such as vitamin A or vitamin E, have been shown to cause serious, irreversible adverse events. We will review these significant adverse events and safety profiles of potentially dangerous antioxidant vitamins.

Vitamin E

Vitamin E is a lipid-soluble vitamin, capable of reaching toxic tissue concentrations through storage in the liver and fatty tissues of the body. In healthy adults, 200–800 mg/day may cause gastrointestinal distress, and 800–1,200 mg/day may induce antiplatelet effects and bleeding disturbances, thrombophlebitis, elevated creatinine, and gonadal dysfunction [54, 55]. In several large, multicenter, randomized trials investigating the potential benefits of vitamin E on prevention of cardiac events; many of these studies described a significant increased risk of congestive heart failure. In the multicenter GISSI-Prevenzione trial studying 11,000 patients with previous myocardial infarction, vitamin E showed no benefit for all study endpoints but a 20% increased risk of developing congestive heart failure [56, 57]. In over 9,500 patients studied under the multicenter Heart Outcomes Prevention Evaluation randomized trial, treatment with vitamin E did not prevent cancer or cardiovascular events but did increase the risk of heart failure [58, 59]. High-dose vitamin E can also synergistically interact with vitamin K to exacerbate bleeding diatheses, especially in patients already taking anticoagulation or antiplatelet therapy [60, 61]. Among 30,000 male smokers, a higher incidence of hemorrhagic stroke was noted in men taking vitamin E [62].

High-dose vitamin E has also been shown to increase the overall cancer and mortality risk. The largest study, a meta-analysis of 19 clinical trials investigating over 135,000 patients, demonstrated that 400 IU/day or higher may increase all-cause mortality [63]. In the Women's Health Study, multivariate analysis demonstrated that vitamin E serum levels were associated with increased risk of both invasive and noninvasive breast cancers [64]. In men, supplementation with vitamin E has been demonstrated to increase risk of prostate cancer, especially in men taking vitamin E in conjunction with other supplements [65].

Vitamin A

Vitamin A is mainly stored in the liver. Vitamin A toxicity ranges from elevated liver function tests to cirrhosis, hepatic fibrosis, and death due to liver failure. Vitamin A has been associated with nausea, blurred vision, anorexia, and mental status changes, as well as electrolyte disorders [66]. In over 2,000 men aged 49–51 years old, risk of fracture was seven times higher in men with elevated serum retinol compared to men with the lowest retinol levels [67]. In a large, randomized, multicenter, double-blind, placebo-controlled trial of more than 29,000 male smokers receiving beta-carotene in Finland, as well as in a study of 18,000 men in the USA, the incidence of lung cancer in these men was 18% higher in men taking beta-carotene supplementation compared to the placebo group [62]. In women, two large studies demonstrated conflicting results in female smokers taking beta-carotene supplementation. In one study, the Women's Health Study, no benefit or harm was noted in the incidence of lung cancer and cardiovascular events, whereas a similar study design in another trial also showed no benefit with a significant increased incidence of mortality from both lung cancer and cardiovascular disease [68, 69].

Vitamin C

Vitamin C is generally well tolerated, but in large doses, such as the several gram doses frequently found in supplements, acute adverse effects can include nausea, vomiting, esophagitis, heartburn, fatigue, insomnia, and diarrhea [70]. Long-term vitamin C intake can induce crystallization of urate, oxalate, cysteine, and other drugs in the urinary tract [71]. In a prospective cohort study of over 45,000 men without history of nephrolithiasis, vitamin C intake may increase risk of stones, and multivariate analysis in men consuming 1,000 mg/day versus those consuming less than the recommended daily allowance showed a significant risk of stone formation [72]. However, the comparison of men taking below the recommended amount versus men taking doses measured in grams could be questioned.

In a study of over 1,900 postmenopausal diabetic women, vitamin C was associated with a dose-related increased risk of coronary artery disease, stroke, and overall cardiovascular mortality [73]. More significantly, in the Los Angeles Atherosclerosis Study, investigating the impact of vitamin C supplementation on more than 500 men and women without symptomatic cardiovascular disease, carotid inner wall thickening was noted in males taking 500 mg of vitamin C per day [74].

While these studies demonstrate a significant increased risk of morbidity and mortality in vitamin C supplementation, Lee et al. directly demonstrated that vitamin C can break down lipids in cell membranes into compounds that act as genotoxins, leading to increased levels of DNA damage [73]. This study is one of the few to directly demonstrate the potential mechanisms by which vitamin C may induce cell injury and decreased cellular function.

Management of Oxidative Stress in Male Infertility

Vitamin/Antioxidant Supplementation

The antioxidants α-tocopherol (vitamin E), ascorbic acid (vitamin C), and the retinoids (vitamin A) are all potent scavengers of ROS. Many studies have investigated the role of these and other antioxidants on improvements in sperm parameters. However, the majority of these studies are uncontrolled, focus on healthy men without infertility, or have indirect endpoints of success. Several other studies are noted due to the quality of their study design and demonstrate compelling evidence regarding efficacy of antioxidants toward improving semen parameters.

Silver et al. surveyed 97 healthy nonsmoking men aged 20–80 years old regarding antioxidant intake using a dietary questionnaire and subsequently examined semen samples [75]. Those with high daily intake of antioxidants were noted to have improved semen quality compared to men with low or moderate intake, thereby demonstrating some correlation between increased dietary antioxidant intake and improved semen parameters.

Keskes-Ammar et al. examined the therapeutic efficacy of increased antioxidant intake on semen parameters [76]. They randomized 54 men to either vitamin E and selenium or vitamin B for 3 months, with examination of semen samples quantifying the lipid peroxidation marker, malondialdehyde (MDA), as well as measurement of serum vitamin E levels. Although only 20 patients completed the study protocol, results indicated that vitamin E and selenium supplementation produced a significant decrease in MDA concentrations with improved sperm motility, whereas vitamin B showed no impact.

Suleiman et al. randomized their cohort of asthenozoospermic men with normal female partners to vitamin E or placebo for 6 months, noting decreased MDA levels and increased motility, as well as increased pregnancy rates in the vitamin E arm [77].

Conversely, Rolf et al. randomized 31 men with asthenospermia to either 2 months of high-dose oral treatment with vitamins C and E or placebo and investigated semen parameters [78]. The authors found no changes in semen parameters during treatment, and no pregnancies were initiated during this period.

Most recently, the best designed trial by Greco et al. examined the impact of increased antioxidant intake in a randomized, prospective manner [79]. A group of 64 infertile men with >15% DNA-fragmented spermatozoa were randomized into two groups to receive either 1 g of vitamin C and E daily or placebo for 2 months. While no differences in basic sperm parameters were noted, the antioxidant cohort demonstrated a significantly reduced percentage of DNA-fragmented spermatozoa. The authors further went on to demonstrate that supplementation with Vitamins E and C significantly increased rates of clinical pregnancy and implantation following ICSI [80].

Although these data from different centers are potentially conflicting, direct comparison of these results is difficult given the varying nature of the dose, duration of treatment, and study end points in each of these trials. Nonetheless, these studies provide compelling evidence toward the efficacy of vitamin antioxidants on improving overall sperm quality and possibly improved pregnancy following ICSI.

Five-Year View and Key Issues

Our understanding of the role of ROS on male fertility continues to increase supported by an expanding literature refining this relationship. The etiology of suboptimal semen quality due to oxidative stress is becoming elucidated. The origin of ROS generation and the etiologies of increased ROS in men with suboptimal sperm quality are increasingly clear, offering multiple pathways for potential therapy.

Nonetheless, more well-designed, randomized controlled trials will be required to assess the potential of these antioxidant regimens. Without further studies to test the treatments of best efficacy, it is difficult to derive cohesive clinical guidelines of therapy from these studies. Nonetheless, the initial data demonstrating efficacy in improving sperm quality and conception rates are indeed encouraging.

References

1. Rowe PJ, Comhaire FH, Hargreave TB, Mahmoud AMA. WHO manual for the standardized investigation, diagnosis and management of the infertile male. Cambridge: Cambridge University Press; 2004.
2. Sharlip ID, Jarow JP, Belker AM, Lipshultz LI, Sigman M, Thomas AJ, et al. Best practice policies for male infertility. Fertil Steril. 2002;77:873–82.
3. Vine MF. Smoking and male reproduction: a review. Int J Androl. 1996;19:323–37.
4. Auger J, Eustache F, Andersen AG, Irvine DS, Jorgensen N, Skakkebaek NE, et al. Sperm morphological defects related to environment, lifestyle and medical history of 1001 male partners of pregnant women from four European cities. Hum Reprod. 2001;16:2710–7.
5. Kenkel S, Rolf C, Nieschlag E. Occupational risks for male fertility: an analysis of patients attending a tertiary referral centre. Int J Androl. 2001;24:318–26.
6. Eskenazi B, Wyrobek AJ, Sloter E, Kidd SA, Moore L, Young S, et al. The association of age and semen quality in healthy men. Hum Reprod. 2003;18:447–54.
7. Lenzi A, Lombardo F, Gandini L, Alfano P, Dondero F. Computer assisted sperm motility analysis at the moment of induced pregnancy during gonadotropin treatment for hypogonadotropic hypogonadism. J Endocrinol Invest. 1993;6:683–6.
8. Agarwal A, Ikemoto I, Loughlin KR. Relationship of sperm parameters with levels of reactive oxygen species in semen specimens. J Urol. 1994;152:107–10.
9. Armstrong JS, Rajasekaran M, Chamulitrat W, Gatti P, Hellstrom WJ, Sikka SC. Characterization of reactive oxygen species induced effects on human spermatozoa movement and energy metabolism. Free Radic Biol Med. 1999;26:869–80.
10. Kodama H, Yamaguchi R, Fukuda J, Kasai H, Tanaka T. Increased oxidative deoxyribonucleic acid damage in the spermatozoa of infertile male patients. Fertil Steril. 1997;68:519–24.
11. Barroso G, Morshedi M, Oehninger S. Analysis of DNA fragmentation, plasma membrane translocation of phosphatidylserine and oxidative stress in human spermatozoa. Hum Reprod. 2000;15:1338–44.
12. Aitken RJ, Harkiss D, Buckingham DW. Analysis of lipid peroxidation mechanisms in human spermatozoa. Mol Reprod Dev. 1993;35:302–15.
13. Kemal Duru N, Morshedi M, Oehninger S. Effects of hydrogen peroxide on DNA and plasma membrane integrity of human spermatozoa. Fertil Steril. 2000;74:1200–7.
14. Smith R, Vantman D, Ponce J, Escobar J, Lissi E. Total antioxidant capacity of human seminal plasma. Hum Reprod. 1996;11(8):1655–60.
15. Agarwal A, Prabhakaran SA, Sikka SC. Clinical relevance of oxidative stress in patients with male factor infertility: evidence-based analysis. AUA Update Series. 2007;26:1–12.
16. Aitken RJ, Ryan AL, Baker MA, McLaughlin EA. Redox activity associated with the maturation and capacitation of mammalian spermatozoa. Free Radic Biol Med. 2004;36:994–1010.
17. de Lamirande E, Tsai C, Harakat A, Gagnon C. Involvement of reactive oxygen species in human sperm acrosome reaction induced by A23187, lysophosphatidylcholine, and biological fluid ultrafiltrates. J Androl. 1998;19:585–94.
18. Tremellen K. Oxidative stress and male infertility—a clinical perspective. Hum Reprod Update. 2008;14:243–58.
19. Ochsendorf FR. Infections in the male genital tract and reactive oxygen species. Hum Reprod Update. 1999;5:399–420.
20. Warren JS, Johnson KJ, Ward PA. Oxygen radicals in cell injury and cell death. Pathol Immunopathol Res. 1987;6:301–15.
21. Agarwal A, Prabakaran S, Allamaneni S. What an andrologist/urologist should know about free radicals and why. Urology. 2006;67:2–8.
22. Saleh RA, Agarwal A. Oxidative stress and male infertility: from research bench to clinical practice. J Androl. 2002;23:737–52.
23. Aitken RJ, Fisher H. Reactive oxygen species and human spermatozoa: the balance of benefit and risk. Bioessays. 1994;16:259–67.

24. Aitken RJ. Free radicals, lipid peroxidation, sperm function. Reprod Fertil Dev. 1995;
7:659–68.
25. Aitken RJ, Baker HW. Seminal leukocytes: passengers, terrorists or good Samaritans? Hum Reprod. 1995;10:1736–9.
26. Tomlinson JM, Barratt CL, Cooke ID. Prospective study of leukocytes and leukocyte subpopulations in semen suggests they are not the cause of a male infertility. Fertil Steril. 1993; 60:1069–75.
27. Christiansen E, Tollefsrud A, Purvis K. Sperm quality in men with chronic abacterial prostatovesiculitis verified by rectal ultrasonography. Urology. 1991;38:545–9.
28. Aitken RJ, Fisher HM, Fulton N, Gomez E, Knox W, Lewis B, et al. Reactive oxygen species generation by human spermatozoa is induced by exogenous NADPH and inhibited by the flavoprotein inhibitors diphenylene iodonium and quinacrine. Mol Reprod Dev. 1997; 47:468–82.
29. Hendin B, Kolletis PN, Sharma RK, Thomas AJ, Agarwal A. Varicocele is associated with elevated spermatozoal reactive oxygen species production and diminished seminal plasma antioxidant capacity. J Urol. 1999;161:1831–4.
30. Shalika S, Dugan K, Smith RD, Padilla SL. The effect of positive semen bacterial and ureaplasma cuture on in-vitro fertilization success. Hum Reprod. 1996;11:2789–92.
31. Sharma RK, Pasqualetto AE, Nelson DR, Thomas AJ, Agarwal A. Relationship between seminal white blood cell counts and oxidative stress in men treated at an infertility clinic. J Androl. 2001;22:575–83.
32. Kao SH, Chao HT, Chen HW, Hwang TI, Liao TL, Wei YH. Increase of oxidative stress in human sperm with lower motility. Fertil Steril. 2008;89(5):1183–90.
33. Saleh RA, Agarwal A, Kandirali E, Sharma RK, Thomas AJ, Nada E, et al. Leukocytospermia is associated with increased reactive oxygen species production by human spermatozoa. Fertil Steril. 2002;78:1215–24.
34. Wolff H. The biologic significance of white blood cells in semen. Fertil Steril. 1995; 63:1143–57.
35. Moskovtsev SI, Willis J, White J, Mullen BM. Leukocytospermia: relationship to sperm deoxyribonucleic acid integrity in patients evaluated for male factor infertility. Fertil Steril. 2007;88(3):737–40.
36. Herbert V. The value of antioxidant supplements vs their natural counterparts. J Am Diet Assoc. 1997;97:375–6.
37. Stanner SA, Hughes J, Kelly CN, Buttriss J. A review of the epidemiological evidence or the "antioxidant hypothesis". Public Health Nutr. 2004;7:407–22.
38. Bjelakovic G, Nikolova D, Simonetti RG, Gluud C. Antioxidant supplements for preventing gastrointestinal cancers. Cochrane Database Syst Rev. 2004;(4):CD004183.
39. Bjelakovic G, Nikolova D, Simonetti RG, Gluud C. Antioxidant supplements for preventing gastrointestinal cancers. Cochrane Database Syst Rev. 2008;(3):CD004183.
40. Bjelakovic G, Nikolova D, Simonetti RG, Gluud C. Antioxidant supplements for prevention of gastrointestinal cancers: a systematic review and meta-analysis. Lancet. 2004;364(9441): 1219–28.
41. Hercberg S, Galan P, Preziosi P, Alfarez MJ, Vazquez C. The potential role of antioxidant vitamins in preventing cardiovascular diseases and cancers. Nutrition. 1998;14:513–20.
42. Bjelakovic G, Nikolova D, Gluud LL, Simonetti RG, Gluud C. Mortality in randomized trials of antioxidant supplements for primary and secondary prevention: systematic review and meta-analysis. JAMA. 2007;197:842–57.
43. Evans HM, Bishop KS. On the existence of a hitherto unrecognized dietary factor essential for reproduction. Science. 1922;56:650–1.
44. Brigelius-Flohe R, Traber MG. Vitamin E: function and metabolism. FASEB J. 1999; 13:1145–55.
45. Esterbauer H, Dieber-Rotheneder M, Striegl G, Waeg G. Role of vitamin E in preventing the oxidation of low-density lipoprotein. Am J Clin Nutr. 1991;53(1 Suppl):314S–21.

46. Kamal-Eldin A, Appelqvist LA. The chemistry and antioxidant properties of tocopherols and tocotrienols. Lipids. 1996;31:671–701.
47. Bowry VW, Ingold KU, Stocker R. Vitamin E in human low-density lipoprotein. When and how this antioxidant becomes a pro-oxidant. Biochem J. 1992;288:341–4.
48. Cooney RV, Franke AA, Harwood PJ, Hatch-Pigott V, Custer LJ, Mordan LJ. Gamma-tocopherol detoxification of nitrogen dioxide: superiority to alpha-tocopherol. Proc Natl Acad Sci USA. 1993;90:1771–5.
49. Comhaire FH, Christophe AB, Zalata AA, Dhooge WS, Mahmoud AM, Depuydt CE. The effects of combined conventional treatment, oral antioxidants and essential fatty acids on sperm biology in subfertile men. Prostaglandins Leukot Essent Fatty Acids. 2000;63:159–65.
50. Scott R, MacPherson A, Yates RW, Hussain B, Dixon J. The effect of oral selenium supplementation on human sperm motility. Br J Urol. 1998;82:76–80.
51. Galatioto GP, Gravina GL, Angelozzi G, Sacchetti A, Innominato PF, Pace G, et al. May antioxidant therapy improve sperm parameters of men with persistent oligospermia after retrograde embolization for varicocele? World J Urol. 2008;26:97–102.
52. Linster CL, Van Schaftingen E, Vitamin C. Biosynthesis, recycling and degradation in mammals. FEBS J. 2007;274:1–22.
53. Mulholland CA, Benford DJ. What is known about the safety of multivitamin-multimineral supplements for the generally healthy population? Theoretical basis for harm. Am J Clin Nutr. 2007;85:318S–22.
54. Bendich A, Machlin LJ. Safety of oral intake of vitamin E. Am J Clin Nutr. 1988;48:612–9.
55. Weber P, Bendich A, Machlin LJ. Vitamin E and human health: rationale for determining recommended intake levels. Nutrition. 1997;13:450–60.
56. Dietary supplementation with n-3 polyunsaturated fatty acids and vitamin E after myocardial infarction: results of the GISSI-Prevenzione trial. Gruppo Italiano per lo Studia della Sopravvivenza nell'Infarto miocardico. Lancet. 1999;354:447–55. http://www.ncbi.nlm.nih.gov/pubmed/10465168.
57. Marchioli R, Levantesi G, Macchia A, Marfisi RM, Nicolosi GL, Tavazzi L, et al. Vitamin E increases the risk of developing heart failure after myocardial infarction: results from the GISSI-Prevenzione trial. J Cardiovasc Med (Hagerstown). 2006;7:347–50.
58. Yusuf S, Dagenais G, Pogue J, Bosch J, Sleight P. Vitamin E supplementation and cardiovascular events in high-risk patients. The Heart Outcomes Prevention Evaluation Study Investigators. N Engl J Med. 2000;342:154–60.
59. Lonn E, Bosch J, Yusuf S, Sheridan P, Pogue J, Arnold JM, et al. Effects of long-term vitamin E supplementation on cardiovascular events and cancer: a randomized controlled trial. JAMA. 2005;293:1338–47.
60. Greenblatt DJ, von Moltke LL. Interaction of warfarin with drugs, natural substances, and foods. J Clin Pharmacol. 2005;45:127–32.
61. Mousa SA. Antithrombotic effects of naturally derived products on coagulation and platelet function. Methods Mol Biol. 2010;663:229–40.
62. The Alpha-Tocopherol, Beta Carotene Cancer Prevention Study Group. The effect of vitamin E and beta carotene on the incidence of lung cancer and other cancers in male smokers. N Engl J Med. 1994;330:1029–35.
63. Miller 3rd ER, Pastor-Barriuso R, Dalal D, Riemersma RA, Appel LJ, Guallar E. Meta-analysis: high-dosage vitamin E supplementation may increase all-cause mortality. Ann Intern Med. 2005;142:37–46.
64. Kabat GC, Kim M, Adams-Campbell LL, Caan BJ, Chlebowski RT, Neuhouser ML, et al. Longitudinal study of serum carotenoid, retinol, and tocopherol concentrations in relation to breast cancer risk among postmenopausal women. Am J Clin Nutr. 2009;90:162–9.
65. Lawson KA, Wright ME, Subar A, Mouw T, Hollenbeck A, Schatzkin A, et al. Multivitamin use and risk of prostate cancer in the National Institutes of Health-AARP Diet and Health Study. J Natl Cancer Inst. 2007;99:754–64.

66. Food and Nutrition Board, Institute of Medicine. Dietary reference intakes for vitamin A, vitamin K, arsenic, boron, chromium, copper, iodine, iron, manganese, molybdenum, nickel, silicon, vanadium, and zinc. Washington, DC: National Academy Press; 2002.
67. Michaelsson K, Lithell H, Vessby B, Melhus H. Serum retinol levels and the risk of fracture. N Engl J Med. 2003;348:287–94.
68. Lee IM, Cook NR, Manson JE, Buring JE, Hennekens CH. Beta-carotene supplementation and incidence of cancer and cardiovascular disease: the Women's Health Study. J Natl Cancer Inst. 1999;91:2102–6.
69. Goodman GE, Thornquist MD, Balmes J, Cullen MR, Meyskens Jr FL, Omenn GS, et al. The Beta-Carotene and Retinol Efficacy Trial: incidence of lung cancer and cardiovascular disease mortality during 6-year follow-up after stopping beta-carotene and retinol supplements. J Natl Cancer Inst. 2004;96:1743–50.
70. Food and Nutrition Board, Institute of Medicine. Dietary reference intakes for vitamin C, vitamin E, selenium, and carotenoids. Washington, DC: National Academy Press; 2000.
71. Levine M, Rumsey SC, Daruwala R, Park JB, Wang Y. Criteria and recommendations for vitamin C intake. JAMA. 1999;281:1415–23.
72. Taylor EN, Stampfer MJ, Curhan GC. Dietary factors and the risk of incident kidney stones in men: new insights after 14 years of follow-up. J Am Soc Nephrol. 2004;15:3225–32.
73. Lee DH, Folsom AR, Harnack L, Halliwell B, Jacobs Jr DR. Does supplemental vitamin C increase cardiovascular disease risk in women with diabetes? Am J Clin Nutr. 2004;80:1194–200.
74. Dwyer JH, Paul-Labrador MJ, Fan J, Shircore AM, Merz CN, Dwyer KM. Progression of carotid intima-media thickness and plasma antioxidants: the Los Angeles Atherosclerosis Study. Arterioscler Thromb Vasc Biol. 2004;24:313–9.
75. Silver EW, Eskenazi B, Evenson DP, Block G, Young S, Wyrobek AJ. Effect of antioxidant intake on sperm chromatin stability in healthy nonsmoking men. J Androl. 2005;26:550–6.
76. Keskes-Ammar L, Feki-Chakroun N, Rebai T, Sahnoun Z, Ghozzi H, Hammami S, et al. Sperm oxidative stress and the effect of an oral vitamin E and selenium supplement on semen quality in infertile men. Arch Androl. 2003;49:83–94.
77. Suleiman SA, Ali ME, Zaki ZM, el-malik EM, Nasr MA. Lipid peroxidation and human sperm motility: protective role of vitamin E. J Androl. 1996;17:530–7.
78. Rolf C, Cooper TG, Yeung CH, Nieschlag E. Antioxidant treatment of patients with asthenozoospermia or moderate oligoastheozoospermia with high dose vitamin C and E: a randomized, placebo-controlled, double blinded study. Hum Reprod. 1999;14:1028–33.
79. Greco E, Iacobelli M, Rienzi L, Ubaldi F, Ferrero S, Tesarik J. Reduction of the incidence of sperm DNA fragmentation by oral antioxidant treatment. J Androl. 2005;26:349–53.
80. Greco E, Romano S, Iacobelli M, Ferrero S, Baroni E, Minasi MG, et al. ICSI in cases of sperm DNA damage: beneficial effect of oral antioxidant treatment. Hum Reprod. 2005;20:2590–4.

Chapter 19
Antioxidant Therapy for the Enhancement of Male Reproductive Health: A Critical Review of the Literature

Kelton Tremellen

Infertility is a condition that affects one in six couples, with impaired sperm quality playing a role in at least half of all cases of infertility. Of even more concern is the evidence suggesting that sperm quality has actually been decreasing over the last 50 years [1, 2], leading to more and more couples requiring expensive fertility treatments such as in vitro fertilization (IVF) and intracytoplasmic sperm injection (ICSI). This trend has prompted researchers to focus more on identifying the underlying causes of male infertility, allowing treatments to be tailored to pathology, rather than a reliance on generic "mechanical" solutions such as ICSI.

While the identifiable causes of male infertility are many and varied (reviewed in Chap. 1), oxidative stress has been identified as a very significant cause. MacLeod [3] was first to link oxidative stress with impaired sperm function when, in 1943, he published his observations that sperm cultured under conditions of high oxygen tension lost their motility, yet in vitro supplementation with the antioxidant catalase could preserve sperm motility. Since this pioneering work, there has been an exponential increase in our knowledge of how oxidative stress may impair male reproductive function and how various treatments may help combat this damage. The focus of this chapter is to critically review the evidence for use of antioxidant supplements to improve male reproductive function.

K. Tremellen, MBBS (Hons.), PhD, FRANZCOG, CREI (✉)
School of Pharmacy and Medical Sciences, University of South Australia,
Repromed, 180 Fullarton Road, Dulwich, SA 5065, Australia
e-mail: ktremellen@repromed.com.au

S.J. Parckattil and A. Agarwal (eds.), *Antioxidants in Male Infertility: A Guide for Clinicians and Researchers*, © Springer Science+Business Media New York 2013

Rationale for Antioxidant Therapy in Male Infertility

Before examining the clinical studies exploring the use of antioxidant supplements in male infertility, one should ask if there is a reasonable scientific basis behind such treatment. To assess the biological plausibility of using antioxidant therapy in the setting of male infertility, three key questions need to be considered.

- Is oxidative stress more common in the infertile population?
- Do in vitro studies suggest a mechanism whereby oxidative stress could impair male reproductive function?
- Do in vitro studies suggest that antioxidant supplementation may restore normal male reproductive function in the presence of oxidative stress?

As is evident from discussions in the preceding chapters, there does appear to be an abundance of evidence supporting the biological rationale behind the use of antioxidant supplements to treat male factor infertility. Infertile men's semen does contain higher levels of reactive oxygen species (ROS) and lower levels of protective antioxidants than fertile men, thereby placing these men's sperm at increased risk of oxidative damage. It has been estimated that between 30 and 80% of infertile men have some evidence of oxidative stress damage to their sperm, even when routine semen analysis results (concentration, motility and morphology) are within the normal WHO prescribed range [4]. Secondly, in vitro studies have confirmed that the direct application of ROS to sperm or the stimulation of sperm's own production of ROS can reduce sperm motility, membrane integrity and DNA quality, all linked with reduced male reproductive capacity. Finally, direct application of antioxidants in vitro can block the harmful effects of ROS on sperm motility and DNA integrity, confirming a causal association between oxidative stress and impaired male reproductive function. In summary, there appears to be a sound scientific rationale to the use of antioxidants to treat male infertility.

Antioxidant Therapy for the Treatment of Male Infertility

A MEDLINE search for the key words antioxidant, sperm and male infertility, combined with a manual search of references contained in several key review papers [4–6] located a total of 31 primary studies exploring the in vivo use of antioxidant supplements for the enhancement of male reproductive performance. Trials with poorly defined treatments such as the use of "general multi-vitamins" or studies that employed botanical preparations with poorly defined antioxidant action were excluded from this review.

With the existence of such a large body of evidence one would expect that definitive conclusions on the value of antioxidant supplements in the treatment of male infertility would be able to be made. Unfortunately this is not the case for several reasons. Firstly, there is a huge variation in the different types and dosages of antioxidants used in the published studies. Secondly, most of the studies are small and therefore underpowered, making meaningful analysis of differences in pregnancy outcomes with antioxidant therapy very difficult. The following discussion group together clinical studies which use a similar antioxidant treatment protocol, facilitating an assessment of which antioxidants may prove to be useful for the treatment of male infertility.

Vitamin E

Vitamin E is an essential fat soluble vitamin, with α-tocopherol being the most common form of vitamin E available in food. Vitamin E is the major chain breaking antioxidant that directly neutralizes superoxide anions, hydrogen peroxide and the hydroxyl radical. As sperm membranes contain abundant phospholipids which are prone to oxidative damage, it is believed that vitamin E plays a critical role in protecting cellular structures from damage caused by free radicals and reactive products of lipid peroxidation. Secondly, vitamin E exhibits some anti-inflammatory activity and therefore may reduce leukocyte initiated sperm oxidative stress.

The recommended dietary allowance (RDA) for vitamin E is suggested to be 15 mg (equivalent to 22.4 IU) of α-tocopherol per day for adult men, with the tolerable upper intake being suggested as 1,000 mg (1,500 IU) by the US National Institute of Health [7]. However, a meta-analysis of 19 clinical trials using long-term vitamin E supplementation in patients with chronic disease has reported that at dosages of 400 IU or greater per day, vitamin E may actually increase overall mortality compared to placebo [8]. Furthermore, it is known to inhibit platelet aggregation and has been linked with an increased risk of haemorrhagic stroke. Therefore its use in infertile men on anticoagulants or at risk of serious haemorrhagic illness is probably contraindicated.

Two studies have analysed the ability of vitamin E to decrease sperm membrane oxidative damage by measurement of sperm malondialdehyde (MDA) levels before and after vitamin E supplementation. Geva et al. [9] reported that 200 mg a day of vitamin E was able to significantly reduce MDA levels within 1 month of therapy, while Suleiman et al. [10] found that the use of 300 mg of vitamin E per day for 6 months also produced a significant drop in MDA levels. Consistent with a reduction in sperm membrane oxidative damage, two studies have also reported an improvement in in vitro sperm fertilization capacity assessed by routine insemination IVF or the use of sperm–zona binding assays [9, 11]. No study to date has analysed the ability of vitamin E monotherapy to improve sperm DNA quality.

Two small non-controlled studies of vitamin E supplementation have reported no effect on sperm count, motility or morphology [12, 13]. In addition, a well-conducted placebo-controlled trial of 3 months therapy with 600 mg of vitamin E per day reported no significant effect on sperm concentration, motility or morphology [11]. Conversely, another randomized controlled trial (RCT) using 6 months of vitamin E (300 mg/day) or placebo reported a statistically significant improvement in sperm motility, but no change in concentration or morphology [10]. However, in this last trial the "drop out" rate for patients in the placebo arm was significantly greater than that seen in the active treatment arm (20 vs. 3 patients, respectively, from a starting number of 55 patients in each study arm). This selective "drop out" from placebo raises the possibility that patients or their treating physicians became unblinded to treatment allocation during the trial, biasing the final results.

No study to date using vitamin E monotherapy for the treatment of male infertility has been adequately powered to analyse pregnancy outcomes. While some studies have reported pregnancies [10, 11], the small number of pregnancies makes clear conclusions impossible. In the Suleiman study 17% of patients allocated to vitamin E therapy achieved a live birth, compared to none in the placebo [10]. However, as previously outlined, the large "drop out" rate in the placebo arm suggests the potential for significant bias, thereby making it impossible to make firm conclusions on the value of Vitamin E to assist pregnancy in the setting of male infertility.

Vitamin C

Vitamin C (ascorbic acid) is an important water soluble antioxidant that competitively protects lipoproteins from peroxyl radical attack, while also enhancing the antioxidant activity of vitamin E by assisting in its recycling. Seminal plasma vitamin C levels are tenfold higher than serum [14], suggesting a very important protective role for vitamin C in the male reproductive tract. The RDA for vitamin C in the adult male is 75 mg, with the tolerable upper intake limit being suggested as 2,000 mg/day [7]. However, the use of high dosages of vitamin C (≥ 1 gm/day) may be harmful since at these high concentrations vitamin C can act as a pro-oxidant and may predispose to kidney stone formation [7, 15].

A small placebo-controlled randomized study of 30 infertile men allocated an equal number of participants to either placebo, 200 mg or 1,000 mg of vitamin C per day for a total of 4 weeks [16]. Both dosages of vitamin C were able to significantly increase seminal plasma vitamin C levels, with the magnitude of the increase being more significant in the 1,000 mg treated group. Sperm motility, morphology and viability all significantly improved within 1 week of vitamin C therapy. While the average sperm concentration doubled on vitamin C, this did not reach statistical significance. More critical analysis of the baseline characteristics in this study suggests that randomization may not have been successful in creating study groups that were equal. For example, at entry the percentage of abnormal sperm morphology was 45, 64 and 62% for the placebo, 200 and 1,000 mg vitamin C groups, respectively. At the end of the study the placebo group abnormal morphology was 41% and the vitamin C groups had decreased to 35 and 36%, a statistically significant decrease. Critical analysis of these results suggests that the two vitamin C group's morphology results were significantly inferior to the placebo at study entry and that following 4 weeks of vitamin C treatment these poor morphology results simply returned to levels equivalent to that seen in the placebo. This raises the possibility of selection bias or at least a "regression to the mean" spontaneous improvement in sperm morphology. Pregnancy outcomes were not reported in this trial, although, in the introduction, the authors comment that a prior unpublished pilot study had achieved a 100% pregnancy rate with vitamin C therapy ($n = 20$ patients).

A larger study that randomly allocated 75 smokers to either a placebo, 200 or 1,000 mg vitamin C per day reported significant improvements in sperm morphology in the 1,000 mg subgroup, but no significant changes in the 200 mg treated group [17]. As these men were not infertile and were not trying for pregnancy, the implications of this study for the infertile population are uncertain.

Combined Vitamin C and Vitamin E Therapy

Two excellent placebo-controlled randomized studies have examined the ability of a combination of vitamins C and E to alter sperm quality. Rolf et al. [18] reported a small RCT in which infertile patients were allocated to either placebo ($n = 16$) or 2 months treatment with 800 mg vitamin E and 1,000 mg vitamin C ($n = 15$). The inclusion criteria for this study were impaired motility, not the presence of confirmed oxidative stress. No significant difference in sperm concentration, motility or morphology was observed during therapy and no direct assessment of oxidative damage was made. Furthermore, no pregnancies were seen in either study group during the treatment period. A similar RCT using 2 months therapy with both 1,000 mg of vitamin C and E daily or placebo also found no significant changes in sperm count, motility or morphology [19]. However, this group did observe a very significant drop in sperm DNA damage. Unfortunately pregnancy outcomes were not reported in this study, but were reported for a non-controlled study using the same treatment protocol by the same clinical group [20]. In this later report, patients who had failed to have a successful pregnancy after at least one cycle of IVF and who had documented elevated levels of sperm DNA damage were given 2 months of vitamins C/E combination therapy before a further cycle of IVF treatment. A total of 76.3% of participants experienced a normalization of their sperm DNA damage and this "improved" subgroup achieved an implantation rate of 19.6%. As the study did not include a concurrent placebo control, firm conclusions on pregnancy effect are not possible.

Several small non-placebo-controlled trials have also examined the effect of vitamins C and E combinations on sperm quality. Kodama et al. [21] was able to show a significant drop in sperm DNA oxidative damage (8-OHdG) and MDA with 2 months of therapy (200 mg vitamin C, 200 mg vitamin E and 400 mg glutathione). They also reported a small but significant increase in sperm concentration, but no effect of antioxidant supplementation on sperm motility or morphology. Menezo [22] observed a significant drop in sperm DNA fragmentation with 2 months of antioxidant therapy (400 mg vitamins C and E per day, plus low dosages of vitamin A, zinc and selenium) but no change in sperm concentration, motility or morphology. Interestingly, these investigators also noted a significant increase in sperm DNA decondensation. They believed that this was due to the high redox potential of vitamin C interfering with the reduction of cystine to two cysteine moieties, thereby opening protamine disulphide bridges. Decondensation of the sperm DNA may make the DNA more susceptible to ROS attack and may interfere with proper embryo development. Menezo, therefore, cautions against the use of antioxidant preparations containing high dosages of vitamin C in infertile men with sperm decondenstation levels exceeding 20% at baseline. Finally, a small placebo-controlled study of 45 infertile men allocated to placebo, vitamin C 5 mg/vitamin E 10 mg/200 mg zinc or zinc alone observed a non-significant trend in improvement in sperm motility and a decrease in MDA in each treatment group [23]. The magnitude of improvement in MDA and motility was similar in the zinc alone group compared to those treated with zinc and vitamins C/E. This observation suggests that the low dosages of vitamins C and E used in this study are likely to be subtherapeutic, with any improvement in sperm quality more likely to reflect the action of zinc.

Overall, the high-quality placebo-controlled studies suggest that vitamins C and E do not produce significant improvements in sperm concentration, motility or morphology. The significant drop in sperm DNA damage seen in two trials [19, 22], together with observations of a drop in 8-OHdG and MDA in a non-placebo-controlled study [21] suggests that vitamins C and E can still have positive reproductive effects even if they do not alter routine sperm parameters. The ability of vitamins C and E to improve pregnancy rates is still debatable until future adequately powered studies are conducted in this area.

Coenzyme Q_{10}

Coenzyme Q_{10} is primarily concentrated in the mitochondria of the sperm mid-piece and plays an important antioxidant and energy production role in sperm. Coenzyme Q_{10} transports electrons from complexes I and II to complex III in the mitochondrial respiratory chain, leading to ATP synthesis in the mitochondrial membrane. In its reduced form (ubiquinol), coenzyme Q_{10} acts as a strong antioxidant preventing lipid peroxidation in biological membranes.

A small non-controlled study involving 38 men with male factor infertility and previous poor fertilization during IVF–ICSI therapy reported on the use of 60 mg of coenzyme Q_{10} per day for a period of 3 months [24]. This study found that coenzyme Q_{10} produced no significant changes in sperm concentration, motility or morphology, yet IVF–ICSI fertilization rates did improved significantly. This study did not measure sperm lipid peroxidation or DNA damage and offered no explanation how coenzyme Q_{10} supplementation may boost fertilization without altering routine sperm parameters.

A large and very well-conducted placebo RCT recently reported on the use of 300 mg coenzyme Q_{10} or placebo per day for a period of 6 months in 212 men with male factor infertility [25]. At this dose of supplementation a significant increase in seminal plasma coenzyme Q_{10} concentration was observed. Furthermore, significant improvements in sperm count and motility were also observed, together with an increase in serum inhibin B levels and a corresponding fall in FSH concentration. This would suggest that coenzyme Q_{10} therapy is capable of enhancing Sertoli cell function, not just sperm function. This study did not report on oxidative endpoints but did report a significant increase in the calcium ionophore induced acrosome reaction, suggesting some improvement in sperm membrane function. Unfortunately no significant difference in pregnancy rates was observed between the placebo and coenzyme Q_{10} supplement groups over a 12-month period of observation. This is not surprising when one recognizes that the magnitude of the statistically significant changes in sperm parameters observed were very small and unlikely to be of clinical significance. For example, total sperm motility after 6 months of coenzyme Q_{10} therapy was 27.6%, compared to 23.1% in the placebo group. While for the coenzyme Q_{10} group this was a statistically significant increase in sperm motility from baseline (22.2%), the final motility result was not significantly different from the placebo and highly unlikely to be of any clinical significance. As only men, who had partners with no evidence for female factor infertility, were enrolled in the study, the lack of differences in pregnancy outcomes in such a large study suggests that coenzyme Q_{10} monotherapy is not of major benefit in assisting in vivo conception.

Selenium

Selenium is an essential trace element required for normal male reproductive function. The antioxidant glutathione peroxidase 4 (GPX-4) is present within sperm and requires the presence of selenium to function. Not only does GPX-4 play an antioxidant role, it is also involved in augmenting sperm chromatin stability by acting as a protein thiol peroxidase. The adult male RDA for selenium is 55 µg/day, with the upper tolerable limit being 400 µg/day [7]. An individual's dietary intake of selenium depends on the selenium content in the local soil where food is grown. Men living in countries such as China where the soil is commonly selenium deficient are more likely to benefit from selenium supplementation. Conversely, excess supplementation of selenium may lead to toxicity and have detrimental effects on sperm quality [26].

Iwanier et al. [27] gave 200 µg of selenium per day to a group of men (33 infertile and 9 fertile) for a period of 2 months and measured sperm quality before and after treatment. The investigators observed a significant increase in seminal plasma selenium concentration and GPX activity during the trial, but no significant improvement in sperm concentration, motility or morphology. In a small placebo RCT ($n = 18$ placebo, 46 active treatment) the supplementation of infertile men exhibiting low sperm motility with 100 µg of selenium (+/− very low dosages of vitamins A, C and E) produced no significant change in sperm concentration but a small significant improvement in motility (20.6–28.2%) [28]. The clinical significance of this improvement is questionable, as no significant difference in pregnancy rates was observed (no pregnancies in the placebo vs. 11% selenium group).

A very large placebo-controlled study randomized 468 infertile men to either placebo, 200 µg/day of selenium, with or without *N*-acetyl-cysteine, for a period of 6 months [29]. Sperm quality and male reproductive hormones were then assessed during supplementation and for a further 6 months. This study observed statistically significant increases in sperm concentration, motility and morphology in all treatment arms, together with an increase in serum inhibin B and testosterone. However, the magnitude of these improvements was again very small and unlikely to be of any clinical significance. Unfortunately pregnancy outcomes were not reported for this study, making it impossible to draw any firm conclusions on the benefits of selenium supplementation to boost pregnancy rates.

Glutathione

Glutathione is an antioxidant released in large amounts by the epididymis that in turn can neutralize the damaging effects of superoxide anions, thereby preventing lipid peroxidation. Two trials by a single group of investigators have examined the effect of glutathione supplementation (600 µg intramuscular alternate days for 2 months) on two separate groups of infertile men. The first trial involved 20 infertile men with likely oxidative stress (past genitourinary tract infection with residual inflammation, varicocele) in a placebo crossover trial design [30]. This study observed no significant changes in sperm concentration, but significant improvements in sperm motility and morphology. These improvements were observed within 1 month of supplementation, suggesting an epididymal rather than a testicular mode of action. A second smaller non-controlled study using identical inclusion criteria examined changes in sperm lipid peroxidation with glutathione treatment [31]. This study observed improvement in all routine sperm parameters and a significant decrease in sperm MDA concentration, confirming an antioxidant effect. Neither study reported pregnancy outcome, making conclusions about the fertility promoting effect of glutathione treatment impossible. However, the requirement for intramuscular administration of glutathione therapy is certainly likely to limit its clinical application.

L-Carnitine

Carnitine is produced in the liver and then passes via the circulation to the epididymis, where it is taken up by the epididymal epithelium and actively transported into the luminal fluid bathing sperm. In the epididymis carnitine is taken up by sperm, where it involves in energy metabolism by transporting fatty acids from the cytosolic compartment to the mitochondrial matrix.

Costa et al. [32] were the first to examine the effects of L-carnitine supplementation in the setting of male infertility. Their study group of 100 infertile men with unexplained impaired motility were given L-carnitine (3 g/day) for a period of 4 months, while measuring changes in sperm function. They reported small but statistically significant improvements in sperm concentration and motility, but no changes in sperm morphology. Lenzi et al. [33] used an active medication/washout/placebo study design to determine if 2 months of L-carnitine therapy (2 g/day) could alter sperm quality. Analysis of the raw outcome data indicated no significant difference in sperm quality after L-carnitine therapy. However, when the researchers excluded several "outliers" from the analysis a borderline statistically significant increase in sperm concentration and motility was reported. The subjective removal of "outliers" to create statistical significance, plus the failure of L-carnitine therapy to improve either epididymal function (alpha-glucosidase) or reduce levels of sperm lipid peroxidation casts significant doubt on whether L-carnitine therapy has any beneficial effect on male reproductive performance.

Vicari et al. [34] studied the ability of L-carnitine in combination with non-steroidal inflammatory medication (NSAID) to alter sperm function in a group of 98 infertile men with confirmed oxidative stress. The use of 2 months pre-treatment with NSAIDs, followed by 2 months of L-carnitine (2 g/day) produced a significant reduction in seminal ROS production and an improvement in sperm motility and viability. A total of 23% of patients on NSAID/L-carnitine therapies achieved pregnancy, but the absence of a control group makes firm conclusions on these therapies effect on pregnancy rates impossible.

N-Acetyl Cysteine

N-acetyl cysteine (NAC) is believed to act as a precursor to glutathione, increasing the tissue concentration of this potent antioxidant. Recently, several good quality placebo-controlled studies have examined the ability of NAC to alter sperm quality in infertile men with presumed oxidative pathology. Galatioto et al. [35] conducted a RCT in which 42 men with oligospermia were allocated to receive either 600 mg NAC a day plus a vitamin–mineral supplement for 3 months or no therapy at all. This small study reported a significant increase in sperm concentration but no change in sperm motility or morphology. A larger placebo-controlled study using 600 mg/day of NAC for a period of 3 months reported no change in sperm concentration or morphology, but a small improvement in motility [36]. Finally, one arm of a multi-therapy RCT compared sperm quality between men with idiopathic male factor infertility on 600 mg NAC per day with placebo [29]. This study reported very minor, although statistically significant, improvements in sperm concentration and morphology but no changes in sperm motility.

The conflicting sperm quality outcomes for these three trials using an identical dose of NAC, and the failure to report pregnancy outcomes makes it impossible to conclude that NAC therapy has any clinically meaningful effect on male reproductive performance.

Miscellaneous Antioxidant Monotherapies

Astaxanthin is a carotenoid extract from the algae *Haematococcus pluvialis* with reported potent antioxidant qualities. A small placebo-controlled RCT reported on the effect of 3 months therapy with this antioxidant in men with idiopathic male factor infertility [37]. Astaxanthin produced no change in sperm concentration or morphology but did produce a significant reduction in seminal ROS levels and improvement in sperm motility. Furthermore, the researchers observed a significant increase in natural or intrauterine insemination-assisted conceptions in the antioxidant-treated group, suggesting that the small improvement in sperm motility was of clinical significance.

Lycopene, an antioxidant found in high concentrations in fruits such as tomatoes and watermelon is a powerful natural antioxidant. A non-controlled trial of 30 men with male factor infertility reported a significant improvement in sperm quality with 3 months of lycopene therapy at a dose of 4 mg/day [38]. However, upon further analysis of this study, it appears that the researchers only analysed sperm outcomes for the 14–20 men who showed an improvement in either sperm concentration, motility or morphology. Such an analysis is obviously flawed since excluding half the study participants who did not respond to treatment is clearly going to result in a significant difference being concluded. Therefore, this study provides no scientific support for the use of lycopene in male factor infertility.

Combination Therapies

The combination of vitamins C and E would appear to be the most commonly studied combinational antioxidant therapies for male factor infertility. However, other unique combinations have been trialled in the hope that using several different antioxidants with different modes of action may be more beneficial than antioxidant monotherapy.

The combination of vitamin E (400 mg/day) and selenium (225 µg/day) has been trialled in a placebo-controlled study of 54 men with male factor infertility [39]. Antioxidant therapy produced a small increase in sperm mobility and a drop in sperm MDA levels, confirming an antioxidant effect. No changes in sperm concentration or morphology were observed, and pregnancy outcomes were not reported. A significant weakness in this study was that out of a total of 54 initial participants, only 20 completed the study. This raises the possibility of bias and makes firm conclusions difficult.

Piomboni et al. [40] performed a controlled study comparing 3 months therapy with an antioxidant combination (β-glucan 20 mg, papaya 50 mg, lactoferrin 97 mg, vitamin C 30 mg, vitamin E 5 mg) or no therapy. They observed a significant improvement in sperm motility, viability and morphology, but no change in sperm DNA quality. Pregnancy outcomes were not reported in this study.

A small uncontrolled study of 33 men reported on the use of a combination of 600 mg NAC, 30 mg β-carotene, 180 mg vitamin E and a mixture of essential fatty acids for a period of 6 months as treatment for male factor infertility [41]. This combination produced no change in sperm concentration, motility or morphology, but a drop in seminal ROS levels and sperm DNA oxidative damage (8-OHdG) was observed, together with an increase in the ionophore induce acrosome reaction. A total off 22.2% of couples who completed the 6-month therapy did successfully conceive, but the absence of a control arm makes it impossible to determine if this is a clinical improvement above non-treatment levels.

A small case series reported on the success of using a combinational antioxidant (β-carotene 5,000 IU, vitamin C 60 mg, vitamin E 30 IU, zinc 15 mg) for the treatment of early embryo loss related to sperm oxidative damage [42]. Out of 17 men screened, 9 men were confirmed to have oxidative stress-related sperm pathology which could be amenable to antioxidant therapy. In six of these nine cases the partners subsequently fell pregnant. When antioxidants had been taken by the male before conception all pregnancies were viable ($n = 4$), whereas all the pregnancies conceived by men who refused antioxidant therapy miscarried. Such a small case series precludes definitive conclusions, yet does suggest that oxidative pathology may be a significant cause of early pregnancy wastage.

One of the most widely studied combinational antioxidants in the field of male infertility is Menevit®. This preparation consists of a combination of several natural antioxidants (vitamin C 100 mg, vitamin E 400 IU, lycopene 6 mg, selenium 26 μg, garlic oil 333 μg) and other ingredients involved in sperm DNA synthesis and packaging (zinc 25 mg, folate 500 mg). Three-month therapy with the Menevit® antioxidant has been reported to produce no significant change in sperm concentration, motility or morphology, but did produce a significant reduction in seminal ROS levels and sperm DNA fragmentation [43]. Interestingly, while a dose of 400 mg of vitamin C has been shown to produce sperm chromatin decondensation by interfering with protamine disulphide bonds [22], the Menevit® antioxidant containing one-quarter the dose of vitamin C has been reported to significantly increase sperm DNA protamination [43]. The Menevit® antioxidant has also been shown to improve pregnancy outcomes when compared with placebo in a RCT of 60 patients undergoing IVF–ICSI treatment [44]. Finally, recent preliminary studies have linked male infertility and sperm oxidative stress with impaired sperm DNA methylation, a possible risk factor for epigenetic disease in the next generation [45]. The treatment of infertile men with 3 months of Menevit® resulted in an improvement in the levels of sperm global DNA methylation [45]. This pilot study will require replication, and large epidemiological studies will need to confirm the link between sperm DNA methylation defects and childhood illness before definitive conclusions can be made regarding the utility of antioxidant supplements to prevent epigenetic disease in the next generation.

Overview of Common Methodological Weaknesses in Antioxidant Trials

Before making a final conclusion on the value of antioxidant therapy to enhance male reproductive function, a brief overview of the common methodological flaws in the previously described studies is warranted. Table 19.1 summarizes the methodological strengths and weaknesses of the placebo-controlled antioxidant trials and should allow the reader to make their own conclusions on the merits of antioxidant supplement therapy for the treatment of male infertility.

Lack of Appropriate Inclusion Criteria

It is obvious that only infertile men experiencing oxidative stress are likely to benefit from antioxidant therapy. Despite this, the vast majority of studies do not actually screen potential study participants for oxidative stress before enrolling only those with confirmed oxidative pathology. If we assume that only half of all infertile men have significant oxidative stress, the indiscriminate enrolment of all infertile men will result in half of the study participants having no significant oxidative pathology and no real chance of improvement in sperm function on antioxidant therapy. This will of course weaken the study power and increase the chance of missing a true biological effect of antioxidant supplementation.

Lack of an Appropriate Control

The most common study design in the field of antioxidant therapy is where patients act as their own historical control, with comparison of sperm quality or pregnancy outcomes before and after antioxidant therapy. While these studies are easy to conduct, they can be fraught with significant bias that can invalidate the study outcomes. One common bias is the so-called regression to the mean phenomenon. When study participants are selected for enrolment in a study by the presence of a single extreme sperm result (e.g., rapidly progressive motility < 25%), there is a natural tendency for the results to normalize on retesting with no active treatment. Sperm parameters such as concentration and motility are prone to large day-to-day intra-individual fluctuations and, therefore, are especially susceptible to this regression to the mean bias. Any study that reports an improvement in sperm motility or concentration when deficiencies in either were used as inclusion criteria for entry into the study has the potential to be biased by regression to the mean. More stable sperm parameters such as morphology and sperm DNA integrity are less prone to this type of bias due to their minimal intra-individual day-to-day variation and may be studied adequately using patients own historical controls.

Table 19.1 Placebo controlled studies examining the effect of antioxidant therapy on male reproductive heath

Study reference	Therapy used per day	Duration of therapy (months)	Oxidative stress as an inclusion criteria	Positive changes in semen quality	Positive changes in sperm OS endpoints	Positive changes in reproductive outcomes
[10]	Vitamin E 300 mg	6	No	↑ motility	↓ MDA	Pregnancy 17% active group vs. 0% placebo
[11]	Vitamin E 300 mg	3	No	Nil	Nil	Improved sperm zona binding
[16]	Vitamin C (200 or 1,000 mg)	1	No	↑ motility, morph and viability	Not tested	Not reported
[18]	Vit E 800 mg, Vit C 1,000 mg	2	No	Nil	Not tested	None
[19]	Vitamin E and C (1,000 mg each)	2	No	Nil	↓ sperm DNA damage	Not reported
[23]	Vit E 10 mg, Vit C 5 mg, zinc 200 mg	3	No	Nil	Trend for ↓ MDA	Not reported
[25]	Coenzyme Q_{10} 300 mg	6	No	↑ conc and motility	Not tested	No difference in pregnancy rates
[28]	Sn 100 µg, Vit A 1 mg, Vit C 10 mg, Vit E 15 mg	3	No	↑ motility	Not tested	No difference in pregnancy rates (11% vs. 0% placebo)
[29]	Sn 200 µg, NAC 600 mg	6	No	↑ conc, motility and morph.	Not tested	Not reported
[30]	Glutathione 600 mg	2	No	↑ motility and morph	Not tested	Not reported
[33]	L-carnitine 2 g	2	No	Nil (raw data analysis)	No change in MDA	No difference
[35]	NAC 600 mg	3	No	↑ sperm conc	Not tested	Not reported
[36]	NAC 600 mg	3	No	↑ motility	Not tested	Not reported
[37]	Astaxanthin 16 mg	3	No	↑ motility	↓ semen ROS	↑ natural + IUI conceptions
[39]	Vitamin E 400 mg, Sn 225 µg	3	No	↑ motility	↓ MDA	Not reported
[40]	Vit C 30 mg, Vit E 5 mg, β-glucan 20 mg, papaya 50 mg, lactoferrin 97 mg	3	No	↑ motility and morph	No change in DNA quality	Not reported
[44]	Menevit® (Vit C, Vit E, Sn, lycopene, folate, zinc and garlic oil)	3	No	Not reported	Not tested	↑ IVF–ICSI conceptions on active antioxidant (38.5% vs. 16% placebo)

OS oxidative stress, *MDA* malondialdehyde, *ROS* reactive oxygen species, *Sn* selenium, *NAC* N-acetyl cysteine, *IUI* intrauterine insemination

Insufficient Sample Size

Unfortunately, the majority of studies examining the effect of antioxidant supplements are relatively small, most containing less than 100 subjects in total. Such small underpowered studies predispose to type II statistical errors where the null hypothesis is not rejected (i.e., no statistical significant difference), despite a true biological effect of treatment being present. For relatively low-probability outcomes such as pregnancy in an infertile cohort, very large sample sizes are required to reach statistical significance. Only large multi-centre studies or a meta-analysis of many similar studies can negate this size weakness and allow for true biological effects of antioxidant therapy to become apparent.

Inappropriate Study Endpoints

Due to their ease of measurement, the majority of male infertility antioxidant studies use sperm parameters such as count, motility and morphology as their primary study endpoint. While this approach has some scientific merit, there are major drawbacks from this approach. Firstly, infertile men are not primarily interested in improving their sperm quality. They and their partner wish to have a child and, therefore, the only clinically relevant primary endpoint should be live birth, not sperm quality. Secondly, the presence of a statistically significant improvement in sperm count, motility and morphology may not have any clinical significance in regard to fertility potential. The link between routine sperm parameters and fertility potential is relatively weak until sperm quality reaches low levels. For example, the ability of an antioxidant therapy to improve average sperm concentration from 40 to 45 million/ml is not likely to be clinically relevant, even if statistical significance has been reached.

Expert Commentary

The current evidence clearly identifies oxidative stress as a cause of impaired sperm function and a significant underlying pathology in many cases of male factor infertility. While many studies have been conducted examining the ability of various antioxidants to improve male reproductive function, it is still unclear if male preconception antioxidant therapy can actually improve a couples chances of becoming parents. Critical analysis of the various higher quality trials suggest that a combination of vitamins C and E can produce a reduction in sperm membrane and DNA oxidation, an increase in sperm IVF capacity but no clinically meaningful improvements in sperm concentration, motility and morphology. The ability of vitamins C and E to boost natural conception is questionable, but may assist in vitro conception. The use of a supplement exceeding 400 IU of vitamin E or 1,000 mg of vitamin C per day is probably not advisable, due to potential general health concerns and the ability of high dose vitamin C to produce sperm DNA decondensation. The addition of other antioxidants such as selenium, lycopene and astaxanthin to a combination of vitamins C and E antioxidant therapy has some possible additional benefit as these ingredients have also been shown to produce meaningful decreases in sperm oxidative damage and improvement in natural and assisted conception. However, evidence supporting the use of other antioxidants such as coenzyme Q_{10}, glutathione, L-carnitine and NAC as effective therapies for male infertility is presently weak.

Five-Year View

Before pre-conception antioxidant therapy becomes routine medical care for the infertile couple, three main issues need to be addressed. Firstly, the present diagnostic tests for oxidative stress are cumbersome and expensive and therefore not available in the majority of infertility clinics. Without the availability of a "quick and easy" test for oxidative stress, many doctors are unwilling to offer empirical antioxidant therapy. Future studies aimed at developing such assays for sperm oxidative stress are urgently required. Secondly, there is a pressing need for large multi-centre trials using a single antioxidant combination therapy to confirm that pre-conception supplementation can boost live birth rates. Without such a definitive trial, antioxidant therapy will be relegated to the "promising but never proven" basket of medical treatments, never receiving widespread medical support. Finally, research suggests that oxidative damage to sperm DNA may result in miscarriage and possibly even affect the health of the next generation [46, 47]. If such inter-generational effects of sperm oxidative damage are confirmed, pre-conception antioxidant supplementation for the male will become standard medical practice, just as pre-conception folate supplementation for the prevention of neural tube defects is standard care for women. If these three goals can be realized, the next 5 years promise to be a very exciting time for the discipline of andrology.

Key Issues

- Oxidative stress is a significant cause of impaired sperm function resulting in infertility, miscarriage and possibly even long-term health consequences for the next generation.
- The present body of evidence surrounding the treatment of male factor infertility with antioxidants is difficult to critically interpret because of less than ideal study design (not screening for oxidative stress at enrolment, sperm quality as a primary endpoint instead of pregnancy and a lack of concurrent placebo controls).

Furthermore, the use of a large number of different types and dosages of antioxidant and the lack of adequately powered studies to analyse pregnancy outcomes precludes definitive conclusions being made.

- Antioxidants such as vitamin E, vitamin C, selenium, lycopene and astaxanthin all appear to have the ability to improve sperm health by reducing seminal ROS levels, decreasing sperm membrane peroxidation and oxidative DNA damage. Furthermore, there is some evidence that these antioxidants may also result in improved natural and in vitro conception.
- Firm conclusions relating to antioxidant therapies ability to improve sperm concentration, motility and morphology is presently impossible due to the abundance of contradictory results and inadequately controlled studies. However, an analysis of the better quality placebo-controlled studies suggests that antioxidants may produce a small improvement in sperm motility but are unlikely to improve sperm concentration or morphology.
- Future studies must use confirmed oxidative stress-related damage to sperm as their inclusion criteria and should have pregnancy outcome as their primary endpoint. These studies must be adequately powered to detect meaningful improvements in pregnancy rates.

References

1. Carlsen E, Giwercman A, Keiding N, Skakkebaek NE. Evidence for decreasing quality of semen during past 50 years. BMJ. 1992;305(6854):609–13.
2. Auger J, Kunstmann JM, Czyglik F, Jouannet P. Decline in semen quality among fertile men in Paris during the past 20 years. N Engl J Med. 1995;332(5):281–5.
3. MacLeod J. The role of oxygen in the metabolism and motility of human spermatozoa. Am J Physiol. 1943;138:512–8.
4. Tremellen K. Oxidative stress and male infertility—a clinical perspective. Hum Reprod Update. 2008;14(3):243–58.
5. Agarwal A, Nallella KP, Allamaneni SS, Said TM. Role of antioxidants in treatment of male infertility: an overview of the literature. Reprod Biomed Online. 2004;8(6):616–27.
6. Lanzafame FM, La Vignera S, Vicari E, Calogero AE. Oxidative stress and medical antioxidant treatment in male infertility. Reprod Biomed Online. 2009;19(5):638–59.
7. Panel of Dietary Antioxidants and Related Compounds, Food and Nutrition Board, Institute of Medicine. Dietary reference intakes for vitamin C, vitamin E, selenium and crotenoids. Washington, DC: National Academy Press; 2000.
8. Miller 3rd ER, Pastor-Barriuso R, Dalal D, Riemersma RA, Appel LJ, Guallar E. Meta-analysis: high-dosage vitamin E supplementation may increase all-cause mortality. Ann Intern Med. 2005;142(1):37–46.
9. Geva E, Bartoov B, Zabludovsky N, Lessing JB, Lerner-Geva L, Amit A. The effect of antioxidant treatment on human spermatozoa and fertilization rate in an in vitro fertilization program. Fertil Steril. 1996;66(3):430–4.
10. Suleiman SA, Ali ME, Zaki ZM, el-Malik EM, Nasr MA. Lipid peroxidation and human sperm motility: protective role of vitamin E. J Androl. 1996;17(5):530–7.
11. Kessopoulou E, Powers HJ, Sharma KK, Pearson MJ, Russell JM, Cooke ID, Barratt CL. A double-blind randomized placebo cross-over controlled trial using the antioxidant vitamin E to treat reactive oxygen species associated male infertility. Fertil Steril. 1995;64(4):825–31.

12. Moilanen J, Hovatta O. Excretion of alpha-tocopherol into human seminal plasma after oral administration. Andrologia. 1995;27(3):133–6.
13. Giovenco P, Amodei M, Barbieri C, Fasani R, Carosi M, Dondero F. Effects of kallikrein on the male reproductive system and its use in the treatment of idiopathic oligozoospermia with impaired motility. Andrologia. 1987;19:238–41.
14. Jacob RA, Pianalto FS, Agee RE. Cellular ascorbate depletion in healthy men. J Nutr. 1992;122(5):1111–8.
15. Wayner DD, Burton GW, Ingold KU. The antioxidant efficiency of vitamin C is concentration-dependent. Biochim Biophys Acta. 1986;884(1):119–23.
16. Dawson EB, Harris WA, Rankin WE, Charpentier LA, McGanity WJ. Effect of ascorbic acid on male fertility. Ann N Y Acad Sci. 1987;498:312–23.
17. Dawson EB, Harris WA, Teter MC, Powell LC. Effect of ascorbic acid supplementation on the sperm quality of smokers. Fertil Steril. 1992;58(5):1034–9.
18. Rolf C, Cooper TG, Yeung CH, Nieschlag E. Antioxidant treatment of patients with asthenozoospermia or moderate oligoasthenozoospermia with high-dose vitamin C and vitamin E: a randomized, placebo-controlled, double-blind study. Hum Reprod. 1999;14(4):1028–33.
19. Greco E, Iacobelli M, Rienzi L, Ubaldi F, Ferrero S, Tesarik J. Reduction of the incidence of sperm DNA fragmentation by oral antioxidant treatment. J Androl. 2005;26(3):349–53.
20. Greco E, Romano S, Iacobelli M, Ferrero S, Baroni E, Minasi MG, Ubaldi F, Rienzi L, Tesarik J. ICSI in cases of sperm DNA damage: beneficial effect of oral antioxidant treatment. Hum Reprod. 2005;20(9):2590–4.
21. Kodama H, Yamaguchi R, Fukuda J, Kasai H, Tanaka T. Increased oxidative deoxyribonucleic acid damage in the spermatozoa of infertile male patients. Fertil Steril. 1997;68(3):519–24.
22. Ménézo YJ, Hazout A, Panteix G, Robert F, Rollet J, Cohen-Bacrie P, Chapuis F, Clément P, Benkhalifa M. Antioxidants to reduce sperm DNA fragmentation: an unexpected adverse effect. Reprod Biomed Online. 2007;14(4):418–21.
23. Omu AE, Al-Azemi MK, Kehinde EO, Anim JT, Oriowo MA, Mathew TC. Indications of the mechanisms involved in improved sperm parameters by zinc therapy. Med Princ Pract. 2008; 17(2):108–16.
24. Lewin A, Lavon H. The effect of coenzyme Q_{10} on sperm motility and function. Mol Aspects Med. 1997;18(Suppl):S213–9.
25. Safarinejad MR. Efficacy of coenzyme Q_{10} on semen parameters, sperm function and reproductive hormones in infertile men. J Urol. 2009;182(1):237–48.
26. Bleau G, Lemarbre J, Faucher G, Roberts KD, Chapdelaine A. Semen selenium and human fertility. Fertil Steril. 1984;42(6):890–4.
27. Iwanier K, Zachara BA. Selenium supplementation enhances the element concentration in blood and seminal fluid but does not change the spermatozoal quality characteristics in subfertile men. J Androl. 1995;16(5):441–7.
28. Scott R, MacPherson A, Yates RW, Hussain B, Dixon J. The effect of oral selenium supplementation on human sperm motility. Br J Urol. 1998;82(1):76–80.
29. Safarinejad MR, Safarinejad S. Efficacy of selenium and/or N-acetyl-cysteine for improving semen parameters in infertile men: a double-blind, placebo controlled, randomized study. J Urol. 2009;181(2):741–51.
30. Lenzi A, Culasso F, Gandini L, Lombardo F, Dondero F. Placebo-controlled, double-blind, cross-over trial of glutathione therapy in male infertility. Hum Reprod. 1993;8(10):1657–62.
31. Lenzi A, Picardo M, Gandini L, Lombardo F, Terminali O, Passi S, Dondero F. Glutathione treatment of dyspermia: effect on the lipoperoxidation process. Hum Reprod. 1994;9(11):2044–50.
32. Costa M, Canale D, Filicori M, D'Iddio S, Lenzi A. L-carnitine in idiopathic asthenozoospermia: a multicenter study. Italian Study Group on Carnitine and Male Infertility. Andrologia. 1994;26(3):155–9.
33. Lenzi A, Lombardo F, Sgrò P, Salacone P, Caponecchia L, Dondero F, Gandini L. Use of carnitine therapy in selected cases of male factor infertility: a double-blind crossover trial. Fertil Steril. 2003;79(2):292–300.

34. Vicari E, La Vignera S, Calogero AE. Antioxidant treatment with carnitines is effective in infertile patients with prostatovesiculoepididymitis and elevated seminal leukocyte concentrations after treatment with nonsteroidal anti-inflammatory compounds. Fertil Steril. 2002;78(6):1203–8.
35. Paradiso Galatioto G, Gravina GL, Angelozzi G, Sacchetti A, Innominato PF, Pace G, Ranieri G, Vicentini C. May antioxidant therapy improve sperm parameters of men with persistent oligospermia after retrograde embolization for varicocele? World J Urol. 2008;26(1):97–102.
36. Ciftci H, Verit A, Savas M, Yeni E, Erel O. Effects of *N*-acetylcysteine on semen parameters and oxidative/antioxidant status. Urology. 2009;74(1):73–6.
37. Comhaire FH, El Garem Y, Mahmoud A, Eertmans F, Schoonjans F. Combined conventional/antioxidant "Astaxanthin" treatment for male infertility: a double blind, randomized trial. Asian J Androl. 2005;7(3):257–62.
38. Gupta NP, Kumar R. Lycopene therapy in idiopathic male infertility—a preliminary report. Int Urol Nephrol. 2002;34(3):369–72.
39. Keskes-Ammar L, Feki-Chakroun N, Rebai T, Sahnoun Z, Ghozzi H, Hammami S, Zghal K, Fki H, Damak J, Bahloul A. Sperm oxidative stress and the effect of an oral vitamin E and selenium supplement on semen quality in infertile men. Arch Androl. 2003;49(2):83–94.
40. Piomboni P, Gambera L, Serafini F, Campanella G, Morgante G, De Leo V. Sperm quality improvement after natural anti-oxidant treatment of asthenoteratospermic men with leukocytospermia. Asian J Androl. 2008;10(2):201–6.
41. Comhaire FH, Christophe AB, Zalata AA, Dhooge WS, Mahmoud AM, Depuydt CE. The effects of combined conventional treatment, oral antioxidants and essential fatty acids on sperm biology in subfertile men. Prostaglandins Leukot Essent Fatty Acids. 2000;63(3):159–65.
42. Gil-Villa AM, Cardona-Maya W, Agarwal A, Sharma R, Cadavid A. Role of male factor in early recurrent embryo loss: do antioxidants have any effect? Fertil Steril. 2009;92(2):565–71.
43. Tunc O, Thompson J, Tremellen K. Improvement in sperm DNA quality using an oral antioxidant therapy. Reprod Biomed Online. 2009;18(6):761–8.
44. Tremellen K, Miari G, Froiland D, Thompson J. A randomised control trial examining the effect of an antioxidant (Menevit) on pregnancy outcome during IVF-ICSI treatment. Aust N Z J Obstet Gynaecol. 2007;47(3):216–21.
45. Tunc O, Tremellen K. Oxidative DNA damage impairs global sperm DNA methylation in infertile men. J Assist Reprod Genet. 2009;26(9–10):537–44.
46. Zini A, Boman JM, Belzile E, Ciampi A. Sperm DNA damage is associated with an increased risk of pregnancy loss after IVF and ICSI: systematic review and meta-analysis. Hum Reprod. 2008;23(12):2663–8.
47. Aitken RJ, Koopman P, Lewis SE. Seeds of concern. Nature. 2004;432(7013):48–52.

Chapter 20
In Vitro Studies of Antioxidants for Male Reproductive Health

Armand Zini and Maria San Gabriel

The detrimental effects of oxidants on spermatozoa were suggested close to 70 years ago with the demonstration that oxygen is sperm toxic. Later studies confirmed the susceptibility of spermatozoa to oxidative stress and the fact that human spermatozoa and semen leukocytes can generate reactive oxygen species (ROS). These observations have led to studies on the role of antioxidants in protecting spermatozoa from oxidative stress in vitro.

The purpose of this chapter is to discuss the rationale for antioxidant therapy in male infertility and evaluate the data on the efficacy of in vitro antioxidant preparations on sperm function. A review of the literature demonstrates a beneficial effect of in vitro antioxidants in protecting spermatozoa from exogenous oxidants and cryopreservation (and subsequent thawing). However, the protective effect of in vitro antioxidants on sperm preparations subjected to endogenous ROS and gentle sperm processing has not been established.

Reactive Oxygen Species and Male Infertility

The relationship between seminal ROS and male infertility is the basis for proposing treatment with antioxidants in these men [1, 2]. High levels of ROS have been detected in the semen of 25% of infertile men but not in the semen of fertile men [3, 4]. Semen ROS levels are inversely related to the probability of achieving a

A. Zini, MD (✉)
Department of Surgery, St. Mary's Hospital,
3830 Lacombe Avenue, Room B270, Montreal, QC, Canada, H3T 1M5
e-mail: ziniarmand@yahoo.com

M. San Gabriel, PhD
Division of Urology, Department of Surgery, Royal Victoria Hospital,
McGill University, Montreal, QC, Canada, H3A 1A1

S.J. Parckattil and A. Agarwal (eds.), *Antioxidants in Male Infertility: A Guide for Clinicians and Researchers*, © Springer Science+Business Media New York 2013

spontaneous pregnancy [5]. Moreover, the levels of sperm DNA oxidation (a marker of oxidative stress) are higher in infertile men compared with fertile men [6, 7]. Semen ROS are generated by spermatozoa (especially, defective or immature) and semen leukocytes [8–12].

In contrast to the pathologic effects of excess ROS production, small amounts of ROS may be necessary for the initiation of critical sperm functions, including capacitation and the acrosome reaction [13–15]. Therefore, there is a finely tuned balance between ROS scavenging and low, physiologic levels of ROS that are necessary for normal sperm function and maturation.

The susceptibility of human spermatozoa to oxidative stress stems primarily from the abundance of unsaturated fatty acids localized within the sperm plasma membrane. These fatty acids provide fluidity necessary for membrane fusion events, such as the acrosome reaction and sperm–egg interaction, and for sperm motility. However, the unsaturated nature of these fatty acids predisposes them to oxidative stress and lipid peroxidation. Once the lipid peroxidation cascade has been initiated, sperm dysfunction (e.g., loss of motility) ensues as a result of accumulation of lipid peroxides on the sperm membrane, depletion of ATP, and oxidative damage to the DNA [16–19]. It has been shown that ROS can cause damage to the sperm DNA, directly or indirectly via production and subsequent translocation of lipid peroxides [19–22].

Semen Antioxidants and Sperm Function

Seminal fluid is an important source of antioxidants (both enzymatic and nonenzymatic) that can protect spermatozoa from oxidative injury [4, 23, 24]. This feature of seminal plasma is of critical importance in view of the inherent susceptibility of spermatozoa to oxidative stress and also because spermatozoa themselves have little cytoplasmic fluid and minimal antioxidant capacity [4]. There are several endogenous antioxidant enzymes in the male reproductive tract and in seminal fluid: superoxide dismutase (SOD), catalase, and glutathione peroxidase (GPX) [4, 23, 25–28]. Moreover, there are several small, nonenzymatic antioxidants (e.g., vitamins C and E, hypotaurine, taurine, L-carnitine, and lycopene) in semen and, in fact, this nonenzymatic fraction represents most of the total seminal antioxidant activity [4, 29].

A number of investigators have proposed that oxidative sperm dysfunction may be secondary to reduced semen antioxidant capacity. However, clinical studies have reported conflicting results in this respect. Several studies have found that seminal antioxidant activity is reduced in infertile men with high levels of seminal ROS (relative to those with normal levels of ROS), whereas others have not shown this [4, 30–32]. Studies have also reported that a deficiency in semen antioxidants is related to sperm dysfunction (including DNA damage), whereas other studies have not observed this relationship [17, 33–37].

There is no evidence to suggest that male infertility is caused by systemic antioxidant or vitamin deficiency. Silver et al. evaluated a group of fertile men and did not identify any relationships between dietary antioxidant intake (vitamins C, E, or β-carotene) and sperm DNA damage [38]. Nonetheless, it is very likely that a subgroup of infertile men may have specific antioxidant deficiency, particularly, vitamin C deficiency [35, 39, 40]. Moreover, infertile men with various lifestyles (smoking, excessive alcohol intake, and dieting) may also be at high risk for antioxidant or vitamin deficiency [41, 42].

In Vitro Antioxidants in Male Infertility

Several studies have examined the role of in vitro antioxidant supplementation in protecting spermatozoa from oxidative injury and resulting sperm dysfunction (i.e., loss of motility and viability). This is clinically relevant as sperm washing is routinely performed prior to ARTs (e.g., intrauterine insemination and in vitro fertilization) and the process may result in the generation of ROS with ensuing sperm dysfunction [43]. During semen processing, spermatozoa are particularly vulnerable to oxidative stress because seminal plasma (rich in antioxidants) has been removed in the process [44, 45]. For assisted reproductive techniques that require the use of spermatozoa with progressive motility (e.g., IUI and IVF), minimizing sperm dysfunction during semen processing is critical for fertilization and subsequent pregnancy.

Recently, a number of studies have examined the role of in vitro antioxidant supplementation in protecting the sperm DNA from oxidative damage because of the concern that unrepaired oxidative sperm DNA damage may be transmitted to the offspring when used in the context of ARTs (e.g., intrauterine insemination and in vitro fertilization) [46]. However, it is important to note that subpopulations of spermatozoa will exhibit variable susceptibility to oxidative stress: the DNA of normal spermatozoa is reportedly less susceptible to gentle processing techniques than the DNA of abnormal or immature spermatozoa [10, 47]. It is likely that the susceptibility of the sperm DNA to oxidative injury is related to the degree of sperm chromatin compaction (i.e., level of protamination) [48, 49]. Experimental (animal) studies suggest that the spermatozoa of infertile men may be more susceptible to oxidative injury in vitro but benefit more so from antioxidants than the spermatozoa of fertile men [50].

Role of In Vitro Antioxidants in Protecting Spermatozoa from Exogenous Reactive Oxygen Species

This is of clinical relevance as many of the semen samples contain leukocytes and these cells have the potential to generate exogenous ROS [51]. Antioxidants such as vitamin E, catalase, and glutathione have been shown to protect sperm motility from the effects of exogenous ROS (Table 20.1) [19, 52]. In contrast, superoxide

Table 20.1 Role of in vitro antioxidants in protecting spermatozoa from the loss of motility and DNA damage due to exogenous ROS

Study	Exogenous ROS	Antioxidant supplement and results
Sperm motility		
de Lamirande (1992)	X + XO	Catalase protects spz from X + XO-induced loss of motility
		SOD, DTT, or GSH less effective in protecting spz motility from ROS
Griveau (1995)	X + XO	Catalase protects spz from X + XO-induced loss of motility
		SOD or mannitol ineffective in protecting spz motility from ROS
Sperm DNA		
Lopes (1998)	X + XO	GSH+hypotaurine protect spz from X + XO-induced DD
		Catalase protects spz from X + XO-induced DD
		n-Acetylcysteine protects spz from X + XO-induced DD
Potts (2000)	H_2O_2 + Fe + ADP	S. plasma (>60%v/v) lowers oxidative spz damage ($\downarrow$DD, LPO)
Sierens (2002)	H_2O_2	Isoflavones, vit C and E protect spz from H_2O_2-induced DD (Isoflavones: genistein, equol). Dose effect noted
Russo (2006)	(1) H_2O_2 (2) Benzopyrene (3) H_2O_2 + Fe + ADP	Propolis lowers oxidative spz damage ($\downarrow$LPO, DD, LDH) (Propolis—a natural resinous hive product)

ADP adenosine diphosphate, *COMET* single-cell gel electrophoresis, *DD* DNA damage, *DFI* DNA fragmentation index, *Fe* iron, *GSH* glutathione, *LDH* lactate dehydrogenase, *LPO* lipid peroxidation, *S. plasma* seminal plasma, *Spz* sperm, *TUNEL* terminal deoxynucleotidyl transferase dUTP nick end labeling, *X* xanthine, *XO* xanthine oxidase

dismutase is less effective in preventing the loss of motility due to exogenous oxidants [19, 52]. Altogether, these data suggest that H_2O_2 is the most sperm-toxic exogenous ROS.

Antioxidants have also been shown to protect the sperm DNA from the effects of exogenous ROS (Table 20.1) [44, 53–55]. This is of clinical relevance as sperm DNA damage may impact on reproductive outcomes after ARTs [56]. Indeed, sperm DNA damage has been associated with reduced pregnancy rates with IUI, and, to a lesser extent with conventional IVF.

Role of In Vitro Antioxidants in Protecting Spermatozoa from Endogenous Reactive Oxygen Species

Spermatozoa can be stimulated to generate ROS using a variety of agents (e.g., NADPH and estrogens) and this ROS production can impair sperm function [57].

Table 20.2 Role of in vitro antioxidant supplements in protecting sperm DNA from stimulated endogenous ROS generation

Study	Assay	ROS stimulant	Antioxidant supplement and results
Twigg (1998)	IS NTL	NADPH	Vit E, SOD, catalase, hypotaurine, albumin all ineffective in protecting spz DNA from endogenous ROS
Anderson (2003)	COMET	Estrogens	Catalase protects spz from estrogen-induced oxidative DD SOD and vit C less effective (Estrogens: equol, daidzein, genistein, DES, E2)
Cemeli (2004)	COMET	Estrogens (1 h 37 C)	Flavonoid (Kaempferol) protects sperm from estrogen-induced oxidative DD
Dobrzynska (2004)	COMET	DES, T3, T4, NA (1 h 37 C)	Flavonoids and catalase protect spz from stimulant-induced oxidative DD (Flavonoids: Kaempferol, Quercetin)

*COMEt al*kaline single-cell gel electrophoresis, *DD* DNA damage, *ISNTL* in situ nick translation assay, *LPO* lipid peroxidation, *NA* noradrenaline, *ROS* reactive oxygen species, *SOD* superoxide dismutase, *Spz* sperm, *T3* triiodothyronine, *T4* thyroxine, *vit* vitamin

In contrast to the beneficial effect of antioxidants in protecting spermatozoa from exogenous ROS, antioxidants appear to be of limited value in protecting spermatozoa from endogenous ROS production [58]. Twigg et al. demonstrated that SOD, catalase, or both are ineffective, whereas albumin is effective in protecting spermatozoa from loss of motility due to endogenous ROS generation [58]. These findings stress the importance of using gentle (brief, little centrifugation) semen processing protocols so as to minimize the production and adverse impact of low levels of endogenous ROS.

Similarly, antioxidants appear to be of limited value in protecting the DNA of normal spermatozoa (with normal chromatin compaction) from endogenous ROS production (e.g., NADPH induced or centrifugation induced) (Table 20.2) [58–61]. In samples with poor morphology and poor sperm chromatin compaction, antioxidants may protect the sperm DNA from endogenous ROS production, as these samples are more vulnerable to oxidative stress [10, 47].

Role of In Vitro Antioxidants in Protecting Spermatozoa from Semen Processing

Several studies have reported on the effects of antioxidants in preventing the decline in sperm motility after semen processing and incubation (Table 20.3). These studies have clinical relevance because it is important to maximize sperm motility prior to assisted reproductive techniques such as IUI and standard IVF. The available studies report conflicting results regarding the effects of antioxidants in preventing

Table 20.3 The effect of in vitro antioxidants on sperm motility during semen processing

Study	Parameter	Semen processing	Antioxidant supplement and results
Griveau (1994)	Motility	1. CF at 400 g × 2 2. Swim-up 3. 24-h Incubation	DTT, Catalase, SOD or GSH improve motility
Zheng (1997)	Motility	2- and 3-h Incubation (fertile and infertile)	Ferulic acid improves sperm motility and reduces LPO
	LPO		Ferulic acid increases sperm cAMP and cGMP
Oeda (1997)	Motility	2-h Incubation	NAC lowers semen ROS levels
	ROS		NAC improves sperm motility
Verma (1999)	Motility	6-h Incubation	Vitamin E lowers sperm LPO and protects spermatozoa from loss of motility
	LPO		
Donnelly (2000)	Motility	Percoll DGC + 4 h incubation	GSH or hypotaurine do not protect spermatozoa from loss of motility
Calamera (2001)	Motility	2–47-h Incubation	Catalase did not protect spermatozoa from loss of motility
	ROS		
Chi (2008)	Motility	Centrifugation (1,000 rpm × 2) + 1 h incubation	EDTA or catalase lower CF-induced sperm ROS
	ROS		EDTA (but not catalase) protects spermatozoa from CF-induced loss sperm motility

CF centrifugation, *COMEt* alkaline single-cell gel electrophoresis, *DD* DNA damage, *DGC* density-gradient centrifugation, *DTT* dithiotreitol, *GSH* glutathione, *LPO* lipid peroxidation, *NAC* N-acetyl-L-cysteine, *ROS* reactive oxygen species, *SOD* superoxide dismutase

the loss of sperm motility during sperm processing such as centrifugation and incubation. Some studies have shown that antioxidants (e.g., vitamin E, glutathione, *n*-acetylcysteine, catalase, and ferulic acid) are effective in reducing ROS levels and in preventing the decline in sperm motility during sperm processing [62–65]. In contrast, other studies have reported that antioxidants (e.g., glutathione and catalase) are ineffective in protecting spermatozoa from the loss of motility during sperm processing [66–68]. It is important to note that sperm samples from infertile men may be more susceptible to oxidative injury (from semen processing) and be afforded greater protection by antioxidants than samples from fertile men [50].

Antioxidants appear to be of limited value in protecting sperm DNA from gentle semen processing (e.g., incubation or density-gradient centrifugation) (Table 20.4) [67–70]. In some cases, antioxidants supplementation in vitro (e.g., combination of vitamins C and E) may cause sperm DNA damage [68, 70].

Table 20.4 Role of in vitro antioxidant supplements in protecting sperm DNA from semen processing

Study	Assay	Semen processing	Antioxidant supplement and results
Hughes (1998)	COMET	Percoll DGC	Vits C, E, or urate lower sperm DD after DGC
			Vits C + E or AC increase sperm DD after DGC
Donnelly (1999)	COMET	Percoll DGC	Vit C or E does not lower baseline sperm ROS and DD
			Vit C or E protect sperm from H_2O_2-induced ROS and DD
			Vits C + E induce sperm DD and increase H_2O_2-induced DD
Donnelly (2000)	COMET	Percoll DGC $\pm$ H_2O_2	GSH, hypotaurine or both do not alter baseline sperm DD
			GSH, hypotaurine or both do not alter sperm motility at 4 h
			GSH and/or hypotaurine lower H_2O_2-induced sperm DD
Chi (2008)	COMET	Centrifugation (1,000 rpm × 2) + 1 h incubation	EDTA or catalase lower centrifugation-induced sperm ROS
			EDTA or catalase lower centrifugation-induced sperm DD
			EDTA or datalase have no protective effect on LPO

AC Acetyl cysteine, *COMEt* alkaline single-cell gel electrophoresis, *DD* DNA damage, *DGC* density-gradient centrifugation, *GSH* glutathione, *LPO* lipid peroxidation, *ROS* reactive oxygen species, *vit* vitamin

Role of In Vitro Antioxidants in Protecting Spermatozoa from Cryopreservation and Thawing

Several studies have evaluated the role of antioxidants in protecting spermatozoa from the loss of motility that occurs following cryopreservation and thawing. Most studies have reported on the use of pentoxifylline (an antioxidant and phosphodiesterase inhibitor). Some studies have shown that pentoxifylline improves post-thaw sperm motility and/or sperm function [71–74], whereas others have demonstrated that this antioxidant does not have a beneficial effect [75]. Other antioxidants (vitamins E and C and rebamipide) have been used to enhance post-thaw motility, however the results have been modest [76, 77].

Several studies have also evaluated the role of antioxidants in protecting sperm DNA from injury following cryopreservation and thawing. Most studies have shown that antioxidants (vitamin C, catalase, resveratrol, and genistein) can protect the sperm DNA from oxidative injury during cryopreservation and subsequent thawing [78–81] (Table 20.5). In contrast, Taylor et al. reported that the antioxidant vitamin E does not protect sperm DNA during cryopreservation [82].

Table 20.5 The role of in vitro antioxidants in protecting human sperm DNA from injury caused by cryopreservation and thawing

Study	Assay	Antioxidant	Effect of antioxidant on cryo-preservation and thawing
Taylor '09	TUNEL	Vitamin E	No effect on sperm DNA integrity Improved post-thaw motility
Li '09	COMET	Catalase or ascorbic acid	Improved sperm DNA integrity Reduced ROS production
Branco '09	COMET	Resveratrol or ascorbic acid	Improved sperm DNA integrity
Martinez-Soto '09	TUNEL	Genistein	Improved sperm DNA integrity Reduced ROS production, improved post-thaw motility
Thompson '09	8-OHdG TUNEL	Genistein	Improved sperm DNA integrity (reduced oxidative damage)

8-OHdG 8-hydroxy-2-deoxyguanosine, *COMEt* alkaline single-cell gel electrophoresis, *ROS* reactive oxygen species, *TUNEL* terminal deoxynucleotidyl transferase dUTP nick end labeling

Taken together, the data suggest that antioxidants are generally effective in protecting spermatozoa from the effects of cryopreservation and thawing. However, the technique of cryopreservation and type of cryoprotectant are also important in improving post-thaw sperm function [83].

Summary

Oxidative stress plays an important role in the pathophysiology of male infertility. The study of in vitro antioxidants is highly relevant in the era of assisted reproduction because of the susceptibility of human spermatozoa to oxidative injury and the vulnerability of these cells during semen processing. Most studies have demonstrated a beneficial effect of in vitro antioxidant supplements in protecting spermatozoa from exogenous oxidants and cryopreservation (with subsequent thawing). In contrast, the effect of these antioxidants in protecting normal spermatozoa from endogenous ROS and gentle sperm processing has not been established conclusively. Additional studies are needed to determine the optimal antioxidant preparation to protect spermatozoa from oxidative stress in vitro.

Expert Commentary

The biological basis for the use of in vitro antioxidants in male infertility is sound and is based on the body of literature showing that sperm dysfunction is strongly related to oxidative stress. Furthermore, the inherent susceptibility of human spermatozoa to oxidative stress is particularly relevant during semen processing as a result of the removal of seminal plasma, a natural antioxidant. Clinical studies of in vitro antioxidants support the use of antioxidants in protecting spermatozoa (particularly abnormal spermatozoa) from exogenous ROS and cryopreservation. However, the optimal antioxidant and concentration has not been established.

Five-Year View

To see a real advance in the field of in vitro antioxidants for male infertility, we need to undertake additional, comparative studies to assess the differential effect of various antioxidants. We also need to undertake studies to better define the differential treatment response between normal (fertile) and subnormal (infertile) semen samples and identify the optimal protocol (type and concentration of antioxidant).

References

1. Agarwal A, Saleh RA. Role of oxidants in male infertility: rationale, significance, and treatment. Urol Clin North Am. 2002;29:817–27.
2. Agarwal A, Sharma RK, Nallella KP, Thomas Jr AJ, Alvarez JG, Sikka SC. Reactive oxygen species as an independent marker of male factor infertility. Fertil Steril. 2006;86:878–85.
3. Iwasaki A, Gagnon C. Formation of reactive oxygen species in spermatozoa of infertile patients. Fertil Steril. 1992;57:409–16.
4. Zini A, de Lamirande E, Gagnon C. Reactive oxygen species in semen of infertile patients: levels of superoxide dismutase-and catalase-like activities in seminal plasma and spermatozoa. Int J Androl. 1993;16:183–8.
5. Aitken RJ, Irvine DS, Wu FC. Prospective analysis of sperm-oocyte fusion and reactive oxygen species generation as criteria for the diagnosis of infertility. Am J Obstet Gynecol. 1991;164:542–51.
6. Kodama H, Yamaguchi R, Fukuda J, Kasai H, Tanaka T. Increased oxidative deoxyribonucleic acid damage in the spermatozoa of infertile male patients. Fertil Steril. 1997;68:519–24.
7. Shen HM, Chia SE, Ong CN. Evaluation of oxidative DNA damage in human sperm and its association with male infertility. J Androl. 1999;20:718–23.
8. Barroso G, Morshedi M, Oehninger S. Analysis of DNA fragmentation, plasma membrane translocation of phosphatidylserine and oxidative stress in human spermatozoa. Hum Reprod. 2000;15:1338–44.
9. Gomez E, Buckingham DW, Brindle J, Lanzafame F, Irvine DS, Aitken RJ. Development of an image analysis system to monitor the retention of residual cytoplasm by human spermatozoa: correlation with biochemical markers of the cytoplasmic space, oxidative stress, and sperm function. J Androl. 1996;17:276–87.
10. Muratori M, Piomboni P, Baldi E, Filimberti E, Pecchioli P, Moretti E, et al. Functional and ultrastructural features of DNA-fragmented human sperm. J Androl. 2000;21:903–12.
11. de Lamirande E, Jiang H, Zini A, Kodama H, Gagnon C. Reactive oxygen species and sperm physiology. Rev Reprod. 1997;2:48–54.
12. Aitken RJ, West K, Buckingham D. Leukocytic infiltration into the human ejaculate and its association with semen quality, oxidative stress, and sperm function. J Androl. 1994;15:343–52.

13. Aitken RJ, Paterson M, Fisher H, Buckingham DW, van Duin M. Redox regulation of tyrosine phosphorylation in human spermatozoa and its role in the control of human sperm function. J Cell Sci. 1995;108(Pt 5):2017–25.
14. de Lamirande E, Gagnon C. Impact of reactive oxygen species on spermatozoa: a balancing act between beneficial and detrimental effects. Hum Reprod. 1995;10 Suppl 1:15–21.
15. Griveau JF, Le Lannou D. Reactive oxygen species and human spermatozoa: physiology and pathology. Int J Androl. 1997;20:61–9.
16. Aitken RJ, Gordon E, Harkiss D, Twigg JP, Milne P, Jennings Z, et al. Relative impact of oxidative stress on the functional competence and genomic integrity of human spermatozoa. Biol Reprod. 1998;59:1037–46.
17. Alvarez JG, Touchstone JC, Blasco L, Storey BT. Spontaneous lipid peroxidation and production of hydrogen peroxide and superoxide in human spermatozoa. Superoxide dismutase as major enzyme protectant against oxygen toxicity. J Androl. 1987;8:338–48.
18. de Lamirande E, Gagnon C. Reactive oxygen species and human spermatozoa. II. Depletion of adenosine triphosphate plays an important role in the inhibition of sperm motility. J Androl. 1992;13:379–86.
19. de Lamirande E, Gagnon C. Reactive oxygen species and human spermatozoa. I. Effects on the motility of intact spermatozoa and on sperm axonemes. J Androl. 1992;13:368–78.
20. Yang MH, Schaich KM. Factors affecting DNA damage caused by lipid hydroperoxides and aldehydes. Free Radic Biol Med. 1996;20:225–36.
21. Aitken RJ, Clarkson JS. Cellular basis of defective sperm function and its association with the genesis of reactive oxygen species by human spermatozoa. J Reprod Fertil. 1987;81:459–69.
22. Lewis SE, Aitken RJ. DNA damage to spermatozoa has impacts on fertilization and pregnancy. Cell Tissue Res. 2005;322:33–41.
23. Jeulin C, Soufir JC, Weber P, Laval-Martin D, Calvayrac R. Catalase activity in human spermatozoa and seminal plasma. Gamete Res. 1989;24:185–96.
24. Gagnon C, Iwasaki A, De Lamirande E, Kovalski N. Reactive oxygen species and human spermatozoa. Ann N Y Acad Sci. 1991;637:436–44.
25. Jow WW, Schlegel PN, Cichon Z, Phillips D, Goldstein M, Bardin CW. Identification and localization of copper-zinc superoxide dismutase gene expression in rat testicular development. J Androl. 1993;14:439–47.
26. Zini A, Schlegel PN. Expression of glutathione peroxidases in the adult male rat reproductive tract. Fertil Steril. 1997;68:689–95.
27. Zini A, Schlegel PN. Catalase mRNA expression in the male rat reproductive tract. J Androl. 1996;17:473–80.
28. Zini A, Schlegel PN. Identification and characterization of antioxidant enzyme mRNAs in the rat epididymis. Int J Androl. 1997;20:86–91.
29. Holmes RP, Goodman HO, Shihabi ZK, Jarow JP. The taurine and hypotaurine content of human semen. J Androl. 1992;13:289–92.
30. Lewis SE, Boyle PM, McKinney KA, Young IS, Thompson W. Total antioxidant capacity of seminal plasma is different in fertile and infertile men. Fertil Steril. 1995;64:868–70.
31. Sanocka D, Miesel R, Jedrzejczak P, Kurpisz MK. Oxidative stress and male infertility. J Androl. 1996;17:449–54.
32. Smith R, Vantman D, Ponce J, Escobar J, Lissi E. Total antioxidant capacity of human seminal plasma. Hum Reprod. 1996;11:1655–60.
33. Aitken RJ, Buckingham DW, Carreras A, Irvine DS. Superoxide dismutase in human sperm suspensions: relationship with cellular composition, oxidative stress, and sperm function. Free Radic Biol Med. 1996;21:495–504.
34. Appasamy M, Muttukrishna S, Pizzey AR, Ozturk O, Groome NP, Serhal P, et al. Relationship between male reproductive hormones, sperm DNA damage and markers of oxidative stress in infertility. Reprod Biomed Online. 2007;14:159–65.
35. Fraga CG, Motchnik PA, Shigenaga MK, Helbock HJ, Jacob RA, Ames BN. Ascorbic acid protects against endogenous oxidative DNA damage in human sperm. Proc Natl Acad Sci USA. 1991;88:11003–6.

36. Song GJ, Norkus EP, Lewis V. Relationship between seminal ascorbic acid and sperm DNA integrity in infertile men. Int J Androl. 2006;29:569–75.
37. Verit FF, Verit A, Kocyigit A, Ciftci H, Celik H, Koksal M. No increase in sperm DNA damage and seminal oxidative stress in patients with idiopathic infertility. Arch Gynecol Obstet. 2006;274:339–44.
38. Silver EW, Eskenazi B, Evenson DP, Block G, Young S, Wyrobek AJ. Effect of antioxidant intake on sperm chromatin stability in healthy nonsmoking men. J Androl. 2005;26:550–6.
39. Fraga CG, Motchnik PA, Wyrobek AJ, Rempel DM, Ames BN. Smoking and low antioxidant levels increase oxidative damage to sperm DNA. Mutat Res. 1996;351:199–203.
40. Hampl JS, Taylor CA, Johnston CS. Vitamin C deficiency and depletion in the United States: the Third National Health and Nutrition Examination Survey, 1988 to 1994. Am J Public Health. 2004;94:870–5.
41. Jacob RA. Assessment of human vitamin C status. J Nutr. 1990;120 Suppl 11:1480–5.
42. Ryle PR, Thomson AD. Nutrition and vitamins in alcoholism. Contemp Issues Clin Biochem. 1984;1:188–224.
43. Aitken RJ, Clarkson JS. Significance of reactive oxygen species and antioxidants in defining the efficacy of sperm preparation techniques. J Androl. 1988;9:367–76.
44. Potts RJ, Notarianni LJ, Jefferies TM. Seminal plasma reduces exogenous oxidative damage to human sperm, determined by the measurement of DNA strand breaks and lipid peroxidation. Mutat Res. 2000;447:249–56.
45. Twigg J, Irvine DS, Houston P, Fulton N, Michael L, Aitken RJ. Iatrogenic DNA damage induced in human spermatozoa during sperm preparation: protective significance of seminal plasma. Mol Hum Reprod. 1998;4:439–45.
46. Aitken RJ. Founders' Lecture. Human spermatozoa: fruits of creation, seeds of doubt. Reprod Fertil Dev. 2004;16:655–64.
47. Said TM, Agarwal A, Sharma RK, Thomas Jr AJ, Sikka SC. Impact of sperm morphology on DNA damage caused by oxidative stress induced by beta-nicotinamide adenine dinucleotide phosphate. Fertil Steril. 2005;83:95–103.
48. Cho C, Willis WD, Goulding EH, Jung-Ha H, Choi YC, Hecht NB, et al. Haploinsufficiency of protamine-1 or -2 causes infertility in mice. Nat Genet. 2001;28:82–6.
49. De Iuliis GN, Thomson LK, Mitchell LA, Finnie JM, Koppers AJ, Hedges A, et al. DNA damage in human spermatozoa is highly correlated with the efficiency of chromatin remodeling and the formation of 8-hydroxy-2′-deoxyguanosine, a marker of oxidative stress. Biol Reprod. 2009;81:517–24.
50. Libman J, Gabriel MS, Sairam MR, Zini A. Catalase can protect spermatozoa of FSH receptor knock-out mice against oxidant-induced DNA damage in vitro. Int J Androl. 2010;33:818–22.
51. Aitken RJ, Buckingham DW, Brindle J, Gomez E, Baker HW, Irvine DS. Analysis of sperm movement in relation to the oxidative stress created by leukocytes in washed sperm preparations and seminal plasma. Hum Reprod. 1995;10:2061–71.
52. Aitken RJ, Buckingham D, Harkiss D. Use of a xanthine oxidase free radical generating system to investigate the cytotoxic effects of reactive oxygen species on human spermatozoa. J Reprod Fertil. 1993;97:441–50.
53. Lopes S, Jurisicova A, Sun JG, Casper RF. Reactive oxygen species: potential cause for DNA fragmentation in human spermatozoa. Hum Reprod. 1998;13:896–900.
54. Russo A, Troncoso N, Sanchez F, Garbarino JA, Vanella A. Propolis protects human spermatozoa from DNA damage caused by benzo[a]pyrene and exogenous reactive oxygen species. Life Sci. 2006;78:1401–6.
55. Sierens J, Hartley JA, Campbell MJ, Leathem AJ, Woodside JV. In vitro isoflavone supplementation reduces hydrogen peroxide-induced DNA damage in sperm. Teratog Carcinog Mutagen. 2002;22:227–34.
56. Zini A, Sigman M. Are tests of sperm DNA damage clinically useful? Pros and cons. J Androl. 2009;30:219–29.
57. Aitken RJ, Fisher HM, Fulton N, Gomez E, Knox W, Lewis B, et al. Reactive oxygen species generation by human spermatozoa is induced by exogenous NADPH and inhibited by the

flavoprotein inhibitors diphenylene iodonium and quinacrine. Mol Reprod Dev. 1997; 47:468–82.

58. Twigg J, Fulton N, Gomez E, Irvine DS, Aitken RJ. Analysis of the impact of intracellular reactive oxygen species generation on the structural and functional integrity of human spermatozoa: lipid peroxidation, DNA fragmentation and effectiveness of antioxidants. Hum Reprod. 1998;13:1429–36.

59. Anderson D, Schmid TE, Baumgartner A, Cemeli-Carratala E, Brinkworth MH, Wood JM. Oestrogenic compounds and oxidative stress (in human sperm and lymphocytes in the Comet assay). Mutat Res. 2003;544:173–8.

60. Cemeli E, Schmid TE, Anderson D. Modulation by flavonoids of DNA damage induced by estrogen-like compounds. Environ Mol Mutagen. 2004;44:420–6.

61. Dobrzynska MM, Baumgartner A, Anderson D. Antioxidants modulate thyroid hormone- and noradrenaline-induced DNA damage in human sperm. Mutagenesis. 2004;19:325–30.

62. Griveau JF, Le Lannou D. Effects of antioxidants on human sperm preparation techniques. Int J Androl. 1994;17:225–31.

63. Oeda T, Henkel R, Ohmori H, Schill WB. Scavenging effect of N-acetyl-L-cysteine against reactive oxygen species in human semen: a possible therapeutic modality for male factor infertility? Andrologia. 1997;29:125–31.

64. Verma A, Kanwar KC. Effect of vitamin E on human sperm motility and lipid peroxidation in vitro. Asian J Androl. 1999;1:151–4.

65. Zheng RL, Zhang H. Effects of ferulic acid on fertile and asthenozoospermic infertile human sperm motility, viability, lipid peroxidation, and cyclic nucleotides. Free Radic Biol Med. 1997;22:581–6.

66. Calamera JC, Fernandez PJ, Buffone MG, Acosta AA, Doncel GF. Effects of long-term in vitro incubation of human spermatozoa: functional parameters and catalase effect. Andrologia. 2001;33:79–86.

67. Chi HJ, Kim JH, Ryu CS, Lee JY, Park JS, Chung DY, et al. Protective effect of antioxidant supplementation in sperm-preparation medium against oxidative stress in human spermatozoa. Hum Reprod. 2008;23:1023–8.

68. Donnelly ET, McClure N, Lewis SE. Glutathione and hypotaurine in vitro: effects on human sperm motility, DNA integrity and production of reactive oxygen species. Mutagenesis. 2000; 15:61–8.

69. Donnelly ET, McClure N, Lewis SE. The effect of ascorbate and alpha-tocopherol supplementation in vitro on DNA integrity and hydrogen peroxide-induced DNA damage in human spermatozoa. Mutagenesis. 1999;14:505–12.

70. Hughes CM, Lewis SE, McKelvey-Martin VJ, Thompson W. The effects of antioxidant supplementation during Percoll preparation on human sperm DNA integrity. Hum Reprod. 1998;13:1240–7.

71. Esteves SC, Sharma RK, Thomas Jr AJ, Agarwal A. Cryopreservation of human spermatozoa with pentoxifylline improves the post-thaw agonist-induced acrosome reaction rate. Hum Reprod. 1998;13:3384–9.

72. Brennan AP, Holden CA. Pentoxifylline-supplemented cryoprotectant improves human sperm motility after cryopreservation. Hum Reprod. 1995;10:2308–12.

73. Bell M, Wang R, Hellstrom WJ, Sikka SC. Effect of cryoprotective additives and cryopreservation protocol on sperm membrane lipid peroxidation and recovery of motile human sperm. J Androl. 1993;14:472–8.

74. Wang R, Sikka SC, Veeraragavan K, Bell M, Hellstrom WJ. Platelet activating factor and pentoxifylline as human sperm cryoprotectants. Fertil Steril. 1993;60:711–5.

75. Check DJ, Kiefer D, Katsoff D, Check JH. Effect of pentoxifylline added to freezing media on subsequent post-thaw hypoosmotic swelling test and other semen parameters. Arch Androl. 1995;35:161–3.

76. Park NC, Park HJ, Lee KM, Shin DG. Free radical scavenger effect of rebamipide in sperm processing and cryopreservation. Asian J Androl. 2003;5:195–201.

77. Askari HA, Check JH, Peymer N, Bollendorf A. Effect of natural antioxidants tocopherol and ascorbic acids in maintenance of sperm activity during freeze-thaw process. Arch Androl. 1994;33:11–5.
78. Branco CS, Garcez ME, Pasqualotto FF, Erdtman B, Salvador M. Resveratrol and ascorbic acid prevent DNA damage induced by cryopreservation in human semen. Cryobiology. 2010;60:235–7.
79. Li Z, Lin Q, Liu R, Xiao W, Liu W. Protective effects of ascorbate and catalase on human spermatozoa during cryopreservation. J Androl. 2010;31:437–44.
80. Martinez-Soto JC, de Dioshourcade J, Gutierrez-Adan A, Landeras JL, Gadea J. Effect of genistein supplementation of thawing medium on characteristics of frozen human spermatozoa. Asian J Androl. 2010;12:431–41.
81. Thomson LK, Fleming SD, Aitken RJ, De Iuliis GN, Zieschang JA, Clark AM. Cryopreservation-induced human sperm DNA damage is predominantly mediated by oxidative stress rather than apoptosis. Hum Reprod. 2009;24:2061–70.
82. Taylor K, Roberts P, Sanders K, Burton P. Effect of antioxidant supplementation of cryopreservation medium on post-thaw integrity of human spermatozoa. Reprod Biomed Online. 2009;18:184–9.
83. Nallella KP, Sharma RK, Allamaneni SS, Aziz N, Agarwal A. Cryopreservation of human spermatozoa: comparison of two cryopreservation methods and three cryoprotectants. Fertil Steril. 2004;82:913–8.

Chapter 21
Sperm Processing and Selection

Sonja Grunewald and Uwe Paasch

The application of assisted reproductive techniques (ART) has provided help to many men seeking to father a child, although the current success rates of these procedures remain suboptimal [1]. Since raw semen cannot be used in most ART, a workup of the ejaculate is needed to extract those sperm that are capable to fertilize the egg. However, the seminal fluid has a high antioxidant capacity, and sperm processing and separation could profoundly increase oxidative stress [2].

High levels of reactive oxygen species (ROS, e.g., superoxide, hydroxyl, hydrogen peroxide, nitric oxide, peroxynitrite) endanger sperm motility, viability, and function by interacting with membrane lipids, proteins, and nuclear and mitochondrial DNA. Normally, there exists a balance between free radical generating and scavenging systems. It is well known that high levels of ROS are generated by immature and abnormal spermatozoa, contaminating leukocytes and sperm processing, for example, excessive centrifugation and cryopreservation/thawing [3–8]. Naturally, high antioxidant levels in seminal plasma are the major scavenging mechanism [9]. This chapter gives an overview on sperm selection techniques and their impact on oxidative stress to the sperm.

S. Grunewald, MD (✉)
Department of Dermatology, Venerology and Allergology,
European Training Center of Andrology, University of Leipzig,
Philipp-Rosenthal-Strasse 23-25, Leipzig 04103, Germany
e-mail: sonja.grunewald@medizin.uni-leipzig.de

U. Paasch, MD, PhD
Division of Dermatopathology, Division of Aesthetics and Laserdermatology,
Department of Dermatology, Venerology and Allergology,
European Training Center of Andrology, University of Leipzig,
Philipp-Rosenthal-Strasse 23-25, Leipzig 04103, Germany
e-mail: uwe.paasch@medizin.um-leipzig.de

S.J. Parekattil and A. Agarwal (eds), *Antioxidants in Male Infertility: A Guide for Clinicians and Researchers*, © Springer Science+Business Media New York 2013

Impact of Sperm Processing and Separation on Oxidative Stress Levels

The Protective Effects of Seminal Plasma

During maturation, the extrusion of the sperm cytoplasm leads to a loss of cytoplasmic enzymes and as a consequence to diminished endogenous repair mechanisms and enzymatic defenses to oxidative stress [8, 10]. This loss of defense mechanisms is compensated by seminal plasma that contains an array of antioxidants acting as free radical scavengers to protect spermatozoa against oxidative stress [7, 11–13].

Enzymatic antioxidants detected in human seminal plasma are superoxide dismutase (SOD), catalase [14], and glutathione peroxidase [15]. In addition, a variety of nonenzymatic antioxidants are present, among them, alpha-tocopherol, ascorbate, glutathione, pyruvate, taurine, hypotaurine, and urate [16].

The removal of seminal fluid during sperm processing and separation procedures leads to a significant reduction of ROS scavenging mechanisms. ROS generation is a major source of sperm DNA damage leading to significantly impaired male fertility [17, 18]. Consequently, many studies investigated the effect of antioxidant supplementation to sperm media during ART procedures [11].

When added in vitro during IVF preparation or as sperm wash media, ascorbic acid (600 mM), alpha-tocopherol (30 and 60 mM), and urate (400 mM) have each been reported to provide significant protection from subsequent sperm DNA damage [19, 20]. Also isoflavones (e.g., genistein and equol) show antioxidant activity and may prevent sperm damage. Compared with ascorbic acid and alpha-tocopherol, genistein was shown to be more potent antioxidant when added to culture media [21].

However, human serum albumin which is routinely added to ART media acts as a powerful antioxidant that prevents oxidative stress-induced damage [22]. This might explain other studies showing no effect of additional antioxidant supplementation of sperm media [10].

Conventional Sperm Selection Methods

Over the last decades, a variety of standard procedures have been developed with certain modifications (conventional selection strategies). These sperm selection techniques can be classified by their basis on centrifugation, filtration, or sperm migration. Among the centrifugation techniques, density gradient centrifugation has been proposed as the gold standard for sperm preparation. The latest developments in sperm selection are focused on the sperm surface combined with or without a standard preparation protocol (see advanced selection strategies).

Simple Sperm Wash

The first sperm separation methods developed embraced one- or two-step washing procedures with subsequent resuspension of the male germ cells [23]. The one-step washing technique is considered a good alternative for processing certain compromised samples [24]. However, simple centrifugation is known to cause definite harm to the cells. In addition, it does not reduce the number of leukocytes or immature sperm cells (producing ROS) while removing the protecting seminal plasma. Therefore, simple sperm wash should not be applied for routine sperm processing.

Density Gradient Centrifugation

Density gradient centrifugation is currently the gold standard technique for sperm preparation. The semen sample is placed on top of a density gradient and centrifuged for 15–30 min. During this procedure, highly motile spermatozoa move actively in the direction of the sedimentation gradient and therefore can reach lower areas quicker than poorly motile or immotile cells. Finally, highly purified motile sperm cells are enriched in the soft pellet at the bottom. This method allows for the enrichment of mature and motile sperm (multiplicative factor of 1.2–2.1) as well as morphologically normal sperm (multiplicative factor of 1.2–1.8) [25]. In principle, continuous or discontinuous gradients are in use for density gradient centrifugation [26, 27]. The former comprises a gradually increasing density toward the bottom of the vial, whereas the latter is characterized by clear boundaries between the different densities of the gradient. Comparison of the discontinuous gradient with other techniques for separation of motile sperm indicated that the discontinuous gradient has advantages in terms of recovery, enhancement of motility, and increased ability to penetrate zona-free hamster ova [28]. In principle, density gradient centrifugation has been demonstrated to be beneficial for all methods of assisted reproduction [29].

Various separation media for density gradient centrifugation have been introduced over time, such as Percoll®—polyvinylpyrrolidone (PVP)-coated silica particles (GE Healthcare Life Sciences, Uppsala, Sweden) [30], Ficoll® (Chalfont St. Giles, UK) [31, 32], Nycodenz (Gentaur, Brussels, Belgium) [33], and dextran-visotrast [34].

Although the discontinuous Percoll® gradient centrifugation significantly reduced the number of seminal bacteria and oxidative stress levels [35], the risk of contamination with endotoxins, possible membrane alterations, and inflammatory responses that could be induced by the insemination of sperm populations contaminated with Percoll® led to its withdrawn from the market for clinical use in assisted reproduction in October 1996 [36]. Replacement products such as IxaPrep® (Medicult, Copenhagen, Denmark), PureSperm® (Sepal Reproductive Devices, Boston, MA), SilSelect® (FertiPro NV, Beernem, Belgium), and Isolate® (Irvine Scientific, Santa Ana, CA) have been introduced [37, 38]. All these less toxic media contain silane-coated silica particles. The quality of sperm prepared with these media seems to be equivalent compared with Percoll® with regard to recovery rate, motility, viability, normal sperm morphology, and velocity [39–41], although there are conflicting reports for motility [42].

Nitric oxide production has been found to be lower using IxaPrep® as a replacement for Percoll®. High levels of nitric oxide adversely affect sperm motility, zona binding, and embryonic development, suggesting that using these newer replacement media offers an overall advantage in ART [43].

Several studies have demonstrated that samples processed by density gradient centrifugation displayed fewer secondary indicators of oxidative stress, for example, membrane changes, disruption of transmembrane mitochondrial membrane potential, in line with activated apoptosis signal transduction and DNA fragmentations [3, 44–46], emphasizing the—although nonspecific—superior selection quality of the procedure.

Glass Wool Filtration

The principle of glass wool filtration for sperm preparation was introduced more than 30 years ago [47, 48]. This technique offers the advantage of processing the whole ejaculate, followed by an additional centrifugation step to remove the seminal plasma. Highly motile spermatozoa are separated from immotile sperm cells by means of densely packed glass wool fibers using gravitational forces and the self-propelled motion of the cells. The efficacy of each filtration run is directly dependent on the properties of the glass wool used [49]. The chemical nature of the glass (i.e., borate, silicate, or quartz), its surface structure, charge, and thickness of the glass wool fibers directly influence filtration efficacy [50].

Potential risks of the technique are damages to the membrane and acrosome or the transmission of glass particles into the filtrate [51]. Glass wool filtration separates human spermatozoa according to motility and size of the sperm head. Sperm head size is closely correlated with the chromatin condensation quality and DNA fragmentation as measured by the sperm chromatin structure assay (SCSA) [45, 52]. In addition, glass wool filtration eliminates up to 90% of leukocytes [49], leading to a significant reduction of ROS in the sample, thereby also contributing to the prevention of sperm DNA damage [53]. A very recent study proved that sperm filtrated through glass wool columns contains significantly lower levels of intracellular H_2O_2 compared to sperm prepared with Percoll® density gradient centrifugation [54]. These findings are underlined by molecular analyses of semen samples filtrated through glass wool, which show significantly reduced activation of apoptosis signaling and DNA fragmentation [45, 54, 55]. Particularly, the glass wool (Code # 112, Manville Fiber Glass Corp., Denver, CO) available as SpermFertil® columns (TransMIT GmbH, Giessen, Germany) has been tested extensively [55] for those subcellular separation effects.

From a clinical perspective, glass wool filtration yields functionally intact spermatozoa of superior quality [56], without affecting fertilization rate and embryo quality in an ICSI program [57]. However, these positive effects are partly related to initial sperm concentration [58].

Swim-Up Procedure

The self-propelled movement of spermatozoa is an essential prerequisite for all migration methods and guarantees a very clean workup. The swim-up procedure uses the active motion of spermatozoa. Intact moving cells swim out of a pellet derived by a simple washing step into an overlaid media for 30–60 min. Highly motile, morphologically intact spermatozoa are enriched in the absence of other cells, proteins, and debris within the supernatant [59]. Antigravitational centrifugation has been proposed to shorten preparation time [60].

The benefit of this method may be limited due to the fact that close cell-to-cell contacts of sperm with each other, debris, and other substances may lead to extensive ROS production and consecutive DNA damage [9], although this could not be verified [61].

To further improve the quality of sperm, a combination of density gradient centrifugation and swim-up is widely used [62] and should overcome the discussed cell-to-cell contacts causing oxidative stress. On a subcellular level, post density gradient centrifugation swim-up was proven to eliminate sperm with activated apoptosis signaling in a routine IVF setting [63].

Other Conventional Sperm Selection Techniques

Over the years, several other sperm selection techniques were introduced, among them, glass bead filtration [64], Sephadex columns (SpermPrep®, ZDL, Lexington, KY) [65], as well as migration-sedimentation [66] and transmembrane migration techniques [67]. None of them is used routinely for sperm preparation in ART procedures due to several limitations and disadvantages compared to the previously described sperm preparation procedures. No data on oxidative stress levels are available for those less known techniques with the exception of one study on the transmembrane migration technique. This sperm preparation technique uses filtration through a membrane filter with cylindrical pores at right angles to the plane of the membrane. Due to a low ratio of the total cross-sectional area of the pores to the overall membrane area, the yield is extremely low. Nevertheless, L4 membranes selective for spermatozoa with normal membrane integrity have been introduced with a simultaneous increase in motility and significant depletion of leukocytes implicating reduced oxidative stress levels [68].

Advanced Sperm Selection Methods

Advanced protocols that allow sperm to be selected according to their ultrastructural morphology [69] or surface charges by electrophoresis [70] overcome the limitations of the classical separation procedures. New insights into the molecular biology of spermatozoa have prompted the development of molecular selection strategies, including hyaluronic acid-mediated sperm selection [71], annexin V magnetic-activated cell sorting (MACS), and annexin V molecular glass wool filtration [55, 72, 73].

Ultrastructural Sperm Selection

The ultrastructural morphology of the sperm head components has been correlated with sperm fertilizing capacity in vitro [74]. The examination is performed in real time using an inverted light microscope equipped with high-power Nomarski optics enhanced by digital imaging to achieve a magnification up to 6,300×. The motile sperm organelle morphology examination (MSOME) method was significantly and positively associated with both fertilization rate and pregnancy outcome [69]. ICSI performed with selected spermatozoa with strictly defined, morphologically normal nuclei significantly improves the incidence of pregnancy in couples with previous ICSI failures [75], particularly when the use of sperm with vacuoles is avoided. Recently, a conductive correlation between an increase in DNA fragmentation and the presence of spermatozoa with large nuclear vacuoles (LNV) was shown. A correlation between a higher fraction of denatured DNA and LNV also was found. These results support the routine selection of spermatozoa by MSOME [76]. On the other hand, the procedure is very time consuming, and although the sperm are placed after density gradient centrifugation in a sperm medium containing human serum albumin, they might be exposed to oxidative stress. Currently, there are no studies available on ROS levels during the MSOME procedure.

Electrophoretic Sperm Isolation

A novel approach to sperm isolation based on electrophoretic sperm separation by size and charge has been described recently [70]. Electrophoresis-based microflow technology for the separation of spermatozoa by size and charge consists of two outer chambers separated from two inner chambers by polyacrylamide restriction membranes with a pore size of 15 kDa. The pore size allows directional movement of competent spermatozoa in the applied electric field and the size exclusion of contaminating cell populations. Large numbers of spermatozoa that are viable and morphologically normal can be selected. The resulting cell population shows a low incidence of DNA damage and contaminating cells and compared favorably with density gradient centrifugation in purity of the sperm population and lack of ROS generation, as well as the viability and morphological integrity of the isolated cells. However, although the method was successfully applied to reduce the percentage of DNA-fragmented sperm before ICSI [77], electrophoresis of spermatozoa is detrimental to their motility [70].

Hyaluronic Acid-Mediated Sperm Selection

Hyaluronic acid-mediated sperm selection is a novel technique that is comparable to sperm-zona pellucida binding. The presence of hyaluronic acid receptor on the plasma membrane of mature acrosome-intact sperm, coupled with hyaluronic acid-coated glass or plastic surfaces, facilitates selection of single mature sperm [71]. The frequencies of sperm with chromosomal disomy are reduced approximately four- to fivefold in hyaluronic acid-selected sperm compared with semen sperm compensating the increase in such abnormalities in intracytoplasmic sperm injection offspring. Hyaluronic acid binding also excludes immature sperm with cytoplasmic extrusion, persistent histones, and DNA chain breaks [78] implicating reduced oxidative stress to the selected sperm. However, no studies are available measuring directly oxidative stress levels before, during, and after the hyaluronic acid binding assay.

Annexin V MACS Separation

The effects of oxidative stress on human sperm comprise impairment of sperm motility, viability, and subcellular function by interacting with membrane lipids, proteins, and nuclear and mitochondrial DNA [79]. In addition, recent studies indicate not only direct effects of ROS on sperm DNA integrity [18, 80, 81] but also activation of parts of the apoptosis signaling cascade as known from somatic cells [82, 83].

Externalization of phosphatidylserine from inner to outer leaflet of the plasma membrane is a main apoptosis event detectable at the sperm surface [84, 85]. Annexin V is a phospholipid-binding protein that has high affinity for PS and lacks the ability to pass through an intact sperm membrane. Therefore, annexin V binding to spermatozoa may be used to label sperm that have compromised membrane integrity and that are less capable to fertilize eggs [85].

Annexin V-conjugated super-paramagnetic microbeads can effectively separate nonapoptotic spermatozoa from those with deteriorated plasma membranes based on the externalization of phosphatidylserine using magnetic-activated cell sorting (MACS). Annexin V MACS separation of sperm yields two fractions: EPS negative (no *externalized* *p*hosphatidyl*s*erine, intact membranes, nonapoptotic) and EPS positive (externalized *p*hosphatidyl*s*erine, apoptotic) which is retained in the magnetic field [72, 73, 86].

Sperm preparation that combines density gradient centrifugation with annexin V MACS enhances the advantages of both methods. While density gradient centrifugation removes immature sperm cells, debris, and leukocytes, the annexin V MACS depletes already damaged sperm cells with membrane changes, activated apoptosis signaling, and (in part) DNA fragmentations [87]. Although it was not measured directly, these results implicate a tremendous reduction of oxidative stress.

This is of clinical relevance as it leads to a selection of sperm showing not only improved motility, viability, and morphology but also superior oocyte penetration and fertilization rates [88, 89]. First clinical application revealed also improved pregnancy rates compared to sperm preparation by density gradient centrifugation only [90].

Annexin V Molecular Glass Wool Separation

Although integrating annexin V MACS into standard semen preparation protocols offers a potentially major advantage, the possibility of an accidental transmission of super-paramagnetic microbeads into eggs cannot be fully excluded. A sperm preparation system using the binding properties of annexin V by avoiding free flotation of super-paramagnetic microbeads in a liquid-phase buffer might help to avoid side effects. The annexin V glass filtration technique is a promising step toward the development of a molecular-based preparation system with an enhanced capability for selecting vital spermatozoa with superior fertilizing capacity. We recently demonstrated the feasibility of combining the classical glass wool filtration method with phosphatidylserine-binding properties of annexin V and a solid-phase molecular filtration system. We investigated the apoptosis markers of sperm following simple wash, glass wool filtration, molecular glass wool filtration, and MACS. We demonstrated that the application of annexin V glass wool may improve the outcome of ART. Our data support the highly efficient filtration capacity of a solid-phase annexin V-coated glass wool filter [55].

Expert Commentary

Immature sperm and leukocytes are main sources of ROS in human semen. In general, sperm separation techniques depleting these cells are able to reduce oxidative stress that may harm the sperm during assisted reproduction techniques. Conventional sperm preparation techniques fulfilling those criteria are density gradient centrifugation and glass wool filtration. The swim-up procedure as well as advanced sperm separation methods, like ultrastructural and electrophoretic sperm selection as well as methods based on binding to hyaluronic acid and annexin V, should be used after density gradient centrifugation or glass wool filtration to prevent longer contacts of mature sperm with immature sperm and leukocytes.

In contrast, the removal of the seminal fluid during sperm processing and separation procedures leads to a significant reduction of ROS scavenging mechanisms. However, human serum albumin in ART media acts as a powerful antioxidant that prevents oxidative stress-induced damage. Thus, any substitution of IVF media with other potential antioxidants may not have additional benefits to improve the success of ART procedures.

Five-Year View

Further development of specific molecular-based sperm selection methods requires careful analysis of oxidative stress levels to avoid side effects. All new sperm separation procedures must include depletion of immature sperm and leukocytes. Possibly, the combination with standard sperm preparation techniques like density gradient centrifugation or glass wool filtration will be still of advantage. The supplementation of sperm preparation and incubation media with human serum albumin or other antioxidants should not be forgotten during the development of such "high-end" techniques.

Key Issues

- Sperm separation from seminal fluid removes also the natural protective antioxidants contained in the seminal fluid. To prevent excessive oxidative stress to the sperm, antioxidants like human serum albumin must be added to sperm preparation and incubation media for assisted reproduction.
- Standard sperm selection techniques like density gradient centrifugation and glass wool filtration, but not swim-up, are able to reduce oxidative stress by depletion of immature sperm and leukocytes.
- Advanced sperm separation techniques focus rather on the depletion of already damaged sperm; until now, a combination with gradient centrifugation or glass wool filtration is advisable.

Acknowledgment The authors are grateful to Prof. emeritus Hans-Juergen Glander for his support and encouragement.

References

1. Society for Assisted Reproductive Technology and American Society for Reproductive Medicine. Assisted reproductive technology in the United States: 2000 results generated from the American Society for Reproductive Medicine/Society for Assisted Reproductive Technology Registry. Fertil Steril. 2004;81:1207–20.
2. Sikka SC. Relative impact of oxidative stress on male reproductive function. Curr Med Chem. 2001;8:851–62.
3. Ollero M, Gil-Guzman E, Lopez MC, Sharma RK, Agarwal A, Larson K, Evenson D, Thomas Jr AJ, Alvarez JG. Characterization of subsets of human spermatozoa at different stages of maturation: implications in the diagnosis and treatment of male infertility. Hum Reprod. 2001;16:1912–21.
4. Mazzilli F, Rossi T, Sabatini L, Pulcinelli FM, Rapone S, Dondero F, Gazzaniga PP. Human sperm cryopreservation and reactive oxygen species (ROS) production. Acta Eur Fertil. 1995;26:145–8.

5. Ludwig M, Kummel C, Schroeder-Printzen I, Ringert RH, Weidner W. Evaluation of seminal plasma parameters in patients with chronic prostatitis or leukocytospermia. Andrologia. 1998;30 Suppl 1:41–7.

6. Iwasaki A, Gagnon C. Formation of reactive oxygen species in spermatozoa of infertile patients. Fertil Steril. 1992;57:409–16.

7. Aitken RJ, Buckingham DW, Brindle J, Gomez E, Baker HW, Irvine DS. Analysis of sperm movement in relation to the oxidative stress created by leukocytes in washed sperm preparations and seminal plasma. Hum Reprod. 1995;10:2061–71.

8. Aitken RJ, West K, Buckingham D. Leukocytic infiltration into the human ejaculate and its association with semen quality, oxidative stress, and sperm function. J Androl. 1994;15:343–52.

9. Twigg J, Irvine DS, Houston P, Fulton N, Michael L, Aitken RJ. Iatrogenic DNA damage induced in human spermatozoa during sperm preparation: protective significance of seminal plasma. Mol Hum Reprod. 1998;4:439–45.

10. Donnelly ET, McClure N, Lewis SE. Antioxidant supplementation in vitro does not improve human sperm motility. Fertil Steril. 1999;72:484–95.

11. Agarwal A, Saleh RA. Role of oxidants in male infertility: rationale, significance, and treatment. Urol Clin North Am. 2002;29:817–27.

12. Lewis SE, Boyle PM, McKinney KA, Young IS, Thompson W. Total antioxidant capacity of seminal plasma is different in fertile and infertile men. Fertil Steril. 1995;64:868–70.

13. Potts RJ, Notarianni LJ, Jefferies TM. Seminal plasma reduces exogenous oxidative damage to human sperm, determined by the measurement of DNA strand breaks and lipid peroxidation. Mutat Res. 2000;447:249–56.

14. Zini A, de Lamirande E, Gagnon C. Reactive oxygen species in semen of infertile patients: levels of superoxide dismutase- and catalase-like activities in seminal plasma and spermatozoa. Int J Androl. 1993;16:183–8.

15. Alvarez JG, Storey BT. Role of glutathione peroxidase in protecting mammalian spermatozoa from loss of motility caused by spontaneous lipid peroxidation. Gamete Res. 1989;23:77–90.

16. Saleh RA, Agarwal A. Oxidative stress and male infertility: from research bench to clinical practice. J Androl. 2002;23:737–52.

17. Twigg J, Fulton N, Gomez E, Irvine DS, Aitken RJ. Analysis of the impact of intracellular reactive oxygen species generation on the structural and functional integrity of human spermatozoa: lipid peroxidation, DNA fragmentation and effectiveness of antioxidants. Hum Reprod. 1998;13:1429–36.

18. Lopes S, Jurisicova A, Sun JG, Casper RF. Reactive oxygen species: potential cause for DNA fragmentation in human spermatozoa. Hum Reprod. 1998;13:896–900.

19. Hughes CM, Lewis SE, McKelvey-Martin VJ, Thompson W. The effects of antioxidant supplementation during Percoll preparation on human sperm DNA integrity. Hum Reprod. 1998;13:1240–7.

20. Geva E, Lessing JB, Lerner GL, Amit A. Free radicals, antioxidants and human spermatozoa: clinical implications. Hum Reprod. 1998;13:1422–4.

21. Sierens J, Hartley JA, Campbell MJ, Leathem AJ, Woodside JV. In vitro isoflavone supplementation reduces hydrogen peroxide-induced DNA damage in sperm. Teratog Carcinog Mutagen. 2002;22:227–34.

22. Armstrong JS, Rajasekaran M, Hellstrom WJ, Sikka SC. Antioxidant potential of human serum albumin: role in the recovery of high quality human spermatozoa for assisted reproductive technology. J Androl. 1998;19:412–9.

23. Edwards RG, Bavister BD, Steptoe PC. Early stages of fertilization in vitro of human oocytes matured in vitro. Nature. 1969;221:632–5.

24. Srisombut C, Morshedi M, Lin MH, Nassar A, Oehninger S. Comparison of various methods of processing human cryopreserved-thawed semen samples. Hum Reprod. 1998;13:2151–7.

25. Glander HJ. Effektivität der Methoden für die Spermienkollektion, -separation und -konzentrierung. Hautnah Derm. 1993;9:52–60.

26. Bolton VN, Braude PR. Preparation of human spermatozoa for in vitro fertilization by isopycnic centrifugation on self-generating density gradients. Arch Androl. 1984;13:167–76.

27. Pousette A, Akerlof E, Rosenborg L, Fredricsson B. Increase in progressive motility and improved morphology of human spermatozoa following their migration through Percoll gradients. Int J Androl. 1986;9:1–13.
28. Berger T, Marrs RP, Moyer DL. Comparison of techniques for selection of motile spermatozoa. Fertil Steril. 1985;43:268–73.
29. Mortimer D, Mortimer ST. Methods of sperm preparation for assisted reproduction. Ann Acad Med Singapore. 1992;21:517–24.
30. Gorus FK, Pipeleers DG. A rapid method for the fractionation of human spermatozoa according to their progressive motility. Fertil Steril. 1981;35:662–5.
31. Bongso A, Ng SC, Mok H, Lim MN, Teo HL, Wong PC, Ratnam S. Improved sperm concentration, motility, and fertilization rates following Ficoll treatment of sperm in a human in vitro fertilization program. Fertil Steril. 1989;51:850–4.
32. Harrison RA. A highly efficient method for washing mammalian spermatozoa. J Reprod Fertil. 1976;48:347–53.
33. Gellert-Mortimer ST, Clarke GN, Baker HW, Hyne RV, Johnston WI. Evaluation of Nycodenz and Percoll density gradients for the selection of motile human spermatozoa. Fertil Steril. 1988;49:335–41.
34. Glander HJ, Schaller J, Ladusch M. [A simple method for separating fresh and cryopreserved human sperm using dextran-visotrast density gradient centrifugation] Eine einfache Methode zur Separierung von frischen und kryokonservierten Humanspermien mittels einer Dextran-Visotrast- Dichtegradientenzentrifugation. Zentralbl Gynakol. 1990;112:91–7.
35. Aitken RJ, Clarkson JS. Significance of reactive oxygen species and antioxidants in defining the efficacy of sperm preparation techniques. J Androl. 1988;9:367–76.
36. Pharmacia Biotech I. Important notice: Percoll® NOT to be used in Assisted Reproduction Technologies in Humans. 1996.
37. Makkar G, Ng HY, Yeung SB, Ho PC. Comparison of two colloidal silica-based sperm separation media with a non-silica-based medium. Fertil Steril. 1999;72:796–802.
38. Sills ES, Wittkowski KM, Tucker MJ, Perloe M, Kaplan CR, Palermo GD. Comparison of centrifugation- and noncentrifugation-based techniques for recovery of motile human sperm in assisted reproduction. Arch Androl. 2002;48:141–5.
39. Chen MJ, Bongso A. Comparative evaluation of two density gradient preparations for sperm separation for medically assisted conception. Hum Reprod. 1999;14:759–64.
40. Claassens OE, Menkveld R, Harrison KL. Evaluation of three substitutes for Percoll in sperm isolation by density gradient centrifugation. Hum Reprod. 1998;13:3139–43.
41. Soderlund B, Lundin K. The use of silane-coated silica particles for density gradient centrifugation in in-vitro fertilization. Hum Reprod. 2000;15:857–60.
42. McCann CT, Chantler E. Properties of sperm separated using Percoll and IxaPrep density gradients. A comparison made using CASA, longevity, morphology and the acrosome reaction. Int J Androl. 2000;23:205–9.
43. Wu TP, Huang BM, Tsai HC, Lui MC, Liu MY. Effects of nitric oxide on human spermatozoa activity, fertilization and mouse embryonic development. Arch Androl. 2004;50:173–9.
44. Barroso G, Taylor S, Morshedi M, Manzur F, Gavino F, Oehninger S. Mitochondrial membrane potential integrity and plasma membrane translocation of phosphatidylserine as early apoptotic markers: a comparison of two different sperm subpopulations. Fertil Steril. 2006;85:149–54.
45. Larson KL, Brannian JD, Timm BK, Jost LK, Evenson DP. Density gradient centrifugation and glass wool filtration of semen remove spermatozoa with damaged chromatin structure. Hum Reprod. 1999;14:2015–9.
46. Said TM, Grunewald S, Paasch U, Glander HJ, Baumann T, Kriegel C, Li L, Agarwal A. Advantage of combining magnetic cell separation with sperm preparation techniques. Reprod Biomed Online. 2005;10:740–6.
47. Paulson JD, Polakoski KL. A glass wool column procedure for removing extraneous material from the human ejaculate. Fertil Steril. 1977;28:178–81.
48. Paulson JD, Polakoski KL, Leto S. Further characterization of glass wool column filtration of human semen. Fertil Steril. 1979;32:125–6.

49. Sanchez R, Concha M, Ichikawa T, Henkel R, Schill WB. Glass wool filtration reduces reactive oxygen species by elimination of leukocytes in oligozoospermic patients with leukocytospermia. J Assist Reprod Genet. 1996;13:489–94.

50. Ford WC, McLaughlin EA, Prior SM, Rees JM, Wardle PG, Hull MG. The yield, motility and performance in the hamster egg test of human spermatozoa prepared from cryopreserved semen by four different methods. Hum Reprod. 1992;7:654–9.

51. Sherman JK, Paulson JD, Liu KC. Effect of glass wool filtration on ultrastructure of human spermatozoa. Fertil Steril. 1981;36:643–7.

52. Henkel RR, Franken DR, Lombard CJ, Schill WB. Selective capacity of glass-wool filtration for the separation of human spermatozoa with condensed chromatin: a possible therapeutic modality for male-factor cases? J Assist Reprod Genet. 1994;11:395–400.

53. Henkel R, Schill WB. Sperm separation in patients with urogenital infections. Andrologia. 1998;30 Suppl 1:91–7.

54. Kim SH, Yu DH, Kim YJ. Apoptosis-like change, ROS, and DNA status in cryopreserved canine sperm recovered by glass wool filtration and Percoll gradient centrifugation techniques. Anim Reprod Sci. 2010;119:106–14.

55. Grunewald S, Miska W, Miska G, Rasch M, Reinhardt M, Glander HJ, Paasch U. Molecular glass wool filtration as a new tool for sperm preparation. Hum Reprod. 2007;22:1405–12.

56. Johnson DE, Confino E, Jeyendran RS. Glass wool column filtration versus mini-Percoll gradient for processing poor quality semen samples. Fertil Steril. 1996;66:459–62.

57. Van den Bergh M, Revelard P, Bertrand E, Biramane J, Vanin AS, Englert Y. Glass wool column filtration, an advantageous way of preparing semen samples for intracytoplasmic sperm injection: an auto-controlled randomized study. Hum Reprod. 1997;12:509–13.

58. Rhemrev J, Jeyendran RS, Vermeiden JP, Zaneveld LJ. Human sperm selection by glass wool filtration and two-layer, discontinuous Percoll gradient centrifugation. Fertil Steril. 1989;51:685–90.

59. Dominguez LA, Burgos MH, Fornes MW. Morphometrical comparison of human spermatozoa obtained from semen and swim-up methodology. Andrologia. 1999;31:23–6.

60. Babbo CJ, Hecht BR, Jeyendran RS. Increased recovery of swim-up spermatozoa by application of "antigravitational" centrifugation. Fertil Steril. 1999;72:556–8.

61. Younglai EV, Holt D, Brown P, Jurisicova A, Casper RF. Sperm swim-up techniques and DNA fragmentation. Hum Reprod. 2001;16:1950–3.

62. Scott Jr RT, Oehninger SC, Menkveld R, Veeck LL, Acosta AA. Critical assessment of sperm morphology before and after double wash swim-up preparation for in vitro fertilization. Arch Androl. 1989;23:125–9.

63. Grunewald S, Reinhardt M, Blumenauer V, Hmeidan AF, Glander HJ, Paasch U. Effects of post-density gradient swim-up on apoptosis signalling in human spermatozoa. Andrologia. 2010;42:127–31.

64. Daya S, Gwatkin RB. Improvement in semen quality using glass bead column. Arch Androl. 1987;18:241–4.

65. Drobnis EZ, Zhong CQ, Overstreet JW. Separation of cryopreserved human semen using Sephadex columns, washing, or Percoll gradients. J Androl. 1991;12:201–8.

66. Yavetz H, Hauser R, Homonnai ZT, Paz GF, Lessing JB, Amit A, Yogev I. Separation of sperm cells by sedimentation technique is not suitable for in vitro fertilization purposes. Andrologia. 1996;28:3–6.

67. Chijioke PC, Crocker PR, Gilliam M, Owens MD, Pearson RM. Importance of filter structure for the trans-membrane migration studies of sperm motility. Hum Reprod. 1988;3:241–4.

68. Agarwal A, Manglona A, Loughlin KR. Improvement in semen quality and sperm fertilizing ability after filtration through the L4 membrane: comparison of results with swim up technique. J Urol. 1992;147:1539–41.

69. Bartoov B, Berkovitz A, Eltes F, Kogosowski A, Menezo Y, Barak Y. Real-time fine morphology of motile human sperm cells is associated with IVF-ICSI outcome. J Androl. 2002;23:1–8.

70. Ainsworth C, Nixon B, Aitken RJ. Development of a novel electrophoretic system for the isolation of human spermatozoa. Hum Reprod. 2005;20:2261–70.

71. Huszar G, Ozkavukcu S, Jakab A, Celik-Ozenci C, Sati GL, Cayli S. Hyaluronic acid binding ability of human sperm reflects cellular maturity and fertilizing potential: selection of sperm for intracytoplasmic sperm injection. Curr Opin Obstet Gynecol. 2006;18:260–7.
72. Grunewald S, Paasch U, Glander HJ. Enrichment of non-apoptotic human spermatozoa after cryopreservation by immunomagnetic cell sorting. Cell Tissue Bank. 2001;2:127–33.
73. Paasch U, Grunewald S, Fitzl G, Glander HJ. Deterioration of plasma membrane is associated with activation of caspases in human spermatozoa. J Androl. 2003;24:246–52.
74. Mashiach R, Fisch B, Eltes F, Tadir Y, Ovadia J, Bartoov B. The relationship between sperm ultrastructural features and fertilizing capacity in vitro. Fertil Steril. 1992;57:1052–7.
75. Bartoov B, Berkovitz A, Eltes F, Kogosovsky A, Yagoda A, Lederman H, Artzi S, Gross M, Barak Y. Pregnancy rates are higher with intracytoplasmic morphologically selected sperm injection than with conventional intracytoplasmic injection. Fertil Steril. 2003;80:1413–9.
76. Franco Jr JG, Baruffi RL, Mauri AL, Petersen CG, Oliveira JB, Vagini LD. Significance of large nuclear vacuoles in human spermatozoa: implications for ICSI. Reprod Biomed Online. 2008;17:42–5.
77. Ainsworth C, Nixon B, Jansen RP, Aitken RJ. First recorded pregnancy and normal birth after ICSI using electrophoretically isolated spermatozoa. Hum Reprod. 2007;22:197–200.
78. Huszar G, Ozenci CC, Cayli S, Zavaczki Z, Hansch E, Vigue L. Hyaluronic acid binding by human sperm indicates cellular maturity, viability, and unreacted acrosomal status. Fertil Steril. 2003;79 Suppl 3:1616–24.
79. Sikka SC, Rajasekaran M, Hellstrom WJ. Role of oxidative stress and antioxidants in male infertility. J Androl. 1995;16:464–8.
80. Barroso G, Morshedi M, Oehninger S. Analysis of DNA fragmentation, plasma membrane translocation of phosphatidylserine and oxidative stress in human spermatozoa. Hum Reprod. 2000;15:1338–44.
81. Moustafa MH, Sharma RK, Thornton J, Mascha E, Abdel-Hafez MA, Thomas Jr AJ, Agarwal A. Relationship between ROS production, apoptosis and DNA denaturation in spermatozoa from patients examined for infertility. Hum Reprod. 2004;19:129–38.
82. Wang X, Sharma RK, Sikka SC, Thomas Jr AJ, Falcone T, Agarwal A. Oxidative stress is associated with increased apoptosis leading to spermatozoa DNA damage in patients with male factor infertility. Fertil Steril. 2003;80:531–5.
83. Aitken RJ, De Iuliis GN. On the possible origins of DNA damage in human spermatozoa. Mol Hum Reprod. 2010;16:3–13.
84. Vermes I, Haanen C, Steffens-Nakken H, Reutelingsperger CP. A novel assay for apoptosis: flow cytometric detection of phosphatidylserine expression of early apoptotic cells using fluorescein labelled Annexin V. J Immunol Methods. 1995;184:39–51.
85. Glander HJ, Schaller J. Binding of annexin V to plasma membranes of human spermatozoa: a rapid assay for detection of membrane changes after cryostorage. Mol Hum Reprod. 1999;5:109–15.
86. Paasch U, Grunewald S, Agarwal A, Glandera HJ. Activation pattern of caspases in human spermatozoa. Fertil Steril. 2004;81 Suppl 1:802–9.
87. Said TM, Paasch U, Grunewald S, Baumann T, Li L, Glander HJ, Agarwal A. Advantage of combining magnetic cell separation with sperm preparation techniques. Reprod Biomed Online. 2005;10:740–6.
88. Said TM, Agarwal A, Grunewald S, Rasch M, Baumann T, Kriegel C, Li L, Glander HJ, Thomas Jr AJ, Paasch U. Selection of nonapoptotic spermatozoa as a new tool for enhancing assisted reproduction outcomes: an in vitro model. Biol Reprod. 2006;74:530–7.
89. Grunewald S, Reinhardt M, Blumenauer V, Said TM, Agarwal A, Abu HF, Glander HJ, Paasch U. Increased sperm chromatin decondensation in selected nonapoptotic spermatozoa of patients with male infertility. Fertil Steril. 2009;92:572–7.
90. Dirican EK, Ozgun OD, Akarsu S, Akin KO, Ercan O, Ugurlu M, Camsari C, Kanyilmaz O, Kaya A, Unsal A. Clinical outcome of magnetic activated cell sorting of non-apoptotic spermatozoa before density gradient centrifugation for assisted reproduction. J Assist Reprod Genet. 2008;25:375–81.

Chapter 22
Antioxidants in Sperm Cryopreservation

Tamer Said and Ashok Agarwal

Cryopreservation of human spermatozoa and achieving successful fertilization via assisted reproductive techniques (ART) has been well established [1]. The indications for sperm cryopreservation are many. The technique could be of help in many scenarios encountered in infertility management. It provides an option for storing spermatozoa while maintaining their functional capabilities. Subsequent uses of the preserved semen include intrauterine insemination, in vitro fertilization (IVF), and intracytoplasmic sperm injection (ICSI). Sperm cryopreservation is the only standardized and most feasible method for fertility preservation in men. Cancer patients often resort to cryopreservation to preserve their fertility prior to treatments such as radiation and chemotherapy. Additionally, men undergoing vasectomy procedures will use this method to maintain fertility [2].

Cryopreservation and thawing exposes spermatozoa to various stresses that could eventually lead to the loss of fertilizing potential. Therefore, several improvements have been made to the process of cryopreservation [3]. Despite various advances in cryopreservation methodology, the recovery rate of functional post-thaw spermatozoa remains to be improved [4]. The use of cryoprotectants such as glycerol, ethylene glycol, dimethyl sulfoxide (DMSO), and 1,2-propanediol (PROH) marked one of the most significant advancements in cryopreservation. Cryoprotectants are low molecular weight, highly permeable chemicals that serve to protect spermatozoa from freeze damage induced by ice crystallization. Cryoprotectants act by decreasing the freezing point of a substance, reducing the amount of salts and solutes present in the liquid phase of the sample, and decreasing ice formation within the spermatozoa [5].

T. Said, MD, PhD (✉)
Andrology Laboratory and Reproductive Tissue Bank, The Toronto Institute
for Reproductive Medicine, Toronto, ON, Canada
e-mail: tsaid@repromed.ca

A. Agarwal, PhD
Center for Reproductive Medicine, Glickman Urological and Kidney Institute, Cleveland
Clinic Foundation, 9500 Euclid Avenue, Desk A19, Cleveland, OH 44195, USA
e-mail: agarwaa@ccf.org

S.J. Parekattil and A. Agarwal (eds.), *Antioxidants in Male Infertility: A Guide
for Clinicians and Researchers*, © Springer Science+Business Media New York 2013

Oxidative stress (OS), resulting from an imbalance between reactive oxygen species (ROS) and antioxidants, is detrimental to human spermatozoa resulting in significant loss of function. Increased ROS production and decreased antioxidant levels is known to occur during sperm cryopreservation and thawing [6, 7]. Therefore, OS does play a role in injury sustained by spermatozoa during cryopreservation. Subsequently, antioxidants that counteract the effects of ROS could be of use in preventing OS-induced cryoinjury.

Oxidative Stress and Male Infertility

Oxidative stress has become the focus of interest as a potential cause of male infertility [8–12]. Under physiological conditions, spermatozoa produce small amounts of ROS, which are needed for capacitation, acrosome reaction, and fertilization [13]. However, excessive amounts of ROS produced by leukocytes and immature spermatozoa can cause damage to the normal spermatozoa by inducing lipid peroxidation and DNA damage [14–16]. The primary product of the spermatozoon's free radical generating system appears to be the superoxide anion, which secondarily dismutase to hydrogen peroxide (H_2O_2) through the catalytic action of superoxide dismutase (SOD) [17]. The combination of superoxide anion and H_2O_2 is potentially harmful, and in the presence of transition metals, it can precipitate the generation of hydroxyl radicals [18]. Sperm damage induced by OS includes membrane and DNA damage leading to necrozoospermia, asthenozoospermia, and DNA fragmentation [19].

Normally, an equilibrium exists between ROS production and antioxidant scavenging activities in the male reproductive tract. However, the production of excessive amounts of ROS in semen may overwhelm the antioxidant defense mechanisms of spermatozoa and seminal plasma, leading to OS [20, 21]. The OS status of an individual can be identified by measuring the ROS levels and antioxidants [22]. ROS levels are usually measured by chemiluminescence method [23], while total antioxidant capacity is measured by enhanced chemiluminescence assay or colorimetric assay [22, 24].

Spermatozoa are naturally surrounded by the seminal plasma, which is well endowed with an array of antioxidants that act as free radical scavengers to protect spermatozoa against OS [25]. This defense mechanism compensates for the loss of sperm cytoplasmic enzymes occurring when the cytoplasm is extruded during spermiation, which in turn diminishes endogenous repair mechanisms and enzymatic defenses. Seminal plasma contains a number of enzymatic antioxidants such as SOD, catalase, and glutathione peroxidase. In addition, it contains a variety of nonenzymatic antioxidants such as vitamin C (ascorbic acid), vitamin E (α-tocopherol), pyruvate, glutathione, and carnitine [26].

Effects of Antioxidants on Spermatozoa In Vitro

Reduction of Reactive Oxygen Species Levels

In vitro supplementation with antioxidants is responsible for decreasing ROS in sperm suspensions. Significant reduction of H_2O_2 was achieved by adding different concentrations of vitamin C (300 and 600 µM) and vitamin E (40 and 60 µM) to the sperm preparation medium [27, 28]. Significant reduction in the release of superoxide anion by 29–72% was also achieved following the addition of 10 mM pentoxifylline [29, 30]. Other studies also showed that pentoxifylline is capable of reducing spermatozoal generation of ROS and subsequent lipid peroxidation in asthenozoospermic men [31, 32]. The addition of *N*-acetyl-L-cysteine (NAC) (1 mg/mL) also effectively reduced ROS levels. It may of importance to note that samples with initially high ROS showed the greatest tendency for reduction of ROS in response to antioxidant supplementation in vitro [33].

Effects on Sperm Motility

Antioxidants counteract lipid peroxidation which has a negative effect on sperm motility [34]. In vitro exposure of spermatozoa to several antioxidants proved to be of benefit in terms of promoting sperm motility. Vitamin C (ascorbate) is one of the main antioxidants in seminal plasma; it is a chain breaking antioxidant that protects the lipoproteins from peroxyl radicals. Data show that vitamin C can preserve sperm motility, yet in a dose-dependant manner. Motility was highest after 6-h of incubation in 800 µM vitamin C. However, motility was decreased with concentrations exceeding 1,000 µM [35]. Vitamin E is another major chain breaking antioxidant that when added in vitro can efficiently protect sperm motility and morphology by suppressing the lipid peroxidation [36]. The effects of supplementation with vitamins C and E on sperm motility are also dose dependant. Higher concentrations of vitamins C and E are not protective against H_2O_2-induced peroxidative damage of motility, instead they increase the damage in both normozoospermic and asthenozoospermic patients [37].

Glutathione (GSH) appears also to have a protective effect on sperm motility. In samples characterized with leukocytospermia, the addition of GSH during sperm Percoll preparation and during 24-h incubation resulted in higher recovery of motile spermatozoa [38]. Similarly, a significant improvement was observed in sperm motility after 2-h of incubation with 1.0 mg/mL NAC [33]. Albumin is another antioxidant/extender that has been extensively used in sperm preparation. Its antioxidant properties are due to its ability to react against peroxyl radicals and prevent the propagation of peroxidative damage in sperm [39, 40]. When albumin was used in sperm preparation media, it resulted in significant improvement in motility and viability compared to Percoll [41]. Other antioxidants that proved to be of benefit to the sperm motility include Coenzyme Q10 (50 µM) [42], hypotaurine, and catalase [43].

Enzymatic antioxidants such as SOD and catalase protect spermatozoa from superoxide anion and H_2O_2. Sperm suspension treated with SOD (400 U/mL) had significantly reduced motility loss and malondialdehyde concentration [44]. Similarly, the addition of catalase (0.008 mg/mL) to sperm suspension offered protection against H_2O_2-induced toxicity [45]. In support, the role of catalase and SOD against sperm-intracellular (mitochondrial and plasma membrane) and -extracellular (leukocytes) ROS and their beneficial effects on sperm motility has been consistently reported [46, 47]. Different concentrations of vitamin E (800 µM, 10 mM) can protect sperm against lipid peroxidation [35, 44]. Similarly, pentoxifylline at the dosage of 3.6 and 7.2 mM was proven to limit lipid peroxidation in asthenozoospermic men [31].

Protection of Sperm DNA Integrity

Sperm preparation protocols that are routinely applied during ART and cryopreservation, involve repeated high-speed centrifugation and the isolation of spermatozoa from the protective antioxidant environment provided by seminal plasma. This has been shown to result in sperm DNA damage via pathways that are mediated by increased ROS generation [48]. Swim-up media supplemented with antioxidants [NAC (0.01 mM), catalase (500 U/mL), reduced GSH (10 mM), and hypotaurine (10 mM)] lead to significant reduction of DNA damage induced by ROS generation [49]. Similarly, albumin in doses from 0.3% to 10% protected sperm DNA integrity by neutralizing peroxides produced during lipid peroxidation [40].

It is critical to consider the approach for adding antioxidants as protective agents for the sperm DNA integrity whether single or in combination. Protection of the sperm DNA against H_2O_2-induced damage was demonstrated by vitamin E and vitamin C individually in both normozoospermic and asthenozoospermic samples [27]. However, when a combination of vitamin C and vitamin E was used for spermatozoa incubation, DNA damage was increased. This may be due to vitamin E and vitamin C acting as pro-oxidants [50].

Oxidative Stress During Cryopreservation

Oxidative stress occurring during sperm cryopreservation may be due to increased ROS production and/or decreased antioxidant scavenging activities. The process of ROS generation during cryopreservation and thawing of spermatozoa has been well documented. Data shows that freezing and thawing of spermatozoa causes an increase in the generation of superoxide radicals. A sudden burst of nitric oxide radicals was also observed during thawing [7]. In samples with initially detectable ROS levels, these levels are further significantly increased after cryopreservation/thawing. On the other hand, when samples with no detectable ROS are subjected cryopreservation/thawing, ROS become detected [51].

The decrease in recovery of motile viable sperm following cryopreservation/thawing may be due to damage caused by OS leading to lipid peroxidation of the sperm membrane. The increase in lipid peroxidation sometimes appears to be more significant than the increase in ROS levels when comparing fresh to cryopreserved/thawed sperm [52]. This was demonstrated by the detection of ROS-induced membrane lipid damage in frozen spermatozoa [53]. It has been also reported that the extent of lipid peroxidation is negatively correlated with post-thaw sperm motility [54]. Thus, cryopreservation does enhance lipid peroxidation in human sperm, and this enhancement may be mediated at least in part by the loss of SOD activity occurring during the process [53].

The cryopreservation process has been shown to diminish the antioxidant activity of the spermatozoa making them more susceptible to the ROS-induced damage. In bovine spermatozoa, levels of antioxidants were diminished during freeze/thaw cycles. Cryopreservation significantly reduced sperm GSH levels by 78% and SOD activity by 50% [6]. In humans, one consistent effect of cryopreservation is loss of the enzymatic activity of the peroxidation defense enzyme, SOD [55].

Recent body of evidence suggests that sperm DNA fragmentation occurs as a result of increased OS during sperm cryopreservation [56]. The alteration in the mitochondrial membrane fluidity that occurs during cryopreservation will lead to rise in mitochondrial membrane potential and the release of ROS. Subsequently, released ROS causes DNA damage in sperm. It has been reported that ROS production by both human sperm and seminal leukocytes increases on cooling to 4°C [57]. Thus, cryopreserved semen samples containing leukocytes may be more prone to DNA fragmentation.

The increase in sperm DNA damage during cryopreservation remains to be fully elucidated. While some studies documented it [4, 58], others found that it does not occur [59, 60]. The oxidative DNA biomarker 8-oxoguanine was recently used to assess oxidative DNA damage. Results showed that oxidative sperm DNA damage increased significantly after cryopreservation/thawing [61].

DNA damage resulting from OS is not limited to only ejaculated sperm. Aerobic incubation of testicular sperm results in a significant increase in DNA fragmentation. DNA fragmentation was noted to be higher in cryopreserved sperm than in fresh testicular sperm, and it was maximal after 4-h of incubation [62]. Therefore, care must be taken to avoid incubating cryopreserved and fresh testicular sperm for prolonged periods of time before ICSI is performed.

ROS-induced DNA damage that occurs during sperm cryopreservation may be further increased by other technical procedures that are concurrently conducted. Current laboratory cryopreservation protocols include freezing of raw semen and freezing of washed sperm without seminal plasma [63]. The removal of the antioxidant-rich seminal plasma by sperm preparation prior to cryopreservation may lead to the deterioration in sperm motility post-thaw, cryosurvival rates, and DNA integrity [58, 64]. However, it is important to note that the decrease in quality in pre-washed frozen-thawed sperm may not result in an actual decrease in cycle fecundity [65]. A potential source of ROS in the ART media during semen preparation is the activation of ROS production by immature spermatozoa by either centrifugation or leukocytes contamination. Recent studies suggest that DNA fragmentation in sperm is induced, for the most part, during sperm transport through the seminiferous tubules and the epididymis [15]. This could be mediated by ROS produced by immature sperm. A similar mechanism occurs in the pellet of centrifuged semen where sperm would be also highly packed.

Antioxidants as In Vitro Supplements During Sperm Cryopreservation

Antioxidants act as the main defense against OS induced by free radicals. Thus, the concept of their integration during the cryopreservation/thawing procedure to protect sperm against OS has been extensively evaluated. The addition of vitamin E and vitamin C along to cryoprotectants during cryopreservation resulted in limited if no preservation to the sperm motility when compared with cryoprotectant alone [66]. In contrast, a recent study tested if the addition of an antioxidant to cryopreservation medium could improve the post-thaw integrity of cryopreserved human spermatozoa. It was found that vitamin E was significantly associated with post-thaw motility but neither sperm viability nor DNA fragmentation was affected [67]. The protective effects reported for vitamin E on post-thaw motility may be due to its ability to counteract lipid peroxidation [68]. The benefits of vitamin E supplementation in the cryoprotectant appear to be most marked in semen samples compromised with higher levels of ROS. These include samples from older men and samples with high prevalence of abnormal forms [67, 69].

It is important to note that in other studies, the preserving effects of antioxidants on sperm DNA integrity following cryopreservation and thawing were reported. Supplementation with the antioxidants ascorbate and catalase with the cryoprotectant pre-freeze resulted in a decrease in ROS levels and sperm DNA damage during cryopreservation/thawing [70]. Similarly, the addition of GSH to the thawing medium resulted in: (1) a higher number of non-capacitated viable spermatozoa, (2) a reduction in ROS generation, (3) lower chromatin condensation, (4) lower DNA fragmentation, (5) higher oocyte penetration rate in vitro, and (6) higher in vitro embryo production compared with control group [71].

The positive impact for adding the antioxidant rebamipide was also validated in an in vitro study. Rebamipide effectively scavenged ROS during sperm processing and cryopreservation. This was manifested by lesser decrease in sperm motility following cryopreservation in sperm exposed to 100 and 300 μmol/L of rebamipide. The levels of ROS and lipid peroxidation in semen were also significantly decreased in proportion to the concentrations of rebamipide both after incubation and after cryopreservation [72].

In support of using antioxidant combinations, a study was performed to evaluate the in vitro supplementation of cryoprotectant media with SOD and catalase using samples from 25 male partners of infertile couples. No significant variation in the recovery of progressive motility after freezing and thawing was seen in the aliquots with added SOD or catalase alone, compared with the control group. On the other hand, a significant improvement in sperm parameter recovery was seen in the aliquot with both SOD and catalase supplementation. This may be due to their combined and simultaneous action on superoxide anion and H_2O_2. Therefore, the combination of SOD and catalase prevented lipid peroxidation of the sperm plasma membrane by ROS and contributed to the recovery of high-quality spermatozoa after freezing–thawing procedures [73].

Expert Commentary

The purpose of this chapter was to discuss the role played by antioxidants in human sperm cryopreservation. Normally, a balance exists between levels of ROS and antioxidant scavenging systems. Disturbance of such balance results in OS, which is known to cause peroxidative damage of the sperm plasma membrane and loss of its motility, viability, and DNA integrity. Cryopreservation and thawing is a widely used technique in conjunction with ART that has been reported to cause OS when applied to human spermatozoa. Moreover, cryopreserved spermatozoa tend to lose their limited antioxidant defenses. Subsequent sperm preparation for ART involves several steps of centrifugation and incubation, which further induces OS and affects ART outcome.

One of the rational strategies to counteract OS is to increase the scavenging capacity of the medium that surrounds spermatozoa. This approach has been documented to improve the recovery of spermatozoa with higher quality and fertilization potential following cryopreservation and thawing. Thus, the use of antioxidants in cryopreservation and post-thaw media should be advised.

Five-Year View

Strong body of evidence currently supports the use of antioxidants in cryoprotectant and post-thaw media to prevent OS during cryopreservation and thawing. However, there is no consensus as to the type, combination and concentrations of antioxidants to be added. Therefore, caution should be exercised as excessive amounts of antioxidants may act paradoxically to damage spermatozoa. Well-controlled studies are still needed to identify the ideal antioxidant combination/concentration to supplement the cryoprotectant and post-thaw media.

Key Issues

- Sperm damage is likely to occur during cryopreservation and thawing due to OS. The occurrence of OS during these processes is due to increased ROS production and decrease in scavenging antioxidants.
- Sperm damage occurring during cryopreservation and thawing is manifested by decrease in motility, viability, and DNA integrity. Such changes will ultimately affect the sperm fertilization potential.
- The use of antioxidants is proven to counteract ROS preventing their damaging effect on the sperm.
- The supplementation of cryoprotectant and post-thaw media with antioxidants prevents to a certain extent the damage inflicted on spermatozoa during cryopreservation and thawing.
- Further studies are still needed to identify the optimum antioxidant supplementation protocol during sperm cryopreservation and thawing.

References

1. Bunge RG, Sherman JK. Fertilizing capacity of frozen human spermatozoa. Nature. 1953;172:767–8.
2. Anger JT, Gilbert BR, Goldstein M. Cryopreservation of sperm: indications, methods and results. J Urol. 2003;170:1079–84.
3. Nawroth F, Rahimi G, Isachenko E, et al. Cryopreservation in assisted reproductive technology: new trends. Semin Reprod Med. 2005;23:325–35.
4. Donnelly ET, Steele EK, McClure N, Lewis SE. Assessment of DNA integrity and morphology of ejaculated spermatozoa from fertile and infertile men before and after cryopreservation. Hum Reprod. 2001;16:1191–9.
5. Royere D, Barthelemy C, Hamamah S, Lansac J. Cryopreservation of spermatozoa: a 1996 review. Hum Reprod Update. 1996;2:553–9.
6. Bilodeau JF, Chatterjee S, Sirard MA, Gagnon C. Levels of antioxidant defenses are decreased in bovine spermatozoa after a cycle of freezing and thawing. Mol Reprod Dev. 2000;55:282–8.
7. Chatterjee S, Gagnon C. Production of reactive oxygen species by spermatozoa undergoing cooling, freezing, and thawing. Mol Reprod Dev. 2001;59:451–8.
8. Sharma RK, Agarwal A. Role of reactive oxygen species in male infertility. Urology. 1996;48:835–50.
9. Pasqualotto FF, Sharma RK, Nelson DR, Thomas AJ, Agarwal A. Relationship between oxidative stress, semen characteristics, and clinical diagnosis in men undergoing infertility investigation. Fertil Steril. 2000;73:459–64.
10. Aitken RJ, Baker MA, Sawyer D. Oxidative stress in the male germ line and its role in the aetiology of male infertility and genetic disease. Reprod Biomed Online. 2003;7:65–70.
11. Wang X, Sharma RK, Gupta A, et al. Alterations in mitochondria membrane potential and oxidative stress in infertile men: a prospective observational study. Fertil Steril. 2003;80 Suppl 2:844–50.
12. Wang X, Sharma RK, Sikka SC, Thomas Jr AJ, Falcone T, Agarwal A. Oxidative stress is associated with increased apoptosis leading to spermatozoa DNA damage in patients with male factor infertility. Fertil Steril. 2003;80:531–5.

13. Griveau JF, Le Lannou D. Reactive oxygen species and human spermatozoa: physiology and pathology. Int J Androl. 1997;20:61–9.
14. Aitken RJ, Gordon E, Harkiss D, et al. Relative impact of oxidative stress on the functional competence and genomic integrity of human spermatozoa. Biol Reprod. 1998;59:1037–46.
15. Ollero M, Gil-Guzman E, Lopez MC, et al. Characterization of subsets of human spermatozoa at different stages of maturation: implications in the diagnosis and treatment of male infertility. Hum Reprod. 2001;16:1912–21.
16. Moustafa MH, Sharma RK, Thornton J, et al. Relationship between ROS production, apoptosis and DNA denaturation in spermatozoa from patients examined for infertility. Hum Reprod. 2004;19:129–38.
17. Alvarez J, Touchstone J, Blasco L, Storey B. Spontaneous lipid peroxidation and production of hydrogen peroxide and superoxide in human spermatozoa. Superoxide dismutase as major enzyme protectant against oxygen toxicity. J Androl. 1987;8:338–48.
18. Aitken RJ, Fisher HM, Fulton N, et al. Reactive oxygen species generation by human spermatozoa is induced by exogenous NADPH and inhibited by the flavoprotein inhibitors diphenylene iodonium and quinacrine. Mol Reprod Dev. 1997;47:468–82.
19. Agarwal A, Said TM, Bedaiwy MA, Banerjee J, Alvarez JG. Oxidative stress in an assisted reproductive techniques setting. Fertil Steril. 2006;86:503–12.
20. Sikka SC, Rajasekaran M, Hellstrom WJ. Role of oxidative stress and antioxidants in male infertility. J Androl. 1995;16:464–8.
21. Sikka SC. Role of oxidative stress and antioxidants in andrology and assisted reproductive technology. J Androl. 2004;25:5–18.
22. Sharma RK, Pasqualotto FF, Nelson DR, Thomas Jr AJ, Agarwal A. The reactive oxygen species-total antioxidant capacity score is a new measure of oxidative stress to predict male infertility. Hum Reprod. 1999;14:2801–7.
23. Kobayashi H, Gil-Guzman E, Mahran AM, et al. Quality control of reactive oxygen species measurement by luminol-dependent chemiluminescence assay. J Androl. 2001;22:568–74.
24. Said TM, Kattal N, Sharma RK, et al. Enhanced chemiluminescence assay vs colorimetric assay for measurement of the total antioxidant capacity of human seminal plasma. J Androl. 2003;24:676–80.
25. Smith R, Vantman D, Ponce J, Escobar J, Lissi E. Total antioxidant capacity of human seminal plasma. Hum Reprod. 1996;11:1655–60.
26. Saleh RA, Agarwal A. Oxidative stress and male infertility: from research bench to clinical practice. J Androl. 2002;23:737–52.
27. Donnelly ET, McClure N, Lewis SE. The effect of ascorbate and alpha-tocopherol supplementation in vitro on DNA integrity and hydrogen peroxide-induced DNA damage in human spermatozoa. Mutagenesis. 1999;14:505–12.
28. Donnelly ET, McClure N, Lewis SE. Glutathione and hypotaurine in vitro: effects on human sperm motility, DNA integrity and production of reactive oxygen species. Mutagenesis. 2000;15:61–8.
29. Gavella M, Lipovac V, Marotti T. Effect of pentoxifylline on superoxide anion production by human sperm. Int J Androl. 1991;14:320–7.
30. Gavella M, Lipovac V. Pentoxifylline-mediated reduction of superoxide anion production by human spermatozoa. Andrologia. 1992;24:37–9.
31. McKinney KA, Lewis SE, Thompson W. The effects of pentoxifylline on the generation of reactive oxygen species and lipid peroxidation in human spermatozoa. Andrologia. 1996;28:15–20.
32. Okada H, Tatsumi N, Kanzaki M, Fujisawa M, Arakawa S, Kamidono S. Formation of reactive oxygen species by spermatozoa from asthenospermic patients: response to treatment with pentoxifylline. J Urol. 1997;157:2140–6.
33. Oeda T, Henkel R, Ohmori H, Schill WB. Scavenging effect of N-acetyl-L-cysteine against reactive oxygen species in human semen: a possible therapeutic modality for male factor infertility? Andrologia. 1997;29:125–31.

34. Jones R, Mann T, Sherins R. Peroxidative breakdown of phospholipids in human spermatozoa, spermicidal properties of fatty acid peroxides, and protective action of seminal plasma. Fertil Steril. 1979;31:531–7.
35. Verma A, Kanwar KC. Human sperm motility and lipid peroxidation in different ascorbic acid concentrations: an in vitro analysis. Andrologia. 1998;30:325–9.
36. Aitken RJ, Clarkson JS. Significance of reactive oxygen species and antioxidants in defining the efficacy of sperm preparation techniques. J Androl. 1988;9:367–76.
37. Donnelly ET, McClure N, Lewis SE. Antioxidant supplementation in vitro does not improve human sperm motility. Fertil Steril. 1999;72:484–95.
38. Parinaud J, Le Lannou D, Vieitez G, Griveau JF, Milhet P, Richoilley G. Enhancement of motility by treating spermatozoa with an antioxidant solution (Sperm-Fit) following ejaculation. Hum Reprod. 1997;12:2434–6.
39. Hong CY, Lee MF, Lai LJ, Wang CP. Effect of lipid peroxidation on beating frequency of human sperm tail. Andrologia. 1994;26:61–5.
40. Twigg J, Fulton N, Gomez E, Irvine DS, Aitken RJ. Analysis of the impact of intracellular reactive oxygen species generation on the structural and functional integrity of human spermatozoa: lipid peroxidation, DNA fragmentation and effectiveness of antioxidants. Hum Reprod. 1998;13:1429–36.
41. Armstrong JS, Rajasekaran M, Hellstrom WJ, Sikka SC. Antioxidant potential of human serum albumin: role in the recovery of high quality human spermatozoa for assisted reproductive technology. J Androl. 1998;19:412–9.
42. Lewin A, Lavon H. The effect of coenzyme Q10 on sperm motility and function. Mol Aspects Med. 1997;18(Suppl):S213–9.
43. Baker HW, Brindle J, Irvine DS, Aitken RJ. Protective effect of antioxidants on the impairment of sperm motility by activated polymorphonuclear leukocytes. Fertil Steril. 1996;65:411–9.
44. Kobayashi T, Miyazaki T, Natori M, Nozawa S. Protective role of superoxide dismutase in human sperm motility: superoxide dismutase activity and lipid peroxide in human seminal plasma and spermatozoa. Hum Reprod. 1991;6:987–91.
45. Gagnon C, Iwasaki A, De Lamirande E, Kovalski N. Reactive oxygen species and human spermatozoa. Ann N Y Acad Sci. 1991;637:436–44.
46. Kovalski NN, de Lamirande E, Gagnon C. Reactive oxygen species generated by human neutrophils inhibit sperm motility: protective effect of seminal plasma and scavengers. Fertil Steril. 1992;58:809–16.
47. Griveau JF, Le Lannou D. Effects of antioxidants on human sperm preparation techniques. Int J Androl. 1994;17:225–31.
48. Zalata A, Hafez T, Comhaire F. Evaluation of the role of reactive oxygen species in male infertility. Hum Reprod. 1995;10:1444–51.
49. Lopes S, Jurisicova A, Sun JG, Casper RF. Reactive oxygen species: potential cause for DNA fragmentation in human spermatozoa. Hum Reprod. 1998;13:896–900.
50. Hughes CM, Lewis SE, McKelvey-Martin VJ, Thompson W. The effects of antioxidant supplementation during Percoll preparation on human sperm DNA integrity. Hum Reprod. 1998;13:1240–7.
51. Mazzilli F, Rossi T, Sabatini L, et al. Human sperm cryopreservation and reactive oxygen species (ROS) production. Acta Eur Fertil. 1995;26:145–8.
52. Kadirvel G, Kumar S, Kumaresan A. Lipid peroxidation, mitochondrial membrane potential and DNA integrity of spermatozoa in relation to intracellular reactive oxygen species in liquid and frozen-thawed buffalo semen. Anim Reprod Sci. 2009;114:125–34.
53. Alvarez JG, Storey BT. Evidence for increased lipid peroxidative damage and loss of superoxide dismutase activity as a mode of sublethal cryodamage to human sperm during cryopreservation. J Androl. 1992;13:232–41.
54. Bell M, Wang R, Hellstrom WJ, Sikka SC. Effect of cryoprotective additives and cryopreservation protocol on sperm membrane lipid peroxidation and recovery of motile human sperm. J Androl. 1993;14:472–8.

55. Lasso JL, Noiles EE, Alvarez JG, Storey BT. Mechanism of superoxide dismutase loss from human sperm cells during cryopreservation. J Androl. 1994;15:255–65.
56. Thomson LK, Fleming SD, Aitken RJ, De Iuliis GN, Zieschang JA, Clark AM. Cryopreservation-induced human sperm DNA damage is predominantly mediated by oxidative stress rather than apoptosis. Hum Reprod. 2009;24:2061–70.
57. Wang AW, Zhang H, Ikemoto I, Anderson DJ, Loughlin KR. Reactive oxygen species generation by seminal cells during cryopreservation. Urology. 1997;49:921–5.
58. Donnelly ET, McClure N, Lewis SE. Cryopreservation of human semen and prepared sperm: effects on motility parameters and DNA integrity. Fertil Steril. 2001;76:892–900.
59. Duru NK, Morshedi MS, Schuffner A, Oehninger S. Cryopreservation-thawing of fractionated human spermatozoa is associated with membrane phosphatidylserine externalization and not DNA fragmentation. J Androl. 2001;22:646–51.
60. Isachenko V, Isachenko E, Katkov II, et al. Cryoprotectant-free cryopreservation of human spermatozoa by vitrification and freezing in vapor: effect on motility, DNA integrity, and fertilization ability. Biol Reprod. 2004;71:1167–73.
61. Zribi N, Chakroun NF, El Euch H, Gargouri J, Bahloul A, Keskes LA. Effects of cryopreservation on human sperm deoxyribonucleic acid integrity. Fertil Steril. 2010;93:159–66.
62. Dalzell LH, McVicar CM, McClure N, Lutton D, Lewis SE. Effects of short and long incubations on DNA fragmentation of testicular sperm. Fertil Steril. 2004;82:1443–5.
63. Saritha KR, Bongso A. Comparative evaluation of fresh and washed human sperm cryopreserved in vapor and liquid phases of liquid nitrogen. J Androl. 2001;22:857–62.
64. Grizard G, Chevalier V, Griveau JF, Le Lannou D, Boucher D. Influence of seminal plasma on cryopreservation of human spermatozoa in a biological material-free medium: study of normal and low-quality semen. Int J Androl. 1999;22:190–6.
65. Wolf DP, Patton PE, Burry KA, Kaplan PF. Intrauterine insemination-ready versus conventional semen cryopreservation for donor insemination: a comparison of retrospective results and a prospective, randomized trial. Fertil Steril. 2001;76:181–5.
66. Askari HA, Check JH, Peymer N, Bollendorf A. Effect of natural antioxidants tocopherol and ascorbic acids in maintenance of sperm activity during freeze-thaw process. Arch Androl. 1994;33:11–5.
67. Taylor K, Roberts P, Sanders K, Burton P. Effect of antioxidant supplementation of cryopreservation medium on post-thaw integrity of human spermatozoa. Reprod Biomed Online. 2009;18:184–9.
68. Verma A, Kanwar KC. Effect of vitamin E on human sperm motility and lipid peroxidation in vitro. Asian J Androl. 1999;1:151–4.
69. Weir CP, Robaire B. Spermatozoa have decreased antioxidant enzymatic capacity and increased reactive oxygen species production during aging in the Brown Norway rat. J Androl. 2007;28:229–40.
70. Li ZL, Lin QL, Liu RJ, Xie WY, Xiao WF. Reducing oxidative DNA damage by adding antioxidants in human semen samples undergoing cryopreservation procedure. Zhonghua Yi Xue Za Zhi. 2007;87:3174–7.
71. Gadea J, Gumbao D, Canovas S, Garcia-Vazquez FA, Grullon LA, Gardon JC. Supplementation of the dilution medium after thawing with reduced glutathione improves function and the in vitro fertilizing ability of frozen-thawed bull spermatozoa. Int J Androl. 2008;31:40–9.
72. Park NC, Park HJ, Lee KM, Shin DG. Free radical scavenger effect of rebamipide in sperm processing and cryopreservation. Asian J Androl. 2003;5:195–201.
73. Rossi T, Mazzilli F, Delfino M, Dondero F. Improved human sperm recovery using superoxide dismutase and catalase supplementation in semen cryopreservation procedure. Cell Tissue Bank. 2001;2:9–13.

Chapter 23
Antioxidants in ICSI

Nicolas Garrido, Sandra García-Herrero, Laura Romany, José Remohí, Antonio Pellicer, and Marcos Meseguer

Male factor infertility can be caused by reasons, either related or not with total sperm production. Among causes of male infertility in cases of normal sperm count and motility, oxidative stress is one of the most relevant processes influencing fertility in vivo or in assisted reproduction treatments' results. This chapter provides the most updated information regarding the oxidative stress situation in sperm and the relevance of antioxidants use in intracytoplasmic sperm injection (ICSI) results.

Male Factor Infertility Relevance and Its Measurement

Male factor infertility is responsible of almost 50% of all cases of infertility affecting approximately 5% of the general population [1]. Male fertility is defined as the ability of a man to impregnate a healthy, fertile woman of reproductive age, although

N. Garrido, PhD (✉)
Andrology Laboratory and Sperm Bank, Instituto Universitario IVI Valencia,
Plaza de la Policía Local 3, Valencia, 46015, Spain
e-mail: nicolas@garrido@ivi.es

S. García-Herrero, PhD
IVIOMICS, Valencia, Spain

L. Romany, MD • M. Meseguer, PhD
Clinical Embryology Laboratory, Instituto Universitario IVI Valencia,
Plaza de la Policía Local 3, Valencia, 46015, Spain

J. Remohí, MD • A. Pellicer, MD
Department of Gynecology and Obstetrics, School of Medicine,
Universidad de Valencia, Valencia, Spain

Assisted Reproduction Unit, Instituto Universitario IVI Valencia,
Universidad de Valencia, Plaza de la Policía Local 3, Valencia, 46015, Spain

S.J. Parekattil and A. Agarwal (eds.), *Antioxidants in Male Infertility: A Guide for Clinicians and Researchers*, © Springer Science+Business Media New York 2013

tagging a male as fertile or infertile is extremely difficult since it can vary in short periods of time and with different partners. These assertions also may be considered from the point of view of a single ejaculate. In this sense, it is interesting to define a sperm sample as able to accomplish a pregnancy or not, instead of defining a male as fertile or infertile [2].

The only accepted tool to estimate the male potential to become a father is the basic sperm analysis as stated by the World Health Organization [3] based on the volume, sperm concentration and percentage of spermatozoa with progressive motility and normal shape. Subsequently, subfertile men can also be defined as those unable to achieve a natural conception and able to conceive with the help of assisted reproduction techniques.

The inability of a man to conceive can be either related with sperm count or related with molecular defects within sperm cells, thus leading to a reproductive failure at different levels. Those related with sperm count, that are frequently associated with genetic defects in the most severe cases, have been successfully treated to a certain extent by the implementation of IVF and ICSI techniques. These assisted reproduction technologies permit the avoidance of natural barriers in the selection of sperm that makes conception in the cases presenting low sperm count impossible and that otherwise would be necessary to select the most adequate sperm to fertilize an egg. Then, the collateral and involuntary harm caused by assisted reproduction could be related to the lack of natural selection, thus being able to create embryos with the wrong sperm cell, thus leading to embryo blockage during development or implantation failure.

Subsequently, the most intriguing male infertility causes are those independent of the total number of sperm cells produced by the testis. These defects are not detected by the routine sperm analysis and are responsible of a huge amount of infertility problems [4].

Apart from the basic sperm analysis, few tests are available to conclude the real possibilities of a male to become a father. From the existing evidences, several factors in sperm seem to be related to male fertility, but none of them seem enough to cause themselves inability to procreate, leading us to the hypothesis that male idiopathic infertility is caused by the combination of different factors. Among them, those related to the reactive oxygen species overload have been demonstrated to be crucial in the last years.

Oxidative Stress and Male Factor Infertility

OS is the disequilibrium between oxidative and antioxidative molecules in a biological system where the oxidants overcome the defensive systems [5] where reactive oxygen species (ROS) are primarily produced by O_2 metabolism in cells living under aerobic conditions, being able to produce interferences or destruction on cell biological functions and properties.

Cells in a biological environment (as ejaculates are) contribute to the maintenance of the oxidative homeostasis by complex systems, and a small and controlled level of ROS is necessary for normal cell function. This control is produced by antioxidants. These molecules are grouped depending on their nature into enzymatic and non-enzymatic or endogenous and exogenous.

Endogenous Sources of Free Radicals

Human semen is a complex mixture of cells comprised within the seminal plasma, including both mature and immature spermatozoa, round cells from different initial steps of the spermatogenesis process, leukocytes and other occasional cell types as epithelial cells. Among them, immature spermatozoa and leukocytes are the main ROS sources. Abnormal spermatozoa, with aberrant cytoplasmic droplet retention, are very important ROS producers since an excess of cytoplasmic enzymes involved in the glucose metabolism (such as glucose-6-phosphate dehydrogenase, NADPH oxidase system and NADH-dependent oxidoreductase) can be found at two different sites: plasma membrane and mitochondria due to the above mentioned cytoplasmic retention. Serial steps of different ROS production and combination results in the formation of distinct ROS such as superoxide anion, hydrogen peroxide and hydroxyl radicals initiate molecular damage by their interaction with cellular macromolecules [5].

Moreover, it has been confirmed that when seminal ejaculate is fractioned by a density gradient, the layer with immature sperm, with the highest percentage of immature cells, is the most ROS-producing group. This ROS production by immature spermatozoa is also directly correlated with the extent of DNA damage to mature sperm, and the higher ROS production, the lower percentage of mature spermatozoa [6].

The second ROS-producer cell type is the immune white cell lineage of the ejaculate. Their presence on the raw semen exerts a part of their defensive activity when activated by the direct production of ROS and the indirect stimulation of ROS production of neighbouring immune cells via soluble factors

Furthermore, two considerations must be done: first, leukocyte concentrations considered normal by WHO criteria can produce damaging ROS levels [7, 8], and second, leukocytes can stimulate sperm ROS production [9]. Overwhelming the protective capacity of the system by the ROS attack provokes an irreparable damage on DNA molecules, acrosome reaction is also deregulated, and finally, sperm/oocyte fusion is disturbed or impeded [10]. Some studies revealed the importance of these phenomena on male fertility since almost 40% of infertile males displayed abnormally increased ROS levels, and human spermatozoa are extremely sensitive to ROS-induced damage due to their particular plasma membrane composition [11, 12].

Exogenous Sources of Free Radicals

Lab Protocols

Centrifugation of a semen sample to select sperm for intrauterine insemination (IUI) or in vitro fertilization (IVF) can aggravate sperm oxidative stress, although it is easily reduced by decreasing the centrifugation time [13, 14], use of swim-up or glass-wool filtration, and limiting the time in which sperm are cultured in media with seminal plasma. Furthermore, culturing sperm under low oxygen tension (5% O_2/95% CO_2 vs. 20% atmospheric O_2 content) has been shown to also improve sperm quality by reducing seminal leukocyte ROS production [15–17]. Avoiding use of cryopreserved sperm for fertilization is also ideal since ROS are produced during freezing and thawing of the sperm, thereby decreasing sperm quality [17]. Sperm preparation media may also be supplemented with a variety of antioxidants to guard against oxidative stress. The addition of catalase/SOD [18], vitamin C [19], vitamin E [20], ferulic acid [21], EDTA [22], glutathione/hypotaurine [23], albumin [24] and *N*-acetyl-cysteine [25] to sperm preparation media has all been shown to protect sperm from oxidative attack. Recently, the use of genistein as antioxidant has been demonstrated to improve sperm quality after freezing [26].

Lifestyle

Smoking results in a 48% increase in seminal leukocyte concentrations and a 107% in seminal ROS [27]. Smokers have decreased levels of seminal plasma antioxidants such as vitamin E [28] and vitamin C [29], placing their sperm at additional risk of oxidative damage, confirmed by the finding of a significant increase in levels of 8-OHdG within smoker's seminal plasma [28] and deficiencies in sperm capacitation [30, 31].

Dietary deficiencies have been linked with sperm oxidative damage by several research groups. The Age and Genetic Effects in Sperm (AGES) study examined the self-reported dietary intake of various antioxidants and nutrients (vitamins C and E, b-carotene, folate and zinc) [32], finding a significant correlation between vitamin C intake and sperm concentration and also in vitamin E intake and total progressively motile sperm and reinforcing previous reports [33]. However, the AGES study did not found a link between low intake of antioxidants and sperm DNA damage [34] against the results of others [35].

Excessive alcohol consumption increases systemic oxidative stress as ethanol stimulates the production of ROS [36, 37]. Within the testicle, this implies a significant reduction in plasma testosterone, increase in serum lipid peroxidation by-products and a drop in antioxidants [38].

Extremes of exercise activity, at both ends of the spectrum, have been linked with oxidative stress; this link is explained by the increased muscle aerobic metabolism creating a large amount of ROS [39]. On the other side, obesity produces oxidative stress as adipose tissue releases proinflammatory cytokines that increase leukocyte production of ROS [40] and heating of the testicle [41] also linked with oxidative stress and reduced sperm quality.

Environment

Phthalates are chemicals used as plastics softener contained in food packaging and personal care products that have been linked with impaired spermatogenesis and increased sperm DNA damage [42, 43]. In rat model, it increases the generation of ROS within the testis and decreases antioxidant levels, impairing spermatogenesis [44].

Several environmental pollutants have been linked with testicular oxidative stress in rodent models, such as lindane [45], methoxychlor and the herbicide dioxin-TCDD [46, 47]. The commonly used preservative sulphur dioxide has also been shown to produce testicular oxidative stress in laboratory animals [48]. Air pollutants such as diesel particulate matter act as potent stimuli for leukocyte ROS generation [49].

Also, heavy metal exposure has reported with a similar effect: cadmium and lead are linked with an increase in testicular oxidative stress [50, 51] and a resultant increase in sperm DNA oxidation [52].

The Control of Free Radicals: The Antioxidants

Seminal plasma is especially relevant to protect spermatozoa against ROS; because of the diminished cytoplasm of sperm decreasing the capacity to retain adequate loads of protective molecules inside the cell, they will depend on the extracellular environment [53].

The SOD family presents three different classes, depending on the catalytic metal at the active site. This enzyme works catalyzing the dismutation of superoxide into hydrogen peroxide and oxygen, with a direct relationship between sperm SOD activity in spermatozoa, but not plasma, and sperm motility [54]. Adding exogenous SOD significantly decreased the loss of motility with time, and the increase of the malonyldialdehyde concentration was initially related with the percentage of immotile cells. These data suggest a significant role for SOD in sperm motility. It seems that lipid peroxidation of human spermatozoa may cause loss of motility and that SOD may inhibit this lipid peroxidation, although some authors are unable to correlate SOD activity with seminal parameters or reproductive success in vivo or in vitro [55, 56].

Catalase has also been found in human spermatozoa and seminal plasma [57] of normal and infertile males and works preventing oxygen-derived free radicals induced damage inactivating H_2O_2 and yielding water and O_2.

Other ROS scavenging enzymes such as glutathione (GPx) have also been measured in seminal plasma and correlated with the fertility status of the male [58]. GPx family of enzymes is composed by several forms, able to detoxify organic or hydrogen peroxides, converting them to stable alcohols or water, thus protecting cells from oxidative damage. The GPx enzymes containing Se (as a selenocysteine on the molecule) need the presence of reduced glutathione (GSH) that restores the oxidized Se.

Coupled to this reaction, glutathione reductase (GR) catalyzes the step from oxidized to reduced glutathione to restore the GSH stock available for GPX. We evaluated the GPX system finding a significant relationship of GPX1 and GPX4 with male infertility [59, 60].

Non-enzymatic protection was described by Alvarez and Storey in classical experiments, where demonstrated in vitro the effect of protection against lipid peroxidation of rabbit spermatozoa of some molecules as taurine, hypotaurine, epinephrine, pyruvate, lactate and bovine serum albumin [61]. Taurine and hypotaurine molecules have been lately found to be present in seminal plasma of infertile males at a different rate and have also been associated with concrete sperm defects [62].

Other non-enzymatic molecules are probably acting in seminal plasma in the scavenging of free radicals, and lots of information regarding their scavenging activity are available about other biological systems, but they have not been yet studied in semen. Some examples are ferritin, alpha lipoic acid, L-ergothioneine, ebselen, etc.

The Main Consequences of OS in Sperm Affecting ICSI Results

DNA Oxidation

We determined the relevance of sperm DNA oxidation as one of the main consequences of OS on embryo quality and reproductive outcome by prospectively studying pairs of oocyte donation cycles, i.e. the same oocyte donors, donating to two recipients, where the only difference between the two treatments was the use of a different sperm sample [63].

Regarding embryo morphology, an important association of embryo asymmetry and increased DNA oxidation was observed. In addition, in the later in vitro phase, those embryos reaching the blastocyst stage were associated with lower sperm DNA oxidation levels (Fig. 23.1).

On the other hand, we observed a minor decrease of DNA oxidation in patients who did not achieve pregnancy, although this difference was not found to be significant. This could be due to embryo selection before transfer, so poor prognosis embryos are no longer chosen. In the absence of such selection, it may be possible that pregnancy could be associated with sperm DNA oxidation.

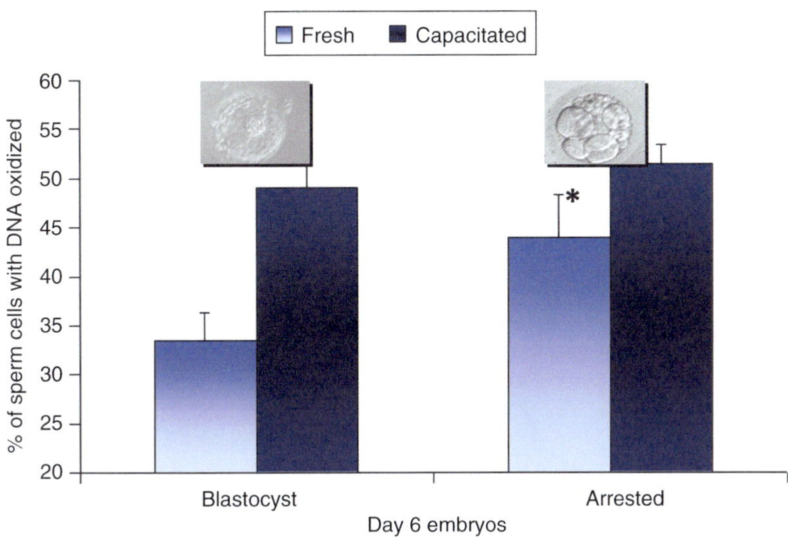

Fig. 23.1 Embryo quality on day 6 depending on the sperm DNA oxidation status

In addition, if we analyse the differences in the IVF outcome parameters of the couples who shared the oocyte cohort (same donor) with the differences in the OXI DNA values, we observed increased and further relationships with embryo quality. Oxidative damage in the DNA is clearly increased in samples with lower sperm motility. An association between early and late embryo quality and sperm DNA oxidation supports the relevance of the hydroxylation of 8-oxoguanine like a biomarker of sperm quality reflecting the free radical damage in human sperm.

We also determined the relevance of sperm DNA oxidation caused by free radicals in sperm retrieved from testicular biopsies, analysing their corresponding assisted reproduction treatments and using ovum donation to standardize female's characteristics. We studied its effect on embryo quality and reproductive success [64].

Testicular cells present a wide variety of types and ploidies (haploids: sperm and round spermatids; diploids: spermatogonia, secondary spermatocytes, Sertoli and Leydig cells, immune cells, myoid cells, fibroblasts, etc.; and tetraploids: primary spermatocytes). To determine cell ploidy, a dual staining with propidium iodide was conducted. This staining permitted the evaluation of cell ploidy and 8-OH staining within each category. Also, the appropriate gates to distinguish between spermatic and non-spermatic haploid cells were created by using shape properties analysed by the flow cytometer.

When the percentage of 8-OhdG + cells is considered within each ploidy group among testicular cells, there is an increase in non-obstructive azoospermia (NOA) in comparison with obstructive azoospermia (OA) when considering only haploid sperm cells. About 4% more haploid cells are presenting oxidized DNA, while there is almost a 1.5% increase in the cells with presence of DNA oxidation in NOA vs.

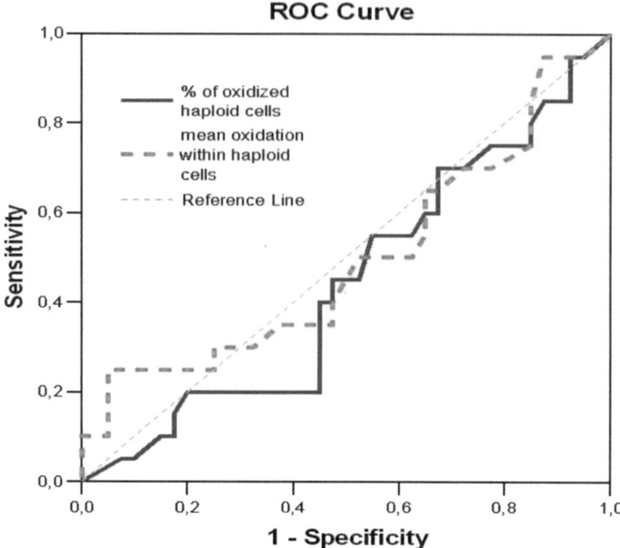

Fig. 23.2 ROC curve analysis of the predictive value of sperm DNA oxidation on pregnancy forecast

OA considering only diploid cells, and only a 0.16% difference in 8-OH staining is found in tetraploid cells between groups, being again more oxidized those sperm from males with NOA.

We found a very low clinical relevance of the status of sperm DNA oxidation on several embryo quality parameters and fertilization rate, early (days 2–3) and late (days 5–6) development, and pregnancy achievement (Fig. 23.2). The studies where DNA oxidation was studied, the employment of ovum donation models to standardize clinical parameters of the female, as well as employing regression analysis controlling possible confounding factors add strength to these results.

DNA Fragmentation

One of the OS consequences is a direct damage to sperm DNA integrity. Male infertility is associated with poor sperm DNA integrity, and it has been suggested that these DNA abnormalities may affect procreation in couples having natural intercourse and in those treated by IUI, IVF and ICSI. The increase in the use of ART has enlarged the emphasis on the sperm chromatin quality.

We prospectively evaluated the predictive value of the SCD test on pregnancy outcome by IUI [65] in couples with non-severe male factor, and to correlate DNA fragmentation with sperm parameters, and found that chromatin dispersion in sperm, as measured by the SCD test, is not correlated with pregnancy outcome in IUI.

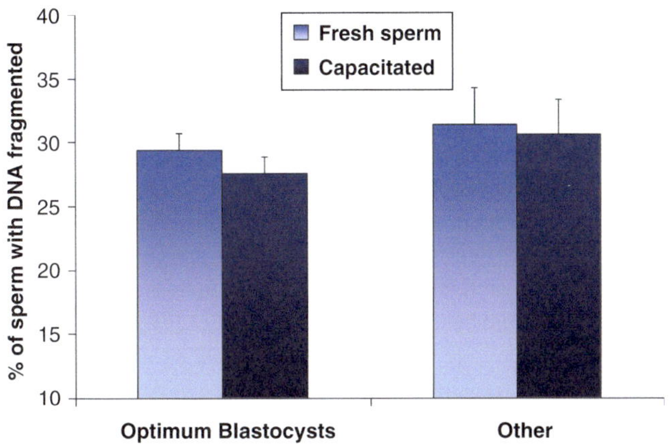

Fig. 23.3 Blastocyst quality depending on the % of sperm with fragmented DNA

However, a significant correlation was found between sperm motility and SCD test values.

In a subsequent work, we also determined the prognostic value of sperm DNA fragmentation levels, as measured by the SCD test, in predicting IVF and ICSI outcome [66]. The degree of DNA fragmentation was inversely correlated with fertilization rate, synchrony of the nucleolar precursor bodies' pattern in pronuclei, embryo ability to achieve blastocyst stage and embryo morphological quality. Because SCD test values were correlated with embryo quality and blastocyst rate, the lack of correlation between sperm DNA fragmentation and pregnancy outcome in IVF might be due to embryo selection before transfer.

Essentially, two interesting details are derived from the results. First, the determination of sperm DNA fragmentation could be of special interest for patients with low gestation rates and low embryonic quality. The DNA damage could then be a possible causal factor. Second, the observation of nucleolar asynchrony in a zygote from a sperm sample with a high DNA fragmentation level could orientate to the possibility of a future low-quality blastocyst. Therefore, this could be an interesting criterion to orientate for embryo selection when the transfer occurs on day 3. In conclusion, the degree of DNA fragmentation, established using the SCD test, appears to be related to the ability of sperm to fertilize as well as the ability of the embryo to achieve the blastocyst stage until day 6 (Fig. 23.3). The correlation of the sperm DNA fragmentation level with embryo health appears quite promising in predicting the quality of the embryo cohort after IVF/ICSI procedures [66].

Recently, we prospectively analysed sperm DNA fragmentation in testicular sperm samples from azoospermic patients, either by spermatogenic failure or by duct obstruction [67]. Levels of fragmentation in testes presented an average of 37.70% of positive spermatozoa. The number of sperm cells recovered per field and motile sperm recovered per field after testicular biopsy was not related with fragmentation, but these levels were associated with defective spermatogenesis (non-obstructive azoospermia), being significantly higher (46.92%) than in patients with normal testicular sperm production (obstructive azoospermia) (35.96%). A moderate relationship between embryo morphological parameters and testicular DNA fragmentation was detected. Nevertheless and like we observed in previous studies, no significant relation was detected with pregnancy outcome. This result suggests that spermatogenesis failure may result in a more severe affectation of sperm DNA integrity. The degree of DNA fragmentation using SCD test is related to the sperm production and embryo quality parameters, but finally, this is not reflected in pregnancy chances, probably due to the embryo selection bias. Our observations reveal that average values are comparable to levels of ejaculated sperm from infertile and cancer patients and higher than sperm donors [68].

Further studies are also needed to determine those mechanisms involved in the increased DNA fragmentation observed in those patients with defective spermatogenesis process. Current research projects are undergoing the study of the direct effect of the oxidative stress on DNA oxidation process produced in testicular sperm cells. This could be the primary source of DNA fragmentation and maybe the administration of antioxidants to the patients could overcome this defect. Nevertheless, reports concerning the clinical usefulness of antioxidants in the treatment of male infertility are controversial. Even more, our results are against post-testicular damage on DNA because we have observed high levels of fragmentation in testicular sperm and even higher in those coming from a non-obstructive azoospermia. In consequence, we are not completely agreed with those that postulate the utility of testicular sperm extraction in patients with high levels of DNA fragmentation combined with severe oligozoospermia. In this situation, spermatogenesis is clearly affected, and in consequence, those sperm cells coming from testes would have also high fragmentation.

Apoptosis

Apoptosis is a noninflammatory response to tissue damage characterized by a series of morphological and biochemical changes [69–72]. In the context of male reproductive tissue, it helps in elimination of abnormal spermatozoa, thus maintaining the nursing capacity of the Sertoli cells [71, 72]. High levels of ROS disrupt the inner and outer mitochondrial membranes, inducing the release of the cytochrome-C protein and activating the caspases and apoptosis. Apoptosis in sperm also may be initiated by ROS-independent pathways involving the cell surface protein Fas. Fas is a type I membrane protein that belongs to the tumour necrosis factor-nerve growth factor receptor family and mediates apoptosis [73]. When Fas ligand or agonistic anti-Fas antibody binds to Fas, apoptosis occurs. On the other hand, bcl-2, the inhibitor gene of apoptosis, protects the cell, most likely by mechanisms that reduce ROS production.

Although the Fas protein often leads to apoptosis, some of the Fas-labelled cells may escape apoptosis through abortive apoptosis. This results in a failure to clear all of the spermatozoa destined for elimination and thus leads to a large population of abnormal spermatozoa in the semen. This failure to clear Fas-positive spermatozoa may be due to a dysfunction at one or more levels. First, the production of spermatozoa may not be enough to trigger apoptosis in men with hypospermatogenesis. In this case, Fas-positive spermatogonia may escape the signal to undergo apoptosis. Second, Fas-positive spermatozoa also may exist because of problems in activating Fas-mediated apoptosis. In this scenario, apoptosis is aborted and fails to clear spermatozoa that are earmarked for elimination by apoptosis [69]. In men with abnormal sperm parameters (oligozoospermia and azoospermia), the percentage of Fas-positive spermatozoa can be as high as 50%. Samples with low sperm concentrations are more likely to have a high proportion of Fas-positive spermatozoa [52].

Mitochondrial exposure to ROS results in the release of apoptosis-inducing factor (AIF), which directly interacts with the DNA and leads to DNA fragmentation. In another study by our group, a positive correlation was demonstrated between increased sperm damage by ROS and higher levels of cytochrome C and caspases 9 and 3, which indicate positive apoptosis in patients with male factor infertility [74]. Activation of caspases 8, 9, 1 and 3 in human ejaculated spermatozoa has been studied to examine the main pathways of apoptosis [75, 76]. Potential functional impact of this phenomenon and possible activation mechanisms were examined by subjecting cells to freezing and thawing, and testing the dependence of caspase activity on membrane integrity [77].

In an earlier study carried out by our group, annexin V staining assay was used to study the externalization of phosphatidylserine, a marker of early apoptosis. It was shown that mature spermatozoa from infertility patients had significantly higher levels of apoptosis compared with the mature spermatozoa from a control group of normal sperm donors [78].

The Effects of Antioxidant Supplementation in ICSI Results

To date, several studies have been published examining the effect of antioxidant treatments on sperm parameters and pregnancy outcome by means of sexual intercourse, but the use of different types and doses of antioxidants and lack of placebos or randomized and controlled studies, together with very small sample sizes, made unable to draw valid conclusions about the benefits of an antioxidant therapy.

Several studies have reported that levels of ROS within semen can be reduced by increasing the protective capacity of seminal plasma with oral antioxidants, such as Astaxanthin [79], carnitine [80] or a combination of antioxidants such as acetylcysteine, b-carotene, vitamin E and essential fatty acids [81]. A randomized control study comparing vitamin E [82, 83] and vitamin E + selenium [84] decreases sperm malonyldialdehyde levels, while the use of vitamin C and vitamin E reported a very significant reduction in sperm DNA damage in other reports [85, 86].

The ability of these changes to improve pregnancy chances is dubious. Suleiman et al. [82] reported that treatment with vitamin E resulted in a significant fall in ROS damage to sperm and an improvement in spontaneous pregnancy rates during the next 6 months (21% pregnancy rate in the vitamin E group vs. 0% in the placebo group), but these results have not been confirmed later.

The only work with an adequate design as randomized and controlled trial available comparing the ability of an antioxidant treatment to improve IVF/ICSI results was published by Tremellen, comparing Menevit with placebo and demonstrating a significant increase in clinical pregnancy rate if the antioxidant was taken for 3 months prior to IVF/ICSI treatment [87].

The main components of Menevit were Vitamins C and E, selenium and lycopene, garlic to reduce seminal leukocyte ROS production and also zinc, selenium and folate to increase protamine and DNA packaging.

Otherwise, there is very little information available about the benefits on having an antioxidant therapy in the male prior to IVF/ICSI treatments, with a design that limited the possibility to draw definitive conclusions [86].

Couples undergoing assisted reproduction treatments due to a prolonged infertility may be benefited from the use of antioxidants in order to improve OS situation in sperm. This hypothesis can be formulated from data supporting a deleterious effect of the ROS in sperm and ICSI treatments, although very few direct evidences are available so far and well-designed randomized controlled trials to demonstrate their effectiveness are needed.

Expert Commentary

Oxidative stress is undoubtedly one of the most prevalent problems contributing to male infertility when infertile males do not present non-severe spermatogenesis impairment. Several molecules and processes are involved, thus forming a complex system, where it is really difficult to measure the OS status of the man and even design the therapies to solve it.

Moreover, these men are investigated regarding infertility causes at the time of attempting assisted reproduction, after they consumed more than 1 year of unprotected intercourse seeking parenthood. This fact makes also relevant to characterize the link between assisted reproduction treatments and results depending on oxidative stress in semen.

Then, it is fundamental to consider the effects of OS in sperm cells as a real difficulty to succeed and consider the possibility of the supplementation of the culture media to treat the biological samples or administering the male antioxidative agents to avoid this damage and improve their chances. Nevertheless, RCTs are needed in order to confirm which antioxidants can effectively improve live birth rates, in both natural conception and after assisted reproduction treatments.

Five-Year View

Actually several scientific efforts are being conducted aiming to establish the way to accurately evaluate the OS situation in a sperm sample and its relevance on the modulation of sperm physiology together with clinical trials aiming to test the effectiveness of several molecules with antioxidant abilities to increase the fertility potential of men susceptible to be affected by OS.

In a recent future, there will be available laboratory tests to determine OS and identify infertile males affected, together with the most convenient antioxidant treatments in each case, which directly will improve conception by either natural or assisted reproduction.

Key Issues

- Oxidative stress is the biochemical situation where the presence of reactive oxygen species overcomes the antioxidant capacity, thus leading to abnormally high amounts of these species causing cellular damage.
- Male infertility has been related to oxidative stress situations in many research works, by means of different origins, processes and systems.
- There are several features of sperm caused by oxidative stress able to be microscopically identified in vivo and others that remain 'occult'.
- When attempting assisted reproduction by ICSI, these 'occult' effects of oxidative stress can be impairing the success chances, given that sperm cells are only selected by their morphology.
- The potential benefits of the antioxidant molecules in these cases are not fully accepted, although theoretically, they can have a positive effect.
- These molecules to scavenge free radicals can be employed either in the male or in the culture media in contact with reproductive cells.
- Further research is needed to develop the adequate diagnostic tools for oxidative stress determination and the design of efficient therapies.

Acknowledgments The authors want to acknowledge all the staff of IVI Valencia, in both the IVF and Andrology laboratory for their support in the research projects during the recent years, especially for the lab technicians.

References

1. McLachlan RI, de Kretser DM. Male infertility: the case for continued research. Med J Aust. 2001;174(3):116–7.
2. Braundmeier AG, Miller DJ. The search is on: finding accurate molecular markers of male fertility. J Dairy Sci. 2001;84(9):1915–25.
3. World Health Organization. WHO laboratory manual for the examination of human semen and sperm-cervical mucus interaction. 4th ed. Cambridge: Cambridge University Press; 1999.

4. Garrido N, Remohi J, Martinez-Conejero JA, Garcia-Herrero S, Pellicer A, Meseguer M. Contribution of sperm molecular features to embryo quality and assisted reproduction success. Reprod Biomed Online. 2008;17(6):855–65.
5. Garrido N, Meseguer M, Simon C, Pellicer A, Remohi J. Pro-oxidative and anti-oxidative imbalance in human semen and its relation with male fertility. Asian J Androl. 2004;6(1): 59–65.
6. Saleh RA, Agarwal A. Oxidative stress and male infertility: from research bench to clinical practice. J Androl. 2002;23(6):737–52.
7. Sharma RK, Pasqualotto AE, Nelson DR, Thomas Jr AJ, Agarwal A. Relationship between seminal white blood cell counts and oxidative stress in men treated at an infertility clinic. J Androl. 2001;22(4):575–83.
8. Sharma RK, Pasqualotto FF, Nelson DR, Thomas Jr AJ, Agarwal A. The reactive oxygen species-total antioxidant capacity score is a new measure of oxidative stress to predict male infertility. Hum Reprod. 1999;14(11):2801–7.
9. Saleh RA, Agarwal A, Kandirali E, et al. Leukocytospermia is associated with increased reactive oxygen species production by human spermatozoa. Fertil Steril. 2002;78(6):1215–24.
10. Agarwal A, Gupta S, Sikka S. The role of free radicals and antioxidants in reproduction. Curr Opin Obstet Gynecol. 2006;18(3):325–32.
11. Padron OF, Brackett NL, Sharma RK, Lynne CM, Thomas Jr AJ, Agarwal A. Seminal reactive oxygen species and sperm motility and morphology in men with spinal cord injury. Fertil Steril. 1997;67(6):1115–20.
12. Sikka SC. Role of oxidative stress and antioxidants in andrology and assisted reproductive technology. J Androl. 2004;25(1):5–18.
13. Shekarriz M, DeWire DM, Thomas Jr AJ, Agarwal A. A method of human semen centrifugation to minimize the iatrogenic sperm injuries caused by reactive oxygen species. Eur Urol. 1995; 28(1):31–5.
14. Shekarriz M, Thomas Jr AJ, Agarwal A. Incidence and level of seminal reactive oxygen species in normal men. Urology. 1995; 45(1):103–7.
15. Griveau JF, Le Lannou D. Influence of oxygen tension on reactive oxygen species production and human sperm function. Int J Androl. 1997;20(4):195–200.
16. Whittington K, Ford WC. The effect of incubation periods under 95% oxygen on the stimulated acrosome reaction and motility of human spermatozoa. Mol Hum Reprod. 1998;4(11): 1053–7.
17. Watson PF. The causes of reduced fertility with cryopreserved semen. Anim Reprod Sci. 2000;60–61:481–92.
18. Rossi T, Mazzilli F, Delfino M, Dondero F. Improved human sperm recovery using superoxide dismutase and catalase supplementation in semen cryopreservation procedure. Cell Tissue Bank. 2001;2(1):9–13.
19. Donnelly ET, McClure N, Lewis SE. The effect of ascorbate and alpha-tocopherol supplementation in vitro on DNA integrity and hydrogen peroxide-induced DNA damage in human spermatozoa. Mutagenesis. 1999;14(5):505–12.
20. Yenilmez E, Yildirmis S, Yulug E, et al. Ham's F-10 medium and Ham's F-10 medium plus vitamin E have protective effect against oxidative stress in human semen. Urology. 2006;67(2):384–7.
21. Zheng RL, Zhang H. Effects of ferulic acid on fertile and asthenozoospermic infertile human sperm motility, viability, lipid peroxidation, and cyclic nucleotides. Free Radic Biol Med. 1997; 22(4):581–6.
22. Gomez E, Aitken J. Impact of in vitro fertilization culture media on peroxidative damage to human spermatozoa. Fertil Steril. 1996; 65(4):880–2.
23. Donnelly ET, McClure N, Lewis SE. Glutathione and hypotaurine in vitro: effects on human sperm motility, DNA integrity and production of reactive oxygen species. Mutagenesis. 2000; 15(1):61–8.
24. Twigg J, Fulton N, Gomez E, Irvine DS, Aitken RJ. Analysis of the impact of intracellular reactive oxygen species generation on the structural and functional integrity of human sperma-

tozoa: lipid peroxidation, DNA fragmentation and effectiveness of antioxidants. Hum Reprod. 1998;13(6):1429–36.

25. Oeda T, Henkel R, Ohmori H, Schill WB. Scavenging effect of N-acetyl-L-cysteine against reactive oxygen species in human semen: a possible therapeutic modality for male factor infertility? Andrologia. 1997;29(3):125–31.

26. Martinez-Soto JC, de DiosHourcade J, Gutierrez-Adan A, Landeras JL, Gadea J. Effect of genistein supplementation of thawing medium on characteristics of frozen human spermatozoa. Asian J Androl. 2010;12(3):431–41.

27. Saleh RA, Agarwal A, Sharma RK, Nelson DR, Thomas Jr AJ. Effect of cigarette smoking on levels of seminal oxidative stress in infertile men: a prospective study. Fertil Steril. 2002;78(3):491–9.

28. Fraga CG, Motchnik PA, Wyrobek AJ, Rempel DM, Ames BN. Smoking and low antioxidant levels increase oxidative damage to sperm DNA. Mutat Res. 1996;351(2):199–203.

29. Mostafa T, Tawadrous G, Roaia MM, Amer MK, Kader RA, Aziz A. Effect of smoking on seminal plasma ascorbic acid in infertile and fertile males. Andrologia. 2006;38(6):221–4.

30. Viloria T, Meseguer M, Martinez-Conejero JA. et al. Fertil Steril: Cigarette smoking affects specific sperm oxidative defense but does not cause oxidative DNA damage in infertile men; 2009.

31. Viloria T, Garrido N, Fernandez JL, Remohi J, Pellicer A, Meseguer M. Sperm selection by swim-up in terms of deoxyribonucleic acid fragmentation as measured by the sperm chromatin dispersion test is altered in heavy smokers. Fertil Steril. 2007;88(2):523–5.

32. Eskenazi B, Kidd SA, Marks AR, Sloter E, Block G, Wyrobek AJ. Antioxidant intake is associated with semen quality in healthy men. Hum Reprod. 2005;20(4):1006–12.

33. Therond P, Auger J, Legrand A, Jouannet P. Alpha-tocopherol in human spermatozoa and seminal plasma: relationships with motility, antioxidant enzymes and leukocytes. Mol Hum Reprod. 1996;2(10):739–44.

34. Silver EW, Eskenazi B, Evenson DP, Block G, Young S, Wyrobek AJ. Effect of antioxidant intake on sperm chromatin stability in healthy nonsmoking men. J Androl. 2005;26(4):550–6.

35. Song GJ, Norkus EP, Lewis V. Relationship between seminal ascorbic acid and sperm DNA integrity in infertile men. Int J Androl. 2006;29(6):569–75.

36. Wu D, Cederbaum AI. Alcohol, oxidative stress, and free radical damage. Alcohol Res Health. 2003;27(4):277–84.

37. Koch OR, Pani G, Borrello S, et al. Oxidative stress and antioxidant defenses in ethanol-induced cell injury. Mol Aspects Med. 2004;25(1–2):191–8.

38. Maneesh M, Dutta S, Chakrabarti A, Vasudevan DM. Alcohol abuse-duration dependent decrease in plasma testosterone and antioxidants in males. Indian J Physiol Pharmacol. 2006;50(3):291–6.

39. Peake JM, Suzuki K, Coombes JS. The influence of antioxidant supplementation on markers of inflammation and the relationship to oxidative stress after exercise. J Nutr Biochem. 2007;18(6):357–71.

40. Singer G, Granger DN. Inflammatory responses underlying the microvascular dysfunction associated with obesity and insulin resistance. Microcirculation. 2007;14(4–5):375–87.

41. Perez-Crespo M, Pintado B, Gutierrez-Adan A. Scrotal heat stress effects on sperm viability, sperm DNA integrity, and the offspring sex ratio in mice. Mol Reprod Dev. 2008;75(1):40–7.

42. Agarwal DK, Maronpot RR, Lamb IV JC, Kluwe WM. Adverse effects of butyl benzyl phthalate on the reproductive and hematopoietic systems of male rats. Toxicology. 1985;35(3):189–206.

43. Srivastava SP, Srivastava S, Saxena DK, Chandra SV, Seth PK. Testicular effects of di-n-butyl phthalate (DBP): biochemical and histopathological alterations. Arch Toxicol. 1990;64(2):148–52.

44. Lee E, Ahn MY, Kim HJ, et al. Effect of di(n-butyl) phthalate on testicular oxidative damage and antioxidant enzymes in hyperthyroid rats. Environ Toxicol. 2007;22(3):245–55.

45. Chitra KC, Sujatha R, Latchoumycandane C, Mathur PP. Effect of lindane on antioxidant enzymes in epididymis and epididymal sperm of adult rats. Asian J Androl. 2001;3(3):205–8.

46. Latchoumycandane C, Chitra KC, Mathur PP. 2,3,7,8-Tetrachlorodibenzo-p-dioxin (TCDD) induces oxidative stress in the epididymis and epididymal sperm of adult rats. Arch Toxicol. 2003;77(5):280–4.

47. Latchoumycandane C, Mathur PP. Induction of oxidative stress in the rat testis after short-term exposure to the organochlorine pesticide methoxychlor. Arch Toxicol. 2002;76(12):692–8.

48. Meng Z, Bai W. Oxidation damage of sulfur dioxide on testicles of mice. Environ Res. 2004;96(3):298–304.

49. Gonzalez-Flecha B. Oxidant mechanisms in response to ambient air particles. Mol Aspects Med. 2004;25(1–2):169–82.

50. Hsu PC, Guo YL. Antioxidant nutrients and lead toxicity. Toxicology. 2002;180(1):33–44.

51. Acharya UR, Acharya S, Mishra M. Lead acetate induced cytotoxicity in male germinal cells of Swiss mice. Ind Health. 2003;41(3):291–4.

52. Xu DX, Shen HM, Zhu QX, et al. The associations among semen quality, oxidative DNA damage in human spermatozoa and concentrations of cadmium, lead and selenium in seminal plasma. Mutat Res. 2003;534(1–2):155–63.

53. Garrido N, Meseguer M, Simon C, Pellicer A, Remohi J. Pro-oxidative and anti-oxidative imbalance in human semen and its relation with male fertility. Asian J Androl. 2004;6(1):59–65.

54. Kobayashi T, Miyazaki T, Natori M, Nozawa S. Protective role of superoxide dismutase in human sperm motility: superoxide dismutase activity and lipid peroxide in human seminal plasma and spermatozoa. Hum Reprod. 1991;6(7):987–91.

55. Hsieh YY, Sun YL, Chang CC, Lee YS, Tsai HD, Lin CS. Superoxide dismutase activities of spermatozoa and seminal plasma are not correlated with male infertility. J Clin Lab Anal. 2002;16(3):127–31.

56. Miesel R, Jedrzejczak P, Sanocka D, Kurpisz MK. Severe antioxidase deficiency in human semen samples with pathological spermiogram parameters. Andrologia. 1997;29(2):77–83.

57. Jeulin C, Soufir JC, Weber P, Laval-Martin D, Calvayrac R. Catalase activity in human spermatozoa and seminal plasma. Gamete Res. 1989;24(2):185–96.

58. Meseguer M, Martinez-Conejero JA, Muriel L, Pellicer A, Remohi J, Garrido N. The human sperm glutathione system: a key role in male fertility and successful cryopreservation. Drug Metab Lett. 2007;1(2):121–6.

59. Meseguer M, Garrido N, Simon C, Pellicer A, Remohi J. Concentration of glutathione and expression of glutathione peroxidases 1 and 4 in fresh sperm provide a forecast of the outcome of cryopreservation of human spermatozoa. J Androl. 2004;25(5):773–80.

60. Garrido N, Meseguer M, Alvarez J, Simon C, Pellicer A, Remohi J. Relationship among standard semen parameters, glutathione peroxidase/glutathione reductase activity, and mRNA expression and reduced glutathione content in ejaculated spermatozoa from fertile and infertile men. Fertil Steril. 2004;82 Suppl 3:1059–66.

61. Alvarez JG, Storey BT. Taurine, hypotaurine, epinephrine and albumin inhibit lipid peroxidation in rabbit spermatozoa and protect against loss of motility. Biol Reprod. 1983;29(3): 548–55.

62. Holmes RP, Goodman HO, Shihabi ZK, Jarow JP. The taurine and hypotaurine content of human semen. J Androl. 1992;13(3):289–92.

63. Meseguer M, Martinez-Conejero JA, O'Connor JE, Pellicer A, Remohi J, Garrido N. The significance of sperm DNA oxidation in embryo development and reproductive outcome in an oocyte donation program: a new model to study a male infertility prognostic factor. Fertil Steril. 2008;89(5):1191–9.

64. Aguilar C, Meseguer M, Garcia-Herrero S, Gil-Salom M, O'Connor JE, Garrido N. Relevance of testicular sperm DNA oxidation for the outcome of ovum donation cycles. Fertil Steril. 2010;94:979–88.

65. Muriel L, Goyanes V, Segrelles E, Gosalvez J, Alvarez JG, Fernandez JL. Increased aneuploidy rate in sperm with fragmented DNA as determined by the sperm chromatin dispersion (SCD) test and fish analysis. J Androl. 2007;28:38–49.

66. Muriel L, Garrido N, Fernandez JL, et al. Value of the sperm deoxyribonucleic acid fragmentation level, as measured by the sperm chromatin dispersion test, in the outcome of in vitro fertilization and intracytoplasmic sperm injection. Fertil Steril. 2006;85(2):371–83.

67. Meseguer M, Santiso R, Garrido N, Gil-Salom M, Remohi J, Fernandez JL. Sperm DNA fragmentation levels in testicular sperm samples from azoospermic males as assessed by the sperm chromatin dispersion (SCD) test. Fertil Steril. 2009;92(5):1638–45.
68. Meseguer M, Santiso R, Garrido N, Fernandez JL. The effect of cancer on sperm DNA fragmentation as measured by the sperm chromatin dispersion test. Fertil Steril. 2008;90(1): 225–7.
69. Sakkas D, Mariethoz E, Manicardi G, Bizzaro D, Bianchi PG, Bianchi U. Origin of DNA damage in ejaculated human spermatozoa. Rev Reprod. 1999;4(1):31–7.
70. Sakkas D, Mariethoz E, St John JC. Abnormal sperm parameters in humans are indicative of an abortive apoptotic mechanism linked to the Fas-mediated pathway. Exp Cell Res. 1999;251(2):350–5.
71. Sinha Hikim AP, Swerdloff RS. Hormonal and genetic control of germ cell apoptosis in the testis. Rev Reprod. 1999;4(1):38–47.
72. Shen HM, Dai J, Chia SE, Lim A, Ong CN. Detection of apoptotic alterations in sperm in subfertile patients and their correlations with sperm quality. Hum Reprod. 2002;17(5): 1266–73.
73. Krammer PH, Dhein J, Walczak H, et al. The role of APO-1-mediated apoptosis in the immune system. Immunol Rev. 1994;142:175–91.
74. Cande C, Cecconi F, Dessen P, Kroemer G. Apoptosis-inducing factor (AIF): key to the conserved caspase-independent pathways of cell death? J Cell Sci. 2002;115(Pt 24):4727–34.
75. Paasch U, Sharma RK, Gupta AK, et al. Cryopreservation and thawing is associated with varying extent of activation of apoptotic machinery in subsets of ejaculated human spermatozoa. Biol Reprod. 2004;71(6):1828–37.
76. Paasch U, Agarwal A, Gupta AK, et al. Apoptosis signal transduction and the maturity status of human spermatozoa. Ann N Y Acad Sci. 2003;1010:486–8.
77. Paasch U, Grunewald S, Agarwal A, Glandera HJ. Activation pattern of caspases in human spermatozoa. Fertil Steril. 2004;81 Suppl 1:802–9.
78. Agarwal A, Said TM. Role of sperm chromatin abnormalities and DNA damage in male infertility. Hum Reprod Update. 2003;9(4):331–45.
79. Comhaire FH, El Garem Y, Mahmoud A, Eertmans F, Schoonjans F. Combined conventional/ antioxidant "Astaxanthin" treatment for male infertility: a double blind, randomized trial. Asian J Androl. 2005;7(3):257–62.
80. Vicari E, La Vignera S, Calogero AE. Antioxidant treatment with carnitines is effective in infertile patients with prostatovesiculoepididymitis and elevated seminal leukocyte concentrations after treatment with nonsteroidal anti-inflammatory compounds. Fertil Steril. 2002;78(6): 1203–8.
81. Comhaire FH, Christophe AB, Zalata AA, Dhooge WS, Mahmoud AM, Depuydt CE. The effects of combined conventional treatment, oral antioxidants and essential fatty acids on sperm biology in subfertile men. Prostaglandins Leukot Essent Fatty Acids. 2000;63(3): 159–65.
82. Suleiman SA, Ali ME, Zaki ZM, el-Malik EM, Nasr MA. Lipid peroxidation and human sperm motility: protective role of vitamin E. J Androl. 1996;17(5):530–7.
83. Kessopoulou E, Powers HJ, Sharma KK, et al. A double-blind randomized placebo cross-over controlled trial using the antioxidant vitamin E to treat reactive oxygen species associated male infertility. Fertil Steril. 1995;64(4):825–31.
84. Keskes-Ammar L, Feki-Chakroun N, Rebai T, et al. Sperm oxidative stress and the effect of an oral vitamin E and selenium supplement on semen quality in infertile men. Arch Androl. 2003;49(2):83–94.
85. Greco E, Iacobelli M, Rienzi L, Ubaldi F, Ferrero S, Tesarik J. Reduction of the incidence of sperm DNA fragmentation by oral antioxidant treatment. J Androl. 2005;26(3):349–53.
86. Greco E, Romano S, Iacobelli M, et al. ICSI in cases of sperm DNA damage: beneficial effect of oral antioxidant treatment. Hum Reprod. 2005;20(9):2590–4.
87. Tremellen K, Miari G, Froiland D, Thompson J. A randomised control trial examining the effect of an antioxidant (Menevit) on pregnancy outcome during IVF-ICSI treatment. Aust N Z J Obstet Gynaecol. 2007;47(3):216–21.

Chapter 24
Antioxidants in IMSI

Monica Antinori

Conventional semen parameters are used routinely by clinicians to obtain a reliable overview of the male reproductive potential. However, in most cases, little information on the fertility status is provided unless semen parameters are evidently abnormal [1, 2]. Among them the best fertilization predictor is morphology as assessed according to strict criteria [3]. Since its introduction [4], several advantages to the outcomes of conventional in vitro fertilization [3, 5], intrauterine insemination [6], and in vivo reproduction have been shown [7]. Therefore, it is clear how a spermatozoon's morphological normality reflects its function, in relation to its ability to reach, recognize, bind to, penetrate, and deliver its genome to the oocyte. Differently, once the sperm is mechanically injected into the oocyte by an intracytoplasmic sperm injection (ICSI) method, and crossed both barriers of the zona pellucida and oolemma, its abnormal morphology does not seem to interfere with its fertilizing capacity. In this respect, most authors do not notice any correlation between ICSI outcomes and the strict morphology of the sperm used for microinjection [8–11]. In patients with a poor prognosis (4% normal sperm morphology) [12], and even in extreme, specific cases of total teratozoospermia [13], globozoospermia [14, 15], and megalozoospermia [16] fertilization can be achieved with ICSI.

Nonetheless major morphological anomalies lead to decreased rates of fertilization, pregnancy, implantation [16, 17], embryo quality [18–20], and blastocyst formation [17, 21]. Hence, during an ICSI procedure, the embryologist selects a motile, normal-looking spermatozoon and discards the most distorted forms. This visual assessment of sperm morphology, limited by its low magnification (200–400×) and concomitant low resolution [17], overlooks minor morphologic defects potentially related to sperm functional impairment. At the same time, since men with oligoasthenozooteratozoospermia were shown to have significantly elevated levels of sperm numerical chromosomal aberrations, and DNA chain fragmentation [22–28],

M. Antinori, MD (✉)
Department of Infertility, RAPRUI Day Surgery, Via Timavo 2, 00193 Rome, Italy
e-mail: monica.antinori@raprui.com

S.J. Parekattil and A. Agarwal (eds.), *Antioxidants in Male Infertility: A Guide for Clinicians and Researchers*, © Springer Science+Business Media New York 2013

and the incidence of chromosome aneuploidy in spermatozoa relates with the severity of sperm defects [29], there is great concern regarding the increased risk of chromosomal abnormalities in infants conceived with ICSI [30–32].

Moreover, although ICSI has provided treatment for new groups of couples with male infertility who were previously untreatable by IVF, at present the resulting pregnancy rates are only between 30 and 45% [33–35], while the European average "take-home baby" rates remain similar (36) to those of a decade ago [37, 38]. The rising demand for the improvement of success rates compels us to reassess male fertility potential through the development of new tests with clinical relevance for each ART procedure.

Conventional light microscopy cannot identify the entire variety of sperm morphological defects, especially in the head structure [39–41]. In 1999, electron microscopy [scanning electron microscopy (SEM) and transmission electron microscopy (TEM)] allowed Bartoov [42] to correctly identify the ultramorphological state of seven sperm subcellular organelles (acrosome, postacrosomal lamina, nucleus, neck, axoneme, mitochondrial sheath, and outer dense fibers) that were found to be highly predictive factors for male fertility potential. Due to the fact that the applied technology was expensive and often not available in conventional laboratories, its application was limited only to those cases in which the male infertility factor could not be clearly identified by routine tests or following repeated ART failures. As for conventional sperm morphology, this new evaluation turned out to be useful only in the context of a reproductive prognosis assessment, considering that the single sperm used for fertilization might not reflect the peculiarity of the analyzed sample. Moreover, being that the evaluation was based on the examination of fixed and stained sperm cells, it did not provide the patient with any information about the single sperm used for ICSI. To solve all these problems at the same time, a few years later the same group developed a new method for a real-time, detailed morphological evaluation of motile spermatozoa. The sperm analysis called motile sperm organellar morphology examination (MSOME) was performed using an invertoscope equipped with interferential contrast Normaski optics that combines maximal optical magnification(100×), magnification selector (×1.5) and a video-coupled magnification to reach a final video magnification of 6,600×. This analysis, developed to allow the visualization of subtle sperm morphological malformations which might remain unnoticed to the embryologist during the routine sperm selection performed prior to microinjection, has been introduced to improve the success of ICSI. Of the six sperm subcellular organelles examined (Fig. 24.1) (acrosome, postacrosomal lamina, neck, mitochondria, tail, and nucleus), the sperm's nucleus turned out to be the most important parameter influencing ICSI outcome [24] particularly in the form of large nuclear vacuoles (LNV) that were proposed to reflect damages in the nuclear DNA content and organization [44].

Sperm DNA integrity is a prerequisite to normal fertilization and transmission of paternal genetic information [45]. Higher levels of nuclear DNA strand breaks are detected in the ejaculated spermatozoa of men with abnormal semen parameters [46, 47] due to a great sensitivity to DNA damage caused by oxidative stress and increased production of reactive oxygen species (ROS) [48].

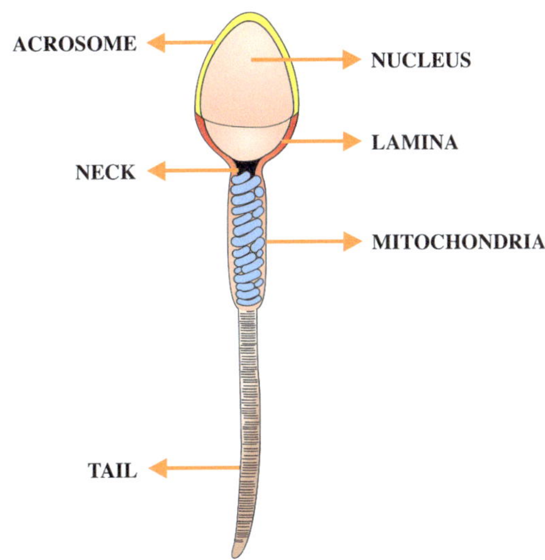

Fig. 24.1 The six subcellular organelles analyzed by MSOME

ROS are active oxidizing agents that render the chromatin vulnerable to external oxidative attacks [49]. An increase in oxidative damage to the sperm membrane, intracellular proteins and DNA, is associated with alterations in signal transduction mechanisms that can affect fertility [50].

Several studies have examined the relationship of sperm nuclear DNA fragmentation with cleavage, embryo quality, and pregnancy rates for both natural [51, 52] and ART conceptions [53–60]. Overall, these studies have suggested that a high content of fragmented DNA may have a negative influence on embryo development and pregnancy rates [61]. Sperm DNA damage further increases the incidence of pregnancy loss after IVF and ICSI [51, 62–64].

For the above reasons, DNA fragmentation can be considered closely related to male-derived repeated ICSI failures, the only marker of such failures that can be objectively and reproducibly diagnosed nowadays [60, 65].

According to the current literature, the incidence of DNA fragmentation in ejaculated spermatozoa can be reduced by oral antioxidant treatment [66–71] and by antioxidant media supplementation [72–74]. The hypothesis that vacuolization of the sperm nucleus may reflect some underlying DNA defects [75] which could impair male fertility potential, such as DNA strand breaks, is a promising perspective considering that, at present, we are not able to offer our patients a selection technique, whereby spermatozoa used for fertilization are preventively tested for DNA integrity. If confirmed, this speculation would enable the verification of potential morphological effects of the antioxidants exogenous administration, validating the further implementation of this therapeutic approach.

Presently, only a few studies have been carried out to investigate the real meaning of nuclear vacuolization and its relationship to DNA status. The opportunity to carry on additional research justifies the application of this new technique which requires specially trained personnel and can be considered extremely time-consuming and expensive, to be routinely inserted in the ART laboratory.

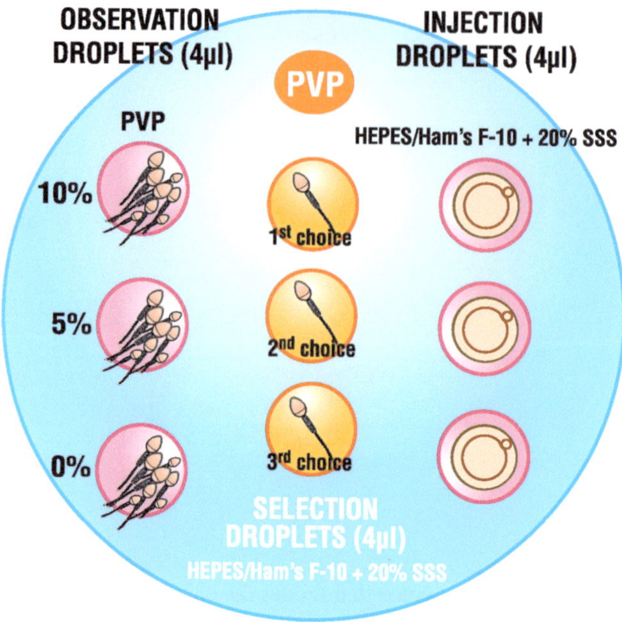

Fig. 24.2 The IMSI Petri dish

Intracytoplasmic Morphologically Selected Sperm Injection Procedure

According to the current literature, a sterile glass-bottomed dish suitable for MSOME evaluation can be prepared as follows (Fig. 24.2).

- On the left side, 4 µl *observation droplets* made up of sperm culture medium containing between 0 and 10% polyvinyl pyrrolidone (PVP) solution. Small bays extruding from the rim of the droplets are created to capture the heads of motile spermatozoa.The temperature of the sperm sample and the PVP concentration are coordinated with the intensity of the sperm motility.
- In the middle, 4 µl *selection droplets* of sperm culture, where selected sperm cells are located after MSOME evaluation. Three distinct drops are made to host spermatozoa with different morphological features.
- On the left side, 4 µl droplets of sperm culture medium that will host the oocytes to be injected in the following ICSI procedure (*injection droplets*), one for each oocyte available for microinjection.
- All microdroplets are placed under sterile liquid paraffin.

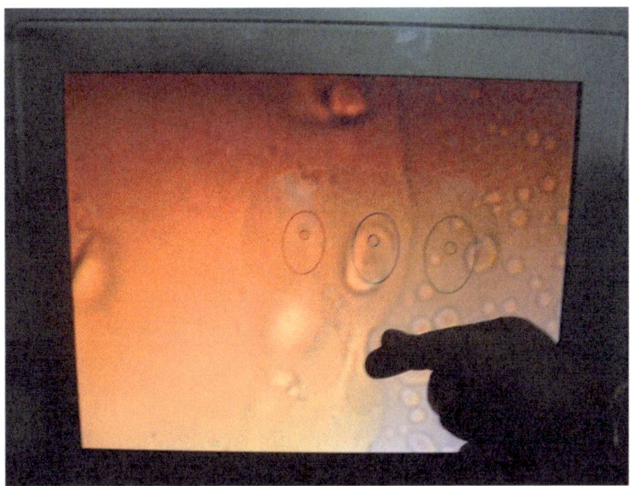

Fig. 24.3 The "chablon" superimposed on the motile sperm to verify its correct size

Motile Sperm Organellar Morphology Examination Criteria and Evaluation Procedure

Based on data collected by electron microscopy [42] that supplied both external and internal information, the MSOME criteria for normally shaped nuclei were defined as size (average length and width to be 4.75 ± 0.28 and 3.28 ± 0.20 μm, respectively), smoothness, symmetry, oval configuration (an extrusion or invagination of the nuclear mass was defined as a regional nuclear shape malformation), and homogeneity of the nuclear chromatin mass containing no more than one vacuole, which occupies less than 4% of the nuclear area (0.78 ± 0.18 μm). Spermatozoa with abnormal head size are excluded by superimposing a transparent celluloid form on the motile examined gametes (Fig. 24.3), representing the correct sperm size, which is calculated by the ratio of expected normal sperm size to the actual size visualized on the monitor screen. Spermatozoa with severe malformations, such as a pin, amorphous, tapered, round, or multinucleated head, which can be identified clearly even by low magnification (200–$400\times$), are not assessed by MSOME. Spermatozoa with a doubtful determination are excluded from selection. To perform a correct sperm evaluation, the embryologist follows each motile single sperm cell with apparent suitability by moving the microscopic stage in the x, y, and z directions until also the smallest details are visualized. Actually some morphological defects, such as large vacuoles, can be revealed only during sperm movement, and therefore motility can be advantageous to the morphological observation. Furthermore, it is relevant to emphasize how a single sperm evaluation is reliable only when it is carried out on a motile sperm cell; on the other hand, static sperm images only allow evaluation of the visible part, leaving some morphological alterations undiscovered.

The sperm selection procedure does not require any computer application since the automated sperm morphology analysis systems available on the market allow only morphology evaluation of immotile sperms on stained slides. On the other hand, two embryologists working together at the same time on the analysis of the same sample, are recommended to minimize the subjective nature of sperm evaluation. Finding normal-looking spermatozoa is variable according to the quality of the semen sample.

Intracytoplasmic Morphologically Selected Sperm Injection Step by Step

Freshly ejaculated semen is subjected to routine morphological selection of motile spermatozoa on the basis of a two-layer density gradient system: 1 mL of postejaculated liquefied semen is placed onto the gradient and centrifuged at $375 \times g$ for 15 min at 25°C. The sperm cell pellet is suspended by adding 3 mL of sperm culture medium and then recentrifuged for 10 min. The supernatant is removed and replaced by sperm culture medium to bring the final concentration of motile sperm cells to about 4×10^6 spermatozoa per milliliter. In severe oligozoospermic cases with sperm density below 1×10^6 spermatozoa per ejaculate, liquefied semen is placed onto 1 mL of the low density layer only, centrifuged as previously mentioned, and the final sperm cell pellet is suspended in 0.1–0.2 mL of sperm culture medium.

The sperm cell suspension obtained after semen preparation is used for real-time high-magnification MSOME [76] that is performed on the observation droplets by means of an inverted microscope (e.g., Olympus IX81, Tokyo, Japan) equipped with Nomarski differential interference contrast optics, an Uplan Apo X 100 oil/1.50 objective lens previously covered by a droplet of immersion oil, and a 0.55 NA condenser lens. The images are captured by a DXC-990P video camera having ½-in., 3-chip power HAD CCD and visualized on a monitor screen with diagonal dimension of 355.6 mm. Calculation of the total magnification is based on four parameters: (1) objective magnification 100×, (2) magnification selector 1.5×, (3) video coupler magnification 0.99 (UPMTV X 0.3, PE X 3.3), and (4) (a) CCD chip diagonal dimension 8 mm and (b) television monitor diagonal dimension for a calculated video magnification (b/a) of 44.45. Thus, total magnification = microscope magnification (150×) × video coupler magnification (0.99×) × video magnification (44.45×) = 6,600×.

Only motile spermatozoa with morphologically normal nuclei are retrieved from the observation droplets and aspirated into a sterilized glass pipette with a 9-μm inner diameter tip. Sperm cells are then placed into the selection droplet and finally used to be injected into the oocytes for the classical ICSI procedure [77]. This procedure is performed using a motorized micropanipulator system (e.g., TransferMan NK2, Eppendorf Germany).

Intracytoplasmic Morphologically Selected Sperm Injection in Assisted Reproductive Technology

Assuming that spermatozoa with severely impaired morphology show reduced fertilization, pregnancy, and implantation rates [16, 17], having identified a variety of morphological anomalies that conventional light microscopy cannot detect at 200–400×, Bartoov [43] developed a new technique for real-time motile sperm morphological evaluation (MSOME) in 2002. The study aimed to determine whether subtle morphological anomalies affected ICSI outcome and identified those that are relevant. Based on the analysis of a total of 10,000 spermatozoa (100 sperm samples and 100 spermatozoa each), it was demonstrated that in routine IVF–ICSI cycles patients who exhibited less than 20% spermatozoa with a morphologically normal nucleus, defined by MSOME, did not achieve any pregnancy. With respect to the ICSI fertilization rate, the morphological normalcy of the entire sperm cell, according to MSOME criteria, showed a positive and significant correlation ($r = 0.52$, $P \leq 0.01$) and a very high predictive value (area under the ROC curve, 88%), whereas no association with pregnancy outcome was found. The morphological normalcy of the sperm nucleus (shape + chromatin content), defined by MSOME, was significantly and positively correlated with both fertilization rate ($r = 0.42$, $P \leq 0.01$) and pregnancy occurrence ($r = 0.38$, $P \leq 0.01$). Even its predictive value turned out to be significantly high (areas under the ROC curve, 72 and 74%, respectively). Hence the author could conclude that sperm nucleus is the most important sperm parameter influencing ICSI outcome.

In 2003 [76], Bartoov's group investigated how microinjection of motile spermatozoa with morphologically normal nuclei improves the ICSI outcome. The technique, that combines MSOME evaluation applied on the single sperm used for ICSI, was named intracytoplasmic morphologically selected sperm injection (IMSI). Fifty IMSI couples were compared to 50 ICSI couples wit the same number of previous ICSI failures (matched cases). Implantation and pregnancy rates after IMSI were significantly higher, and the abortion rate was significantly lower, compared to the current ICSI trial ($F = 18.0$, $P \leq 0.01$; $\chi^2 = 4.4$, $P \leq 0.01$; and $\chi^2 = 4.4$, $P \leq 0.05$). In addition, the IMSI attempt produced a significantly higher value of top embryo percentage, compared to the current ICSI treatment ($F = 6.5, P \leq 0.01$). Even 12 unmatched IMSI cases with over eight previous failed routine ICSI attempts (9.1 ± 1.2 ICSI cycles in average) achieved a 50% pregnancy rate after one IMSI trial. The obtained results demonstrated that IMSI improves significantly the success rate in couples with previous ICSI failures.

To exclude that the increased pregnancy outcome was linked to the sperm preparation technique adapted for IMSI and not to the nuclear morphology of the selected spermatozoa special, in 2005 Berkovitz [44] published a comparative study between IVF and IMSI cycles involving 38 transfers of embryos derived from "second best" morphologically evaluated sperm cells (negative group) versus 38 derived from morphologically normal nuclei (positive group). Comparison between the groups revealed that fertilization rate, percentage of top embryos, and implantation rates were significantly higher in the positive group than in the negative group.

Out of six pregnancies achieved in the negative group, four turned into a first trimester missed abortion. Interestingly, three missed abortion cases occurred when microinjection was conducted with spermatozoa exhibiting LNV, whereas in the other abortion case the sperm cells exhibited combined malformations: large vacuoles associated with narrow formed head shape.

Thus, implantation and pregnancy achieved by ICSI seem associated with morphological nuclear normalcy of the sperm. Nonetheless spermatozoa with a morphologically abnormal nucleus show low fertility potential, even if some with certain nuclear abnormalities may still be able to produce pregnancy following ICSI.

This result confirmed previous reports [78, 79] that had already shown a clear negative association between the existence of sperm nuclear vacuoles and natural male fertility potential, and led the author to assume that within the category of specific morphological malformations the existence of large vacuoles in the sperm nuclei indicates more damage to the nuclear DNA content and organization than nuclear shape or size impairment.

The impact of sperm with normal nuclear shape but LNV on pregnancy outcome compared to those with strictly defined morphologically normal nuclei, including shape and content, was investigated in 2006 by Berkovitz [75]. The pregnancy rate per cycle in the experimental group was significantly lower, and the early spontaneous abortion rate per pregnancy significantly higher, than those of the control group (18 versus 50%, Pearson's Chi-square = 6.4 and 80 versus 7%, Pearson's Chi-square = 10.9, respectively, $P = 0.01$).

MSOME revealed that the ejaculates of males routinely referred for ICSI exhibit on average 30–40% spermatozoa with a vacuolated nucleus. This sperm malformation, identifiable as a pregnancy risk factor on the basis of the previous findings, can easily be missed by the standard selection prior to ICSI, and have, therefore, a chance to be chosen for microinjection of at least 30%.

A subsequent enlarged study by the same group [80] confirmed all the previous findings as follows: pregnancy rate was significantly higher and the abortion rate significantly lower following IMSI compared with ICSI attempts (χ^2 = 20.1, $P \leq 0.01$ and χ^2 = 5.1, $P \leq 0.03$, respectively). Furthermore, IMSI provided a higher percentage of top quality embryos with a better implantation rate than ICSI.

A comparison between a "best group," in which embryos were obtained from microinjection exclusively performed using spermatozoa with intact nuclei, and a "second best group," in which only sperm cells with minimal impairment were used for microinjection, since no "best" sperm cells were available in those cases, demonstrated that fertilization rate, percentage of top embryos, implantation, pregnancy, and delivery rates per cycle were significantly higher, and the abortion rate was significantly lower in the "best" group than in the "second best" one (F = 10.5, $P \leq 0.01$; F = 4.6, $P \leq 0.03$; F = 23.4, $P \leq 0.01$; χ^2 = 15.5, $P \leq 0.05$; χ^2 = 19.6, $P \leq 0.01$; and χ^2 = 5.5, $P \leq 0.02$, respectively).

The authors restricted the application of this new procedure to cases with over two previous implantation failures. Actually, according to recent publications, those couples seem to have the worst reproductive prognosis with a dramatic reduction in pregnancy and implantation rates as against couples with no or one previous failed

IVF attempts [81, 82]. Hence Antinori [83] designed a prospective randomized controlled protocol to assess the potential advantages of the IMSI procedure in the treatment of patients with severe oligoasthenoteratozoospermia regardless of their previous failed ICSI attempts, followed by a subgroup splitting according to the number of previous failed attempts (Subgroup *A*: no previous attempts; Subgroup *B*: 1 previous failed attempt; Subgroup *C*: ≥2 previous failed attempts). The comparisons between the two different techniques were made in terms of pregnancy, abortion, and implantation rates.

Pregnancy and implantation rates resulted statistically better in IMSI than ICSI cycles (PR: 39.2 versus 26.5%; $P = 0.004$) (IR: 17.3 versus 11.3%; $P = 0.007$).

However, cases with two or more failed attempts benefited most from IMSI, with a statistically significant doubling of pregnancy rate (12.9 versus 29.8%; $P = 0.017$) and a remarkable 50% reduction in the abortion rate (17 versus 35%). Comparisons did not show any statistical difference in terms of abortions but the clinical trend was clearly in favor of the IMSI method in cases with two or more previous failed attempts. Based on the above results, it is likely that in those couples the male factor could be featured by semen impairment, undetected by conventional diagnostic tools, thus reducing the effectiveness of previous ICSI treatments.

Intracytoplasmic Morphologically Selected Sperm Injection and DNA Fragmentation

When strict criteria were originally introduced [84], it was not already possible to correlate poor sperm morphology with fragmented DNA [85, 86], whereas later reports found that abnormal spermatozoa negatively correlates with DNA integrity [72], especially in the case of head malformations [87–89]. The potential relationship between sperm shape and genetic integrity has become very relevant with the introduction of ICSI, which gives chances of fertilization even to those male gametes affected by severe malformations [13, 90, 91] and might overlook some subtle defects because of the low magnification and low resolution of its sperm morphology assessment. In both cases, there is a great concern about the fact that morphologically abnormal spermatozoa, which were shown to have significantly elevated levels of sperm numerical chromosomal aberrations, ROS production, and DNA chain fragmentation [46, 47] would participate to impair fertilization, embryogenesis, or fetal development and nonetheless to the birth of infants with higher prevalence of chromosomal abnormalities and birth defects compared to natural conception [92].

The introduction of a new visual method applied on conventional ICSI technique, called IMSI, that clearly identifies sperm characteristics, undetected by conventional microscopy, allows investigation into their relationship with ICSI outcome that provide reliable evidence that a morphologically normal sperm nucleus is the most important sperm parameter showing high correlation with both fertilization and pregnancy occurrence [43]. Based on preliminary unpublished data by Bartoov' s group, which reported a significant negative correlation between the size of the nuclear vacuoles and chromatin stability assessed by the sperm chromatin structure assay (SCSA) and according to Lee [93], who demonstrated that no increase in chromosome aberrations was found in spermatozoa with large or small heads, it has been proposed that the existence of large sperm vacuoles in the sperm nuclei indicates more damage to nuclear DNA content and organization than nuclear shape or size impairment [44]. Furthermore, LNV injection resulted in a normal early embryonic development (normal fertilization, development of top-quality embryos, and implantation) followed by an impaired embryo survival (low pregnancy and high abortion rates) [75].

To verify that the LNV in the sperm cell reflect some underlying chromosomal or DNA defect, sperm cells with and without large vacuoles were recommended be selected from the same ejaculate and examined by different biochemical methods from an external analytic system [75]. Therefore, a recent paper from Hazout [94] compared the outcomes of 125 couples with at least two previous ICSI failures and an undetected female infertility factor that underwent conventional and high-magnification ICSI in two sequential attempts. Following sperm injection into the oocytes without nuclear alterations a double pregnancy rate and a 50% decrease in the abortion rate were recorded as against similar cases treated by conventional ICSI. In 72 out of 125 patients involved in the study, the degree of sperm DNA fragmentation was determined by TUNEL and the outcomes of high-magnification ICSI were compared in cases with different sperm DNA fragmentation degrees. However, this test was not performed directly with the sperm samples used for ICSI. A marked rise in clinical implantation and birth rates was observed in patients with normal (<30%), moderately (30–40%), and highly (>40%) increased percentage of DNA-fragmented spermatozoa in the ejaculate.

To stress the above assumptions, Franco [95] evaluated the extent of DNA fragmentation (TUNEL assay) and the presence of denatured single-stranded or normal double-stranded DNA (acridine orange fluorescence method; AOT) in spermatozoa with LNV selected by high magnification compared with those with normal nucleus. The percentage of positive DNA fragmentation was significantly higher ($P < 0.0001$) in LNV spermatozoa (29.1%) than in NN spermatozoa (15.9%). Similarly, the percentage of denatured-stranded DNA was significantly higher ($P < 0.0001$) in the former (67.9%) than in the latter (33.1%).

So far a direct correlation in DNA quality has not been tested in single-selected spermatozoa. With that in mind as their major aim, Garolla [96] analyzed the chromatin structure (sperm DNA integrity by acridine orange; DNA fragmentation by TUNEL assay) and sperm aneuploidies (FISH test) in ten patients affected by severe testicular damage (severe oligozoospermia) on single immotile sperm cells morphologically selected by high-magnification microscopy (13×,161). From the sample of each patient, ten spermatozoa with normal morphology and no vacuoles (group A) and ten spermatozoa with normal morphology and at least one large head vacuole (group B) were selected. Single cells from group A showed a more physiological status of DNA integrity and DNA fragmentation than cells from group B. Furthermore, FISH analysis showed that no chromosomal alteration was present in cells from group A. Moreover, the authors reported that considering together spermatozoa with normal morphology and both presence and absence of large head vacuoles the mean results (data not shown) from all tests were significantly better with respect to those of unselected cells performed in the first part of the study (all $P < 0.001$).

These results seem to suggest a strong relationship between high-magnification morphology and the DNA status of spermatozoa and the chromatinic origin of nuclear vacuoles visualized by MSOME. Based on technical limits of differential interference contrast (DIC),which does not allow intracellular evaluation [97–99], since to detect chromatin vacuoles the evaluation has to be performed at 20,000× magnification by electron microscopy, and because of their main localization, in the anterior part of the sperm head, the acrosomal origin of these vacuoles was theorized [100]. The first experiment of this study consisted of MSOME evaluation on immotile spermatozoa followed by acrosomal status assessment of the same spermatozoon using pisum sativum agglutinin (PSA)–fluorescein isothiocyanate (FITC). The complete acrosome reaction corresponded in most of the cases (70.9%) to spermatozoa of regular shape and absent or slight vacuolization, whereas those sperms with incomplete or missing acrosome reaction showed 60.7% of vacuole presence. The second experiment involved ten patients whose immotile sperms were analyzed according to MSOME before and after the acrosome had been induced by ionophore A23587. Vacuole-free spermatozoa increased from 41.2 to 63.8% ($P > 0.005$) with a concomitant rise of the acrosome-reacted gamete from 17.4 + 7.8 to 36.1 + 12.7 ($P < 0.001$).The last part of the study was performed on motile acrosome-reacting spermatozoa that were analyzed by MSOME. It was possible to visualize large protruding bleds that become similar to vacuoles when seen upfront as well as a sort of invagination that look like a vacuole in the following image. The author came to the conclusion that the vacuole-free spermatozoa microinjected during IMSI are mostly acrosome-reacted spermatozoa.

Expert Commentary

This chapter was designed to provide practical guidelines and clinical application data of a new method of sperm morphological selection recently introduced to increase ART success in overcoming severe male infertility. In the last two decades, male infertility diagnosis has been based on conventional sperm parameters of questionable clinical value and other tests that investigate properties of sperm function that have been perceived useless after ICSI introduction. This was valid especially regarding strict morphological criteria, since it was demonstrated that even sperm with major malformations can obtain pregnancies and healthy deliveries. Moreover, most of these tests investigate the entire sperm population rather than providing information about the single sperm that would be employed in the conventional ICSI technique.

Even if a rising number of studies have reported IMSI as having remarkable clinical advantages in terms of fertilization, embryo quality, pregnancy occurrence, and prosecution until delivery, this new method continues to be debated regarding its routine application in the ART laboratory. Although, currently, IMSI has not been standardized and requires further validation, one promising perspective is the potential correlation between MSOME sperm nuclear malformations of the male gamete and its abnormal DNA status in terms of fragmentation. The future confirmation of this hypothesis warrants the investment of great quantities of human and technical resources needed to enable a reliable identification of only those spermatozoa that possess low levels of DNA damage in their nuclei for assisted conception purposes. Consequently this research would provide explanations regarding:

- Unexplained sterility
- Repeated abortions
- Repeated implantation failures.

Five-Year View

In light of its confirmed effectiveness and prospective reliability concerning DNA fragmentation, ultramorphological selection could be applied to demonstrate if, and how, antioxidants play a role in male reproductive potential. Hence, new antioxidant therapies with different morphological targets, at different concentrations could be tested and modified according to the attained quality of nuclear morphology, as well as the corresponding implantation and pregnancy rates.

The main challenges resulting from this research are:

- The number of microinjected oocytes/patient could be reduced in relation with improved fertilization ability of selected spermatozoa.
- It would be possible to decrease the number of embryos/transfer and the consequent risk of going through multiple pregnancy, due to the greater implantation potential of those embryos.
- Higher pregnancy rates would enable to reduce the number of ART attempts to achieve pregnancy and consequently hormonal intakes and costs.

Key Issues

- IMSI allows the selection, under 6,600× magnification, of a best motile sperm to be injected into the oocyte.
- According to current literature, IMSI provides better results than ICSI in defeating severe male infertility.
- Among the different malformation identified by MSOME, those affecting nuclear structure, such as vacuoles, demonstrated to be highly correlated with a male reproductive prognosis impairment.

- Nuclear vacuoles has been proposed to be morphological signs of DNA fragmentation. At present, the few published data are limited and in some cases discordant, at the point that we are still far from the clear identification of their meaning.
- Further studies are necessary to come to an adequate standardization of this new technique to clarify what are the biological mechanisms involved and give enlarged confirmations of effectiveness.

Acknowledgment The author gratefully acknowledge the help of Mrs Stella Antinori in the preparation of the manuscript.

References

1. Dumpy BC, Neal LM, Cooke ID. The clinical value of conventional semen analysis. Fertil Steril. 1989;51:324–9.
2. Aitkin RJ, Irvine DS, Wu FC. Prosecute analysis of spermoocyte fusion and reactive oxygen species generation as catena for the diagnosis of infertility. Am J Obstet Gynecol. 1991;164:542–51.
3. Vawda AI, Gunby J, Younglai EV. Semen parameters as predictors of in-vitro fertilization: the importance of strict criteria morphology. Hum Reprod. 1996;11:1445–50.
4. Kruger TF, Menkveld R, Stander FSH, Lombard CJ, Van der Merwe JP, van Zyl JA, et al. Sperm morphologic features as a prognostic factor in vitro fertilization. Fertil Steril. 1986;46:1118–23.
5. Grow DR, Oehninger S, Seltman HJ, Toner JP, Swanson RJ, Kruger TF, et al. Sperm morphology as diagnosed by strict criteria: probing the impact of teratozoospermia on fertilization rate and pregnancy outcome in a large in vitro fertilization population. Fertil Steril. 1994;62:559–67.
6. Burr RW, Siegberg R, Flaherty SP, Wang X-J, Matthews CD. The influence of sperm morphology and the number of motile sperm inseminated on the outcome of intrauterine insemination combined with mild ovarian stimulation. Fertil Steril. 1996;65:127–32.
7. Eggert-Kruse W, Schwartz H, Rohr G, Demirakca T, Tilgen W. Runnebaum sperm morphology assessment using strict criteria and male fertility under in-vivo conditions of conception. Hum Reprod. 1996;11:139–46.
8. Oehninger S, Veeck L, Lanzendorf S, Maloney M, Toner J, Muasher S. Intracytoplasmic sperm injection: achievement of high pregnancy rates in couples with severe male factor infertility is dependent primarily upon female not male factors. Fertil Steril. 1995;64:977–81.
9. Kupker W, Schulze W, Diedrich K. Ultrastructure of gametes and intracytoplasmic sperm injection: the significance of sperm morphology. Hum Reprod. 1998;13 Suppl 1:99–106.
10. Host E, Ernst E, Lindenberg S, Smidt-Jensen S. Morphology of spermatozoa used in IVF and ICSI from oligozoospermic men. Reprod Biomed Online. 2001;3:212–5.
11. Celik-Ozenci C, Jakab A, Kovacs T, Catalanotti J, Demir R, Bray-Ward P, Ward D, Huszar G. Sperm selection for ICSI: shape properties do not predict the absence or presence of numerical chromosomal aberrations. Hum Reprod. 2004;19:2052–9.
12. Sukcharoen N, Sithipravej T, Promviengchai S, Chinpilas V, Boonkasemsanti W. Sperm morphology evaluated by computer (IVOS) cannot predict the fertilization rate in vitro after intracytoplasmic sperm injection. Fertil Steril. 1998;69:564–8.
13. Tasdemir I, Tasdemir M, Tavukcuog S, Kahraman S, Biberog K. Effect of abnormal sperm head morphology on the outcome of intracytoplasmic sperm injection in humans. Hum Reprod. 1997;12:1214–7.

14. Liu J, Nagy Z, Joris H, Tournaye H, Devroey P, Van Steirteghem A. Successful fertilization and establishment of pregnancies after intracytoplasmic sperm injection in patients with globozoospermia. Hum Reprod. 1995;10:626–9.
15. Battaglia DE, Koehler JK, Klein NA, Tucker MJ. Failure of oocyte activation after intracytoplasmic sperm injection using round-headed sperm. Fertil Steril. 1997;68:118–22.
16. Kahraman S, Akarsu C, Cengiz G, Dirican K, Sozen E, Can B, Guven C, Vanderzwalmen P. Fertility of ejaculated and testicular megalohead spermatozoa with intracytoplasmic sperm injection. Hum Reprod. 1999;14:726–30.
17. De Vos A, Van De Velde H, Joris H, Verheyen G, Devroey P, Van Steirteghem A. Influence of individual sperm morphology on fertilisation, embryo morphology, and pregnancy outcome of intracytoplasmic sperm injection. Fertil Steril. 2003;79:42–8.
18. Cohen J, Alikani M, Malter H, et al. Partial zona dissection or subzonal sperm insertion: microsurgical fertilization alternatives based on evaluation of sperm and embryo morphology. Fertil Steril. 1991;56:696–706.
19. Parinaud J, Mieusset R, Vieitez G, Labal B, Richoilley G. Influence of sperm parameters on embryo quality. Fertil Steril. 1993;60: 888–92.
20. Loutradi KE, Tarlatzis BC, Goulis DG, Zepiridis L, Pagou T, Chatziioannou E, et al. The effects of sperm quality on embryo development after intracytoplasmic sperm injection. J Assist Reprod Genet. 2006;23:69–74.
21. Miller JE, Smith TT. The effect of intracytoplasmic sperm injection and semen parameters on blastocyst development in vitro. Hum Reprod. 2001;16:918–24.
22. Huszar G, Vigue L. Incomplete development of human spermatozoa is associated with increased creatine phosphokinase concentration and abnormal head morphology. Mol Reprod Dev. 1993;34:292–8.
23. Aitken J, Krausz C, Buckingham D. Relationships between biochemical markers for residual sperm cytoplasm, reactive oxygen species generation, and the presence of leukocytes and precursor germ cells in human sperm suspensions. Mol Reprod Dev. 1994;39:268–79.
24. Bernardini L, Borini A, Preti S, Conte N, Flamigni C, Capitanio GL, Venturini PL. Study of aneuploidy in normal and abnormal germ cells from semen of fertile and infertile men. Hum Reprod. 1998;13:3406–13.
25. Rubes J, Lowe X, Moore II D, Perreault S, Slott V, Evenson D, Selevan SG, Wyrobek AJ. Smoking cigarettes is associated with increased sperm disomy in teenage men. Fertil Steril. 1998;70:715–23.
26. Twigg JP, Irvine DS, Aitken RJ. Oxidative damage to DNA in human spermatozoa does not preclude pronucleus formation at intracytoplasmic sperm injection. Hum Reprod. 1998;13:1864–71.
27. Sakkas D, Mariethoz E, Manicardi G, Bizzaro D, Bianchi PG, Bianchi U. Origin of DNA damage in ejaculated human spermatozoa. Rev Reprod. 1999;4:31–7.
28. Griffin DK, Hyland P, Tempest HG, Homa ST. Safety issues in assisted reproduction technology: should men undergoing ICSI be screened for chromosome abnormalities in their sperm? Hum Reprod. 2003;18:229–35.
29. Carrell DT, Emery BR, Wilcox AL, Campbell B, Erickson L, Hatasaka HH, Jones KP, Peterson CM. Sperm chromosome aneuploidy as related to male factor infertility and some ultrastructure defects. Arch Androl. 2004;50:181–5.
30. Rubio C, Simon C, Blanco V, Vidal F, Minguez Y, Egozcue J, et al. Implications of sperm chromosome abnormalities in recurrent miscarriage. J Assist Reprod Genet. 1999;16:253–8.
31. Van Steirteghem A, Bonduelle M, Devroey P, Liebaers I. Follow up of children born after ICSI. Hum Reprod Update. 2002;8:111–6.
32. Hansen M, Kurinczuk JJ, Bower C, Webb S. The risk of major birth defects after intracytoplasmic sperm injection and in vitro fertilization. N Engl J Med. 2002;346:725–30.
33. Kuczynski W, Dhont M, Grygoruk C, Grochowski D, Wolczynski S, Szamatowicz M. The outcome of intracytoplasmic injection of fresh and cryopreserved ejaculated spermatozoa—a prospective randomized study. Hum Reprod. 2001;16:2109–13.

34. Stolwijk AM, Wetzels AM, Braat DD. Cumulative probability of achieving an ongoing pregnancy after in-vitro fertilization and intracytoplasmic sperm injection according to a woman's age, subfertility diagnosis and primary or secondary subfertility. Hum Reprod. 2000;15: 203–9.
35. Olivius K, Friden B, Lundin K, Bergh C. Cumulative probability of live birth after three in vitro fertilization/intracytoplasmic sperm injection cycles. Fertil Steril. 2002;77:505–10.
36. European IVF-monitoring programme (EIM), for the European Society of Human Reproduction and Embryology (ESHRE) Assisted reproductive technology in Europe, Results generated from European registers by ESHRE. Human reproduction 2002;21: 1680–97.
37. Van Steirteghem AC, Liu J, Joris H, Nagy Z, Janssenswillen C, Tournaye H, Derde MP, Van Assche E, Devroey P. Higher success rate by intracytoplasmic sperm injection than by subzonal insemination. Report of a second series of 300 consecutive treatment cycles. Hum Reprod. 1993;8:1055–60.
38. Harari O, Bourne H, McDonald M, Richings N, Speirs AL, Johnston WIH, Baker HWG. Intracytoplasmic sperm injection—a major advance in the management of severe male subfertility. Fertil Steril. 1995;64:360–8.
39. Glezerman M, Bartoov B. Semen analysis. In: Insler V, Lunenfeld B, editors. Infertility: male and female. Edinburgh: Churchill Livingstone; 1993. p. 285–315.
40. Piomboni P, Strehler E, Capitani S, Collodel G, De Santo M, Gambera L, Moretti E, Baccetti B, Sterzic K. Submicroscopic mathematical evaluation of spermatozoa in assisted reproduction, in vitro fertilization (notulae seminologicae 7). J Assist Reprod Genet. 1996;13:635–46.
41. Zamboni L. The ultrastructural pathology of the spermatozoan as a course of infertility: the role of electron microscopy in the evaluation of sperm quality. Fertil Steril. 1987;48: 711–34.
42. Bartoov B, Eltes F, Reichart M, Langzam J, Lederman H, Zabludovsky N. Quantitative ultramorphological analysis of human sperm: fifteen years of experience in the diagnosis and management of male factor infertility. Arch Androl. 1999;43(1): 13–25.
43. Bartoov B, Berkovitz A, Eltes F, Kogosowski A, Menezo Y, Barak Y. Real-time fine morphology of motile human sperm cells is associated with IVF-ICSI outcome. J Androl. 2002;23:1–8.
44. Berkovitz A, Eltes F, Yaari S, Katz N, Barr I, Fishman A, Bartoov B. The morphological normalcy of the sperm nucleus and pregnancy rate of intracytoplasmic injection with morphologically selected sperm. Hum Reprod. 2005;20:185–90.
45. Agarwal A, Said TM. Role of sperm chromatin abnormalities and DNA damage in male infertility. Hum Reprod Update. 2003;9:331–45.
46. Irvine DS, Twigg JP, Gordon EL, Fulton N, Milne PA, Aitken RJ. DNA integrity in human spermatozoa: relationships with semen quality. J Androl. 2000;21:33–44.
47. Seli E, Moffatt O, Kayisli UA, Nijs M, Ombelet W and Sakkas D. Apoptosis in testis of normal and azoospermic males: a Fas mediated phenomenon. Annual meeting of the society for gynecologic investigation, Los Angeles, CA, 2002.
48. Aitken RJ, De Iuliis GN. Origins and consequences of DNA damage in male germ cells. Reprod Biomed Online. 2007;14:727–33.
49. Aitken RJ, De Iuliis GN, McLachlan RI. Biological and clinical significance of DNA damage in the male germ line. Int J Androl. 2008;32(1):46–56. ISSN 0105-6263.
50. Sikka A, Rajasekaran M, Hellstrom W. Role of oxidative stress and antioxidants in male infertility. J Androl. 1995;16:464–8.
51. Evenson DP, Jost LK, Marshall D, Zinaman MJ, Clegg E, Purvis K, de Angelis P, Claussen OP. Utility of the sperm chromatin structure assay as a diagnostic and prognostic tool in the human fertility clinic. Hum Reprod. 1999;14:1039–49.
52. Spano M, Bonde JP, Hjollund HI, Kolstad HA, Cordelli E, Leter G. Sperm chromatin damage impairs human fertility. The Danish First Pregnancy Planner Study Team. Fertil Steril. 2000;73:43–50.

53. Morris ID, Ilott S, Dixon L, Brison DR. The spectrum of DNA damage in human sperm assessed by single cell gel electrophoresis (Comet assay) its relationship to fertilization and embryo development. Hum Reprod. 2002;17:990–8.
54. Benchaib M, Braun V, Lornage J, Hadj S, Salle B, Lejeune H, Guerin JF. Sperm DNA fragmentation decreases the pregnancy rate in an assisted reproductive technique. Hum Reprod. 2003;18:1023–8.
55. Larson-Cook KL, Brannian JD, Hansen KA, Kasperson KM, Aamold ET, Evenson DP. Relationship between the outcomes of assisted reproductive techniques and sperm DNA fragmentation as measured by the sperm chromatin structure assay. Fertil Steril. 2003;80: 895–902.
56. Loft S, Kold-Jensen T, Hjollund NH, Giwercman A, Gyllemborg J, Ernst E, Olsen J, Scheike T, Poulsen HE, Bonde JP. Oxidative DNA damage in human sperm influences time to pregnancy. Hum Reprod. 2003;18:1265–72.
57. Bungum M, Humaidan P, Spano M, Jepson K, Bungum L, Giwercman A. The predictive value of sperm chromatin structure assay (SCSA) parameters for the outcome of intrauterine insemination, IVF and ICSI. Hum Reprod. 2004;19:1401–8.
58. Gandini L, Lombardo F, Paoli D, Caruso F, Eleuteri P, Leter G, Ciriminna R, Culasso F, Dondero F, Lenzi A, et al. Full-term pregnancies achieved with ICSI despite high levels of sperm chromatin damage. Hum Reprod. 2004;19:1409–17.
59. Seli E, Gardner DK, Schoolcraft WB, Moffatt O, Sakkas D. Extent of nuclear DNA damage in ejaculated spermatozoa impacts on blastocyst development after in vitro fertilization. Fertil Steril. 2004;82:378–83.
60. Tesarik J, Greco E, Mendoza C. Late, but not early, paternal effect on human embryo development is related to sperm DNA fragmentation. Hum Reprod. 2004;19:611–5.
61. Smith R, Kaune H, Parodi D, Madariaga M, Rios R, Morales I, Castro A. Increased sperm DNA damage in patients with varicocele: relationship with seminal oxidative stress. Hum Reprod. 2006;21(4):986–93.
62. Borini A, Tarozzi N, Bizzaro D, Bonu MA, Fava L, Flamigni C, Coticchio G. Sperm DNA fragmentation: paternal effect on early post-implantation embryo development in ART. Hum Reprod. 2006;21:2876–81.
63. Lin MH, Kuo-Kuang Lee R, Li SH, Lu CH, Sun FJ, Hwu YM. Sperm chromatin structure assay parameters are not related to fertilization rates, embryo quality, and pregnancy rates in in vitro fertilization and intracytoplasmic sperm injection, but might be related to spontaneous abortion rates. Fertil Steril. 2007;90:352–9.
64. Zini A, Boman JM, Belzile E, Ciampi A. Sperm DNA damage is associated with an increased risk of pregnancy loss after IVF and ICSI: systematic review and metaanalysis. Hum Reprod. 2008;23:2663–8.
65. Tesarik J. Paternal effects on cell division in the human preimplantation embryo. Reprod Biomed Online. 2005;10:370–5.
66. Suleiman SA, Ali ME, Zaki ZM, el-Malik EM, Nasr MA. Lipid peroxidation and human sperm motility: protective role of vitamin E. J Androl. 1996;17:530–7.
67. Kodama H, Yamaguchi R, Fukuda J, Kasai H, Tanaka T. Increased oxidative deoxyribonucleic acid damage in the spermatozoa of infertile male patients. Fertil Steril. 1997;68:519–24.
68. Geva E, Lessing JB, Lerner-Geva L, Amit A. Free radicals, antioxidants and human spermatozoa: clinical implications. Hum Reprod. 1998;13:1422–4.
69. Comhaire FH, Christophe AB, Zalata AA, Dhooge WS, Mahmoud AM, Depuydt CE. The effects of combined conventional treatment, oral antioxidants and essential fatty acids on sperm biology in subfertile men. Prostaglandins Leukot Essent Fatty Acids. 2000;63: 159–65.
70. Keskes-Ammar L, Feki-Chakroun N, Rebai T, Sahnoun Z, Ghozzi H, Hammami S, Zghal K, Fki H, Damak J, Bahloul A. Sperm oxidative stress and the effect of an oral vitamin E and selenium supplement on semen quality in infertile men. Arch Androl. 2003;49:83–94.

71. Greco E, Scarselli F, Iacobelli M, Rienzi L, Ubaldi F, Ferrero S, Franco G, Anniballo N, Mendoza C, Tesarik J. Efficient treatment of infertility due to sperm DNA damage by ICSI with testicular spermatozoa. Hum Reprod. 2005;20:226–30.
72. Lopes S, Jurisicova A, Sun JG, Casper RF. Reactive oxygen species: potential cause for DNA fragmentation in human spermatozoa. Hum Reprod. 1998;13(4):896–900.
73. Krausz C, Mills C, Rogers S, et al. Stimulation of oxidant generation by human sperm suspensions using phorbol esters and formyl peptides: relationships with motility and fertilization in vitro. Fertil Steril. 1994;62:599–605.
74. Lenzi A, Picardo M, Gandini L, et al. Glutathione treatment of dyspermia: effect on the lipoperoxidation process. Hum Reprod. 1994;9:2044–50.
75. Berkovitz A, Eltes F, Ellenbogen E, Peer S, Feldberg D, Bartoov B. Does the presence of nuclear vacuoles in human sperm selected for ICSI affect pregnancy outcome? Hum Reprod. 2006;21:1787–90.
76. Bartoov B, Berkovitz A, Eltes F, Kogosovsky A, Yagoda A, Lederman H, Artzi S, Gross M, Barak Y. Pregnancy rates are higher with intracytoplasmic morphologically selected sperm injection than with conventional intracytoplasmic injection. Fertil Steril. 2003;80:1413–9.
77. Palermo G, Joris H, Devroey P, Van Steirteghem A. Pregnancies after intracytoplasmic injection of single spermatozoon into an oocyte. Lancet. 1992;340:17.
78. Bartoov B, Eltes F, Pansky M, Langzam J, Reichart M, Soffer Y. Improved diagnosis of male fertility potential via a combination of quantitative ultramorphology and routine semen analyses. Hum Reprod. 1994;9:2069–75.
79. Mundy AJ, Ryder TA, Edmonds DK. A quantitative study of sperm head ultrastructure in subfertile males with excess sperm precursors. Fertil Steril. 1994;61:751–4.
80. Berkovitz A, Eltes F, Lederman H, Peer S, Ellenbogen A, Feldberg B, Bartoov B. How to improve IVF–ICSI outcome by sperm selection. Reprod Biomed Online. 2006;12:634–8.
81. Shapiro BS, Richter KS, Harris DC, Daneshmand ST. Dramatic declines in implantation and pregnancy rates in patients who undergo repeated cycles of in vitro fertilization with blastocyst transfer after one or more failed attempts. Fertil Steril. 2001;76:538–42.
82. Silberstein T, Trimarchi JR, Gonzalez L, Keefe D, Blazar AS. Pregnancy outcome in in vitro fertilization decreases to a plateau with repeated cycles. Fertil Steril. 2005;84:1043–5.
83. Antinori M, Licata E, Dani G, Cerusico C, Versaci C, D'Angelo D, Antinori S. Intracytoplasmic morphologically selected sperm injection :a prospective randomized trial. Reprod Biomed Online. 2008;16:835–41.
84. Kruger TF, Acosta AA, Simmons KF, Swanson JR, Matta JF, Oehninger S. Predictive value of sperm morphology in in vitro fertilization. Fertil Steril. 1988;49:112–7.
85. Martin RH, Rademaker A. The relationship between sperm chromosomal abnormalities and sperm morphology in humans. Mutat Res. 1988;207:159–64.
86. Rosenbusch B, Strehler E, Sterzik K. Cytogenetics of human spermatozoa: correlations with sperm morphology and age of fertile men. Fertil Steril. 1992;58:1071–2.
87. Sailer BL, Jost LK, Evenson DP. Bull sperm head morphometry related to abnormal chromatin structure and fertility. Cytometry. 1996;24:167–73.
88. Virro MR, Larson-Cook KL, Evenson DP. Sperm chromatin structure assay (SCSA) parameters are related to fertilization, blastocyst development, and ongoing pregnancy in in vitro fertilization and intracytoplasmic sperm injection cycles. Fertil Steril. 2004;81:1289–95.
89. Vicari E, de Palma A, Burrello N, Longo G, Grazioso C, Barone N, Zahi M, D'Agata Check JH, Graziano V, Cohen R, et al. Effect of an abnormal sperm chromatin structural assay (SCSA) on pregnancy outcome following (IVF) with ICSI in previous IVF failures. Arch Androl. 2005;51:121–4.
90. Nagy ZP, Liu J, Joris H, et al. The result of intracytoplasmic sperm injection is not related to any of the three basic sperm parameters. Hum Reprod. 1995;10:1123–9.
91. McKenzie LJ, Kovanci E, Amato P, et al. Pregnancy outcome of in vitro fertilization/intracytoplasmic sperm injection with profound teratospermia. Fertil Steril. 2004;82:847–9.

92. Bonduelle M, Aytoz A, Van Assche E, et al. Incidence of chromosomal aberrations in children born after assisted reproduction through intracytoplasmic sperm injection. Hum Reprod. 1998;13: 781–2.

93. Lee JD, Kamiguchi Y, Yanagimachi R. Analysis of chromosome constitution of human spermatozoa with normal and aberrant head morphologies after injection into mouse oocytes. Hum Reprod. 1996;11:1942–6.

94. Hazout A, Dumont-Hassan M, Junca AM, Bacrie PC, Tesarik J. High-magnification ICSI overcomes paternal effect resistant to conventional ICSI. Reprod Biomed Online. 2006;12: 19–25.

95. Franco Jr JG, Baruffi RL, Mauri AL, et al. Significance of large nuclear vacuoles in human spermatozoa: implications for ICSI. Reprod Biomed Online. 2008;17:42–5.

96. Garolla A, Fortini D, Menegazzo M, et al. High-power microscopy for selecting spermatozoa for ICSI by physiological status. Reprod Biomed Online. 2008;17:610–6.

97. Hoffman R, Gross L. Reflected light differential-interference microscopy: principles, use and image interpretation. J Microsc. 1970;91:149–72.

98. Hoffman R, Gross L. Demodulation contrast microscope. Nature. 1975;254:586–8.

99. Padawer J. The Nomarski interference-contrast microscope. An experimental basis for image interpretation. J R Microsc Soc. 1968;88:305–49.

100. Kacem O, Sifer C, Barraud-Lange V, Ducot B, De Ziegler D, Poirot C, Wolf JP. Sperm nuclear vacuoles, assessed by motile sperm organellar morphological examination, are mostly of acrosomal origin. Reprod Biomed Online. 2010;20:132–7.

Chapter 25
Extended Embryo Culture Supplementation

Alex C. Varghese, Eulalia Pozo-Guisado, Ignacio S. Alvarez,
and Francisco Javier Martin-Romero

Reactive oxygen and nitrogen species are generated by diverse enzyme activities, and they act as modulators of many physiological functions. However, due to the intrinsic reactivity of these species, they can trigger undesired reactions threatening `nisms that counteract these reactive species, by means of scavenging, chelation, or modification of reactive species. These mechanisms constitute the antioxidant system, and the imbalance between the generation of reactive oxygen species (ROS) and the antioxidant system is known as oxidative stress. Oxidative stress is often the origin of a large number of diseases, including some cases of male and female infertility. However, the handling and in vitro culture of gametes and embryos during assisted reproductive techniques generate a significant level of oxidative stress. This oxidative stress is associated to the culture conditions because gametes and embryos are not within their physiological environment, but in a much more oxidative milieu. This chapter reviews the recent knowledge regarding the role of reactive oxygen and nitrogen species on reproductive physiology. We also focus on the strategies that researches have considered to neutralize the oxidative stress that develops in parallel to the in vitro culture and cryopreservation. Basic studies using mammalian oocytes

A.C. Varghese, PhD (✉)
Montreal Reproductive Centre, 2110, Boul Decarie,
Montreal, QC, Canada, H4A 3J3
e-mail: alexcv2008@gmail.com; alex@lifeinvitro.com

E. Pozo-Guisado, PhD • F.J. Martin-Romero, PhD
Department of Biochemistry and Molecular Biology,
School of Life Sciences, University of Extremadura,
Avenida De Elvas S/N, 06006, Badajoz, Spain
e-mail: epozo@unex.es; fjmartin@unex.es

I.S. Alvarez, PhD
Department of Cell Biology, School of Life Sciences,
University of Extremadura, Avenida de Elvas s/n, 06006, Badajoz, Spain
e-mail: ialvarez@unex.es

S.J. Parckattil and A. Agarwal (eds.), *Antioxidants in Male Infertility: A Guide for Clinicians and Researchers*, © Springer Science+Business Media New York 2013

have been designed to investigate the benefits of the use of antioxidants during in vitro culture, and this chapter summarizes the most important findings regarding the supplementation of culture media to minimize the harmful effects of oxidative stress. However, an intense line of investigation is required to transfer the recent knowledge to the particular conditions of the human embryo to ensure high rates of successful IVF cycles.

Role of Reactive Species During Oogenesis

Many of the physiological processes in the ovary function are influenced by ROS and reactive nitrogen species (RNS), including folliculogenesis and oocyte maturation. Regarding oogenesis, it is known that members of the *Bcl-2* gene family are expressed in ovarian granulosa cells during follicular maturation, this expression being controlled by the follicle-stimulating hormone (FSH) [1]. FSH prevents apoptosis in granulosa cells in vitro in the same extent as some antioxidants, either enzymatic or nonenzymatic, such as superoxide dismutase (SOD), ascorbic acid, or *N*-acetyl-L-cysteine. In this regard, granulosa cells from rats primed with equine chorionic gonadotropin (eCG), which promotes antral follicular growth and survival, show an upregulation of the expression of extracellular SOD (ecSOD) isoforms and Mn-SOD, although the expression of Cu/Zn-SOD, glutathione peroxidase (GPx), or catalase is not influenced by gonadotropin priming [1]. In sum, gonadotropins support granulosa cell survival in developing follicles through the activation of antioxidant defenses, strongly strengthening the hypothesis that ROS/RNS modulate the kinetics of the folliculogenesis.

Physiological Role of Superoxide and Hydrogen Peroxide

ROS/RNS play a physiological role during ovulation, as suggested by the finding that the perfusion of in vitro cultured ovaries with SOD or catalase, delays ovulation [2]. In fact, the ovary and uterus of cycling and pregnant mice generate NADPH-dependent superoxide [3], and both ovarian and uterine NADPH-dependent superoxide production are likely to be luteinizing hormone (LH) inducible [4, 5]. Therefore, it is possible that ovulation could be associated with a significant increase in ROS levels, and these reactive species are generated by different cells. Macrophages, neutrophilic granulocytes, and T lymphocytes are present in the ovary at ovulation. There is an increase in the level of macrophages and neutrophilic granulocytes in the medullar region and in the thecal layer as the ovulatory period progresses [6], and macrophages and neutrophils in the ovary could be a major source of significant amounts of ROS during ovulation [7].

The superoxide generation can eventually lead to an increase in the hydrogen peroxide (H_2O_2) concentration, due to the presence of different isoforms of SOD in developing antral follicles. The location of these isoforms has been described recently, and cumulus–oocyte complexes (COCs) exhibit a compartmentalized and varying distribution of SOD1 (or Cu, Zn-SOD), SOD2 (or Mn-SOD), and SOD3 (extracellular or ecSOD) protein expression. SOD1, SOD2, and SOD3 proteins and activities are found in high levels in the follicular fluid from small follicles, while SOD3 protein is more abundant in oocytes and cumulus cells from large follicles relative to small follicles [8]. Regardless, SOD2 is the predominant isoform expressed in the ooplasm, while SOD3 is the main SOD type in cumulus cells. SOD1 shows enhanced nuclear accumulation in oocytes [8]. It is important to highlight that oocytes or COCs accumulate the diverse SOD isoforms during folliculogenesis to neutralize potential oxidative bursts, like the suggested during ovulation [7].

Role of Nitric Oxide

Nitric oxide (NO·) is biologically produced form L-arginine in a reaction catalyzed by the nitric oxide synthase (NOS). There are three isoforms of the NOS: NOS1, or neuronal constitutive NOS (nNOS); NOS2, the inducible NOS (iNOS); and NOS3, endothelial constitutive NOS (eNOS). They are all expressed in the ovary [9–11] and the oviduct [12], and NOS has been immunolocalized in thecal and stromal cells of the ovary during follicular development and ovulation [10]. NO· synthesis increases during follicular development [13] and a parallel increase of nitrites and nitrates in the follicular fluid has been reported, as a direct consequence of the upregulated NO· synthesis [14]. Moreover, the NO· synthesis kinetics correlates well with estradiol concentration, suggesting that NO· is an important signaling molecule during folliculogenesis. The role of NO· as endocrine regulator is supported by the significant reduction in the folliculogenesis rate and the production of mature oocytes by aminoguanidine and L-NMMA, two well-known NOS inhibitors [15]. In contrast, sodium nitroprusside (SNP), a NO· donor, reverses the effects of the NOS inhibitors, further supporting the conclusion that the production of NO· by NOS is required for the follicle development. However, the production of NO· during folliculogenesis and ovulation shows a relevant spatiotemporal dynamics. The concentration of nitrate/nitrite (NO· metabolites) in preovulatory follicles is high before hCG injection but then decreases after hCG stimulation [16]. Accordingly, NO· donors prevent germinal vesicle breakdown (GVBD) and inhibitors of iNOS counteract this prevention [17, 18]. Expression of eNOS, mainly localized in the thecal layer, increases after hCG priming [9, 11, 17, 19], and iNOS expression, largely found in granulosa cells, significantly decreases after hCG injection, reducing the levels of NO· in the preovulatory follicular fluid. Thus, NO· levels are reflecting significant alterations of iNOS expression, but not for eNOS in preovulatory follicles [17]. The iNOS-produced NO· is an inhibitor of the oocyte maturation, because it induces an increase in cGMP concentration in preovulatory follicles, leading to an increase in the cGMP concentration in the oocyte via gap junctions, where it plays a key role in the meiotic arrest of oocytes [20]. cGMP keeps the meiotic arrest of preovulatory oocytes, increasing cAMP levels by the inhibition of the phosphodiesterase activity and by the activation of cGMP-dependent protein kinase [20], demonstrating that the iNOS–NO·–cGMP pathway modulates meiotic progression of the oocyte.

The dual effect of NO· is also observed with maturing mammalian oocytes in vitro. High concentrations of SNP or *S*-nitroso-*N*-acetylpenicillamine (SNAP) in culture induce the blockade of the meiotic progression at MI, and these arrested MI oocytes remain at this stage even after eliminating the NO· donor from the culture [21, 22]. On the contrary, SNP, within the nano- to low micromolar range, increases cytoplasmic maturation [21, 23] and the percentage of blastocyst rates [21]. There is some controversy in the recent data from studies using NO· donors, since micromolar SNP has been shown to induce embryotoxicity by reducing the glucose and pyruvate uptake and by depleting the levels of essential amino acids, leading to a much lower developmental rate [24]. The major reason for the contradictory data could be that the NO· concentration produced by NO· donors, which depends on the decomposition time, is strongly influenced by the redox status in the cytosolic compartment, or by the presence of other reactive species. Thus, it is absolutely required to study further the effect of ROS/RNS after a meticulous determination of the ROS/RNS-releasing kinetics from donors in every experimental condition. These methods are available from the recent literature and they are easy to adapt to particular experimental conditions. This is the case for the quantification of peroxynitrite, a strong oxidant and nitrating agent formed after the reaction of NO· with superoxide anion. Decomposition of SIN-1, a peroxynitrite releasing agent, can be continuously monitored, with a sensitivity lower to 0.1 μM, from the kinetics of NADH fluorescence quenching [25], giving the opportunity to calculate the concentration of the donor required for the exposure of oocytes/embryos to specific peroxynitrite concentrations.

Endothelium-derived NOS is a key modulator of oocyte meiotic maturation in vitro, as it has been described that ovaries from eNOS-knockout (eNOS-KO) mice contain a smaller amount of COCs, relative to wild-type mice, and that in vitro maturation of COCs from eNOS-KO mice results in a high percentage of abnormal MI oocytes with a low rate of fully mature oocytes [26]. Inhibition of NOS activity, attained with L-NAME, during in vitro maturation leads to an increase in apoptosis during embryo development, supporting a role for NO· in the meiotic progression of the mammalian oocyte [27].

In addition, NO· is probably related with implantation, as iNOS is differentially expressed in pre-, peri-, and postimplantation blastocysts. The enhanced NO· production, supported by the upregulation of iNOS, would act as a vasodilator and an angiogenic mediator [28]. However, it is known that embryo development is downregulated under high NO· concentrations in vivo and in vitro [29]. Finally, the eNOS-KO mice show severe defects in different aspects of reproduction, such as ovulation, fertilization, and early embryo development, further demonstrating the physiological role of NO· [30].

Oxidative Stress in Fertilization and Preimplantation Development

Role of Reactive Oxygen Species at Fertilization

In some marine invertebrate species, fertilization is accompanied by a significant increase in the rate of ROS/RNS formation in eggs, producing a respiratory burst [31–36]. After insemination, a rise in $[Ca^{2+}]_i$ takes place in the zygote, similarly to other species, which induces the secretion of the cortical granules content into the perivitelline space [37]. In addition, there is a calcium-dependent activation of PKC that slightly increases the intracellular pH (pH_i) through the activation of the Na^+/H^+ antiporter. Both the PKC activation and the increase in the pH_i are required for the subsequent activation of Udx1, a plasma membrane protein with NADPH oxidase activity that produces H_2O_2 [38]. The function of this increased production of H_2O_2 is to drive the formation of dityrosyl bonds to harden the fertilization envelope and block polyspermy [39]. Thus, the oxidative burst observed in invertebrates plays a well-known physiological role during the first stages of fertilization. However, a similar oxidative burst in mammalian oocytes at fertilization has not been reported.

It has been suggested that the lipid peroxidation has an enhancing effect on the ability of human spermatozoa to bind to zona pellucida, by a mechanism that can be reverted by α-tocopherol [40], suggesting a possible physiological role for the ROS generated by human spermatozoa in mediating sperm–zona interaction. The lipid peroxidation is indicative of an oxidative burst in spermatozoa, and the generation of superoxide has been demonstrated in sperm cells [41, 42]. Mammalian oocytes have been found to produce superoxide, this production being inhibited by SOD and diphenyleneiodonium (DPI), therefore suggesting that superoxide is generated by a NADPH oxidase activity in oocytes [41]. During the fusion of gametes at fertilization the measured production of superoxide is somehow diminished, probably due to the SOD release from gametes [41], weakening any potential physiological role of the oocyte superoxide at fertilization.

Although the occurrence of a sustained increase in ROS generation at fertilization is unlikely, a physiological role of some of these reactive species in the cell signaling in embryos has been suggested. This is the case for H_2O_2 in the blastocysts. Hydrogen peroxide in the blastocele fluid triggers apoptosis in the trophectoderm, while inner cell mass cells are protected from this oxidative-triggered apoptosis by a mechanism dependent on reduced glutathione (GSH) [43]. Thus, the balance of H_2O_2/GSH has a role in early development for the maintenance of the balance between inner cell mass and trophectoderm.

NO', which plays a role during oocyte maturation, embryonic development, and implantation, has a signaling role at fertilization. Although it has been reported that the concentration of intracellular NO' does not change, globally or locally, during sperm-induced calcium waves [44], the role of NO' remains controversial, since Goud et al. observed that SNAP prevents deterioration of oocytes in culture, extending the temporal window for optimal fertilization, while NOS inhibitors reverse this action [45]. Those authors propose that the role of NO• in oocytes at fertilization is closely related with the regulation of calcium waves. The transient increase in the NO• concentration within the oocyte leads to the activation of guanylyl cyclase, and the increased cGMP levels would trigger the phosphorylation of inositol 1,4,5-trisphosphate receptor at the endoplasmic reticulum, which in turn regulates Ca^{2+} release from the ER. Thus, NO• would be required for the optimal generation of calcium waves, and the insufficient availability of NO• may accelerate oocyte aging.

Oxidative Burst in Embryos

The role of ROS as signal molecules at early embryo development is controversial. While many works reported the inhibition of embryo development under exposure to ROS (reviewed in [46]), a considerable oxidative burst has been monitored in the mouse embryos during blastocyst hatching [47]. The blastocyst hatching, i.e., the emergence of the mammalian blastocysts from their glycoprotein envelope previous to the implantation, generates ROS for a short period of time. This observation is supported by the induction of the hatching by the treatment of blastocysts with extracellular superoxide, within the low micromolar range, an experimental approach that shows no detrimental effects on the viability of the embryo. In fact, this level of superoxide (1–1.5 μM) is close to that observed in peri-hatching blastocyst suspension, and supports the hypothesis that superoxide has a key role in cell signaling at peri-hatching stages. Conversely, superoxide scavengers (*N-t*-butyl-α-phenyl nitrone, SOD, and menadione) inhibit the hatching of blastocysts in vitro, and the implantation in vivo, further strengthening the potential role of superoxide [47]. However, the molecular mechanism underlying the superoxide generation at this stage of the early development remains unknown.

As stated above, NO• is related with implantation. Inducible NOS is expressed in pre-, peri-, and postimplantation blastocysts with a differential profile, and the NO• production helps in the implantation while acting as vasodilator and angiogenic mediator [28]. However, it has been demonstrated that high concentrations of NO• inhibit development in vivo and in vitro [29], showing that the excess of NO• is harmful for embryo development.

On the other hand, the superoxide-dependent oxidative burst in embryos is probably limited to this particular stage of the development. A similar increase in other ROS, such as H_2O_2, has been found in the transition from the two- to four-cell stages, but it reflects, at least in part, the consequences of the exposure of embryos to in vitro culture conditions. Thus, the rise of H_2O_2 levels in the transition to the two- and four-cell stages is much reduced for in vivo developed embryos [48]. The increase of H_2O_2 observed in vitro is also involved in the two-cell block that has been reported in embryos developed in vitro from several mouse strains.

Sensitivity of Embryos to Oxidative Stress

The preimplantation embryo development, i.e., between one-cell and blastocyst stage, is highly sensitive to oxidative stress [7, 49, 50]. The oxygen tension in the female reproductive organ varies during the preimplantation stage, although it is always significantly lower than the atmospheric concentration. While this tension is $pO_2 \sim 5–10\%$ in the oviduct [51], the uterus shows a lower O_2 tension [52]. The decreasing O_2 tension suggests that embryos develop in healthy conditions under low O_2 concentrations, and that the almost anoxic conditions that surround the trophectoderm at the moment of implantation are not harmful for the developing embryo. In this regard, a number of reports demonstrate that the rate of in vitro development to the blastocyst stage increases when pO_2 is lowered to 5–10% in culture [53–57], and it is assumed that the benefits of the low O_2 tension culture are due to a probable lower generation of ROS in these experimental conditions. At the onset of compaction in vivo, embryos increase ATP production [51]. This metabolic switch is characterized by the increase in glycolytic activity and the dependence on ATP generated by glycolysis during preimplantation development, i.e., the preferred use of glucose as major energy substrate, rather than pyruvate [58]. The metabolic shift at the compaction stage is associated with a shift in the embryo redox state that accommodates the embryo to a more reduced environment in vivo, with decreasing O_2 concentration in the oviduct–uterus transition.

ROS have been associated with detrimental effects during maturation and early cleavage, since they account for alterations in the segregation of chromosomes during meiosis, the blockade of embryos in the two-cell stage, and low pregnancy rates [59, 60]. ROS are also responsible for an increased rate of cell death in both oocytes and embryos [50], and the H_2O_2 generation rate in fragmented embryos developed in vitro is significantly higher compared to non-fragmented embryos and unfertilized oocytes, while apoptosis is usually observed in fragmented embryos, but it is absent in non-fragmented embryos [49, 50]. ROS are also responsible for an increase of cell death in spermatozoa, and for severe molecular and biochemical alterations in oocytes such as lipid peroxidation [61, 62] and disruption of the intracellular calcium homeostasis [63, 64]. In this regard, we have shown that extracellular H_2O_2, within the micromolar range, enhances Ca^{2+} influx through store-operated calcium channels, impairing calcium homeostasis in human oocytes [64]. This impairment could eventually lead to a decrease in fertilization rates.

Role of Glutathione in Early Development

The tripeptide glutathione (γ-L-glutamyl-L-cysteinyl-glycine) is the most abundant thiol in mammalian cells. Reduced glutathione (GSH) is an important regulator of the intracellular redox state, and helps in the protection of cells against oxidative damage. Consequently, a depletion of the intracellular pool of GSH has been observed in cells under intensive oxidative insult [65]. Glutathione metabolism of early embryos is dependent on the developmental stage [66–68]. Although glutathione consumption and synthesis increase during oocyte maturation, early development is characterized by a significant decrease of glutathione metabolism. GSH content decreases approximately tenfold from that in the unfertilized oocyte to 0.12 pmol/blastocyst, representing an estimated change in concentration from 7 to 0.7 mM [66]. The GSH content falls quite rapidly, i.e., by 20–25% at fertilization and by approximately 45% by the late two-cell and early four-cell stages [69]. In parallel, NAD(P)H levels remain constant during oocyte maturation, but decrease after fertilization, concomitantly with GSH levels. NADPH is required for the GSH recycling by the glutaredoxin–glutathione reductase system (Grx–GR) and the thioredoxin system, suggesting that the restricted NADPH availability may be responsible of the GSH production after fertilization [68]. Moreover, the lowered GSH level is consistent with a diminished de novo synthesis of GSH after fertilization, compared with the high ATP-dependent de novo synthesis during oocyte maturation [67, 70].

Antioxidant Supplementation in Culture Media and Outcomes

Reactive Oxygen Species Generated by Culture Media

As stated above, the presence of ROS in the fluids and organs involved in the reproductive processes has been well documented in vivo and in vitro. The sources for these ROS in vivo are mainly the follicular fluid and the tubal and uterine milieu where gametes and embryos undergo maturation, fertilization, and early development [46, 71, 72]. During IVF, the gametes and embryos are not in their physiological environment but in culture media. Although culture media composition differs significantly, almost all commercial media are supplemented with serum or serum synthetic replacements, albumin [73], and other molecules that may potentially generate reactive species. Among these molecules we find HEPES buffer, metal chelators, ethylenediaminetetraacetic acid (EDTA), and ferric and cupric salts. Therefore, the medium itself is a putative source of ROS [74–76], and the contribution of this external source to the overall oxidative stress in gametes and embryos should not be considered as negligible.

The most important ROS generated in this manner are superoxide anion, hydroxyl radical, alkyl hydroperoxide, and hydrogen peroxide [74, 77–79]. In buffers and culture media with ferric or cupric salts or with molecules that have been shown to have photodynamic activities, such as flavins, the exposure to visible light and the mixing with atmospheric oxygen may generate significant amounts of superoxide [46, 78].

The effects of ROS on oocytes and early embryos have been tested experimentally, and we have described above the detrimental effects of elevated levels of ROS on oocyte maturation and early development. To gain knowledge on the effect of ROS on these biological processes, most of the studies have been developed on the basis of the addition of fluxes or single bolus of ROS to the culture medium. However, it should be considered that ROS can be chemically produced by buffers and enriched culture media, with superoxide anion, hydroxyl radical, hydroxide anion, and hydrogen peroxide, being the most important ROS generated [74, 77–79]. Serum and serum replacements include oxidases that usually enhance the production of ROS in buffers [46] and commercial media used during IVF generate ROS at different rates depending on the composition, i.e., different brands generate diverse rates of ROS [74, 76]. Common culture media used in IVF are able to produce levels of ROS high enough to damage human oocytes, being easily detectable with ROS-sensitive dyes, like H_2DCF-DA, dihydroethidium, or Amplex red combined with horseradish peroxidase. As we mentioned, superoxide is one of the major ROS generated by the culture media, but many other ROS are derived from superoxide, and they can be detected in significant levels. This is the case for H_2O_2. The production of H_2O_2 in buffers and media used for culturing human oocytes can be as high as 1–15 μM/h, i.e., reaching subtoxic levels that may account for decreased rates of fertilization, or early embryo development [74]. Interestingly, the amount of H_2O_2 produced by follicular fluid, and measured following the same experimental procedure, is extremely low and not significantly different when compared to phosphate-buffered saline buffers. Since H_2O_2 is one of the reactive species involved in the initial steps of lipid peroxidation in biological membranes [61], and taking into consideration that micromolar H_2O_2 induces lipid peroxidation in other cell types [80], we have reported that lipid peroxidation of COCs cultured following a protocol that mimics human IVF protocols is significantly higher compared to COCs in follicular fluid, and that lipid peroxidation can be prevented with the supplementation of the culture medium with either α-tocopherol or catalase [74].

Exposure of human oocytes to extracellularly added H_2O_2, within the micromolar range, enhances Ca^{2+} influx through store-operated calcium channels, and this Ca^{2+} overload leads to a sustained increase of the intracellular free Ca^{2+} concentration ($[Ca^{2+}]_i$) and eventually to the deregulation of the Ca^{2+} homeostasis [64]. Because Ca^{2+} signaling is tightly regulated in the mature oocyte, and the progression from fertilized oocyte to one-cell embryo requires the controlled generation of repetitive and transient increases of the $[Ca^{2+}]_i$, known as calcium waves, H_2O_2 may impairs the cytosolic Ca^{2+} spiking at fertilization [63]. Thus, fluxes of micromolar H_2O_2, generated by culture media, could severely affect Ca^{2+} signaling in human IVF during extended cultures, as the accumulated oxidative damage originated by culture media may not be neutralized by oocytes. In fact, this is the assumed explanation for the deficient generation of calcium waves in aged oocytes. The culture-induced aging of oocytes impairs Ca^{2+} oscillations patterns [81], similarly to what is found in H_2O_2-treated oocytes, leading in both cases to a poor embryo development [82]. In parallel, oocytes exposed to H_2O_2 concentrations within the micromolar range show a deficient readjusting of the intracellular ATP concentration at fertilization [83]. As a consequence of the extracellular oxidative stress generated by in vitro culture protocols with long incubation times in IVF media (at least 6–8 h), a partial but significant depletion in oocyte GSH content has been found, which is not observed when the incubation time is shorter than 2 h, suggesting that a long exposure to the oxidative stress associated with in vitro culture is required to induce this partial depletion in the intracellular pool of GSH [74]. Since GSH reacts with reactive species such as superoxide anion [84] and singlet oxygen [85], a decreased concentration of GSH promotes nonselective disulfide bond formation within proteins [86], having tremendous effects on cell physiology and endangering cell viability, enhancing the effects of a sustained oxidative stress, risking oocyte fertilization and even oocyte viability.

Consequently, we can conclude that exposure of oocytes and embryos to in vitro culture conditions should be considered as a low intensity, but long-lasting oxidative insult, and it seems reasonable to suggest that the proper management of the period time of incubation of oocytes in the culture medium could improve oocyte quality, thereby increasing the success rate of the IVF cycle. For this reason, the future design of culture media and protocols for IVF should consider the role of ROS generation by these media. Although some antioxidants show a rapid decay in cell-free buffers at physiological pH (e.g., ascorbate), the addition of combined lipophilic and hydrosoluble antioxidants arises as a reasonable method for decreasing the impact of the oxidative stress triggered by the culture media.

Addition of Antioxidants to the Culture Medium: Reduced Glutathione

Reduced glutathione represents the oocyte's main nonenzymatic defense against oxidative stress. The data regarding the way in which the in vitro culture conditions affect GSH levels in embryos are not consistent, although it is accepted that in vitro developed embryos show lower GSH levels when compared with in vivo developed embryos [66]. Contradictory data are found when the effect of the addition of extracellular GSH to the culture medium shows either no effect [69] or the improvement in the development through the two-cell block to the morula or blastocyst stages [66, 87, 88]. However, diverse treatments designed to modify the GSH concentration within oocytes or embryos reveal that this intracellular ROS scavenger is a key regulator of both the oocyte maturation and the embryo early development. Thus, the inhibition of GSH synthesis reduces the development of bovine embryos through the eight-cell block to the blastocyst stage [89], and the treatment with t-butyl hydroperoxide (tBH) to induce the depletion in GSH levels significantly blocks development in the two-cell stage [66]. Conversely, the treatment of mammalian oocytes with the flavonoid anthocyanin during IVM that leads to the increase in GSH levels and significant lowering of intracellular ROS generation is accompanied by higher rates of blastocyst formation after parthenogenetic activation or somatic cell nuclear transfer (SCNT) [90].

The addition of GSH to the culture medium (~1 mM) has also been tested during in vitro maturation of mammalian oocytes, increasing significantly the rate of fertilization [91] and the proportion of oocytes undergoing cleavage and morula/blastocyst development [92]. In all cases, GSH was used in the micromolar to low millimolar range, and the success in the observed parameters strongly suggest that oocytes and embryos undergo oxidative stress during in vitro culture, which can be prevented by supplementation with ROS scavengers. The addition of micromolar cysteine increases the content of GSH in oocytes during IVM, but has no effect on sperm penetration, pronuclear formation, or blastocyst formation [93].

The addition of cysteine and cystine, for de novo synthesis of GSH, triggers the increase of the oocyte GSH content, and represents a classic strategy to improve the maturation rate in porcine oocytes [94, 95]. However, a better strategy to increase intracellular GSH levels, without stimulating the γ-glutamyl cycle, is the esterification of GSH to increase the loading of GSH into cells in culture. In this sense, it has been reported recently that the use of extracellularly added GSH ethyl ester does not affect fertilization, or day 3 cleavage rate, but increases blastocyst total cell number [96]. Thus, GSH ethyl ester represents an effective approach to elevate oocyte GSH in vitro and to improve blastocyst cell number.

α-Tocopherol and Ascorbate

The active form of vitamin E, α-tocopherol, is one of the major antioxidants that protects mammalian cells against lipid peroxidation. The recycling of α-tocopherol in cell membranes is achieved by a direct mechanism using intracellular ascorbate [97]. Thus, the cooperation of both antioxidants prevents lipid peroxidative damage due to oxidative stress in culture. Moreover, the concentration of α-tocopherol in COC membranes significantly decreases during IVM, but remains constant in the presence of ascorbic acid in the culture media [98]. Once again, there is some controversy with the recent data regarding the effect of the addition of α-tocopherol to the IVM medium on the subsequent percentage of blastocysts obtained after IVF. Some studies found that the addition of α-tocopherol has no positive effect [98] or even a detrimental effect on fertilization rates in bovine oocytes [99].

Vitamin C or ascorbic acid has long been recognized to be one of the most relevant antioxidants in mammals. Because ascorbic acid has a pK_a value of 4.1 [100], ascorbate is the ionic form of ascorbic acid predominant at physiological pH. The combined addition of both α-tocopherol and ascorbate decreases the rate of development, thus suggesting that high levels of α-tocopherol may impair the acquisition of oocyte developmental competence [98]. On the contrary, using a similar mammalian model of study, it has been reported that 100–400 µM α-tocopherol in the oocyte maturation media increased the rates of cleavage, morula, and blastocyst [101]. Moreover, 100 µM α-tocopherol is found to be beneficial for improving embryo quality by decreasing the number of apoptotic cells in the blastocyst and improving the tolerance of embryos to freezing–thawing cycles [102, 103]. Interestingly, there is some consensus in the use of this concentration of α-tocopherol (100 µM) for the embryo culture [101, 102, 104], as it yields higher rates of blastocyst development, decreasing the number of apoptotic nuclei. Also, the addition of ascorbate along with α-tocopherol does not seem to be beneficial to embryo development [98, 104], although the addition of ascorbate alone (100 μM) reduces the number of apoptotic cells significantly [104]. However, all these studies were carried out in animal models and the blastocyst formation rate was strongly dependent on the concentrations of both the antioxidants. The particular conditions for human embryo culture require further investigation to set the optimal concentrations of both antioxidants with a significant effect on blastocyst formation, although the mentioned reports have narrowed this range to 50–200 μM for either α-tocopherol or ascorbate.

Superoxide Dismutase and Catalase

Superoxide and H_2O_2 are generated by cell-free culture medium, under atmospheric O_2 tension [74]. It has been reported that the addition of ecSOD to the culture medium decreases the intracellular oxidative stress in other cell types [105, 106], and constitutes a potential strategy to be used with oocytes and embryos in culture for assisted reproductive techniques. The dismutation of superoxide however leads to the increased levels of H_2O_2, and the combined use of both SOD and catalase should be considered to completely remove these ROS from the culture.

The probable beneficial effects of the addition of SOD to the embryo culture are supported by the finding that human follicular cells express a number of antioxidant enzymes, including SOD, and this expression negatively correlates with age [107]. In addition, fertilization and cleavage rates correlate with levels of SOD and catalase in the human follicular fluid [108]. The effect of the addition of SOD to the embryo culture has been studied in a mammalian animal model, but the improving of the developmental rate is significant only in high glucose media [109], i.e., SOD protects cells from ROS generation in high glucose conditions. Similarly, when bovine oocytes are matured in vitro in the presence of 10–1,000 U/ml SOD, the developmental competence of the oocytes after IVF is not improved [110]. This lack of SOD effectiveness is also found when SOD is added to a defined culture medium [synthetic oviductal fluid (SOF) + BSA] and the development to the morula and blastocyst stages is monitored [92], or when SOD is added to the synthetic medium KSOM [111]. There are some reports that show the attenuation of the two-cell block for mouse embryos when the cultured medium is supplemented with SOD, expanding the blastocyst formation in a basic synthetic medium but with no improvement of fertilization rate [112, 113].

Heavy Metal Chelation

As we stated above, heavy metals are mediators of ROS generation, mainly through Haber–Weiss reactions. This is the major reason for the requirement of heavy metals chelation in culture media for oocytes and embryos, and several studies have addressed this important question. Jinno et al. [114] reported more than two decades ago the efficiency of the addition of EDTA (10 μM) in the composition of culture media for mammalian oocytes, enhancing the development of embryos derived from oocytes matured in vitro, both to two-cell embryos and to blastocysts. Mouse oocytes and embryos have let us know that the requirement of EDTA is higher in embryos compared to oocytes, and that the increase of EDTA increases blastocysts frequency and day-4 hatching in a low-glucose Earle's balanced salt solution [115]. The optimal concentration of EDTA in the modified Ham's F-10 medium was studied in the 10–100 μM range, strongly supporting the development of in vivo conceived mouse zygotes to the blastocyst stage and increasing the implantation rate, especially when 100 μM EDTA was used [116]. This concentration of EDTA, either alone or in combination with hemoglobin, decreases the accumulation of ROS in porcine embryos, reducing the incidence of apoptosis, demonstrating that EDTA improves mammalian embryo development [117]. Similar conclusions were achieved with human embryos when the HTF medium was modified for the inclusion of EDTA and glutamine, further supporting a key role for heavy metal chelation during handling and culture of embryos in assisted reproductive techniques [118].

Other Antioxidants

The beneficial properties of other compounds, in most cases with radical scavenging properties, have been studied thoroughly in mammalian oocytes, although the information using human oocytes in IVF cycles is much more restricted. Taurine (1 mM) and melatonin (10–50 μM) improve embryo development in vitro [119]. Epigallocatechin-3-gallate, a polyphenolic compound, increases fertilization rates in porcine oocytes when this catechin is added to the IVF medium, although the enhancing effect is found in a narrow range of micromolar concentrations [120], and the efficacy of this supplement should be tested in other species.

Selenium is an inorganic element present in some enzymes with antioxidants activities (reviewed in [121]). The absence of selenium in the diet leads to several diseases, shortens life span, and has a significant effect in fertilization [121, 122]. As a consequence selenium supplementation, usually as sodium selenite, is required in synthetic culture media, although the level of selenium in culture medium needs to be addressed carefully. High concentrations (10 μM or higher) of selenium are toxic because selenium replaces sulfur in many enzyme active sites, modifying the chemistry of the catalyzed reactions. Within the nanomolar range, selenium in the diet of laboratory animals normalizes fertilization [122]. As a supplement of embryo culture media selenite increases levels of GPx, which is a selenoprotein, and reduces levels of caspase 3, improving development rates and preventing apoptosis in embryos [123].

Oxygen Tension

An interesting point regarding oxidative stress and in vitro handling of gametes and embryos during assisted reproductive techniques is the O_2 tension during in vitro culture. In mammals, early embryo development takes place in vivo in a low-oxygen environment (<10%) that may serve to protect the embryo from free radical damage. Culture conditions with defined media are usually carried out under humidified atmosphere of 5% CO_2: 95% air. Under these conditions the partial pressure of O_2 is ~150 mmHg, which is equivalent to ~20% O_2 [124]. Exposure of early embryos to atmospheric oxygen concentrations (20%) may explain reduced viability and the increased rate of fragmentation in embryos [53]. Although no significant differences have been found between 5 and 20% O_2 in the rate of human fertilization and embryo development at day 2 or 3, higher rates of blastocyst formation has been reported with lower O_2 tension at day 5–6. Therefore, it is believed that low O_2 concentrations may exert a beneficial effect only during the later stages of preimplantation development [54]. This conclusion is further supported by extending the culture of mammalian oocytes in 5% O_2 for 7 days in vitro, because the development to the blastocyst stage is significantly higher and the H_2O_2 generation by these embryos is much lower when compared to that measured with 20% O_2 culture [55]. In mammalian models of study, similar results have been reported culturing rabbit embryos in low O_2 (5–10%) [57], bovine embryos [125], or mouse embryos [126] in 5% O_2, suggesting a role for redox regulation during preimplantation development. However, the implantation rate and embryo viability after intrauterine transplantation to pseudopregnant females do not show significant differences for embryos cultured in low or atmospheric oxygen [126].

Antioxidants During Cryopreservation of Embryos

The ability to cryopreserve embryos without critical loss of viability has a profound effect on the success of assisted conception techniques. However, the survival of cryopreserved in vitro produced embryos, as measured either by post-warming survival in culture or by established pregnancies after embryo transfer, has lagged behind that of in vivo-derived embryos. Since oocyte/embryo plasma membranes contain significant amounts of polyunsaturated fatty acids (PUFA), they are particularly vulnerable to oxidative attack. It has been reported that lipid peroxidation of membrane phospholipids is adversely involved in embryo development. Some reports have indicated that cryopreservation can damage the antioxidant enzymes that protect against lipid peroxidation and that freeze–thaw stress can be modified by incubating the embryo in the presence of inhibitors of membrane lipid peroxidation [127]. These results suggest the possibility that the process of cryopreservation induces the production of ROS or alters the antioxidant enzyme potential of oocytes, leading to lipid peroxidation of the plasma membrane and resulting in reduced survival potential by a perturbation of membrane structure and permeability. Loss of cell membrane function via lipid peroxidation might interfere with transport systems such as pH regulatory systems on the cell membrane, and disruption of organelle membranes could affect transport systems such as mitochondrial transport systems essential for oxidative phosphorylation—the major energy-generating pathway of the early embryo [128]. Cells contain antioxidants such as GSH and SOD to protect against the production of oxygen radicals. However, it has been shown in sperm that the levels of these antioxidants are reduced by >50% following cryopreservation [129].

In addition, it is possible that loss of survival and fertilization competence following oocyte cryopreservation is also mediated by the mechanism of cytotoxic action of peroxynitrite and NO$^{\bullet}$. Supplementation of 50 IU/ml of SOD or the concomitant addition of SOD and hemoglobin to the freezing and thawing media has been shown to improve survival and fertilization of mouse oocytes [130]. It has been suggested that peroxynitrite, formed by the interaction of superoxide and NO$^{\bullet}$, may exert a cytotoxic effect on mouse metaphase II oocytes during cryopreservation. In addition, inclusion of LBP (*Lycium barbarum* polysaccharide) in the vitrification solution has shown to reduce the production of ROS, thereby preventing plasma membranes from lipid peroxidation and stabilizing membrane structure and permeability of porcine oocytes [131].

The work by Lane et al. demonstrates that including 0.1 mM ascorbate when cryopreserving mouse cleavage-stage and blastocyst-stage embryos is beneficial to subsequent embryo development and maintenance of normal cell function [128]. Ascorbate assists embryo development by stimulating development of the ICM following cryopreservation. Ascorbate is a very potent hydrophilic antioxidant that is able to scavenge H_2O_2, superoxide anion, hydroxyl free radical, and singlet oxygen [132]. Additionally, ascorbate is found in follicular fluid [133], indicating that it may have a physiological role as an antioxidant in oocyte and embryo development. The beneficial effects of ascorbate were most evident in mouse embryos that were slow frozen compared with those that were vitrified, which substantiates the fact that the damage from oxygen radicals is greater after slow freezing. Ascorbate also reduced H_2O_2 generation significantly among vitrified embryos but failed to do so in the slow-frozen ones. These results indicate that the slow-freezing procedure augments the production of H_2O_2 considerably more than the ultrarapid vitrification procedure. Peng et al. evaluated the effect of α-tocopherol on blastocyst development and subsequent cryosurvival of the somatic cell nuclear transferred ovine embryos [102]. α-Tocopherol (100 μg/ml) was added to the culture medium for the SCNT embryos, and the blastocysts from the α-tocopherol and untreated groups were then freeze–thawed, and their cryosurvival was assessed by in vitro culture for 48 h. The addition of α-tocopherol to the culture medium significantly decreased the apoptotic cell number (3.4% vs. 5.5%) and significantly increased the cryosurvival of SCNT blastocysts (66.8% vs. 50.7%). Future studies on antioxidative enzymes and NO$^{\bullet}$ scavengers may lead to a better understanding of the biochemical processes that occur during oocyte/embryo cryopreservation. Estimating the total antioxidant capacity (TAC) and measuring ROS levels in the follicular fluid of retrieved oocytes will help select patients whose gametes require antioxidant supplementation during cryopreservation and subsequent in vitro cultures. The implication that ROS-mediated damage to oocyte developmental competence and embryo viability in infertile patients have raised concerns and need further research to identify the pathology behind this condition [134].

The expression of various biomarkers of oxidative stress such as SOD (both Cu/Zn-SOD and Mn-SOD), GPx, glutamyl synthetase, and lipid peroxides has been demonstrated in normal cycling human ovaries [134]. A delicate balance exists between ROS and antioxidant enzymes in ovarian tissue. Since hypoxic conditions following retransplantation of ovarian tissues induce ROS generation and the freeze–thaw cycle depletes the tissue's antioxidant capacity, antioxidant treatment might arguably be warranted. Studies of bovine ovarian tissue transplantation showed that ascorbate reduced apoptosis [135].

Another molecule with potent antioxidant activity is resveratrol. Studies are required for its effect on embryo freezing. However, when embryos produced by in vitro fertilization were incubated with 0.5 µM resveratrol, the treatment led to higher frequencies of blastocyst formation (8.6% vs. 13.3%) and elevated total cell numbers (37.1 ± 2.4 vs. 43.2 ± 1.7) by the end of the 7-day culture period ($p < 0.05$). The results indicate that 0.5 µM resveratrol during culture has a positive effect on early embryonic development of porcine embryos [136]. When embryos produced by in vitro fertilization were incubated with 0.5 µM resveratrol, the treatment led to higher frequencies of blastocyst formation (8.6% vs. 13.3%) and elevated total cell number (37.1 ± 2.4 vs. 43.2 ± 1.7) by the end of the 7-day culture period ($p < 0.05$). The results indicate that 0.5 µM resveratrol during culture has a positive effect on early embryonic development of porcine embryos. More studies are required to find the optimal candidate antioxidants and the required concentration that could nullify the deleterious effect of oxidative stress associated with embryo cryopreservation.

Five-Year View and Key Issues

From what we have stated regarding oxidative stress it should not be inferred that the complete elimination of ROS is a requirement for the success in IVF cycles. ROS/RNS play a physiological role in many aspects of female reproduction, including folliculogenesis, ovulation, as well as fertilization, early embryo development, and implantation. Thus, every culture condition intended to diminish the occurrence of ROS/RNS should be carefully studied and clinically evaluated. We have reviewed in this chapter the recent research focused on the use of antioxidants as supplements of culture media, and we have shown that most of the studies have used mammalian models (mouse, pig, and bovine oocytes). There is though a long way to transfer this knowledge to human-assisted reproductive techniques, i.e., oocyte in vitro maturation, IVF and embryo culture, and cryoconservation. Enriched culture media are well-known producers of ROS/RNS upon exposure of the media to daylight and atmospheric oxygen [74, 79]. This finding can be explained also by the presence in the media of riboflavin or amine pyridine nucleotides, or even glucose plus metals, which can lead to the photochemical production of superoxide and singlet oxygen [78, 137, 138]. The generation of superoxide enhances the formation of H_2O_2, especially when HEPES buffer or other amines are present in the medium. Then, H_2O_2 may react with superoxide (Haber–Weiss reaction) to produce hydroxyl radicals and peroxyl radicals [78], amplifying the production of radicals and reactive species by chain reactions. In this scenario, a plausible strategy to neutralize the oxidative stress induced by the culture medium could be the drastic reduction of the concentration in those metabolites not required by oocytes/embryos. In this regard, the requirement of glucose increases during early development, and the combination of glucose and metals act as an enhancer of ROS production (see above). For this reason, EDTA needs to be increased in cultured media for embryos, compared to what is found for oocytes.

In addition to EDTA, GSH has been successfully used as culture media supplement. However, GSH ethyl ester arises as an alternative for GSH loading in oocytes. In fact, GSH ethyl ester has been used to increase GSH levels in oocytes during IVM, an experimental approach that increases blastocyst cell number [96, 139]. Although addition of α-tocopherol, within the micromolar range improved IVM, fertilization, and blastocysts rates, the effects of the combination of ascorbate and α-tocopherol are still obscure. We have reviewed here the recent data and it has been proved that the presence of both antioxidants does not sustain embryo viability. One explanation could be that ascorbate is oxidized rapidly at physiological pH to dehydroascorbate (DHA) and ascorbate free radical (AFR), and cells need to recycle the oxidized forms of ascorbate, to keep high intracellular levels [140]. Both AFR and DHA are recycled by coupling to other cellular redox systems, being $NAD(P)H/NAD(P)^+$ and GSH/GSSG, particularly relevant to this end (reviewed in [141]). Recycling of ascorbate at the AFR oxidation stage is advantageous for living cells, because DHA is unstable at physiological pH (half-life of approximately 6 min) undergoing irreversible ring opening to form 2,3-diketo-1-gulonic acid. Intracellular ascorbate recycling from AFR and DHA in cells is achieved at the expense of NAD(P)H oxidation, and is mostly carried out by specific NADH- and NADPH oxidases [141]. However, this recycling requires the consumption of ATP, and the excessive drop in ATP levels could block oocyte maturation or early development. Besides, in the absence of DHA recycling to ascorbate, DHA can rapidly react with many other dithiol systems, including dithiols in unfolded or partially folded proteins [142], with likely adverse consequences.

Although this chapter does not review the recent bibliography regarding clinical trials to counteract infertility, it should be highlighted that one of the most promising therapies to this end is the oral administration of dietary antioxidants, like the combination of α-tocopherol and selenium [143], further supporting a role of antioxidants in the overall treatment of infertility.

There is still an open question regarding the effect of short-term mild oxidative stress on fertilization and development rates. In this sense, data from recent studies suggest that a short-term osmotic stress during maturation of mammalian oocytes improves embryo development [144, 145], and short-term exposure of oocytes to micromolar H_2O_2 results in a significant blastocyst yield, without altering fertilization rate or the GSH content [146]. However, it is required to address this phenomenon in human embryos.

In conclusion, current protocols for handling and in vitro culture of gametes and embryos generate a significant oxidative stress which may risk the outcome of the IVF cycle. The shortening of incubation times in pro-oxidant culture media and the appropriate addition of antioxidants that have been reported to work well in the improvement of embryo development, such as GSH (as its derivative GSH ethyl ester), α-tocopherol, and EDTA as heavy metal chelator, will lead to the significant reduction of oxidative stress, without affecting the viability of gametes and embryos. The concentration of these antioxidants and the stage of addition need to be addressed carefully for human embryos, but the recent literature showed narrowed ranges of concentrations for all these antioxidants when mammalian embryos were used.

Acknowledgments Funded by Grant PDT08A021 of the Junta de Extremadura—Fondo Europeo de Desarrollo Regional (FEDER), and Grant BFU2008-00104 of the Spanish Ministerio de Ciencia e Innovación.

References

1. Tilly JL, Tilly KI. Inhibitors of oxidative stress mimic the ability of follicle-stimulating hormone to suppress apoptosis in cultured rat ovarian follicles. Endocrinology. 1995;136(1):242–52.
2. Miyazaki T, et al. Effect of inhibition of oxygen free radical on ovulation and progesterone production by the in-vitro perfused rabbit ovary. J Reprod Fertil. 1991;91(1):207–12.
3. Jain S, et al. NADPH dependent superoxide generation in the ovary and uterus of mice during estrous cycle and early pregnancy. Life Sci. 2000;66(12):1139–46.
4. Carlson JC, et al. Stimulation of progesterone secretion in dispersed cells of rat corpora lutea by antioxidants. Steroids. 1995;60(3):272–6.
5. Sawada M, Carlson JC. Intracellular regulation of progesterone secretion by the superoxide radical in the rat corpus luteum. Endocrinology. 1996;137(5):1580–4.
6. Brannstrom M, Mayrhofer G, Robertson SA. Localization of leukocyte subsets in the rat ovary during the periovulatory period. Biol Reprod. 1993;48(2):277–86.
7. Fujii J, Iuchi Y, Okada F. Fundamental roles of reactive oxygen species and protective mechanisms in the female reproductive system. Reprod Biol Endocrinol. 2005;3:43.
8. Combelles CM, et al. Profiling of superoxide dismutase isoenzymes in compartments of the developing bovine antral follicles. Reproduction. 2010;139(5):871–81.
9. Jablonka-Shariff A, Olson LM. Hormonal regulation of nitric oxide synthases and their cell-specific expression during follicular development in the rat ovary. Endocrinology. 1997;138(1):460–8.
10. Zackrisson U, et al. Cell-specific localization of nitric oxide synthases (NOS) in the rat ovary during follicular development, ovulation and luteal formation. Hum Reprod. 1996; 11(12):2667–73.
11. Van Voorhis BJ, et al. Expression and localization of inducible and endothelial nitric oxide synthase in the rat ovary. Effects of gonadotropin stimulation in vivo. J Clin Invest. 1995;96(6):2719–26.

12. Lapointe J, et al. Hormonal and spatial regulation of nitric oxide synthases (NOS) (neuronal NOS, inducible NOS, and endothelial NOS) in the oviducts. Endocrinology. 2006; 147(12):5600–10.
13. Rosselli M, et al. Circulating nitrite/nitrate levels increase with follicular development: indirect evidence for estradiol mediated NO release. Biochem Biophys Res Commun. 1994; 202(3):1543–52.
14. Anteby EY, et al. Human follicular nitric oxide pathway: relationship to follicular size, oestradiol concentrations and ovarian blood flow. Hum Reprod. 1996;11(9):1947–51.
15. Shukovski L, Tsafriri A. The involvement of nitric oxide in the ovulatory process in the rat. Endocrinology. 1994;135(5):2287–90.
16. Nakamura Y, et al. Nitric oxide inhibits oocyte meiotic maturation. Biol Reprod. 2002; 67(5):1588–92.
17. Yamagata Y, et al. Alterations in nitrate/nitrite and nitric oxide synthase in preovulatory follicles in gonadotropin-primed immature rat. Endocr J. 2002;49(2):219–26.
18. Dave S, Farrance DP, Whitehead SA. Evidence that nitric oxide inhibits steroidogenesis in cultured rat granulosa cells. Clin Sci (Lond). 1997;92(3):277–84.
19. Nakamura Y, et al. Changes in nitric oxide synthase activity in the ovary of gonadotropin treated rats: the role of nitric oxide during ovulation. Endocr J. 1999;46(4):529–38.
20. Tornell J, Billig H, Hillensjo T. Regulation of oocyte maturation by changes in ovarian levels of cyclic nucleotides. Hum Reprod. 1991;6(3):411–22.
21. Viana KS, et al. Effect of sodium nitroprusside, a nitric oxide donor, on the in vitro maturation of bovine oocytes. Anim Reprod Sci. 2007;102(3–4):217–27.
22. Schwarz KR, et al. Influence of nitric oxide during maturation on bovine oocyte meiosis and embryo development in vitro. Reprod Fertil Dev. 2008;20(4):529–36.
23. Bilodeau-Goeseels S. Effects of manipulating the nitric oxide/cyclic GMP pathway on bovine oocyte meiotic resumption in vitro. Theriogenology. 2007;68(5):693–701.
24. Orsi NM. Embryotoxicity of the nitric oxide donor sodium nitroprusside in preimplantation bovine embryos in vitro. Anim Reprod Sci. 2006;91(3–4):225–36.
25. Martin-Romero FJ, et al. Fluorescence measurements of steady state peroxynitrite production upon SIN-1 decomposition: NADH versus dihydrodichlorofluorescein and dihydrorhodamine 123. J Fluoresc. 2004;14(1):17–23.
26. Jablonka-Shariff A, Olson LM. Nitric oxide is essential for optimal meiotic maturation of murine cumulus-oocyte complexes in vitro. Mol Reprod Dev. 2000;55(4):412–21.
27. Schwarz KR, et al. Consequences of nitric oxide synthase inhibition during bovine oocyte maturation on meiosis and embryo development. Reprod Domest Anim. 2010;45(1):75–80.
28. Saxena D, et al. Increased appearance of inducible nitric oxide synthase in the uterus and embryo at implantation. Nitric Oxide. 2000;4(4):384–91.
29. Barroso RP, et al. Nitric oxide inhibits development of embryos and implantation in mice. Mol Hum Reprod. 1998;4(5):503–7.
30. Pallares P, et al. Disruption of the endothelial nitric oxide synthase gene affects ovulation, fertilization and early embryo survival in a knockout mouse model. Reproduction. 2008;136(5):573–9.
31. Turner E, Somers CE, Shapiro BM. The relationship between a novel NAD(P)H oxidase activity of ovoperoxidase and the CN resistant respiratory burst that follows fertilization of sea urchin eggs. J Biol Chem. 1985;260(24):13163–71.
32. Heinecke JW, Shapiro BM. Respiratory burst oxidase of fertilization. Proc Natl Acad Sci USA. 1989;86(4):1259–63.
33. Schomer B, Epel D. Redox changes during fertilization and maturation of marine invertebrate eggs. Dev Biol. 1998;203(1):1–11.
34. Heinecke JW, et al. A specific requirement for protein kinase C in activation of the respiratory burst oxidase of fertilization. J Biol Chem. 1990;265(14):7717–20.
35. Heinecke JW, Shapiro BM. The respiratory burst oxidase of fertilization. A physiological target for regulation by protein kinase C. J Biol Chem. 1992;267(12):7959–62.

36. Schomer Miller B, Epel D. The roles of changes in NADPH and pH during fertilization and artificial activation of the sea urchin egg. Dev Biol. 1999;216(1):394–405.
37. Steinhardt RA, Epel D. Activation of sea-urchin eggs by a calcium ionophore. Proc Natl Acad Sci USA. 1974;71(5):1915–9.
38. Wong JL, Creton R, Wessel GM. The oxidative burst at fertilization is dependent upon activation of the dual oxidase Udx1. Dev Cell. 2004;7(6):801–14.
39. Foerder CA, Shapiro BM. Release of ovoperoxidase from sea urchin eggs hardens the fertilization membrane with tyrosine crosslinks. Proc Natl Acad Sci USA. 1977;74(10):4214–8.
40. Aitken RJ, Clarkson JS, Fishel S. Generation of reactive oxygen species, lipid peroxidation, and human sperm function. Biol Reprod. 1989;41(1):183–97.
41. Miesel R, Drzejczak PJ, Kurpisz M. Oxidative stress during the interaction of gametes. Biol Reprod. 1993;49(5):918–23.
42. Ellis JA, Mayer SJ, Jones OT. The effect of the NADPH oxidase inhibitor diphenyleneiodonium on aerobic and anaerobic microbicidal activities of human neutrophils. Biochem J. 1988;251(3):887–91.
43. Pierce GB, Parchment RE, Lewellyn AL. Hydrogen peroxide as a mediator of programmed cell death in the blastocyst. Differentiation. 1991;46(3):181–6.
44. Hyslop LA, et al. Simultaneous measurement of intracellular nitric oxide and free calcium levels in chordate eggs demonstrates that nitric oxide has no role at fertilization. Dev Biol. 2001;234(1):216–30.
45. Goud PT, et al. Nitric oxide extends the oocyte temporal window for optimal fertilization. Free Radic Biol Med. 2008;45(4):453–9.
46. Guerin P, El Mouatassim S, Menezo Y. Oxidative stress and protection against reactive oxygen species in the pre-implantation embryo and its surroundings. Hum Reprod Update. 2001;7(2):175–89.
47. Thomas M, et al. A programmed oxyradical burst causes hatching of mouse blastocysts. J Cell Sci. 1997;110(Pt 14):1597–602.
48. Nasr-Esfahani MH, Aitken JR, Johnson MH. Hydrogen peroxide levels in mouse oocytes and early cleavage stage embryos developed in vitro or in vivo. Development. 1990;109(2):501–7.
49. Johnson MH, Nasr-Esfahani MH. Radical solutions and cultural problems: could free oxygen radicals be responsible for the impaired development of preimplantation mammalian embryos in vitro? Bioessays. 1994;16(1):31–8.
50. Yang HW, et al. Detection of reactive oxygen species (ROS) and apoptosis in human fragmented embryos. Hum Reprod. 1998;13(4):998–1002.
51. Leese HJ. Metabolic control during preimplantation mammalian development. Hum Reprod Update. 1995;1(1):63–72.
52. Fischer B, Bavister BD. Oxygen tension in the oviduct and uterus of rhesus monkeys, hamsters and rabbits. J Reprod Fertil. 1993;99(2):673–9.
53. Burton GJ, Hempstock J, Jauniaux E. Oxygen, early embryonic metabolism and free radical-mediated embryopathies. Reprod Biomed Online. 2003;6(1):84–96.
54. Dumoulin JC, et al. Effect of oxygen concentration on human in-vitro fertilization and embryo culture. Hum Reprod. 1999;14(2):465–9.
55. Kitagawa Y, et al. Effects of oxygen concentration and antioxidants on the in vitro developmental ability, production of reactive oxygen species (ROS), and DNA fragmentation in porcine embryos. Theriogenology. 2004;62(7):1186–97.
56. Thompson JG, et al. Effect of oxygen concentration on in-vitro development of preimplantation sheep and cattle embryos. J Reprod Fertil. 1990;89(2):573–8.
57. Li J, Foote RH. Culture of rabbit zygotes into blastocysts in protein-free medium with one to twenty per cent oxygen. J Reprod Fertil. 1993;98(1):163–7.
58. Houghton FD, et al. Oxygen consumption and energy metabolism of the early mouse embryo. Mol Reprod Dev. 1996;44(4):476–85.
59. Hu Y, et al. Effects of low O2 and ageing on spindles and chromosomes in mouse oocytes from pre-antral follicle culture. Hum Reprod. 2001;16(4):737–48.

60. Bedaiwy MA, et al. Differential growth of human embryos in vitro: role of reactive oxygen species. Fertil Steril. 2004;82(3):593–600.
61. Agarwal A, Saleh RA, Bedaiwy MA. Role of reactive oxygen species in the pathophysiology of human reproduction. Fertil Steril. 2003;79(4):829–43.
62. Tarin JJ. Potential effects of age-associated oxidative stress on mammalian oocytes/embryos. Mol Hum Reprod. 1996;2(10):717–24.
63. Takahashi T, et al. Impact of oxidative stress in aged mouse oocytes on calcium oscillations at fertilization. Mol Reprod Dev. 2003;66(2):143–52.
64. Martin-Romero FJ, et al. Store-operated calcium entry in human oocytes and sensitivity to oxidative stress. Biol Reprod. 2008;78(2):307–15.
65. Shivakumar BR, Kolluri SV, Ravindranath V. Glutathione and protein thiol homeostasis in brain during reperfusion after cerebral ischemia. J Pharmacol Exp Ther. 1995;274(3): 1167–73.
66. Gardiner CS, Reed DJ. Status of glutathione during oxidant-induced oxidative stress in the preimplantation mouse embryo. Biol Reprod. 1994;51(6):1307–14.
67. Gardiner CS, Reed DJ. Synthesis of glutathione in the preimplantation mouse embryo. Arch Biochem Biophys. 1995;318(1):30–6.
68. Dumollard R, et al. Regulation of redox metabolism in the mouse oocyte and embryo. Development. 2007;134(3):455–65.
69. Nasr-Esfahani MH, Johnson MH. Quantitative analysis of cellular glutathione in early preimplantation mouse embryos developing in vivo and in vitro. Hum Reprod. 1992;7(9): 1281–90.
70. Luberda Z. The role of glutathione in mammalian gametes. Reprod Biol. 2005;5(1):5–17.
71. Pasqualotto EB, et al. Effect of oxidative stress in follicular fluid on the outcome of assisted reproductive procedures. Fertil Steril. 2004;81(4):973–6.
72. Bedaiwy MA, et al. Relationship between oxidative stress and embryotoxicity of hydrosalpingeal fluid. Hum Reprod. 2002;17(3):601–4.
73. Blake D, et al. Protein supplementation of human IVF culture media. J Assist Reprod Genet. 2002;19(3):137–43.
74. Martin-Romero FJ, et al. Contribution of culture media to oxidative stress and its effect on human oocytes. Reprod Biomed Online. 2008;17(5):652–61.
75. Esfandiari N, et al. Protein supplementation and the incidence of apoptosis and oxidative stress in mouse embryos. Obstet Gynecol. 2005;105(3):653–60.
76. Miguel-Lasobras EM, et al. Oxidative stress in human oocytes during IVF handling. Fertil Steril. 2004;82(Supp 2):S56–7.
77. Cohen G. The fenton reaction. In: Greenwald RA, editor. Handbook of methods for oxygen radical research. Boca Raton: CRC Press; 1987. p. 55–64.
78. Michelson AM. Photochemical production of oxy radicals. In: Greenwald RA, editor. Handbooks of methods for oxygen radical research. Boca Raton: CRC Press; 2000. p. 71–5.
79. Grzelak A, Rychlik B, Bartosz G. Light-dependent generation of reactive oxygen species in cell culture media. Free Radic Biol Med. 2001;30(12):1418–25.
80. Gutierrez-Martin Y, et al. Alteration of cytosolic free calcium homeostasis by SIN-1: high sensitivity of L-type Ca2+ channels to extracellular oxidative/nitrosative stress in cerebellar granule cells. J Neurochem. 2005;92(4):973–89.
81. Igarashi H, et al. Aging-related changes in calcium oscillations in fertilized mouse oocytes. Mol Reprod Dev. 1997;48(3):383–90.
82. Takahashi T, et al. Poor embryo development in mouse oocytes aged in vitro is associated with impaired calcium homeostasis. Biol Reprod. 2009;80(3):493–502.
83. Igarashi H, et al. Aged mouse oocytes fail to readjust intracellular adenosine triphosphates at fertilization. Biol Reprod. 2005;72(5):1256–61.
84. Winterbourn CC, Metodiewa D. The reaction of superoxide with reduced glutathione. Arch Biochem Biophys. 1994;314(2):284–90.
85. Devasagayam TP, et al. Activity of thiols as singlet molecular oxygen quenchers. J Photochem Photobiol B. 1991;9(1):105–16.

86. Cumming RC, et al. Protein disulfide bond formation in the cytoplasm during oxidative stress. J Biol Chem. 2004;279(21):21749–58.
87. Legge M, Sellens MH. Free radical scavengers ameliorate the 2-cell block in mouse embryo culture. Hum Reprod. 1991;6(6):867–71.
88. Ozawa M, et al. Addition of glutathione or thioredoxin to culture medium reduces intracellular redox status of porcine IVM/IVF embryos, resulting in improved development to the blastocyst stage. Mol Reprod Dev. 2006;73(8):998–1007.
89. Takahashi M, et al. Effect of thiol compounds on in vitro development and intracellular glutathione content of bovine embryos. Biol Reprod. 1993;49(2):228–32.
90. You J, et al. Anthocyanin stimulates in vitro development of cloned pig embryos by increasing the intracellular glutathione level and inhibiting reactive oxygen species. Theriogenology. 2010;74:777–85.
91. Fukui Y, et al. Fertilizability and developmental capacity of individually cultured bovine oocytes. Theriogenology. 2000;53(8):1553–65.
92. Luvoni GC, Keskintepe L, Brackett BG. Improvement in bovine embryo production in vitro by glutathione-containing culture media. Mol Reprod Dev. 1996;43(4):437–43.
93. Viet Linh N, et al. Effects of cysteine during in vitro maturation of porcine oocytes under low oxygen tension on their subsequent in vitro fertilization and development. J Reprod Dev. 2009;55(6):594–8.
94. Grupen CG, Nagashima H, Nottle MB. Cysteamine enhances in vitro development of porcine oocytes matured and fertilized in vitro. Biol Reprod. 1995;53(1):173–8.
95. Bing YZ, et al. In vitro maturation and glutathione synthesis of porcine oocytes in the presence or absence of cysteamine under different oxygen tensions: role of cumulus cells. Reprod Fertil Dev. 2002;14(3–4):125–31.
96. Curnow EC, et al. Developmental potential of bovine oocytes following IVM in the presence of glutathione ethyl ester. Reprod Fertil Dev. 2010;22(4):597–605.
97. May JM, Qu ZC, Mendiratta S. Protection and recycling of alpha-tocopherol in human erythrocytes by intracellular ascorbic acid. Arch Biochem Biophys. 1998;349(2):281–9.
98. Dalvit G, et al. Effect of alpha-tocopherol and ascorbic acid on bovine oocyte in vitro maturation. Reprod Domest Anim. 2005;40(2):93–7.
99. Marques A, et al. Effect of alpha-tocopherol on bovine in vitro fertilization. Reprod Domest Anim. 2010;45(1):81–5.
100. Bors W, Buettner GR. The vitamin C radical and its reactions. In: Packer L, Fuchs J, editors. Vitamin C in health and disease. New York: Marcel Dekker, Inc; 1997. p. 75–94.
101. Natarajan R, Shankar MB, Munuswamy D. Effect of alpha-tocopherol supplementation on in vitro maturation of sheep oocytes and in vitro development of preimplantation sheep embryos to the blastocyst stage. J Assist Reprod Genet. 2010;27:483–90.
102. Peng XR, Liu T, Zhang Y. Addition of alpha-tocopherol to culture medium improves the quality and cryosurvival of nuclear-transferred ovine embryos. J Reprod Dev. 2008;54(6):403–7.
103. Hossein MS, et al. Temporal effects of alpha-tocopherol and L-ascorbic acid on in vitro fertilized porcine embryo development. Anim Reprod Sci. 2007;100(1–2):107–17.
104. Jeong YW, et al. Antiapoptotic and embryotrophic effects of alpha-tocopherol and L-ascorbic acid on porcine embryos derived from in vitro fertilization and somatic cell nuclear transfer. Theriogenology. 2006;66(9):2104–12.
105. Martin-Romero FJ, Garcia-Martin E, Gutierrez-Merino C. Inhibition of oxidative stress produced by plasma membrane NADH oxidase delays low-potassium-induced apoptosis of cerebellar granule cells. J Neurochem. 2002;82(3):705–15.
106. Martin-Romero FJ, Garcia-Martin E, Gutierrez-Merino C. Involvement of free radicals in signalling of low-potassium induced apoptosis in cultured cerebellar granule cells. Int J Dev Biol. 1996;(Suppl 1):197S–8S.
107. Carbone MC, et al. Antioxidant enzymatic defences in human follicular fluid: characterization and age-dependent changes. Mol Hum Reprod. 2003;9(1):639–43.

108. Pasqualotto EB, et al. The role of enzymatic antioxidants detected in the follicular fluid and semen of infertile couples undergoing assisted reproduction. Hum Fertil (Camb). 2009;12(3): 166–71.
109. Iwata H, et al. Effects of antioxidants on the development of bovine IVM/IVF embryos in various concentrations of glucose. Theriogenology. 1998;50(3):365–75.
110. Blondin P, Coenen K, Sirard MA. The impact of reactive oxygen species on bovine sperm fertilizing ability and oocyte maturation. J Androl. 1997;18(4):454–60.
111. Liu Z, Foote RH, Yang X. Development of early bovine embryos in co-culture with KSOM and taurine, superoxide dismutase or insulin. Theriogenology. 1995;44(5):741–50.
112. Nonogaki T, et al. Protection from oxidative stress by thioredoxin and superoxide dismutase of mouse embryos fertilized in vitro. Hum Reprod. 1991;6(9):1305–10.
113. Nonogaki T, et al. Effects of superoxide dismutase on mouse in vitro fertilization and embryo culture system. J Assist Reprod Genet. 1992;9(3):274–80.
114. Jinno M, Sandow BA, Hodgen GD. Enhancement of the developmental potential of mouse oocytes matured in vitro by gonadotropins and ethylenediaminetetraacetic acid (EDTA). J In Vitro Fert Embryo Transf. 1989;6(1):36–40.
115. Hentemann M, Bertheussen K. New media for culture to blastocyst. Fertil Steril. 2009;91(3):878–83.
116. Mehta TS, Kiessling AA. The developmental potential of mouse embryos conceived in Ham's F-10 medium containing ethylenediaminetetraacetic acid. Fertil Steril. 1993;60(6): 1088–93.
117. Kim JH, et al. Embryotrophic effects of ethylenediaminetetraacetic acid and hemoglobin on in vitro porcine embryos development. Theriogenology. 2006;66(2):449–55.
118. Quinn P. Enhanced results in mouse and human embryo culture using a modified human tubal fluid medium lacking glucose and phosphate. J Assist Reprod Genet. 1995;12(2):97–105.
119. Manjunatha BM, et al. Effect of taurine and melatonin in the culture medium on buffalo in vitro embryo development. Reprod Domest Anim. 2009;44(1):12–6.
120. Spinaci M, et al. Effects of epigallocatechin-3-gallate (EGCG) on in vitro maturation and fertilization of porcine oocytes. Theriogenology. 2008;69(7):877–85.
121. Hatfield DL, editor. Selenium: its molecular biology and role in human health. Boston: Kluwer; 2001.
122. Martin-Romero FJ, et al. Selenium metabolism in drosophila: selenoproteins, selenoprotein mRNA expression, fertility, and mortality. J Biol Chem. 2001;276(32):29798–804.
123. Uhm SJ, et al. Selenium improves the developmental ability and reduces the apoptosis in porcine parthenotes. Mol Reprod Dev. 2007;74(11):1386–94.
124. Sullivan M, Galea P, Latif S. What is the appropriate oxygen tension for in vitro culture? Mol Hum Reprod. 2006;12(11):653.
125. Liu Z, Foote RH. Development of bovine embryos in KSOM with added superoxide dismutase and taurine and with five and twenty percent O2. Biol Reprod. 1995;53(4):786–90.
126. Umaoka Y, et al. Developmental potentiality of embryos cultured under low oxygen tension with superoxide dismutase. J In Vitro Fert Embryo Transf. 1991;8(5):245–9.
127. Tarin JJ, Trounson AO. Effects of stimulation or inhibition of lipid peroxidation on freezing-thawing of mouse embryos. Biol Reprod. 1993;49(6):1362–8.
128. Lane M, Maybach JM, Gardner DK. Addition of ascorbate during cryopreservation stimulates subsequent embryo development. Hum Reprod. 2002;17(10):2686–93.
129. Bilodeau JF, et al. Levels of antioxidant defenses are decreased in bovine spermatozoa after a cycle of freezing and thawing. Mol Reprod Dev. 2000;55(3):282–8.
130. Dinara S, et al. Effects of supplementation with free radical scavengers on the survival and fertilization rates of mouse cryopreserved oocytes. Hum Reprod. 2001;16(9):1976–81.
131. Huang J, et al. Effect of sugars on maturation rate of vitrified-thawed immature porcine oocytes. Anim Reprod Sci. 2008;106(1–2):25–35.
132. Meister A. On the antioxidant effects of ascorbic acid and glutathione. Biochem Pharmacol. 1992;44(10):1905–15.

133. Paszkowski T, Clarke RN. The graafian follicle is a site of L-ascorbate accumulation. J Assist Reprod Genet. 1999;16(1):41–5.
134. Agarwal A, Gupta S, Sharma RK. Role of oxidative stress in female reproduction. Reprod Biol Endocrinol. 2005;3:28.
135. Kim SS. Ovarian tissue banking for cancer patients. To do or not to do? Hum Reprod. 2003;18(9):1759–61.
136. Lee K, et al. Effect of resveratrol on the development of porcine embryos produced in vitro. J Reprod Dev. 2006;56(3):330–5.
137. Cunningham ML, et al. Superoxide anion is generated from cellular metabolites by solar radiation and its components. Free Radic Biol Med. 1985;1:381–5.
138. Wells-Knecht KJ, et al. Mechanism of autoxidative glycosylation: identification of glyoxal and arabinose as intermediates in the autoxidative modification of proteins by glucose. Biochemistry. 1995;34(11):3702–9.
139. Curnow EC, et al. Bovine in vitro oocyte maturation as a model for manipulation of the gamma-glutamyl cycle and intraoocyte glutathione. Reprod Fertil Dev. 2008;20(5):579–88.
140. May JM. Is ascorbic acid an antioxidant for the plasma membrane? FASEB J. 1999;13(9):995–1006.
141. Martin-Romero FJ, S.G. Pandalai, et al. Molecular biology of mammalian AFR reductases. In: Recent research developments in molecular biology. Kerala: Research Signpost; 2004. pp. 29–52.
142. Saaranen MJ, et al. The role of dehydroascorbate in disulfide bond formation. Antioxid Redox Signal. 2010;12(1):15–25.
143. Westphal LM, et al. A nutritional supplement for improving fertility in women: a pilot study. J Reprod Med. 2004;49(4):289–93.
144. Pribenszky C, et al. Increased stress tolerance of matured pig oocytes after high hydrostatic pressure treatment. Anim Reprod Sci. 2008;106(1–2):200–7.
145. Lin L, et al. Osmotic stress induced by sodium chloride, sucrose or trehalose improves cryotolerance and developmental competence of porcine oocytes. Reprod Fertil Dev. 2009;21(2):338–44.
146. Vandaele L, et al. Short-term exposure to hydrogen peroxide during oocyte maturation improves bovine embryo development. Reproduction. 2010;139(3):505–11.

Chapter 26
Best Practice Guidelines for the Use of Antioxidants

Francesco Lanzafame, Sandro La Vignera, and Aldo E. Calogero

Oxidative stress (OS), an imbalance between the production of radical oxygen species (ROS) and antioxidant scavenging activities in which the former prevails [1], causes male and female infertility. The role of OS in the pathophysiology of human sperm function has been extensively explored. Indeed, spermatozoa are extremely sensitive to ROS because of their high content of polyunsaturated fatty acids (PUFA) and their limited ability to repair deoxyribonucleic acid (DNA) damage [2, 3]. Therefore, the administration of many antioxidants has been proposed in the attempt to improve sperm quality.

Treatments varied over the years involving the use of many different compounds, such as carnitines, phosphatidylcholine, kallikrein, pentoxifylline, vitamins A, C, and E, etc. [4]. The administration of antioxidants to infertile men represents a great challenge for the andrologist. Indeed, a correct and complete diagnostic workup should not be ignored, because different andrological diseases may respond to antioxidant administration in a different manner [5]. Furthermore, it should be reminded that no standardized markers have been developed which may help to identify those patients who may benefit from a scavenging treatment. Additionally, reliable, prognostic, and not expensive tests to evaluate the effects of ROS exposure or to determine the total antioxidant capacity (TAC) are not yet available for the clinical practice.

The efficacy of antioxidant administration would positively benefit from the use of markers that can reliable measure OS before treatment and/or of markers which evaluate the damage caused by OS on the sperm membrane and DNA. Many studies have not taken into account the measurement of OS, a primary endpoint, and its possible improvement after treatment. Moreover, diseases which impair fertility have often a subclinical development with few or no symptoms and/or signs;

F. Lanzafame, MD (✉)
Centro Territoriale di Andrologia, Siracusa, Italy

S. La Vignera, MD • A.E. Calogero, MD
Department of Medical and Pediatrics Sciences, University of Catania, Catania, Italy
e-mail: sandrolavignera@unict.it; acaloger@unict.it

S.J. Parekattil and A. Agarwal (eds.), *Antioxidants in Male Infertility: A Guide for Clinicians and Researchers*, © Springer Science+Business Media New York 2013

consequently, the patients consult the andrologist after a long time from their onset. This often causes an irreparable OS-induced damage in spermatozoa. Therefore, the first step before antioxidant treatment is prescribed is to consider the clinical history and laboratory and instrumental data to understand if a given patient is suitable for a scavenging treatment or whether a different therapeutic strategy should be undertaken. A suitable strategy would be to eradicate all causes that increase ROS production and/or reduce seminal plasma scavenging action.

Regardless of the discrepant findings reported [6, 7], antioxidant treatment seems to be helpful both in vitro and in vivo to ameliorate sperm quality. Experimental data in laboratory and farm animals support this statement [8, 9]. Glutathione (GSH) administration plays a fundamental action in improving sperm motility and consequently in enhancing fertilization in asthenozoospermic bulls with varicocele and in rabbits with dispermy due to cryptorchidism [10]. In lead-injected mice, vitamin C, given at a concentration equivalent to the human therapeutic dose (10 mg/kg body weight), significantly decreases the concentration of testicular malondialdehyde (MDA), an important marker of OS, with a concurrent improvement in sperm concentration and a significant decline in the percentage of abnormal spermatozoa. Vitamin E (100 mg/kg body weight) and vitamin C have a comparable scavenging power, but the later has a poorer effectiveness. Given together at the above indicated dosages, they induce the most important fall in the content of MDA in lead-treated mice with a concomitant increase of sperm concentration and amelioration of sperm morphology [11]. An analogous protective effect of vitamin E has been shown in mice with mercury-induced decrease of sperm count and function [12]. The presence of an elevated quantity of α-tocopheryl acetate in the rabbit diet significantly enhances the semen amount of vitamin E and its oxidative firmness subsequent to cryoconservation [13].

Thus, many studies carried out in animal models suggest a possible successful use of antioxidants in humans. Unfortunately, contrasting evidences have been published from several uncontrolled trials, often performed to sustain the efficacy of some type of treatment even if its usefulness is not yet confirmed [14]. Heavy smokers [15] and infertile patients [16] who received an antioxidant supplementation ameliorate sperm quality. In addition, antioxidants improve the fertilizing capability of healthy men with elevated seminal ROS concentration [17] and also increase the fertilization rate of fertile normozoospermic men with low fertilization rates in previous IVF cycles, by significantly decreasing the levels of MDA [18].

Despite many studies describe positive results following administration of antioxidants on sperm parameters, there is no well-defined scavenging approach during OS, and often the experimental design is not double blind and/or placebo controlled. In addition, nonhomogenous cohorts of patients have been enrolled in some studies. Finally, a large number of compounds have been used, but for many of them scanty evidence have been published. All this makes the scientific literature very heterogeneous with a consequent difficulty to get an ultimate conclusion, as also suggested by Patel and Sigman [19].

Because of the difficulty to clearly distinguish which antioxidant can play a better role to reduce OS generation and/or to prevent the OS-mediated sperm damage,

Table 26.1 List of antioxidants reviewed in this chapter

Antioxidants
Ascorbic acid (vitamin C)
α-Tocopherol (vitamin E)
Ascorbic acid (vitamin C) plus α-tocopherol (vitamin E)
α-Tocopherol (vitamin E) plus selenium
Glutathione
L-Carnitine plus L-acetyl-carnitine
Coenzyme Q10
Lycopene
Pycnogenol
N-acetyl-cysteine
Vitamin A and vitamin E
Pentoxifylline
Selenium
Shao-Fu-Zhu-Yu-Tang
Astaxanthin
Lepidium meyenii
α-Linolenic acid and lignans
Vitamin C and E, lycopene, selenium, folic acid, garlic oil plus zinc
Morindae officinalis extract

Table 26.2 Evidence classification of the National Clinical Guidelines for Type 2 Diabetes (the Royal College of General practitioners, Effective Clinical Practice Unit, ScHAAR University of Sheffield) used in this chapter

Evidence classification
Ia   Evidence from meta-analysis of randomized controlled trials
Ib   Evidence from at least one randomized controlled trial
IIa   Evidence from at least one controlled study without randomization
IIb   Evidence from at least one other type of quasi-experimental study
III   Evidence from nonexperimental descriptive studies, such as comparative studies, correlation studies, and case–control studies
IV   Evidence from expert committee reports or opinions and/or clinical experience of respected authorities

Adapted from [82]

we decided to use an evidence-based medicine (EBM) method to better understand the role of the various antioxidants for the treatment of infertile men (Table 26.1). To accomplish this, the National Clinical Guidelines for Type 2 Diabetes, formulated by the Royal College of General practitioners, Effective Clinical Practice Unit, ScHAAR University of Sheffield (http://www.nice.org.uk/nicemedia/live/10911/28998/28998.pdf) were used as they seem more suitable for pharmacological trials. These guidelines classify evidences and recommendations as indicated in Tables 26.2 and 26.3.

Table 26.3 Recommendations of the National Clinical Guidelines for Type 2 Diabetes (the Royal College of General practitioners, Effective Clinical Practice Unit, ScHAAR University of Sheffield) used in this chapter

Recommendation grading
A Directly based on category I evidence
B Directly based on category II evidence, or extrapolated recommendation from category I evidence
C Directly based on category III evidence, or extrapolated recommendation from category I or II evidence
D Directly based on category IV evidence, or extrapolated recommendation from category I, II, or III evidence

From [83], with permission

Ascorbic Acid

Ascorbic acid (vitamin C) is ten times higher in the seminal plasma than in serum [20]. It is an effective scavenger if peroxyl radicals are in an aqueous phase [21], but does not have the some powerful scavenging action within membrane lipids [22]. The amount of vitamin C in the seminal plasma decreases significantly when the concentration of ROS increases [23]. Also in leucocytospermic samples, the concentrations of seminal ascorbic acid are significantly depleted. When this occurs, a significantly higher sperm DNA fragmentation index (DFI) has been found compared with semen samples with normal or high levels of ascorbic acid [24]. Interestingly, vitamin C plays an antioxidant action at low concentrations, but it can start auto-oxidation processes at higher concentrations [25]. Moreover, in humans, the vitamin C plasma saturation occurs at daily dose of 1 g. Higher amounts could promote the development of kidney stones, because of the enhanced excretion of oxalate [26].

The administration of vitamin C (1 g/day) increases ascorbic acid level by 2.2-fold [27]. In addition, it has been reported that seminal plasma vitamin C concentrations positively correlates with the number of normal spermatozoa, in a controlled clinical trial [28] (IIa). In earlier studies, vitamin C (1 g/day) supplementation has been proposed to ameliorate the sperm quality in infertile men [15] (III), [29] (Ib). Sperm parameters also increases with a higher vitamin C intake, as shown by the higher sperm concentration and total progressive motile sperm count (TPMS) [30] (IIb). In a placebo-controlled study, vitamin C given to heavy smokers at a dose of 200 or 1,000 mg/day for 4 months improved sperm parameters. The group that took the dose of 1,000 mg/day had a higher increase [29] (Ib). In addition, vitamin C safeguards human spermatozoa from endogenous oxidative DNA damage [31] (IIb).

α-Tocopherol

In a single-blinded study, eight patients treated with 100 mg of α-tocopherol (vitamin E) tid for 4 months did not show any sperm parameter improvement [32] (IIa). While the administration of vitamin E, at a dose of 100 mg three times per day, produced a slight increase in seminal plasma vitamin E concentration. In a study performed on 15 subjects, the number of spermatozoa, the percentage of sperm with forward motility, the half-life of the percentage displaying forward motility, and the rate of swollen spermatozoa in hypo-osmotic medium did not show any significant enhancement during vitamin E administration. The authors explained the lack of effects on these parameters with the small increase of vitamin E achieved in the seminal plasma. They hypothesized that higher doses of vitamin E may be more effective [33] (Ib). When in infertile men, vitamin E is administered at doses ranging between 300 and 1,200 mg/day for 3 weeks, seminal plasma vitamin E levels increase weakly [34]. The sperm α-tocopherol concentration is independent from the concentration or the total amount present in the seminal plasma. On the other hand, the percentage of motile spermatozoa relates significantly with sperm α-tocopherol content [35].

Many trials have been conducted to ameliorate sperm parameters of infertile men by vitamin E administration. In a double-blind randomized, placebo-controlled, crossover trial, 30 healthy men with elevated semen ROS concentrations and healthy female partners were given vitamin E (600 mg/day) or placebo for 3 months. Vitamin E increased significantly blood serum α-tocopherol concentrations and sperm function evaluated by the zona-binding assay [17] (Ia). Some other reports utilized lower doses of vitamin E. For example, a single-blinded study took into account eight patients receiving 300 mg/day of vitamin E, divided in three daily doses of 100 mg each, for 4 months. Patients receiving α-tocopherol did not show any improvement [32] (IIa). A placebo-controlled, double-blind study showed that the elevated sperm MDA in asthenozoospermic and oligoasthenozoospermic men decreased significantly after vitamin E administration which also improved sperm motility in asthenozoospermic patients. In addition, 11 of 52 wives (21%) of the treated group got pregnant during the 6-month treatment; 9 of them had a normal term deliveries, while 2 aborted in the first trimester. No pregnancy was reported in the placebo group [36] (IIa). Moreover, elevated MDA concentrations significantly dropped to normal levels, and the fertilization rate per cycle increased significantly following administration of 200 mg/day of vitamin E for 3 months, in a prospective study conducted in 15 fertile normozoospermic men. The elevated MDA concentrations significantly decreased to normal levels and the fertilization rate per cycle increased significantly after 1 month of treatment [18] (IIa). Furthermore, an elevated consumption of daily nutrients with scavenging potential (food and nutraceutical complements such as zinc, folate, vitamins C and E, and β-carotene) proposed to 97 healthy, nonsmoking men, showed that the vitamin E intake correlated with the highest progressive motility and TPMS [30] (IIb).

Ascorbic Acid and α-Tocopherol

Ascorbic acid (vitamin C) and α-tocopherol (vitamin E) may be administered together to decrease the peroxidative injury on spermatozoa, taking advantage of their hydrophilicity and lipophilicity, respectively. In addition, if these compounds act directly on spermatozoa to prevent ROS-induced damage, the improvement could be rapid, given that the two vitamins reach spermatozoa both within the epididymis and following ejaculation.

A double-blind, placebo-controlled, randomized trial has been performed in asthenozoospermic or moderate oligoasthenozoospermic men. Vitamins C (1 g) and E (800 mg) were prescribed simultaneously for 2 months, but no improvement of semen parameters was reported [37] (Ib). These unsatisfactory findings match with the findings of other studies [32, 33], but diverge from other published data [18, 38]. It is also possible that the duration of the treatment was too short to produce an effect, particularly if the action occurs within the testis.

Sixty-four patients with idiopathic infertility and an increased ($\geq$15%) proportion of spermatozoa with DNA fragmentation were randomly divided into two groups: one was given vitamins C (1 g) and E (1 g) daily and the other one, placebo. After a 2 months of treatment, the proportion of DNA-fragmented spermatozoa decreased significantly in the antioxidant-treated group, while no variation was detected in the placebo group [39] (Ib). An additional trial was performed on 38 patients with a raised ($\geq$15%) percentage of DNA-fragmented spermatozoa in the ejaculate. They were prescribed vitamins C (1 g) and E (1 g) daily for 2 months following one ICSI cycle failure. In 29 of them (76%), the scavenging therapy led to a decline in the proportion of DNA-fragmented spermatozoa and a successful ICSI attempt with a higher clinical pregnancy (48.2% vs. 6.9%) and implantation (19.6% vs. 2.2%) rates [40] (IIb).

α-Tocopherol and Selenium

Few studies have been performed using the association between vitamin E and selenium [41, 42]. A trial was conducted in nine oligoasthenoteratozoospermic patients who were prescribed vitamin E (400 mg) plus selenium (100 μg) daily for 1 month. Thereafter, selenium supplementation was increased to 200 μg/day for the next 4 months. This kind of association produced a significant improvement of sperm motility, morphology, and vitality [41] (Ib). The other study, using the same association, was performed in 28 men who were given vitamin E (400 mg) and selenium (225 μg) daily for 3 months. Other 26 patients assumed vitamin B (4.5 g/day) for the same length of time, as control. The administration of vitamin E and selenium resulted in a significant reduction in MDA concentrations and an enhancement of sperm kinetic parameters [42] (Ib).

Glutathione

GSH is one of the most commonly used drugs; thanks to its antitoxic and scavenging action in different diseases. Although it cannot cross cell membranes, its concentration increases in biological fluids following a systemic intake. GSH is able to reach the seminal plasma and to play an action at this level. Here, it safeguards spermatozoa from ROS attack; hence, GSH may play a beneficial function in several andrological diseases, particularly during male genital tract inflammation [16].

GSH (600 mg/day i.m.) has been prescribed to 11 patients with dyspermia associated with different andrological diseases in a 2-month pilot trial. Sperm kinetics improved, particularly in men with male accessory gland infections (MAGI) and in men with varicocele [43] (III), two circumstances wherein ROS or other noxious substance may play a pathogenic role. Following these encouraging findings, the same investigators conducted a placebo-controlled, double-blind, crossover study on infertile men experiencing unilateral varicocele and amicrobial MAGI. The patients were allocated to treatment with GSH, 600 mg i.m. on alternate days, or placebo ampoules. Men who received GSH showed higher sperm number, motility, kinetic parameters, and percentage of normal forms. These effects on sperm motility and morphology lasted for some time after the treatment was discontinued. The authors hypothesized that these findings may relate to a post-spermatocyte action of GSH, since the length of the treatment did not cover the full length of a complete spermatogenesis [16] (Ib). This kind of sperm modification can be partially corrected by GSH administration when cell membrane injury is not too critical [44] (IIa).

The above reported data indicate that, at least to some extent, the beneficial effect of GSH is suitable for the biochemical changes in membrane organization and its following defensive action on the lipid components of the cell membrane. The decline of lipoperoxide levels in seminal plasma let to consider that GSH minimizes the consequence of lipoperoxidation generated by vascular or inflammatory diseases.

Carnitines

Carnitines are involved in many metabolic pathways in several cellular organelles. These compounds play a primary function in sperm maturation within the male genital organs and a relevant role in the metabolism of spermatozoa by furnishing immediately accessible energy to be utilized by spermatozoa. This positively correlates with sperm motility and concentration [45]. An increase of sperm progressive motility occurs simultaneously to L-carnitine augmentation and storage in the epididymal lumen [46].

Several different kinds of studies (controlled, uncontrolled, human, and animal) have been carried out to evaluate the potential application of carnitines as scavenging molecules. In 1992, a study was conducted on the male partners of 20 couples affected by idiopathic oligoasthenozoospermia (concentration $<20 \times 10^6$ spermatozoa/ml, progressive motility <50%) who were given 4 g/day of L-acetyl-carnitine for 2 months. No significant effect on sperm concentration, total motility, and morphology resulted, whereas a significant improvement of progressive motility (21.7 ± 3.2% vs. 38.2 ± 4.7) was appreciated [47] (IIb). Afterwards, a multicentre open study was performed on 100 men with idiopathic asthenozoospermia.

L-carnitine was administered orally at the dose of 1 g three times per day for 4 months with a significant improvement of several sperm kinetic parameters [48] (IIb). Another study came to similar results, giving an oral solution of L-carnitine (1 g) three times a day for 3 months, to 47 patients with idiopathic asthenozoospermia [49] (IIb). A review article proposed carnitines treatment as an alternative method in the broader medical treatment of patients with infertility due to OS [50].

Some clinical evidence suggests that a selective group of infertile men, those with prostato-vesiculo-epididymitis (PVE), benefit from carnitines administration, since antimicrobial and/or nonsteroidal anti-inflammatory drugs, although effective to eliminate microbial infection, have a poor scavenging action [51] (Ib). Another study conducted on 98 men with PVE and leukocytospermia showed that carnitine scavenging treatment was totally successful once they were pretreated with nonsteroidal anti-inflammatory compounds [52] (Ib).

In a placebo-controlled, double-blind, crossover trial, L-carnitine was capable to enhance sperm parameters, even if it was unsuccessful to reduce LPO concentrations. These findings suggested an incomplete action of L-carnitine to counteract the ROS attack [53] (Ib). The same group proposed a double-blind, randomized, placebo-controlled trial. They gave a combined treatment with L-carnitine (2 g/day) and L-acetyl-carnitine (1 g/day) or placebo to 60 infertile males with oligo-asthenoteratozoospermia. All sperm parameters improved, but the most important enhancement was found in both progressive and total sperm motility particularly in men with the highest degree of asthenozoospermia [54] (Ib). Another placebo-controlled study conducted also in patients with oligoasthenoteratozoospermia showed that the same treatment improved sperm concentration, motility, and morphology, particularly when cinnoxicam (1 suppository every 4 days) was added [55] (Ib). Furthermore, 60 patients with asthenozoospermia were enrolled in a double-blind clinical trial with L-carnitine (3 g/day), L-acetyl-carnitine (3 g/day), a combination of L-carnitine (2 g/day) plus L-acetyl-carnitine (1 g/day), or placebo, for 6 months. Total and forward motility, including kinetic parameters analyzed by computer-assisted sperm analysis, improved in men receiving either L-acetyl-carnitine alone or in association with L-carnitine. The total oxyradical scavenging capacity of the semen towards hydroxyl and peroxyl radicals also improved and correlated with the enhancement of sperm kinetics. Patients with lower motility and total oxyradical scavenging capacity of the seminal fluid had more chances of responding to the treatment [56] (Ib). In another trial, L-carnitine (2 g/day) and L-acetyl-carnitine (1 g/day) were given orally tid for 3 months to 90 men with oligoasthenozoospermia. In the treatment group, ten female partners (11.6%) achieved pregnancy, whereas only two pregnancies (3.7%) were recorded in the control group. Moreover, their percentage of forward and total motile spermatozoa increased significantly [57] (Ib). In the trial lead by De Rosa and colleagues, 66 patients with <50% motility receiving L-carnitine (1 g/day) and L-acetyl-carnitine (500 mg tid), for 6 months, had a significant increase in sperm total motility, viability, membrane integrity, and linearity of sperm movement, both after 3 and 6 months of treatment, and in the ability to penetrate the cervical mucus increased after 6 months [58] (IIb). Twenty-one patients with infertility and with sperm motility ranging from 10 to 50% were given carnitines (2 g of L-carnitine and 1 g of L-acetyl-carnitine per day) orally for 6 months, but differently from the other studies, no significant effects on sperm motility resulted [59] (Ib). In a further trial, L-carnitine (2 g/day) and L-acetyl-carnitine (1 g/day) were administered for 3 months in men with PVE and increased ROS production. Carnitines showed to be a successful treatment once seminal leukocytes were within the normal range [60] (IIb).

On the light of the many studies exploring the effects of carnitines on sperm parameters, a systematic review has been recently published. The meta-analysis compared L-carnitine and/or L-acetyl-carnitine treatment to placebo reported significant improvement in total and forward sperm motility, atypical sperm cells, and pregnancy rate. No significant difference has been found in sperm concentration [61] (Ia).

Coenzyme Q10

Coenzyme Q10 (CoQ10) is a lipid-soluble constituent of the respiratory chain. Ubiquinol is the reduced form and the active one. It behaves as a powerful scavenger in some biological components, for instance lipoproteins and membranes. The concentrations of reduced and oxidized forms of CoQ10 (ubiquinol/ubiquinone) and of hydroperoxide have been measured in the seminal plasma and seminal fluid of 32 infertile men. A positive correlation between ubiquinol concentration and sperm count has been observed, whereas a negative correlation was reported between sperm count and ubiquinol concentration or hydroperoxide levels. An important correlation between sperm concentration, motility, and seminal fluid ubiquinol-10 content has been found, whereas, in total fluid, an inverse correlation between ubiquinol/ubiquinone ratio and the severity of teratozoospermia has been reported. These findings indicate that ubiquinol-10 impedes hydroperoxide occurrence in seminal fluid and in seminal plasma [62].

CoQ10 has been given orally at the dose of 60 mg/day to 17 men with low fertilization rate after ICSI for male infertility for an average of 103 days previously the subsequent ICSI procedure. The results showed a significant enhancement of the fertilization rate [63] (IIb).

In the human seminal fluid, CoQ10 has been found at relevant concentrations and it shows a direct association with sperm concentrations and kinetics. Differently, in men with varicocele, despite a higher proportion of CoQ10 in the seminal plasma, the correlation with sperm motility was not observed [64]. Elevated CoQ10 levels have been found in spermatozoa of oligozoospermic and asthenozoospermic patients without varicocele. This correlation was not detected in men with varicocele, who additionally showed slightly lower intracellular absolute concentrations of CoQ10. Higher intracellular levels could be linked to a spermatozoa protective system. In men with varicocele, this kind of system could be inadequate, leading to an excessive susceptivity to OS [64].

Very recently a double-blind, randomized trial has been carried out in 60 infertile patients with idiopathic asthenozoospermia. Patients underwent a double-blind therapy with CoQ10 (200 mg/day) or placebo for 6 months. After treatment, CoQ10 and ubiquinol raised appreciably in seminal plasma as well as in spermatozoa. Interestingly, spermatozoa improved their motility. Men with a poorer sperm motility and lower concentrations of CoQ10 had a statistically significant more elevated chance to better respond to its administration [65] (Ib).

Lycopene

Lycopene is an element of human redox defensive system against oxidative stress. Oral lycopene administration appears to have a function in the treatment of patients with idiopathic infertility. Following the administration of 2 g of lycopene, twice a day, for 3 months, a significant increase occurs in the sperm number and motility, but the sperm concentration increase is present only in men with a sperm concentration >5 million/ml [66] (IIb).

Pycnogenol

Pycnogenol is a substance obtained from the bark of the "Pinus maritima." Pycnogenol's constituents inhibit cyclooxygenases that release inflammatory prostaglandins [67]. A study has been conducted in subfertile men who were administered pycnogenol (200 mg/day), for 3 months. The results showed a mean sperm morphology improvement by 38% of the pretreatment values and the mannose receptor binding assay score augmented by 19% [68] (IIb).

Other Compounds

N-Acetyl-Cysteine or Vitamin A Plus Vitamin E and Essential Fatty Acids

An open, prospective study, conducted in 27 infertile men who were given a combined oral antioxidants treatment with *N*-acetyl-cysteine (NAC) or vitamin A plus vitamin E and essential fatty acids, showed an increase of sperm concentration in oligozoospermic patients. Moreover, this treatment significantly reduced ROS and 8-OH-dG production, and in the mean time, it increased the percentage of acrosome-reacted spermatozoa, the quantity of PUFA in phospholipids, and sperm membrane [69] (IIb). Very recently, 120 idiopathic infertile men were randomly given NAC alone (600 mg/day orally) or placebo for 3 months. NAC increased semen volume and sperm motility as well as semen viscosity [70] (Ib).

Pentoxifylline

Spermatozoa from 15 patients with asthenozoospermia and high ROS levels were treated in vitro with pentoxifylline to evaluate the effects of this compound on ROS generation and sperm movement. Pentoxifylline was able to reduce the production of ROS by spermatozoa, and it slowed down the in vitro decline of the curvilinear velocity and the beat cross frequency for 6 h. These same 15 patients and 18 asthenozoospermic patients, whose spermatozoa did not generate ROS at steady state, were then prescribed pentoxifylline at two distinct doses (300 and 1,200 mg daily) to validate its in vivo outcome on ROS generation, sperm kinetics, and sperm fertilizing competence. Pentoxifylline administration had no effects on spermatozoon-induced ROS formation, and it did not show any effect on sperm motility and fertilizing capacity. Nevertheless, it increased motility and beat cross frequency at the dose of 1,200 mg daily [71].

Selenium

Selenium supplementation has been given alone to 33 subfertile men for 3 months, but it did not produced any improvement of sperm count, motility, and morphology [72] (IIa). Subsequently, a trial was performed on 69 asthenozoospermic patients who received either placebo, selenium alone, or selenium plus vitamins A, C, and E daily for 3 months. Treatment did not show any improvement of sperm concentration, while sperm motility increased in both selenium-treated groups. This study showed that oral selenium administration is effective especially in patients with a low selenium [73] (Ib). Recently, a clinical trial investigated the usefulness of selenium (200 µg) and/or NAC (600 mg) in 468 infertile men with idiopathic oligoasthenoteratozoospermia for 6 months. This treatment showed to be effective on all sperm parameters measured and a clear correlation between seminal plasma selenium concentrations, NAC, and semen characteristics [74] (Ib).

Shao-Fu-Zhu-Yu-Tang

Shao-Fu-Zhu-Yu-Tang has been proposed to have antiaging and sperm scavenging properties. Its administration, for 60 days to 36 patients with chronic prostatitis, revealed a significant increase in sperm motility as evaluated by computer-assisted semen analysis [75] (IIb).

Zinc, Folic Acid, Astaxanthin, and Acetyl-Carnitine

Sperm parameters ameliorated following the intake of a mixture of zinc and folic acid, or the antioxidant astaxanthin, or a so-called energy-providing combination including (acetyl)-carnitine (Proxeed®). Furthermore, a double-blind study showed that the latter two compounds increase spontaneous or intrauterine insemination-assisted conception rates [76] (Ib). Astaxanthin appears to act significantly to decrease ROS and inhibin B concentrations and to increase sperm linear velocity and pregnancy rate [76].

Lepidium meyenii

The extracts of the Peruvian plant *Lepidium meyenii* appeared to be useful to increase the sperm number and the percentage of normal forms in an uncontrolled trial [77] (IIb).

α-Linolenic Acid and Lignans

Linseed oil includes α-linolenic acid and lignans. α-linolenic acid adjusts the poor intake of omega-3 essential fatty acids that is connected with reduced sperm motility among patients with fertility problems [78] (IV).

Vitamin C and Vitamin E, Lycopene, Selenium, Folic Acid, Garlic Oil, and Zinc

Menevit®, an antioxidant preparation combining vitamins C and E, lycopene, selenium, folic acid, garlic oil, and zinc, has been prescribed to 60 couples with severe male infertility for 3 months, in a prospective randomized, double-blind, placebo-controlled trial, before undergoing an IVF cycle. Men who assumed Menevit® had a significant improvement of the pregnancy rate (38.5%) compared to the men who assumed placebo (16% pregnancy) [79] (Ib).

Morindae Officinalis Extract

Morindae officinalis extract, taken at the concentrations of 0.25 or 0.5 g/ml, showed to be more effective than vitamin C in enhancing SOD vitality of sperm suspension and in decreasing MDA concentration. It has been shown to take part in a defensive action in the ROS-mediated damage of sperm membrane. Moreover, at higher dosage (0.5 mg/ml), Morindae officinalis particularly safeguards sperm membrane function [80].

Zinc

Zinc therapy has been shown valuable in decreasing OS, sperm apoptosis, and DFI in asthenozoospermic men. Zinc associated with vitamin E or with vitamin E plus vitamin C did not result in any further significant effect [81].

Expert Commentary

Many studies have been performed using different antioxidant compounds with the aim to improve semen parameters. Unfortunately the endpoints taken into account by these studies are often different and this does not help in understanding the efficacy of a given antioxidant. Moreover, it should be kept in mind that any andrological disease, independently of the OS, may be reversible or not according to the degree of the damage that has developed at the time of the therapeutical intervention. A prolonged exposure to OS can also cause an extensive damage that, over the time, can compromise the efficiency of the male accessory glands on sperm function. This represents an additional bias for many trials that have not considered the duration of the disease. All these reasons make the scavenging therapy a great challenge for the andrologist.

Bearing this in mind, we attempted a primary distinction dividing the antioxidants into compounds which play positive effects and compounds which play negative effects, as reported in Table 26.4. Using an EBM method, we proposed that some compounds may be considered as first-line treatment, because of the extensive investigation and the higher EBM evidences. These include vitamins C and E and carnitines. The efficacy of other antioxidants is not yet supported by a sufficient number of studies. These include pycnogenol, lycopene, etc., which need additional controlled trials. Other scavenging molecules, such as CoQ10 and GSH, can be proposed as second-line treatment because of the well-done, though few, studies performed on them. Nevertheless, also for these compounds studies that can clarify the dark points previously analyzed are welcome.

Five-Year View and Key Issues

Two major issues need, in the next future, to be further implemented to allow a clear evaluation of the true effectiveness of the antioxidant treatment in the infertile men. First of all, studies should be carried out in homogeneous cohorts of patients. This requires a careful andrological screening aimed at exactly diagnosing the disease which increases the oxidative stress. The second issue relates to the development of more precise and hopefully inexpensive and non-cumbersome methods to estimate the oxidative stress in the semen samples. Finally, keeping these issues in mind,

Table 26.4 Summary of the evidences and grading of the recommendations of the effects of each antioxidant used alone or combination on sperm quality and function, according to the National Clinical Guidelines for Type 2 Diabetes (the Royal College of General practitioners, Effective Clinical Practice Unit, ScHAAR University of Sheffield)

| | Classification of evidences | | |
| | Positive effects | Any or negative effects | |
Compound			Grading of recommendations
Vitamin C			
Dawson et al. [15]	III		B
Fraga et al. [31]	IIb		C
Dawson et al. [29]	Ib		A
Thiele et al. [28]	IIa		B
Eskenazi et al. [30]	IIb		B
Vitamin E			
Giovenco et al. [32]		IIa	B
Moilanen et al. [33]		Ib	A
Kessopoulou et al. [17]	Ia		A
Suleiman et al. [36]	IIa		B
Geva et al. [18]	IIa		B
Eskenazi et al. [30]	IIb		B
Vitamin C plus vitamin E			
Rolf et al. [37]		Ib	A
Greco et al. [39]	Ib		A
Greco et al. [40]	IIb		B
Vitamin E plus selenium			
Vezina et al. [41]	Ib		A
Keskes-Ammar et al. [42]	Ib		A
N-acetyl-cysteine plus vitamin E			
Comhaire et al. [69]	IIb		
Selenium plus N-acetyl-cysteine			
Safarinejad and Safarinejad [74]	Ib		
N-acetyl-cysteine			
Ciftci et al. [70]	Ib		
Glutathione			
Lenzi et al. [43]	III		C
Lenzi et al. [16]	Ib		A
Carnitines			
Moncada et al. [47]	IIb		B
Costa et al. [48]	IIb		B
Vitali et al. [49]	IIb		B
Vicari et al. [51]	Ib		A
Vicari and Calogero [60]	IIb		A
Vicari et al. [52]	Ib		A
Lenzi et al. [53]	Ib		A
Lenzi et al. [54]	Ib		A
Cavallini et al. [55]	Ib		A
Balercia et al. [56]	Ib		A

(continued)

Table 26.4 (continued)

Compound	Classification of evidences		Grading of recommendations
	Positive effects	Any or negative effects	
Li et al. [57]	Ib		B
De Rosa et al. [58]	IIb		A
Sigman et al. [59]		Ib	A
Zhou et al. [61]	Ia		B
Coenzyme Q10			
Lewin and Lavon [63]	IIb		B
Balercia et al. [65]	Ib		A
Lycopene			
Gupta and Kumar [66]	IIb		B
Pycnogenol			
Roseff [68]	IIb		B
Selenium			
Iwanier and Zachara [72]		IIa	B
Scott [73]	Ib		A
Shao-Fu-Zhu-Yu-Tang			
Yang et al. [75]	IIb		B
Astacarox®			
Comhaire et al. [76]	Ib		A
Proxeed®			
Comhaire et al. [76]	Ib		A
Lepidium meyenii			
Gonzales et al. [77]	IIb		B
Linseed oil			
Comhaire and Mahmoud [78]	IV		None
Menevit®			
Tremellen et al. [79]	Ib		A

there is an absolute need of additional double-blind, placebo-controlled, randomized, crossover, multicenter clinical trials to gain more information about the effectiveness of an antioxidant (or a combination of them) over another one in men with infertility due to an increased oxidative stress.

References

1. Sikka SC. Relative impact of oxidative stress on male reproductive function. Curr Med Chem. 2001;8:851–62.
2. Griveau JF, Le Lannou D. Reactive oxygen species and human spermatozoa: physiology and pathology. Int J Androl. 1997;20:61–9.
3. Shen H, Ong C. Detection of oxidative DNA damage in human sperm and its association with sperm function and male infertility. Free Radic Biol Med. 2000;28:529–36.

4. Lanzafame F, Chapman MG, Guglielmino A, et al. Pharmacological stimulation of sperm motility. Hum Reprod. 1994;9:192–9.
5. Vicari E. Effectiveness and limits of antimicrobial treatment on seminal leukocyte concentration and related reactive oxygen species production in patients with male accessory gland infection. Hum Reprod. 2000;15:2536–44.
6. Ten J, Vendrell FJ, Cano A, et al. Dietary antioxidant supplementation did not affect declining sperm function with age in the mouse but did increase head abnormalities and reduced sperm production. Reprod Nutr Dev. 1997;37:481–92.
7. Ménézo YJ, Hazout A, Panteix G, et al. Antioxidants to reduce sperm DNA fragmentation: an unexpected adverse effect. Reprod Biomed Online. 2007;14:418–21.
8. Chew BP. Effects of supplemental β-carotene and vitamin A on reproduction in swine. J Anim Sci. 1993;71:247–52.
9. Luck MR, Jeyaseelan I, Scholes RA. Ascorbic acid and fertility. Biol Reprod. 1995;52:262–6.
10. Tripodi L, Tripodi A, Mammi C, et al. Pharmacological action and therapeutic effects of glutathione on hypokinetic spermatozoa for enzymatic-dependent pathologies and correlated genetic aspects. Clin Exp Obstet Gynecol. 2003;30:130–6.
11. Mishra M, Acharya UR. Protective action of vitamins on the spermatogenesis in lead-treated Swiss mice. J Trace Elem Med Biol. 2004;18:173–8.
12. Rao MV, Sharma PS. Protective effect of vitamin E against mercuric chloride reproductive toxicity in male mice. Reprod Toxicol. 2001;15:705–12.
13. Castellini C, Lattaioli P, Bernardini M, et al. Effect of dietary alpha-tocopheryl acetate and ascorbic acid on rabbit semen stored at 5 degrees C. Theriogenology. 2000;54:523–33.
14. Agarwal A, Said TM. Carnitines and male infertility. Reprod Biomed Online. 2004;8:376–84.
15. Dawson EB, Harris WA, Rankin WE, et al. Effect of ascorbic acid on male fertility. Ann N Y Acad Sci. 1987;498:312–23.
16. Lenzi A, Culasso F, Gandini L, et al. Placebo-controlled, double blind, cross-over trial of glutathione therapy in male infertility. Hum Reprod. 1993;8:1657–62.
17. Kessopoulou E, Powers HJ, Sharma KK, et al. A double-blind randomized placebo cross-over controlled trial using the antioxidant vitamin E to treat reactive species associated male infertility. Fertil Steril. 1995;64:825–31.
18. Geva E, Bartoov B, Zabludovsky N, et al. The effect of antioxidant treatment on human spermatozoa and fertilization rate in an in vitro fertilization program. Fertil Steril. 1996;66:430–4.
19. Patel SR, Sigman M. Antioxidant therapy in male infertility. Urol Clin North Am. 2008;35:319–30.
20. Jacob RA, Pianalto FS, Agee RE. Cellular ascorbate depletion in healthy men. J Nutr. 1992;122:1111–8.
21. Frei B, England L, Ames BN. Ascorbate is an outstanding antioxidant in human blood plasma. Proc Natl Acad Sci USA. 1989;86:6377–81.
22. Doba T, Burton GW, Ingold KU. Antioxidant and co-antioxidant activity of vitamin C. The effect of vitamin C, either alone or in the presence of vitamin E or a water-soluble vitamin E analogue, upon the peroxidation of aqueous multilamellar phospholipid liposomes. Biochim Biophys Acta. 1985;835:298–303.
23. Lewis SE, Sterling ES, Young IS, et al. Comparison of individuals antioxidants of sperm and seminal plasma in fertile and infertile men. Fertil Steril. 1997;67:142–7.
24. Song GJ, Norkus EP, Lewis V. Relationship between seminal ascorbic acid and sperm DNA integrity in infertile men. Int J Androl. 2006;29:569–75.
25. Wayner DD, Burton GW, Ingold KU. The antioxidant efficiency of vitamin C is concentration-dependent. Biochim Biophys Acta. 1986;884:119–23.
26. Levine M, Conry-Cantilena C, Wang Y, et al. Vitamin C pharmacokinetics in healthy volunteers: evidence for a recommended dietary allowance. Proc Natl Acad Sci USA. 1996;93:3704–9.

27. Wen Y, Cooke T, Feely J. The effect of pharmacological supplementation with vitamin C on low-density lipoprotein oxidation. Br J Clin Pharmacol. 1997;44:94–7.
28. Thiele JJ, Friesleben HJ, Fuchs J, et al. Scorbic acid and urate in human seminal plasma: determination and interrelationships with chemiluminescence in washed semen. Hum Reprod. 1995;10:110–5.
29. Dawson EB, Harris WA, Teter MC, et al. Effect of ascorbic acid supplementation on the sperm quality of smokers. Fertil Steril. 1992;58:1034–9.
30. Eskenazi B, Kidd SA, Marks AR, et al. Antioxidant intake is associated with semen quality in healthy men. Hum Reprod. 2005;20:1006–12.
31. Fraga CG, Motchnik PA, Shigenaga MK, et al. Ascorbic acid protects against endogenous oxidative DNA damage in human sperm. Proc Natl Acad Sci USA. 1991;88:11003–6.
32. Giovenco P, Amodei M, Barbieri C, et al. Effects of kallikrein on the male reproductive system and its use in the treatment of idiopathic oligozoospermia with impaired motility. Andrologia. 1987;19 Spec No:238–41.
33. Moilanen J, Hovatta O, Lindroth L. Vitamin E levels in seminal plasma can be elevated by oral administration of vitamin E in infertile men. Int J Androl. 1993;16:165–6.
34. Moilanen J, Hovatta O. Excretion of alpha-tocopherol into human seminal plasma after oral administration. Andrologia. 1995;27:133–6.
35. Therond P, Auger J, Legrand A, et al. Alpha-tocopherol in human spermatozoa and seminal plasma: relationships with motility, antioxidant enzymes and leukocytes. Mol Hum Reprod. 1996;2:739–44.
36. Suleiman SA, Ali ME, Zaki ZM, et al. Lipid peroxidation and human sperm motility: protective role of vitamin E. J Androl. 1996;17:530–7.
37. Rolf C, Cooper TG, Yeung CH, et al. Antioxidant treatment of patients with asthenozoospermia or moderate oligoasthenozoospermia with high-dose vitamin C and vitamin E: a randomized, placebo-controlled, double-blind study. Hum Reprod. 1999;14:1028–33.
38. De Lamirande E, Gagnon C. Reactive oxygen species and human spermatozoa. I. Effects on the motility of intact spermatozoa and on sperm axonemes. J Androl. 1992;13:368–78.
39. Greco E, Iacobelli M, Rienzi L, et al. Reduction of the incidence of sperm DNA fragmentation by oral antioxidant treatment. J Androl. 2005;26:349–53.
40. Greco E, Romano S, Iacobelli M, et al. ICSI in cases of sperm DNA damage: beneficial effect of oral antioxidant treatment. Hum Reprod. 2005;20:2590–4.
41. Vézina D, Mauffette F, Roberts KD, et al. Selenium-vitamin E supplementation in infertile men. Effects on semen parameters and micronutrient levels and distribution. Biol Trace Elem Res. 1996;53:65–83.
42. Keskes-Ammar L, Feki-Chakroun N, Rebai T, et al. Sperm oxidative stress and the effect of an oral vitamin E and selenium supplement on semen quality in infertile men. Arch Androl. 2003;49:83–94.
43. Lenzi A, Lombardo F, Gandini L, et al. Glutathione therapy for male infertility. Arch Androl. 1992;29:65–8.
44. Lenzi A, Picardo M, Gandini L, et al. Glutathione treatment of dyspermia: effect on the lipoperoxidation process. Hum Reprod. 1994;9:2044–50.
45. Tang LF, Jiang H, Shang XJ, et al. Seminal plasma levocarnitine significantly correlated with semen quality. Zhonghua Nan Ke Xue. 2008;14:704–8.
46. Jeulin C, Soufir JC, Marson J, et al. Acetylcarnitine and spermatozoa: relationship with epididymal maturation and motility in the boar and man. Reprod Nutr Dev. 1988;28:1317–27.
47. Moncada ML, Vicari E, Cimino C, et al. Effect of acetyl carnitine treatment in oligoasthenospermic patients. Acta Eur Fertil. 1992;23:221–4.
48. Costa M, Canale D, Filicori M, et al. L-carnitine in idiopathic asthenozoospermia: a multicenter study. Andrologia. 1994;26:155–9.
49. Vitali G, Parente R, Melotti C. Carnitine supplementation in human idiopathic asthenospermia: clinical results. Drugs Exp Clin Res. 1995;21:157–9.
50. Dokmeci D. Oxidative stress, male infertility and the role of carnitines. Folia Med (Plovdiv). 2005;47:26–30.

51. Vicari E, Rubino C, De Palma A, et al. Antioxidant therapeutic efficiency after the use of carnitine in infertile patients with bacterial or non bacterial prostato-vesiculo-epididymitis. Arch Ital Urol Androl. 2001;73:15–25.
52. Vicari E, La Vignera S, Calogero AE. Antioxidant treatment with carnitines is effective in infertile patients with prostatovesiculoepididymitis and elevated seminal leukocyte concentrations after treatment with nonsteroidal anti-inflammatory compounds. Fertil Steril. 2002;78:1203–8.
53. Lenzi A, Lombardo F, Sgrò P, et al. Use of carnitine therapy in selected cases of male factor infertility: a double-blind crossover trial. Fertil Steril. 2003;79:292–300.
54. Lenzi A, Sgrò P, Salacone P, et al. A placebo-controlled double-blind randomized trial of the use of combined L-carnitine and L-acetyl-carnitine treatment in men with asthenozoospermia. Fertil Steril. 2004;81:1578–84.
55. Cavallini G, Ferraretti AP, Gianaroli L, et al. Cinnoxicam and L-carnitine/acetyl-L-carnitine treatment for idiopathic and varicocele associated oligoasthenospermia. J Androl. 2004;25:761–70.
56. Balercia G, Regoli F, Armeni T, et al. Placebo-controlled double-blind randomized trial on the use of L-carnitine, L-acetylcarnitine, or combined L-carnitine and L-acetylcarnitine in men with idiopathic asthenozoospermia. Fertil Steril. 2005;84:662–71.
57. Li Z, Chen GW, Shang XJ, et al. A controlled randomized trial of the use of combined L-CARNITINE and acetyl-L-carnitine treatment in men with oligoasthenozoospermia. Zhonghua Nan Ke Xue. 2005;11:761–4.
58. De Rosa M, Boggia B, Amalfi B. Correlation between seminal carnitine and functional spermatozoal characteristics in men with semen dysfunction of various origins. Drugs R&D. 2005;6:1–9.
59. Sigman M, Glass S, Campagnone J, et al. Carnitine for the treatment of idiopathic asthenospermia: a randomized, double-blind, placebo-controlled trial. Fertil Steril. 2006;85:1409–14.
60. Vicari E, Calogero AE. Effects of treatment with carnitines in infertile patients with prostato-vesiculo-epididymitis. Hum Reprod. 2001;16:2338–42.
61. Zhou X, Liu F, Zhai S. Effect of L-carnitine and/or L-acetyl-carnitine in nutrition treatment for male infertility: a systematic review. Asia Pac J Clin Nutr. 2007;16 Suppl 1:383–90.
62. Alleva R, Scararmucci A, Mantero F, et al. Protective role of ubiquinol content against formation of lipid hydroperoxide in human seminal fluid. Mol Aspects Med. 1997;18:S221–8.
63. Lewin A, Lavon H. The effect of coenzyme Q10 on sperm motility and function. Mol Aspects Med. 1997;18:S213–9.
64. Mancini A, Conte G, Milardi D, et al. Relationship between sperm cell ubiquinone and seminal parameters in subjects with and without varicocele. Andrologia. 1998;30:1–4.
65. Balercia G, Buldreghini E, Vignini A, et al. Coenzyme Q10 treatment in infertile men with idiopathic asthenozoospermia: a placebo-controlled, double-blind randomized trial. Fertil Steril. 2009;91:1785–92.
66. Gupta NP, Kumar R. Lycopene therapy in idiopathic male infertility: a preliminary report. Int Urol Nephrol. 2002;34:369–72.
67. Baumann J, Wurm G, von Bruchhausen F. Prostaglandin synthetase inhibition by flavonoids and phenolic compounds in relation to their O_2—scavenging properties. Arch Pharm (Weinheim). 1980;313:330–7.
68. Roseff SJ. Improvement in sperm quality and function with French maritime pine tree bark extract. J Reprod Med. 2002;47:821–4.
69. Comhaire FH, Christophe AB, Zalata AA, et al. The effects of combined conventional treatment, oral antioxidants and essential fatty acids on sperm biology in subfertile men. Prostaglandins Leukot Essent Fatty Acids. 2000;63:159–65.
70. Ciftci H, Verit A, Savas M, et al. Effects of N-acetylcysteine on semen parameters and oxidative/antioxidant status. Urology. 2009;74:73–6.

71. Okada H, Tatsumi N, Kanzaki M, et al. Formation of reactive oxygen species by spermatozoa from asthenospermic patients: response to treatment with pentoxifylline. J Urol. 1997;157:2140–6.
72. Iwanier K, Zachara BA. Selenium supplementation enhances the element concentration in blood and seminal fluid but does not change the spermatozoal quality characteristics in subfertile men. J Androl. 1995;16:441–7.
73. Scott R, MacPherson A, Yates RW, et al. The effect of oral selenium supplementation on human sperm motility. Br J Urol. 1998;82:76–80.
74. Safarinejad MR, Safarinejad S. Efficacy of selenium and/or N-acetyl-cysteine for improving semen parameters in infertile men: a double-blind, placebo controlled, randomized study. J Urol. 2009;181:741–51.
75. Yang CC, Chen JC, Chen GW, et al. Effects of Shao-Fu-Zhu-Yu-Tang on motility of human sperm. Am J Chin Med. 2003;31:573–9.
76. Comhaire FH, El Garem Y, Mahmoud A, et al. Combined conventional/antioxidant "Astaxanthin" treatment for male infertility: a double blind, randomized trial. Asian J Androl. 2005;7:257–62.
77. Gonzales GF, Cordova A, Gonzales C, et al. *Lepidium meyenii* (Maca) improved semen parameters in adult men. Asian J Androl. 2001;3:301–3.
78. Comhaire FH, Mahmoud A. The role of food supplements in the treatment of the infertile man. Reprod Biomed Online. 2003;7:385–91.
79. Tremellen K, Miari G, Froiland D, et al. A randomised control trial examining the effect of an antioxidant (Menevit) on pregnancy outcome during IVF-ICSI treatment. Aust N Z J Obstet Gynaecol. 2007;47:216–21.
80. Yang X, Zhang YH, Ding CF, et al. Extract from Morindae officinalis against oxidative injury of function to human sperm membrane. Zhongguo Zhong Yao Za Zhi. 2006;31:1614–7.
81. Omu AE, Al-Azemi MK, Kehinde EO, et al. Indications of the mechanisms involved in improved sperm parameters by zinc therapy. Med Princ Pract. 2008;17:108–16.
82. Agency for Health Care Policy and Research. Acute pain management: operative or medical procedures and trauma. Rockville: Agency for Health Care Policy and Research/US Department of Health and Human Services, Public Health Service; 1992.
83. Eccles M, et al. North of England evidence based guideline development project: guideline for angiotensin converting enzyme inhibitors in primary care management of adults with symptomatic heart failure. BMJ. 1998;316:1369.

Chapter 27
Harmful Effects of Antioxidant Therapy

Adam F. Stewart and Edward D. Kim

Oxidative stress has an integral role in the pathophysiology of most human diseases. With a rapidly aging population, increased attention and study have been directed toward the use of antioxidant therapy. The appeal is that these agents are considered "natural" substances and are associated with a healthy diet. The hypothesis has been that decreasing oxidative stress may prevent disease processes such as cancer or coronary heart disease [1, 2]. Because much of the general population use is in relatively healthy patients, it is critically important that these supplements are free of toxicity and side effects.

While initial studies of antioxidant supplementation suggested a beneficial role in disease prevention, more recent clinical trials and a meta-analysis have questioned the benefit of these therapies. Several studies have suggested that excess supplementation may in fact be harmful [3–6]. Recent attention has also focused on the use of antioxidants for the treatment of male infertility. The focus of this chapter is the potentially harmful effects of antioxidant therapy.

Risks of Dietary Antioxidants

Certain vegetables have high contents of oxalic acid, phytic acid, and tannins. These relatively strong reducing acids may have antinutrient effects by binding to dietary minerals in the gastrointestinal tract and diminishing their absorption [7, 8]. Calcium and iron deficiencies are not uncommon in developing countries where less meat is eaten, and there is high consumption of phytic acid from beans and unleavened

A.F. Stewart, MD (✉) • E.D. Kim, MD
Division of Urology, Department of Surgery, University of Tennessee Medical Center,
1928 Alcoa Highway, Suite 222, Knoxville, TN 37920, USA
e-mail: afstewart@utmck.edu; ekim@utmck.edu

S.J. Parekattil and A. Agarwal (eds.), *Antioxidants in Male Infertility: A Guide for Clinicians and Researchers*, © Springer Science+Business Media New York 2013

Table 27.1 Dietary antioxidants

Foods	Reducing acid present
Cocoa bean and chocolate, spinach, turnip, and rhubarb	Oxalic acid
Whole grains, maize, legumes	Phytic acid
Tea, beans, cabbage	Tannins

whole grain bread [9]. In modern, industrialized nations where balanced diets are more common, the adverse effects of excessive dietary antioxidant intake are minimal. Table 27.1 lists foods containing oxalic acid, phytic acid, and tannins.

Oxalic Acid

Oxalic acid impairs calcium absorption by forming an insoluble salt of calcium oxalate. Cases of calcium deficiency have been associated with a high content of oxalates in foods [10]. A high level of oxalate intake constitutes a health risk for infants and metabolically disposed adults. Spinach is among the vegetables richest in oxalate. Sweet potatoes and peanut greens are also high in oxalic acid [11].

Phytic Acid

Phytic acid is a strong inhibitor of iron absorption in both infants and adults [12]. Iron and zinc deficiencies are widespread in infants and young children in developing countries where vegetable protein sources are often mixed with cereals. This iron deficiency in infants can lead to reduced psychomotor and mental development. Complementary foods increase the protein content and improve the protein quality of cereal-based foods. Cereals and common legumes, such as soybean, mung bean, black bean, lentils, and chick peas, are high in phytic acid. Decreasing phytic acid by 90% (approximately 100 mg/100 g dried product) would be expected to increase iron absorption about twofold. Complete enzymatic degradation of phytic acid with cooking methods such as blanching has been recommended for at-risk populations [7, 11].

Tannins

Tannins, which include condensed tannins (proanthocyanidins) and derived tannins, belong to the flavonoid family [13]. Tannins are found in a wide variety of foods, that is, apples, berries, chocolate, red wines, and nuts. Derived tannins are formed during food handling and processing and are found primarily in black and oolong teas, red wine, and coffee. Flavonoids and tannins are quite sensitive to oxidative enzymes and cooking conditions.

Condensed tannins inhibit herbivore digestion by binding to consumed plant proteins and making them more difficult for animals to digest and by interfering with protein absorption and digestive enzymes. Tannins have traditionally been considered antinutritional, but it is now known that their beneficial or antinutritional properties depend upon their chemical structure and dosage. If ingested in excessive quantities, tannins inhibit the absorption of minerals such as iron, which may, if prolonged, lead to anemia [14]. In sensitive individuals, a large intake of tannins may cause bowel irritation, kidney irritation, liver damage, irritation of the stomach, and gastrointestinal pain.

Others

Nonpolar antioxidants such as eugenol, a major component of oil of cloves, have toxicity limits that can be exceeded with the misuse of undiluted essential oils. Toxicity associated with high doses of water-soluble antioxidants such as ascorbic acid is less of a concern as these compounds can be excreted rapidly in urine.

Risk of Antioxidant Supplements

It is well established that certain amounts of antioxidants, vitamins, and minerals are required in the diet. However, the benefit, dosing requirements, and risk profile of most antioxidant supplements are largely unknown. When used for disease prevention, the doses are severalfold greater than the recommended daily allowance (RDA). The hypothesis that antioxidant supplements can prevent diseases has been proven false by researchers. In spite of this information, many companies manufacture and sell dietary supplements with antioxidants in a variety of different formulations. Common ones include the "ACES" (Vitamins A, C, E, and selenium), resveratrol (found in grape seeds and knotweed roots), and herbs like green tea and jiaogulan.

The potential for harmful effects of antioxidant therapy has been suggested, such as in the β-Carotene and Retinol Efficacy Trial (CARET) which was a randomized, double-blinded, placebo-controlled chemoprevention trial in 18,314 men and women at high risk of developing lung cancer [15]. The study was initiated due to the observation of other studies that found people who have high serum β-carotene concentrations had lower rates of lung cancer [15]. The hypothesis of the CARET study was that these antioxidants would decrease the risk of lung cancer in an already high-risk population. Subjects were treated for up to 6 years. This study demonstrated that smokers who ingested a combination of 30 mg β-carotene and 25,000 IU retinyl palmitate (vitamin A) taken daily had 28% more lung cancer and

Table 27.2 Observed side effects with supplemental antioxidants

Antioxidant metabolite	Recommended daily allowance (RDA)	Reported side effects
Glutathione	250 mg/day or 600 mg IM QOD for male infertility	Acute: gastrointestinal disturbances
Carotenes	15–30 mg/day	Acute: skin color changes
		Chronic: possible increased risk of death and certain cancers
α-Tocopherol (vitamin E)	22.4 IU/day	Acute: headache, fatigue, muscle weakness, creatinuria
		Chronic: impaired bone mineralization, increased bleeding, cardiovascular disease; increased overall mortality
Ascorbic acid (vitamin C)	75–90 mg/day	Acute: diarrhea
		Chronic: hyperoxaluria, urinary stone formation, iron overload
Ubiquinol (coenzyme Q)	60–90 mg/day	Acute: gastrointestinal disturbances, heartburn, abdominal discomfort
		Chronic: hemorrhagic toxicity
Selenium	55 mcg/day	Acute: fatigue, gastrointestinal disturbances, skin rashes, irritability
		Chronic: concern for diabetes, loss of hair and nails, neuropathy
Melatonin	10 mg/day (bedtime)	Acute: diarrhea, rash, dizziness, headache, heartburn, nausea
		Chronic: sleep disturbance
Zinc	8–11 mg/day	Acute: gastrointestinal disturbance, anosmia (intranasal)
		Chronic: concern for increased risk prostate cancer, copper deficiency, suppression of immune system, anemia

17% more deaths than placebo subjects. The CARET intervention was stopped 21 months early because of clear evidence of no benefit and substantial evidence of possible harm.

Other studies have found similar findings of adverse events. Table 27.2 lists observed side effects of supplemental antioxidants. The α-Tocopherol (Vitamin E) β-Carotene Cancer Prevention Study Group (ATBC) reported on a randomized, double-blind, placebo-controlled primary prevention trial [16]. The objective was to determine whether daily supplementation with vitamin E, β-carotene, or both would reduce the incidence of lung cancer and other cancers. A total of 29,133 male smokers 50–69 years of age from southwestern Finland were randomly assigned to one of four regimens: α-tocopherol (50 mg/day) alone, β-carotene (20 mg/day) alone, both α-tocopherol and β-carotene, or placebo. These patients were followed for 5–8 years. There was no reduction in the incidence of lung cancer among male smokers after 5–8 years of dietary supplementation with vitamin E. Those men given β-carotene had an 18% increase in the incidence of lung cancer compared to placebo.

There was also an increased number of deaths due to ischemic heart disease and lung cancer in the β-carotene group compared to placebo. The vitamin E group had an increased incidence of death due to hemorrhagic stroke and an increased incidence of other cancers compared to placebo. While these data suggest that there may be harmful effects of these supplements, the authors state that further studies would need to be performed in order to validate these results [16].

Observation of these adverse effects was not limited to smokers. Bjelakovic's meta-analysis from 2007 included 68 randomized trials with 232,606 participants. This publication showed that treatment with β-carotene, vitamin A, and vitamin E may increase all-cause mortality and the potential roles of vitamin C and selenium on mortality may need further study [3].

These results were later confirmed by the same authors with an additional publication using the Cochrane Colla-boration methodology [3]. In this systematic review, several key findings were noted: (1) β-carotene, vitamin A, and vitamin E given singly or combined with other antioxidant supplements appeared to significantly increase mortality, (2) there was no evidence that vitamin C increases longevity, (3) selenium tended to reduce mortality, and (4) trials with inadequate bias control overestimated intervention effects [17–20]. It should be noted that only all-cause, not the cause of the increased mortality, was assessed. It is likely that increased cancer and cardiovascular mortality are the main reasons for the increased all-cause mortality [21, 22].

Several other publications have disagreed with the Bjelakovic meta-analysis [17, 21, 23, 24] and reported no effect on all-cause mortality. The Supplementation en Vitamines et Mineraux Antioxydants (SU.VI.MAX) study by Hercberg et al. was a randomized, double-blind, placebo-controlled primary prevention trial. A total of 13,017 participants took a single daily capsule of a combination of 120 mg of ascorbic acid, 30 mg of vitamin E, 6 mg of β-carotene, 100 mcg of selenium, and 20 mg of zinc or a placebo. After a mean of 7.5 years, there were no major differences found between the groups in total cancer incidence, ischemic cardiovascular disease incidence, or all-cause mortality [23].

Miller et al. performed a meta-analysis on the dose–response relationship between vitamin E supplementation and total mortality by evaluating randomized, controlled trials. Vitamin E doses ranged from 16.5 to 2,000 IU/day, and there were 135,967 who took vitamin E alone or in combination with other vitamins and minerals. While the results showed that there very well may be an increased risk of all-cause mortality with high doses of vitamin E (greater than or equal to 400 IU/day), lower doses did not reveal this same concern [24].

Although Bjelakovic et al. found no compelling evidence that antioxidant supplements have a significant beneficial effect on primary or secondary prevention of colorectal adenoma formation, in their meta-analysis of eight randomized clinical trials comparing antioxidant supplements with placebo or no intervention, they found no statistically significant effects of supplementation with β-carotene, vitamins A, C, E, and selenium alone or in combination. Antioxidant supplements seemed to increase the development of colorectal adenoma in three low-bias risk trials (1.2, 0.99–1.4) and significantly decrease its development in five high-bias risk trials

(0.59, 0.47–0.74). There was also no significant difference between the intervention groups regarding adverse events including mortality (0.82, 0.47–1.4) [17].

The mechanism of the possible negative impact of antioxidant supplements is speculative. First, it is known that oxidative stresses are a part of the pathogenesis of different chronic diseases; however, could the oxidative stress be the cause of the chronic disease or the chronic disease causing the oxidative stress [25]? Second, some essential defense mechanisms, such as phagocytosis, detoxification, and apoptosis, depend on free radicals. If impaired, a negative impact on homeostasis may ensue [26–28]. Third, unlike prescription drugs, antioxidant supplements are not put through the same thorough toxicity studies in order to be sold to consumers [29]. A better understanding of the mechanisms and actions of antioxidants toward specific disease processes is needed [30].

Finally, if antioxidants reduce the redox stress in cancer cells, then they may decrease the effectiveness of chemotherapy and radiation therapy. However, other researchers argue that the antioxidants would reduce the unintentional side effects of the cancer treatment and increase survival times [31, 32].

β-Carotene

α-Carotene, β-carotene, and β-cryptoxanthin are provitamin A carotenoids. In the human body, these carotenoids can be converted to retinol (vitamin A). The essential function of carotenoids is that of provitamin A carotenoids (α-carotene, β-carotene, and β-cryptoxanthin) to serve as a source of vitamin A. Because of its vitamin A activity, β-carotene may be used to provide all or part of the vitamin A in multivitamin supplements. The vitamin A activity of β-carotene from supplements is much higher than that of β-carotene from foods [33].

As previously mentioned, the use of β-carotene was tested for its ability to prevent lung cancer in two large trials, the ATBC trial and the CARET trial. Surprisingly, an increased incidence of lung cancer was observed in the study groups. In CARET, it was not feasible to distinguish whether β-carotene or vitamin A was to blame for the negative results. In ATBC, there was a clear distinction that β-carotene was responsible for the increased incidence of lung cancers and increased overall mortality. Of note, there was no benefit of preventing other cancers, including gastric, pancreatic, breast, bladder, colorectal, and prostate cancer as well as leukemia, mesothelioma, and lymphoma [15, 16].

A large randomized, double-blind, placebo-controlled trial of β-carotene (50 mg on alternate days) involved 22,071 United States male physicians. The results after 12 years showed practically no early or late differences in the overall incidence of malignant neoplasms, cardiovascular disease, or in overall mortality. At initial glance, it seemed there was an increased incidence of thyroid cancer (16 vs. 2) and bladder cancer (62 vs. 41) in the β-carotene versus placebo group; however, after adjustment for multiple comparisons, neither of these differences was statistically significant. Overall, the only adverse side effects reported in the β-carotene group were yellowing of the skin and upset stomach [34].

Two other trials [35, 36] studied the ability of β-carotene to prevent nonmelanoma skin cancer. Neither found a beneficial effect on subsequent skin cancer incidence or reported any adverse effects of β-carotene supplementation.

The Women's Health Study was a large study of 39,876 healthy American women over 45 years old which found no effect of β-carotene on cancer incidence, but there was a suggestion of increased stroke risk during the study duration of 4.1 years (2.1 years treatment plus another 2.0 years follow-up). While it did not show statistical significance, the number of women who suffered a stroke was 61 (0.31%) for the β-carotene group versus 43 (0.22%) for the placebo group [37].

Minor side effects associated with the use of β-carotene include yellowing of the skin, also known as hypercarotenemia, when doses of greater than 30 mg/day are used for more than several weeks. This side effect is reversible upon cessation and has been observed in patients with photosensitivity disorders using these doses. Infrequently, mild gastrointestinal distress with gas and bloating may be seen.

Carotenemia is the ingestion of excessive amounts of vitamin A precursors in food, mainly carrots. It is manifested by a yellow–orange coloring of the skin. This differs from jaundice because the sclerae are still white in carotenemia. Other than the cosmetic effect, carotenemia has no adverse consequences because the conversion of carotenes to retinol is not sufficient to cause toxicity [38].

Tocopherols and Tocotrienols

Vitamin E, also known as α-tocopherol, refers to a set of eight related tocopherols and tocotrienols which are fat-soluble vitamins with antioxidant properties. Adequate amounts of this vitamin are typically present in Western diets. Multivitamins often contain about 30 international units (IU) of vitamin E, but supplements often contain 200, 400, or 1,000 IU. While research suggests that taking vitamin E supplements may boost immune systems and prevent heart disease and some types of cancer [39], large amounts of vitamin E may increase the risk for bleeding problems and death.

Miller et al. published a meta-analysis in 2005 that included 135,967 adults who had participated in 19 placebo-controlled studies of over a 1-year duration [24]. Approximately 60% of subjects had heart disease or risk factors for heart disease. Vitamin E in amounts of 400 IU or more daily for longer than 1 year increased the risk for death compared with placebo or no treatment. Limitations of the study were that trials which tested high amounts of vitamin E often involved older adults with chronic diseases. Therefore, findings from these trials may not apply to younger adults. Also, multivitamin combinations rather than vitamin E alone were often studied. This meta-analysis also did not find the exact lowest amount of vitamin E that was associated with increased risk for death.

In the HOPE and HOPE-TOO trials, the daily administration of 400 IU of natural source vitamin E for a median of 7 years had no clear impact on fatal and nonfatal cancers, major cardiovascular events, or deaths [39]. Unexpectedly, a consistent increase in the risk of heart failure was observed. A regression analysis identified vitamin E as an independent predictor of heart failure and supportive mechanistic evidence from an echocardiographic substudy of the HOPE trial found that vitamin E decreased left ventricular ejection fraction. Based on these findings, the authors recommended that vitamin E supplements should not be used in patients with vascular disease or diabetes mellitus.

A double-blind, placebo-controlled trial by Hemila et al. evaluated 652 Dutch subjects aged greater than or equal to 60 years [40]. These authors identified a greater severity of respiratory infections among participants supplemented with 200 mg vitamin E daily than among those not given vitamin E. These findings suggest that some population groups may be harmed by vitamin E supplementation. In contrast, Hathcock et al. supported the safety of vitamin E supplementation. They concluded that "at present, the evidence is not convincing that vitamin E supplementation up to the UL (i.e., the tolerable upper intake level, or 1,000 mg/day) increases the risk of death due to cardiovascular disease or other causes" [41].

Adults should consider avoiding taking vitamin E preparations in amounts of 400 IU or more. In November 2004, the American Heart Association stated that high amounts of vitamin E can be harmful. Taking 400 IU/day, or higher, may increase the risk of death. Taking smaller amounts, such as those found in a typical multivitamin, was not harmful.

Ascorbic Acid

Ascorbic acid, also known as vitamin C, is a monosaccharide antioxidant that is found in plants and animals. It functions specifically as a substrate for the antioxidant enzyme ascorbate peroxidase. Reactive oxygen species can be neutralized by ascorbic acid because it is a reducing agent [42, 43]. In humans, vitamin C is required for the synthesis of collagen. It is also a component of blood vessels, tendons, ligaments, and bone. Vitamin C also plays an important role in the synthesis of the neurotransmitter norepinephrine. Also, vitamin C is required for the synthesis of carnitine, a small molecule that is essential for the transport of fat into cellular organelles called mitochondria where the fat is converted to energy [44].

In a 15-year study of postmenopausal women, Lee et al. found that diabetic women who reported taking at least 300 mg/day of vitamin C from supplements were at significantly higher risk of death from coronary heart disease and stroke than those who did not take vitamin C supplements. Overall, vitamin C supplement use was not associated with a significant increase in cardiovascular disease mortality in the cohort as a whole [45]. Although a number of observational studies have found that higher dietary intakes of vitamin C are associated with lower cardiovascular disease risk, randomized controlled trials have not found antioxidant supplementation that included vitamin C to reduce the risk of cardiovascular disease in diabetic or other high-risk individuals [46].

Some studies have attempted to reveal if vitamin C supplementation would benefit athletes. While there does not seem to be an increased demand for vitamin C in athletes, there is the idea that if vitamin C is taken, it can allow the athlete a longer more strenuous exercise with less muscle damage. In fact, some research has found that amounts of vitamin C as high as 1,000 mg inhibits recovery theoretically by causing a decrease in mitochondria production and hampering endurance capacity [47].

Excessive doses of vitamin C not absorbed by the gastrointestinal tract can lead to mild diarrhea and indigestion. Large doses of ascorbic acid over prolonged periods can lead to urinary oxalate stone formation, although this effect is minimal and inconsistent [48, 49].

Glutathione

Glutathione is a cysteine-containing peptide made in human cells from specific amino acids. Glutathione is an endogenous intracellular antioxidant. Glutathione has a thiol group in its molecular structure which gives it antioxidant properties that allows it to be reversibly oxidized and reduced [50, 51]. Glutathione is touted by some to be the most important cellular antioxidant due to its high concentration and its main role in keeping the cell's redox state. Thorough literature review has failed to find any reported adverse effects of taking glutathione [52].

Melatonin

Melatonin is a unique antioxidant in that it can easily cross cell membranes including the blood–brain barrier. Another reason it is unique is because it does not undergo redox cycling which allows the antioxidant to undergo repeated reduction and oxidation. This repeated reduction and oxidation functions as a prooxidant and may allow the formation of free radicals [53, 54].

The recommended dose for melatonin is 10 mg by mouth at bedtime. Melatonin has been reported to cause sleep disruption, daytime fatigue, irritability, mood changes, depression, paranoia, hyperglycemia, headaches, dizziness, abdominal cramps, chest pain, and even tachycardia or seizures at higher doses [55, 56]. Several drug interaction precautions should be noted. First, there is caution with the use of systemic steroids and melatonin due to the interference with immunosuppressive activity of the steroid. Second, there is a caution with the use of ginkgo biloba due to the increased risk of seizures. Third, there is a caution with the use of melatonin and other CYP1A2 substrates. Lastly, a caution should be given with concomitant use of any CNS depressing drugs, sedatives, or hypnotics [56].

Antioxidant Nutrients: Selenium and Zinc

Selenium and zinc, commonly referred to as antioxidant nutrients, have no antioxidant action themselves and are instead required for the activity of some antioxidant enzymes. Selenium protects against oxidative damage by means of selenium-dependent proteins called selenoproteins including glutathione peroxidase. At serum levels of 70–90 ng/mL, a maximum level of activity is reached for the selenoproteins with the possible exception of one named selenoprotein P. The dietary intake of selenium in the USA is enough so that 99% of Americans have a serum selenium level greater than 90 ng/mL [57].

The Selenium and Vitamin E Cancer Prevention Trial (SELECT) was a large randomized, placebo-controlled trial set up to evaluate the potential benefit of selenium and vitamin E for the prevention of prostate cancer. Over 35,000 men enrolled and were divided into four groups (selenium, vitamin E, selenium + vitamin E, or placebo). After a mean follow-up of 5.46 years, there was no significant effect on the prevention of prostate cancer or any other prespecified cancer end points. However, in the selenium alone group, there was a statistically insignificant increased risk of type 2 diabetes mellitus. Further prospective, randomized studies would be needed to delineate the effect of supplemental and dietary selenium on the risk for developing diabetes. Because of the lack of benefit on prostate cancer and the potential risk of therapy, this trial was terminated [58].

While long-term use of zinc supplements at the upper limit of tolerability (40 mg/day) in adults is not considered unsafe, there are some common adverse effects of excessive zinc intake. These include metallic taste, nausea, vomiting, abdominal cramping, urinary tract infection, and diarrhea. Extended intake of amounts above the tolerable upper intake level may suppress immunity, decrease high-density lipoprotein cholesterol levels, and cause hypochromic microcytic anemia and copper deficiency [59, 60]. Interestingly, Leitzmann et al. evaluated zinc intake and the risk of prostate cancer in the Health Professionals Follow-up Study [61]. Results showed that in the 46,974 adult men studied, there was a 2.3 increased relative risk of advanced prostate cancer in men using elemental zinc in amounts of 100 mg/day or more. There was not an associated risk of prostate cancer in men who consumed less than 100 mg/day. While the authors could not rule out residual confounding by supplemental calcium intake or some unmeasured correlate of zinc supplement use, the evidence that chronic zinc ingestion above 100 mg/day may play a role in prostate carcinogenesis justifies further investigation.

Zinc may alter the way the body processes some drugs and other vitamins and minerals. For example, it may inhibit the absorption of tetracyclines, penicillamine, and quinolones. On the other hand, the absorption of zinc can be impaired by iron supplements and phytates, which are found in grains and legumes. Therefore, zinc supplements should be taken at least 2 h from iron and phytate ingestion [60].

Expert Commentary

Antioxidant supplements are widely used with the belief their use may improve health and have beneficial effects on disease prevention. These supplements are used in addition to the adequate amounts obtained in the typical Western diet. Recent meta-analyses and large-scale placebo-controlled trials suggest that long-term antioxidant supplements such as β-carotene, vitamin A, and vitamin E may increase overall all-cause mortality. The significance of these adverse effects is controversial as other meta-analyses, using many of the same studies, have provided mixed results depending on the criteria used for study inclusion. Although speculative, it is likely that increased cancer risk and cardiovascular disease risks are the main reasons for the increased mortality. Long-term indiscriminate use of antioxidant supplements should be avoided as the true benefit cannot be determined without further study.

Five-Year View

Although antioxidant supplements have been extensively studied, further large-scale randomized clinical trials with sufficient safety analyses will be necessary to determine their true long-term safety profile. Short-term use appears to be without significant adverse events. While supplements are not subject to the rigorous study required for FDA labeling of pharmaceutical agents, numerous clinical trials of their efficacy in specific disease states are ongoing as indicated by a search of http://www.clinicaltrials.gov. Some insight into harmful effects can be obtained from these studies, although clinical safety is usually a secondary end point of such investigations.

Key Issues

- Antioxidant supplements are increasingly used in the general population. Very high doses of some antioxidants, both dietary and as supplements, may have harmful long-term effects.
- β-Carotene, vitamin A, and vitamin E given singly or combined with other antioxidant supplements may increase all-cause mortality. Meta-analyses on this topic have yielded mixed results.
- Although speculative, it is likely that increased cancer and cardiovascular mortality are the main reasons for the increased all-cause mortality seen with β-carotene, vitamin A, and vitamin E.

Acknowledgment We acknowledge Joy Nicely and Kathy Gribble for manuscript preparation.

References

1. Halliwell B. Antioxidant defense mechanisms: from the beginning to the end (of the beginning). Free Radic Res. 1999;31:261–72.
2. Willcox JK, Ash SL, Catignani GL. Antioxidants and prevention of chronic disease. Crit Rev Food Sci Nutr. 2004;44:275–95.
3. Bjelakovic G, Nikolova D, Gluud LL, Simonetti RG, Gluud C. Mortality in randomized trials of antioxidant supplements for primary and secondary prevention: systematic review and meta-analysis. JAMA. 2007;297(8):842–57.
4. Bjelakovic G, Nikolova D, Simonetti RG, Gluud C. Antioxidant supplements for preventing gastrointestinal cancers. Cochrane Database Syst Rev. 2004;1(4):CD004183.
5. Bjelakovic G, Nikolova D, Simonetti RG, Gluud C. Antioxidant supplements for prevention of gastrointestinal cancers: a systematic review and meta-analysis. Lancet. 2004;364:1219–28.
6. Stanner SA, Hughes J, Kelly CN, Buttriss J. A review of the epidemiological evidence for the "antioxidant hypothesis". Public Health Nutr. 2004;7:407–22.
7. Hurrell R. Influence of vegetable protein sources on trace element and mineral bioavailability. J Nutr. 2003;133(9):2973S–7S.
8. Hunt J. Bioavailability of iron, zinc, and other trace minerals from vegetarian diets. Am J Clin Nutr. 2003;78(3 Suppl):633S–9S.
9. Gibson R, Perlas L, Hotz C. Improving the bioavailability of nutrients in plant foods at the household level. Proc Nutr Soc. 2006;65(2):160–8.
10. Kelsay JL. Effect of oxalic acid on bioavailability of calcium. In: Kies C, editor. Nutritional bioavailability of calcium. Washington, DC: American Chemical Society; 1985.
11. Mosha TC, Gaga HE, Pace RD, Laswai HS, Mtebe K. Effect of blanching on the content of antinutritional factors in selected vegetables. Plant Foods Hum Nutr. 1995;47:361–7.
12. Hallberg L, Brune M, Rossander L. Iron absorption in man: ascorbic acid and dose-dependent inhibition by phytate. Am J Clin Nutr. 1989;49:140–4.
13. Beecher G. Overview of dietary flavonoids: nomenclature, occurrence and intake. J Nutr. 2003;133(10):3248S–54S.
14. Brune M, Rossander L, Hallberg L. Iron absorption and phenolic compounds: importance of different phenolic structures. Eur J Clin Nutr. 1989;43(8):547–57.
15. Omenn GS, Goodman GE, Thornquist MD, et al. Risk factors for lung cancer and for intervention effects in CARET, the Beta-Carotene and Retinol Efficacy Trial. J Natl Cancer Inst. 1996;88(21):1550–9.
16. Heinonen OP, Huttuten JK, Albanes D, et al. The effect of vitamin E and beta carotene on the incidence of lung cancer and other cancers in male smokers. The Alpha-Tocopherol, Beta Carotene Cancer Prevention Study Group. N Engl J Med. 1994;330(15):1029–35.
17. Bjelakovic G, Nagorni A, Nikolova D, Simonetti RG, Bjelakovic M, Gluud C. Meta-analysis: antioxidant supplements for primary and secondary prevention of colorectal adenoma. Aliment Pharmacol Ther. 2006;24:281–91.
18. Moher D, Pham B, Jones A, et al. Does quality of reports of randomized trials affect estimates of intervention efficacy reported in meta-analysis. Lancet. 1998;352:609–13.
19. Schulz KF, Chalmers I, Hayes RJ, Altman DG. Empirical evidence of bias: dimensions of methodological quality associated with estimates of treatment effects in controlled trials. JAMA. 1995;273:408–12.
20. Kjaergard LL, Villumsen J, Gluud C. Reported methodologic quality and discrepancies between large and small randomized trials in meta-analyses. Ann Intern Med. 2001;135:982–9.
21. Caraballoso M, Sacristan M, Serra C, Bonfill X. Drugs for preventing lung cancer in healthy people. Cochrane Database Syst Rev. 2003;2:CD002141.
22. Vivekananthan DP, Penn MS, Sapp SK, Hsu A, Topol EJ. Use of antioxidant vitamins for the prevention of cardiovascular disease: meta-analysis of randomized trials. Lancet. 2003;361:2017–23.

23. Hercberg S, Galan P, Preziosi P, et al. The SU.VI.MAX Study: a randomized, placebo-controlled trial of the health effects of antioxidant vitamins and minerals. Arch Intern Med. 2004;164(21):2335–42.
24. Miller E, Pastor-Barriuso R, Dalal D, Riemersma R, Appel L, Guallar E. Meta-analysis: high-dosage vitamin E supplementation may increase all-cause mortality. Ann Intern Med. 2005;142(1):37–46.
25. Halliwell B. Free radicals, antioxidants, and human disease: curiosity, cause, or consequence? Lancet. 2000;344:721–4.
26. Salganik RI. The benefits and hazards of antioxidants: controlling apoptosis and other protective mechanisms in cancer patients and the human population. J Am Coll Nutr. 2001;20(5 Suppl):464S–72S.
27. Simon HU, Haj-Yehia A, Levi-Schaffer F. Role of reactive oxygen species (ROS) in apoptosis induction. Apoptosis. 2000;5:415–8.
28. Kimura H, Sawada T, Oshima S, Kozawa K, Ishioka T, Kato M. Toxicity and roles of reactive oxygen species. Curr Drug Targets Inflamm Allergy. 2005;4:489–95.
29. Bast A, Haenen GR. The toxicity of antioxidants and their metabolites. Environ Toxicol Pharmacol. 2002;11:251–8.
30. Ratnam DV, Ankola DD, Bhardwaj V, Sahana DK, Kumar MN. Role of antioxidants in prophylaxis and therapy: a pharmaceutical perspective. J Control Release. 2006;113:189–207.
31. Seifried H, McDonald S, Anderson D, Greenwald P, Milner J. The antioxidant conundrum in cancer. Cancer Res. 2003;63(15): 4295–8.
32. Lawenda BD, Kelly KM, Ladas EJ, Sagar SM, Vickers A, Blumberg JB. Should supplemental antioxidant administration be avoided during chemotherapy and radiation therapy? J Natl Cancer Inst. 2008;100(11):773–83.
33. Institute of Medicine, Food and Nutrition Board. Beta-carotene, other carotenoids. Dietary reference intakes for vitamin C, vitamin E, selenium, and carotenoids. Washington, DC: National Academy; 2000. p. 325–400.
34. Hennekens CH, Buring JE, Manson JE, et al. Lack of effect of long-term supplementation with beta carotene on the incidence of malignant neoplasms and cardiovascular disease. N Engl J Med. 1996;334:1145–9.
35. Green A, Williams G, Neale R, et al. Daily sunscreen application and betacarotene supplementation in prevention of basal-cell and squamous-cell carcinomas of the skin: a randomized controlled trial. Lancet. 1999;354:723–9.
36. Greenberg ER, Baron JA, Karagas MR, et al. Mortality associated with low plasma concentration of beta carotene and the effect of oral supplementation. JAMA. 1996;275:699–703.
37. Lee IM, Cook NR, Manson JE, Buring JE, Hennekens CH. Beta-carotene supplementation and incidence of cancer and cardiovascular disease: the Women's Health Study. J Natl Cancer Inst. 1999;91:2102–6.
38. Penniston KL, Tanumihardjo S. The acute and chronic toxic effects of vitamin A. Am J Clin Nutr. 2006;83:191–201.
39. Lonn E, Bosch J, Yusuf S, et al. Effects of long-term vitamin E supplementation on cardiovascular events and cancer: a randomized controlled trial. JAMA. 2005;293:1338–47.
40. Hemila H. Potential harm of vitamin E supplementation [letter]. Am J Clin Nutr. 2005;82(5):1141–2.
41. Hathcock JN, Azzi A, Blumberg J, et al. Vitamins E and C are safe across a broad range of intakes. Am J Clin Nutr. 2005;81:736–45.
42. Padayatty S, Katz A, Wang Y, et al. Vitamin C as an antioxidant: evaluation of its role in disease prevention. J Am Coll Nutr. 2003;22(1):18–35.
43. Linster CL, Van Schaftingen E. Vitamin C biosynthesis, recycling and degradation in mammals. FEBS J. 2007;274(1):1–22.
44. Carr AC, Frei B. Toward a new recommended dietary allowance for vitamin C based on antioxidant and health effects in humans. Am J Clin Nutr. 1999;69(6):1086–107.

45. Lee DH, Folsom AR, Harnack L, Halliwell B, Jacobs Jr DR. Does supplemental vitamin C increase cardiovascular disease risk in women with diabetes? Am J Clin Nutr. 2004;80(5): 1194–200.
46. Waters DD, Alderman EL, Hsia J, et al. Effects of hormone replacement therapy and antioxidant vitamin supplements on coronary atherosclerosis in postmenopausal women: a randomized controlled trial. JAMA. 2002;288(19):2432–40.
47. Mastaloudis A, Traber M, Carstensen K, Widrick J. Antioxidants did not prevent muscle damage in response to an ultramarathon run. Med Sci Sports Exerc. 2006;38(1):72–80.
48. Peake J. Vitamin C: effects of exercise and requirements with training. Int J Sport Nutr Exerc Metab. 2003;13(2):125–51.
49. Massey LK, Liebman M, Kynast-Gales SA. Ascorbate increases human oxaluria and kidney stone risk. J Nutr. 2005;135(7): 1673–7.
50. Meister A. Glutathione metabolism and its selective modification. J Biol Chem. 1988; 263(33):17205–8.
51. Meister A. Glutathione-ascorbic acid antioxidant system in animals. J Biol Chem. 1994; 269(13):9397–400.
52. Meister A, Anderson M. Glutathione. Annu Rev Biochem. 1983;52:711–60.
53. Reiter RJ, Carneiro RC, Oh CS. Melatonin in relation to cellular antioxidative defense mechanisms. Horm Metab Res. 1997;29(8): 363–72.
54. Tan DX, Manchester LC, Reiter RJ, Qi WB, Karbownik M, Calvo JR. Significance of melatonin in antioxidative defense system: reactions and products. Biol Signals Recept. 2000;9(3–4):137–59.
55. Taylor SR, Weiss JS. Review of insomnia pharmacotherapy options for the elderly: implications for managed care. Popul Health Manag. 2009;12(6):317–23.
56. Buscemi N, Vandermeer B, Hooton N, et al. Efficacy and safety of exogenous melatonin for secondary sleep disorders and sleep disorders accompanying sleep restriction: meta-analysis. BMJ. 2006;332(7538):385–93.
57. Bleys J, Navas-Acien A, Guallar E. Selenium and diabetes: more bad news for supplements. Ann Intern Med. 2007;147(4):271–2.
58. Lippman SM, Klein EA, Goodman PJ, et al. Effect of selenium and vitamin E on risk of prostate cancer and other cancers: the Selenium and Vitamin E Cancer Prevention Trial (SELECT). JAMA. 2009;301(1):39–51.
59. Fosmire GJ. Zinc toxicity. Am J Clin Nutr. 1990;51(2):225–7.
60. Saper RB, Rash R. Zinc: an essential micronutrient. Am Fam Physician. 2009;79(9):768–72.
61. Leitzmann MF, Stampfer MJ, Wu K, Colditz GA, Willet WC, Giovannucci EL. Zinc supplement use and risk of prostate cancer. J Natl Cancer Inst. 2003;95(13):1004–7.

Index